ECG Time Series Variability Analysis

ECG Time Series Variability Analysis
Analysis
Engineering and Medicine

Edited by
Herbert F. Jelinek, David J. Cornforth,
and Ahsan H. Khandoker

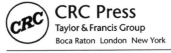

CRC Press
Taylor & Francis Group
Boca Raton London New York

CRC Press is an imprint of the
Taylor & Francis Group, an **informa** business

CRC Press
Taylor & Francis Group
6000 Broken Sound Parkway NW, Suite 300
Boca Raton, FL 33487-2742

First issued in paperback 2019

© 2018 by Taylor & Francis Group, LLC
CRC Press is an imprint of Taylor & Francis Group, an Informa business

No claim to original U.S. Government works

ISBN-13: 978-1-4822-4347-5 (hbk)
ISBN-13: 978-0-367-87015-7 (pbk)

Library of Congress Cataloging-in-Publication Data

Visit the Taylor & Francis Web site at
http://www.taylorandfrancis.com

and the CRC Press Web site at
http://www.crcpress.com

Contents

Contents

Preface

The nexus between engineering and biological science including medicine is a rich area of scientific endeavor in terms of understanding physiological and pathophysiological processes. Advances in computer technology and medical instrumentation have led to opportunities to improve data acquisition, signal processing, and analysis. Much has been written about heart rate variability (HRV) with more to come as engineers, computer scientists, physicists, mathematicians, and clinicians unravel its mysteries. Cardiac rhythms are complex and reflect the physiological or pathophysiological neural control and feedback mechanisms over time. HRV is a statistical measure of the changes in heart rate or the inter-beat intervals over time, and may be obtained from recordings as short as 10 seconds or several days in length. However, clinical diagnostic/therapeutic utility and the usefulness of HRV are still being debated in the literature and are limited in application.

Automated stratification of cardiovascular diseases by HRV of patients at rest provides an additional clinical tool with high accuracy and reliability that does not require patient participation and can be corrected for age and gender. Recordings of HRV can be obtained from a person either in a supine or sitting position or while on a head-up tilt device. In all cases, short recordings with no active participation required provide a highly useful tool in clinical settings.

It is not the intention of this book to provide detailed descriptions of the methods associated with preprocessing of the heart rate time series and related analytical methods, but rather to provide an overview of the field from an engineering and medical perspective, describing the current state of the art applied to understanding pathophysiological processes in disease and disease progression. This book aims to describe the complex time series of the heart rate and how to interpret results for a better understanding of information obtained by the diverse methods applied in HRV analysis and its role in health and disease.

Developing engineering solutions allows clinical science and medical diagnostics to move forward and improve patient care by identifying often asymptomatic disease progression early. HRV analysis has progressed from applying simple time-domain- and frequency-domain–based methodology to applying more complex algorithms toward discovering better and more meaningful descriptors of the inherent variability of the heart rate over time and its meaning. Some of these algorithms are discussed in the following chapters. Biosignal processing and analysis remains an exciting field as it continues to expand, providing novel measures relevant to diverse fields such as biomedical engineering, computing, physics, mathematics, and medicine, to name a few. Linear methods of time and frequency analysis have given way to nonlinear analysis such as fractal geometry and entropy-based methods. These include multiscale entropy, where the scaled measures are thought to provide additional useful information. In many cases, these have led to the identification of subtle changes in the HRV associated with pathological processes even though the physiological meaning is yet to be found.

For any analysis to provide meaningful results, the method applied has to match the data to be analyzed. Hence the basis for HRV can be placed at the bidirectional regulatory mechanisms of the autonomic nervous system (ANS). Parasympathetic input acts as a heart rate brake, slowing heart rate, whereas the sympathetic component or withdrawing of the parasympathetic input of the ANS increases heart rate. The ANS is further regulated by the brainstem, subcortical, and cortical areas, with which it essentially has a closed loop. Anxiety, depression, and schizophrenia are examples of cortical pathologies that affect HRV. Parkinson's disease and brainstem pathology as well as peripheral pathophysiology such as associated with diabetes further change the heart rate pattern. These changes in HRV or the specific HRV results are not specific for a particular pathology but hint at a change away from body homeostasis that can be used for supporting a clinical diagnosis and interpretation with involvement of the ANS as well as an indicator of treatment effectiveness.

The first chapter of the book provides historical context and an introduction to basic biosignals analysis, including some recent advances in HRV algorithm development. It is intended mainly for physicians to familiarize themselves with this area of inquiry. The remaining chapters provide biological and clinical examples of how various HRV measures are applied in biology and specifically in autonomic neuroscience, exercise physiology, cardiac function, renal disease, mental health, fetal health, and pediatrics. The key difference from contemporary HRV-related books is that the current book provides additional insights into the pathophysiological link between physiologically understandable mathematical indices of HRV and ANS function in health and disease.

MATLAB® is a registered trademark of The MathWorks, Inc. For product information, please contact:

The MathWorks, Inc.
3 Apple Hill Drive
Natick, MA 01760-2098
USA Tel: 508-647-7000
Fax: 508-647-7001
Email: info@mathworks.com
Web: www.mathworks.com

Editors

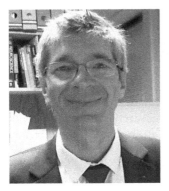

Dr. Herbert F. Jelinek is an associate professor with the School of Community Health, Charles Sturt University, Australia. He received his Bachelor of Science (Hons) in Human Genetics and Psychology from the University of New South Wales, Sydney, followed by a Graduate Diploma in Neuroscience from the Australian National University, Canberra, and his PhD in Medicine from the University of Sydney, Australia. He is an honorary clinical associate professor with Clinical Medicine, Macquarie University in Sydney. His main area of research is in the nexus between genetics, neurophysiology, and engineering. He has been organizing a rural diabetes complications screening research project for over 10 years in Australia and has published widely in ECG signal processing, diabetic retinopathy image analysis, and data mining as well as in genetics and inflammatory/oxidative stress biomarkers associated with diabetes disease progression. Within the area of biosignals processing, he is developing algorithms for accurate diagnostics using short time series that are of value for clinical practice. His current research interests include neurogenetics of diabetes and cognitive function. He is a member of the IEEE Biomedical Engineering Society.

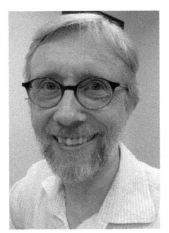

Dr. David J. Cornforth is a researcher and educator working in machine learning applied to health informatics. He holds a Bachelor of Science in Electrical Engineering from Nottingham Trent University, UK, and a PhD in Computer Science from the University of Nottingham, UK. His research experience includes heart rate variability analysis, vessel segmentation of retinal images, neuron modeling, and pattern recognition approaches for detecting diabetes and dementia. He over 130 peer-reviewed published articles. Previously, he has worked as a researcher and educator at Charles Sturt University, the University of New South Wales, and the Commonwealth Scientific and Industrial Research Organisation (CSIRO), and in the New South Wales Public Health Unit.

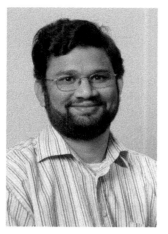

Ahsan H. Khandoker is an associate professor of biomedical engineering at Khalifa University in Abu Dhabi, UAE. He received a Doctor of Engineering in Electronic and Physiological Engineering from the Muroran Institute of Technology, Muroran, Japan, in 2004 and then completed a postdoctoral fellowship in the department of Electrical and Electronic Engineering at the University of Melbourne, Australia, in 2011. He has published over 60 peer-reviewed journal articles and more than 90 conference papers. His research fields of interests include physiological signal processing and modeling in fetal cardiac disorders, sleep disordered breathing, diabetic neuropathy, neuropsychiatric diseases, and human gait dysfunction and he is passionate about research helping clinicians to noninvasively diagnose diseases at an early stage. He has also worked with several Australian and Japanese medical device manufacturing industries, as well as with hospitals as a Research Consultant focusing on the integration of technology in clinical settings. He extensively collaborates with researchers at the University of Melbourne, Australia; Tohoku University, Japan; and the Children's National Medical Center, Washington, DC.

Contributors

Helmut Ahammer
Institute of Biophysics
Medical University of Graz
Graz, Austria

Robert Arnold
Institute of Biophysics
Medical University of Graz
Graz, Austria

Ian J. Baguley
Associate Professor, Brain Injury
 Rehabilitation Service
Westmead Hospital
Westmead, New South Wales, Australia

Dragana Bajić
Division of Communications and Signal
 Processing
Department of Power, Electronica and
 Communications
Faculty of Technical Sciences
University of Novi Sad
Novi Sad, Serbia

Karl-Jürgen Bär
Psychiatric Brain and Body Research
 Group Jena
Department of Psychiatry and
 Psychotherapy
University Hospital,
 Friedrich-Schiller-University
Jena, Germany

Riccardo Barbieri
Department of Electronics, Informatics and
 Bioengineering
Politecnico di Milano
Milano, Italy

Mathias Baumert
School of Electrical and Electronic
 Engineering
University of Adelaide
North Terrace
Adelaide, South Australia, Australia

Aparecida M. Catai
Department of Physiotherapy
Federal University of São Carlos
São Carlos, Brazil

Luca Citi
School of Computer Science and Electronic
 Engineering
University of Essex
Colchester, UK

Tom Collins
Physiotherapy Department
St Vincent's Hospital Melbourne
Fitzroy, Victoria, Australia

David J. Cornforth
School of Electrical Engineering and
 Computing
University of Newcastle
Callaghan, New South Wales, Australia

Goran Dimić
Division of Communications
Institute Mihajlo Pupin
University of Belgrade
Belgrade, Serbia

Luca Faes
Department of Physics and BIOtech
University of Trento
Trento, Italy

Ann K. Goodchild
Department of Biomedical Sciences
Faculty of Medicine and Health Sciences
Macquarie University
North Ryde, New South Wales, Australia

Beata Graff
Hypertension Unit, Department of
    Hypertension and Diabetology Medical
University of Gdańsk
Gdańsk, Poland

Grzegorz Graff
Faculty of Applied Physics and
    Mathematics
Gdańsk University of Technology
Gdańsk, Poland

Marcin Gruchała
1st Chair and Clinic of Cardiology
Medical University of Gdańsk
Gdańsk, Poland

Brett D. Hambly
Discipline of Pathology and Bosch Institute
University of Sydney
Sydney, New South Wales, Australia

Cara Hildreth
Department of Biomedical Sciences
Faculty of Medicine and Health Sciences
Macquarie University
North Ryde, New South Wales, Australia

Olaf Hoos
Julius Maximilians University
Faculty of Human Sciences
Sports Center
Wuerzburg, Germany

Kuno Hottenrott
Martin Luther University Halle-Wittenberg
Institute of Sport Science
Halle (Saale), Germany

Heikki V. Huikuri
Medical Research Center
University Hospital and University
    of Oulu
Oulu, Finland

Md. Hasan Imam
Department of Electrical and Electronic
    Engineering
University of Melbourne
Melbourne, Australia

Nina Japundžić-Žigon
Department of Pharmacology, Clinical
    Pharmacology and Toxicology
School of Medicine
University of Belgrade
Belgrade, Serbia

Herbert F. Jelinek
School of Community Health
Charles Sturt University
Albury, New South Wales, Australia

Agnieszka Kaczkowska
Faculty of Applied Physics and
    Mathematics
Gdańsk University of Technology
Gdańsk, Poland

Divya Sarma Kandukuri
Department of Biomedical Sciences
Faculty of Medicine and Health Sciences
Macquarie University
North Ryde, New South Wales, Australia

Chandan Karmakar
Centre for Pattern Recognition and Data
    Analytics (PRaDA)
Department of Electrical and Electronic
    Engineering
Deakin University
The University of Melbourne
Melbourne, Victoria, Australia

A. H. Kemp
University Hospital and Faculty of
    Medicine
University of São Paulo
São Paulo, Brazil

and

School of Psychology and Discipline of
    Psychiatry
University of Sydney
Sydney, New South Wales, Australia

Ahsan H. Khandoker
Department of Electrical and Electronic
    Engineering
The University of Melbourne
Australia

and

Department of Biomedical Engineering
Khalifa University of Science, Technology
    and Research
Abu Dhabi, United Arab Emirates

Hosen Kiat
Clinical Medicine
Faculty of Medicine and Health Sciences
Macquarie University
North Ryde, New South Wales, Australia

Yoshitaka Kimura
Advanced Interdisciplinary Biomedical
    Engineering
Tohoku University Graduate School of
    Medicine
Sendai, Japan

Alexander Koenig
Sensory-Motor Systems Lab
Department of Health Sciences and
    Technology
Spinal Cord Injury Center
Balgrist University Hospital
University of Zurich
Zurich, Switzerland

Pekka Kuoppa
Department of Applied Physics
University of Eastern Finland
Kuopio, Finland

Jukka A. Lipponen
Department of Applied Physics
University of Eastern Finland
Kuopio, Finland

Tatjana Lončar-Turukalo
Division of Communications and Signal
    Processing
Department of Power, Electronics and
    Communications
Faculty of Technical Sciences
University of Novi Sad
Novi Sad, Serbia

Yaxin Lu
Discipline of Pathology and Bosch
    Institute
University of Sydney
Sydney, New South Wales, Australia

Danuta Makowiec
Institute of Theoretical Physics and
    Astrophysics
University of Gdańsk
Gdańsk, Poland

Faezeh Marzbanrad
Department of Electrical and Computer
    Systems Engineering
Monash University
Clayton, Victoria, Australia

Slade Matthews
Discipline of Pharmacology
University of Sydney
Sydney, Australia

Michael Mayrhofer-Reinhartshuber
Institute of Biophysics
Medical University of Graz
Graz, Austria

Branislav Milovanović
Department of Internal
    Medicine—Cardiology
School of Medicine
University of Belgrade
Belgrade, Serbia

Mario Minichiello
School of Design Communication and IT
University of Newcastle
Callaghan, New South Wales, Australia

Ethan Ng
Discipline of Pathology and Bosch
    Institute
University of Sydney
Sydney, New South Wales, Australia

Giandomenico Nollo
Department of Industrial Engineering and
    BIOtech
University of Trento
IRCS PAT-FBK
Trento, Italy

Melissa T. Nott
Occupational Therapy Lecturer
School of Community Health
Charles Sturt University
Sydney, New South Wales, Australia

Marimuthu Palaniswami
Department of Electrical and Electronic
    Engineering
University of Melbourne
Parkville, Victoria, Australia

Brigitte Pelzmann
Institute of Biophysics
Medical University of Graz
Graz, Austria

Juha S. Perkiömäki
Medical Research Center
University Hospital and University
    of Oulu
Oulu, Finland

Jacqueline K. Phillips
Department of Biomedical Sciences
Faculty of Medicine and Health Sciences
Macquarie University
North Ryde, New South Wales, Australia

Alberto Porta
Department of Biomedical Sciences for
    Health
Department of Cardiothoracic Surgery
University of Milan
Vascular Anesthesia and Intensive Care,
    IRCCS Policlinico San Donato
Milano, Italy

D. S. Quintana
NORMENT, KG Jebsen Centre for
    Psychosis Research
Institute of Clinical Medicine
Division of Mental Health and Addiction
University of Oslo
Oslo University Hospital
Oslo, Norway

Robert Riener
Sensory-Motor Systems Lab
Department of Health Sciences and
    Technology
Spinal Cord Injury Center
Balgrist University Hospital
University of Zurich
Zurich, Switzerland

Jane Russell
Discipline of Psychiatry
Sydney Medical School
Northside Clinic Eating Disorders Program
University of Sydney
Sydney, New South Wales, Australia

Olivera Šarenac
Department of Pharmacology, Clinical
    Pharmacology and Toxicology
School of Medicine
University of Belgrade
Belgrade, Serbia

Steffen Schulz
Department of Medical Engineering and
     Biotechnology
Ernst-Abbe-Hochschule Jena
University of Applied Sciences
Jena, Germany

Ian Spence
Discipline of Pharmacology
Sydney Medical School
Sydney University
Sydney, New South Wales, Australia

Zbigniew R. Struzik
RIKEN Brain Science Institute
Wako, Japan

and

Graduate School of Education
The University of Tokyo
Tokyo, Japan

and

Institute of Theoretical Physics and
Astrophysics
University of Gdańsk
Gdańsk, Poland

Anielle C. M. Takahashi
Department of Physiotherapy
Federal University of São Carlos
São Carlos, Brazil

Mikhail Tamayo
Discipline of Pathology and Bosch Institute
University of Sydney
Sydney, New South Wales, Australia

Mika P. Tarvainen
Department of Applied Physics
Department of Clinical Physiology and
     Nuclear Medicine
University of Eastern Finland
Kuopio University Hospital
Kuopio, Finland

Jasha W. Trompf
Discipline of Pathology and Bosch Institute
University of Sydney
Sydney, New South Wales, Australia

Gaetano Valenza
Bioengineering and Robotics Research
     Centre "E. Piaggio" and Department of
     Information Engineering
University of Pisa
Pisa, Italy

Anne Voigt
School of Community Health
Charles Sturt University
Discipline of Pathology and Bosch Institute
University of Sydney
Sydney, New South Wales, Australia

Andreas Voss
Department of Medical Engineering and
     Biotechnology
Ernst-Abbe University of Applied Sciences
Jena, Germany

Joanna Wdowczyk
1st Chair and Clinic of Cardiology
Medical University of Gdańsk
Gdańsk, Poland

Dorota Wejer
Institute of Theoretical Physics and
     Astrophysics
University of Gdańsk
Gdańsk, Poland

Marta Zarczyńska-Buchowiecka
1st Chair and Clinic of Cardiology
Medical University of Gdańsk
Gdańsk, Poland

Yuling Zhou
Rural Clinical School
University of New South Wales
Sydney, New South Wales, Australia

Klaus Zorn-Pauly
Institute of Biophysics
Medical University of Graz
Graz, Austria

1

Introduction to ECG Time Series Variability Analysis: A Simple Overview

Herbert F. Jelinek, David J. Cornforth, and Ahsan H. Khandoker

CONTENTS

Physiological rhythms or oscillations are the manifestation of a complex physiological system. The clinical community has long recognized that alterations in physiological rhythms are associated with disease and therefore have clinical value. Oscillations in cardiovascular systems are reflected in electrocardiogram (ECG) time series variability. For example, beat to beat variability in heart rate or heart rate variability (HRV) analysis has experienced a tremendous increase in interest from both the engineering community and medical profession, as well as from the social science, economic, and health sectors. What follows is a brief overview of the chapters included in this book, noting that each chapter was a team effort by the various laboratories around the globe that work in this field. This book is organized to provide a historical overview of the domain by Andreas Voss in Chapter 2 and a basic overview of HRV analysis and review of the basics of biosignal processing by Dragana Bajić and her coauthors in Chapter 3. Chapter 3 is aimed at readers who are new to this field or who need an overview of the basic concepts. From these introductory chapters, the book moves on to provide some groundbreaking computational applications by Gaetano Valenza and colleagues (Chapter 4) as well as the laboratory of Alberto Porta and colleagues in Chapter 5. Danuta Makowiec and coauthors discuss how graph theory may be applied to HRV analysis in Chapter 6. Many of these applications require on-site coding and Mika Tarvainen introduces Kubios in Chapter 7, which is a shareware program available from the World Wide Web that provides the opportunity to investigate biosignals processing and obtain the fundamental time and frequency domain measures as well as some nonlinear attributes of the biosignals. This software includes preprocessing options and time and frequency domain analysis as well as nonlinear HRV analysis options, for those that require a user-friendly application for HRV analysis. The remainder of the book then concentrates on several areas of clinical applications with the aim to introduce the reader to the utility of HRV. In some cases, other biosignal variability analysis methods are discussed, such as blood pressure and electroencephalogram (EEG) analysis, which can be coupled to heart rate tachograms. An important aspect of the clinical chapters is the inclusion by the authors of explanations of why they used the algorithms and they also propose more advanced methods that address the research problem better.

Thus, in Chapter 8, David Cornforth and Herbert Jelinek ask the question of how complexity measures deepen our understanding of pathophysiological processes associated with cardiac rhythm. Chapter 9, by Tatjana Lončar-Turukalo et al., is the first chapter to address biosignal coupling between blood pressure and HRV. Chandan Karmakar and coauthors then take the reader, in Chapter 10, back to a fundamental aspect of heart rate and its variability by discussing the tone-entropy feature at multiple scales.

This book does not only address how to classify or identify cardiac rhythm pathology but also covers how HRV can be used to assess the effects of training in sport and as a means of staying healthy, which is discussed in Chapter 11 by Kuno Hottenrott and Olaf Hoos. Using HRV to assess the patient response to a virtual reality neurological rehabilitation is the subject of Chapter 12, by Herbert Jelinek et al., while HRV compared to traditional outcome measures in cardiac rehabilitation is covered by Hosen Kiat's group in Chapter 13. In Chapter 14, Ian Baguley and Melissa Nott examine changes in autonomic nervous system function in acute brain injury. Chapters 15 by Andrew Kemp and Daniel Quintana and Chapter 16 by Karl-Jürgen Bär and Andreas Voss discuss psychiatric disorders and HRV. Ahsan Khandoker, in Chapter 17, presents the recent progress in fetal ECG and fetal HRV technique. Chapter 18, by Janice Russell and Ian Spence, reviews HRV analysis in anorexia nervosa and eating disorders in general. In Chapter 19, Juha Perkiömäki and Heikki Huikuri discuss applying HRV in clinical practice following an acute myocardial infarction. Matthias Baumert outlines HRV analysis in cardiac control during normal and hypertensive pregnancy (Chapter 20). Jaqueline Phillips and Cara Hildreth then introduce, in Chapter 21, telemetry use in animal models of kidney disease. The last chapter then reaches the cellular level and investigates beat-to-beat variability in cardiomyocytes covered by Helmut Ahammer and colleagues from Graz.

However, before any biosignal analysis takes place, a number of issues have to be considered, which are briefly outlined below.

1.1 Preliminary Considerations When Measuring HRV

Methodological considerations form the crux of any research as they are a big part of using HRV as a tool in clinical practice. The number of methods proposed over the last 50 years has risen dramatically as our understanding of the physiology and pathophysiology of cardiac rhythm has grown. Time domain, frequency domain, and nonlinear methods of HRV analysis have to be chosen carefully depending on the information about the biosignal that is required.

A standard ECG signal is shown in Figure 1.1. This type of signal has been exhaustively studied and the diagnostic value of the different features is well established. The QRS complex, with R being the peak of the wave or fiducial point, is used as a surrogate point to the p-wave peak in determining the interbeat time for HRV analysis.

For HRV analysis, several preprocessing considerations have to be met. Noises in the recording and ectopic beats have to be removed. How do we deal with removed or missing beats? Manual selection of noise and ectopics is time consuming and also less likely to lead to identical outcomes if repeated. Therefore, automated preprocessing algorithms

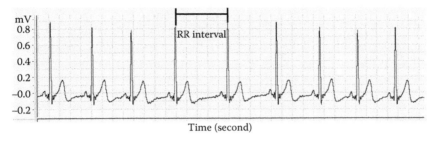

FIGURE 1.1
Normal ECG signal showing the RR interval.

have been proposed (Marzbanrad et al. 2013; Karlsson et al. 2012; Kim et al. 2009; Thuraisingham 2006; Wessel et al. 2000; Sapoznikov et al. 1992). RR intervals are events that are not evenly spaced and therefore for some HRV analysis, especially frequency domain analysis, resampling is required and consequently the resampling frequency becomes important (Clifford and Tarassenko 2005; Struzik and Hayano 2006; Moody 1993). Current algorithms for HRV analysis tend to be applied to tachograms with reduced sampling frequency in order to minimize the data size, increase analysis speed, or as a prerequisite for evenly distributed data, while retaining high clinical accuracy (Grant et al. 2011). Resampling frequencies that have been applied for HRV analysis vary between 1 and 10 Hz with low sampling frequencies possibly leading to a loss of information. In addition, the resampling frequency also affects the HRV results in particular frequency domain measures (Singh et al. 2004). Choosing an appropriate resampling frequency is not only a function of the Nyquist frequency of the signal of interest but also of the HRV analysis employed (Abubaker et al. 2014). Within the context of preprocessing and resampling, the length of the recording also needs to be considered. In clinical practice, 10-second, 12-lead ECGs are routinely recorded in addition to longer Holter recordings, which are usually recorded for between 24 and 72 hours. However, recording lengths of 2, 5, 10, 20, or 30 minutes as well as 2 hours are not uncommon and are often a function of the HRV method used (Smith et al. 2013; Kemp et al. 2012; Grant et al. 2011; Dekker et al. 2000; de Bruyne et al. 1999; Sinnreich et al. 1998; Saul et al. 1988). HRV algorithms such as very low frequency power (VLF) or approximate entropy (ApEn) may not be suitable for use with very short recording periods although when applying even these in clinical practice, they may be sufficiently robust to provide useful information for the clinician (Jelinek et al. 2014). Teich et al. have shown that some measures provide reliable results using recordings of only a few minutes (Teich et al. 2001). In addition, when comparing HRV results, recording lengths need to be of the same duration. Automated preprocessing to remove noise and ectopic beats, resampling, and consideration of length of recording all play an important role in obtaining meaningful results in clinical practice and research. Finally, testing for stationarity is a step often neglected. Biological signals are inherently nonstationary and measures such as the correlation dimension or power spectral analysis are strongly influenced by the nonstationarity of the signal. To address this point rather than determining the extent of nonstationarity, it is suggested that when applying the power spectral analysis using a fast Fourier transform, 5-minute segments are analyzed and averaged to avoid nonstationarity features. One reason for this is that there is currently a lack of understanding relating to what constitutes too much nonstationarity when applying HRV measures that are sensitive to this characteristic of biosignals. One solution is to divide a tachogram into segments and determine the average of the segments. A measure of nonstationarity is a large standard deviation difference between the two segments (Palazzolo et al. 1998; Gao et al. 2013; Camargo et al. 2013; Pacheco et al. 2012; Chen et al. 2002; Żebrowski et al. 1999; Lempel and Ziv 1976).

1.2 HRV Methods: A Short Introduction

The interval between successive R peaks is known as the RR interval (inverse of heart rate). RR intervals are obtained from the recorded ECG and the RR variation can be subjected to further analysis through a variety of algorithms in order to yield variables with good discriminant power, based on the difference of RR interval variability with respect to the total recording interval (Pan and Tompkins 1985; Karlsson et al. 2012; Kim et al. 2009; Marzbanrad et al. 2013; Storck et al. 2001; Thuraisingham 2006). For the purposes of further analysis, the RR interval is expressed as the time between beats (measured in milliseconds), and this can be plotted against time to produce the graph shown in Figure 1.2, which illustrates the natural variation of RR intervals over a recording period. The extent of variation is indicative of a healthy cardiac system, as the heart rate is continuously varied to adapt to current needs of oxygenation and perfusion. It is the absence of such a variation that can indicate cardiac disease, especially arrhythmia and risk of sudden cardiac death (Friedman et al. 1975; Huikuri et al. 2003; Kong et al. 2011; Lane et al. 2005; Lombardi et al. 2001; Mäkikallio et al. 2005; Myerburg 2001; Sabir et al. 2013; Singer et al. 1988).

HRV analysis is a simple, sensitive, and noninvasive method for measuring cardiac rhythm and refers to the beat-to-beat variation in heart rate. It is the result of complex interactions between the autonomic nervous system, endocrine influences, and vasomotor and respiratory centers (Kautzner and Camm 1997; Chandra et al. 2003; Thayer et al. 2010; Porges 2007). A variety of measures can be derived from this, and fall into the three categories of time series measures, frequency domain measures, and complex or nonlinear measures. The analysis of HRV, applying time and frequency domain analysis, has been the subject of extensive work (Akselrod et al. 1981; Billman et al. 2015; Schroeder et al. 2004; Liu et al. 2003; Brennan et al. 2002a; Agelink et al. 2001; Umetani et al. 1998; Stein et al. 1994;

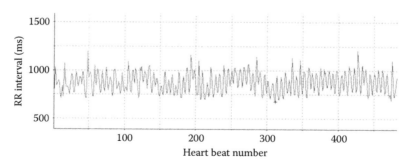

FIGURE 1.2
Normal RR interval graph.

Kleiger et al. 1992; Bigger et al. 1992a). These methods have either focused on the magnitude of RR interval fluctuations around its mean, or on the magnitude of fluctuations in given frequency bands. More recent work has addressed the nonlinearity and nonstationarity characteristics of the ECG signal and development of suitable methods such as those based on Poincaré plot analysis and entropy as well as fractal analysis (TFESC 1996; Cerutti et al. 2009; Cornforth et al. 2015; Cysarz et al. 2000; Goldberger and West 1987; Ho et al. 2011; Hu et al. 2010; Karmakar et al. 2009; Lerma et al. 2003; Lombardi 2000; Peng et al. 1995; Pincus 1991; Porta et al. 2007; Richman and Moorman 2000; Skinner et al. 2011; Stanley et al. 1999; Stein et al. 2005; Teich et al. 2001; Thuraisingham and Gottwald 2006; Voss et al. 2007; Wessel et al. 2000). All of these can be derived from the RR interval time series through suitable mathematical functions.

HRV provides information only on the changes in the interval length between heartbeats over the length of the recording. It is noninvasive and easy to obtain from an ECG recording of any length and with most ECG recording equipment.

For example, an estimate of HRV using the standard deviation of RR intervals (SDRRs) found that this is higher in well-functioning hearts but can be decreased in coronary artery disease, congestive heart failure, and diabetic neuropathy (Kleiger et al. 1987). Although time and frequency domain analysis are useful in disease detection, when only a simple derived measure is required, such as the SDRRs, it is often no better than the average heart rate and in fact contains less information for risk prediction after acute myocardial infarction (Perkiömäki 2011; Reed et al. 2005; Mäkikallio et al. 2005; de Bruin et al. 2005; Anderson and Horne 2005; Huikuri et al. 2003; Abildstrom et al. 2003; Mäkikallio et al. 2001; Odemuyiwa et al. 1991). This indicates that more advanced measures of HRV should be explored, which enable risk prediction based on single-patient RCG recordings. Some of the measures derived from the RR interval fluctuations are now discussed.

1.3 Time Domain Measures of HRV

Time domain measures include the mean and SDRRs recorded. The number of pairs of successive intervals that differ by more than 50 ms, divided by the total number of intervals, yields a parasympathetic measure (pNN50%). The root mean square of successive differences (RMSSD) and the triangular index (Triang. index) are also parasympathetic measures. The triangular interpolation of the interval histogram (TINN) is the estimated width of the density distribution. This is believed to be sensitive to physical and emotional load or to the intensity of the sympathetic nervous system tone.

The Poincaré plot is a visual representation of the time series and is constructed by plotting each consecutive RR interval as a point where $y = RR(t)$ and $x = RR(t-1)$. From this plot, a fitted ellipse leads to estimating SD1 (short-term correlation) and SD2 (long-term correlation) (Figure 1.3; Kamen and Tonkin 1995; Tulppo et al. 1996; Brennan et al. 2002b). An extension is the recurrence plot, which represents a sequence of length n as a point in n-dimensional space, then represents similar pairs as points on a two-dimensional space. The recurrence rate (REC) is the density of these similar points, determinism (DET) is the percentage of recurring points, identified by diagonal lines, and *Lmean* is the mean length of diagonal lines exceeding a threshold (Javorka et al. 2008; Chua et al. 2008).

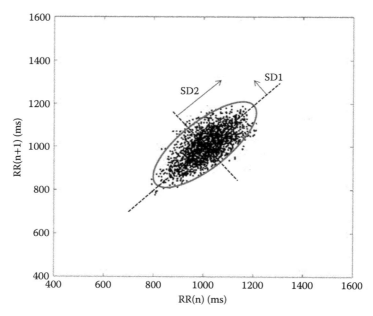

FIGURE 1.3
Poincaré plot for a sequence of RR intervals allows the estimation of SD1 and SD2.

1.4 Frequency Domain Measures of HRV

Frequency domain methods divide the spectral distribution into very low, low, and high frequency regions (Figure 1.4). Low frequency power (LF) is believed to be indicative of both parasympathetic and sympathetic activity, high frequency power (HF) is indicative of parasympathetic activity, and VLF amplitude is closely connected with psycho-emotional state and the functional condition of the brain (TFESC 1996). Other work has shown the importance of VLF—range analysis, and that the capacity of VLF fluctuations of HRV is a sensitive indicator of management of metabolic processes and reflects deficit energy states (Kuusela et al. 2003; Bigger et al. 1992b). The ratio of low to high frequency components, which is indicative of sympathovagal balance, may also be calculated as well as the total power (TFESC 1996). Any component of the power spectrum may also be divided by the total power, to express it in normalized units (n.u.).

1.5 Nonlinear Measures of HRV

The variation in cardiac rhythm has mainly been suggested to be of nonlinear deterministic nature rather than due to stochastic noise. Nonlinear methods include a vast sample of biosignal processing algorithms. Examples are detrended fluctuation analysis (DFA),

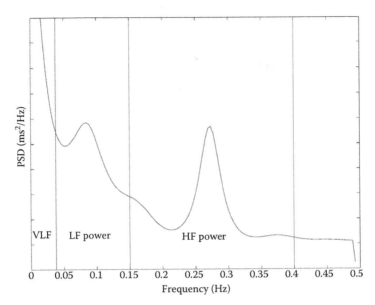

FIGURE 1.4
Power spectrum of RR intervals showing VLF, LF, and HF regions.

fractal dimension, symbolic dynamics, and entropy measures such as sample entropy, Renyi entropy, and the Lyapunov exponent. DFA is an estimate of the fractal correlation of the RR interval series; it provides an exponent expressing short-term correlations (*alpha1*) and another expressing long-term correlations (*alpha2*). Some of these measures are presented in other chapters of this book.

1.6 Clinical Utility of HRV

There is no consensus that any single technique is the single best means of characterizing and differentiating HRV signals in physiology from pathology; rather, investigators agree that multiple techniques should be performed simultaneously to facilitate comparison between methods, techniques, and studies. Before the measurement of HRV can be considered to be of any clinical value, however, therapeutic interventions are needed in the patients who present with abnormal values. Ongoing research should provide important information, for example, whether antiarrhythmic therapy or antidepressant therapy can improve HR variability in patients with arrhythmia or depression. The measurement of HRV by various methods remains a fascinating research subject but not yet a routine clinical tool. If the intensive research into various aspects of HRV continues to increase exponentially as it has done during the last decade, it is possible that the measurement of HRV methods will become a routine clinical procedure comparable with the measurement of blood pressure or plasma cholesterol in the not-too-distant future.

References

Abildstrom, S.Z., B.T. Jensen, E. Agner, C. Torp-Pedersen, O. Nyvad, K. Wachtell, M.M. Ottesen, and J.K. Kanters. 2003. Heart rate versus heart rate variability in risk prediction after myocardial infarction. *Journal of Cardiovascular Electrophysiology* 14:168–173.

Abubaker, H.B., A.H. Khandoker, H.S. Alsafar, and H.F. Jelinek. 2014. Comparison of different se-sampling rates of RR intervals for diabetes classification. ESGCO 2014, Trento, Italy, pp. 239–240.

Agelink, M.W., R. Malessa, B. Baumann, T. Majewski, F. Akila, T. Zeit, and D. Ziegler. 2001. Standardized tests of heart rate variability: Normal ranges obtained from 309 healthy humans, and effects of age, gender and heart rate. *Clinical Autonomic Research* 11:99–108.

Akselrod, S., D. Gordon, F. Ubel, D. Shannon, A. Barger, and R. Cohen. 1981. Power spectrum analysis of heat rate fluctuation: A quantitative probe of beat-to-beat cardiovascular control. *Science* 213:220–222.

Anderson, J.L., and B.D. Horne. 2005. Nonlinear heart rate variability: A better ECG predictor of cardiovascular risk. *Journal of Cardiovascular Electrophysiology* 16:21–23.

Bigger, J.T., Jr., J.L. Fleiss, R.C. Steinman, L.M. Rolnitzky, R.E. Kleiger, and J.N. Rottman. 1992a. Correlations among time and frequency domain measures of heart period variability two weeks after acute myocardial infarction. *American Journal of Cardiology* 69(9):891–898.

Bigger, J.T., Jr., J.L. Fleiss, R.C. Steinman, L.M. Rolnitzky, R.E. Kleiger, and J.N. Rottman. 1992b. Frequency domain measures of heart period variability and mortality after myocardial infarction. *Circulation* 85(1):164–171.

Billman, G.E., H.V. Huikuri, J. Sacha, and K. Trimmel. 2015. An introduction to heart rate variability: Methodological considerations and clinical applications. *Frontiers in Physiology* 6. doi: 10.3389/fphys.2015.00055.

Brennan, M., P. Kamen, and M. Palaniswami. 2002a. New insights into the relationship between Poincare plot geometry and linear measures of heart rate variability. Istanbul, Turkey: IEEE-EMBS, 25–28 October 2001. http://www.dtic.mil/cgi-bin/GetTRDoc?AD=ADA411633&Location=U2&doc=GetTRDoc.pdf.

Brennan, M., M. Palaniswami, and P. Kamen. 2002b. Poincaré plot interpretation using a physiological model of HRV based on a network of oscillators. *American Journal of Physiology: Heart and Circulatory Physiology* 283(5):H1873–H1886.

Camargo, S., M. Riedl, C. Anteneodo, N. Wessel, and J. Kurths. 2013. Diminished heart beat nonstationarities in congestive heart failure. *Frontiers in Physiology: Computational Physiology and Medicine* 4. doi: 10.3389/fphys.2013.00107.

Cerutti, S., D. Hoyer, and A. Voss. 2009. Multiscale, multiorgan and multivariate complexity analyses of cardiovascular regulation. *Philosophical Transactions of the Royal Society A: Mathematical, Physical and Engineering Sciences* 367(1892):1337–1358. doi: 10.1098/rsta.2008.0267.

Chandra, T., D.B. Yeates, and L.B. Wong. 2003. Heart rate variability analysis—Current and future trends. *Business Briefing Global Health Care* 1:1–5.

Chen, Z., P.C. Ivanov, K. Hu, and H. Eugene Stanley. 2002. Effect of nonstationarities on detrended fluctuation analysis. *Physical Review E* 65:041107/1–041107/13.

Chua, K.C., V. Chandran, U.R. Acharya, and C.M. Lim. 2008. Computer-based analysis of cardiac state using entropies, recurrence plots and Poincare geometry. *Journal of Medical Engineering and Technology* 32(4):263–272. doi: 10.1080/03091900600863794.

Clifford, G.D., and L. Tarassenko. 2005. Quantifying errors in spectral estimates of HRV due to beat replacement and resampling. *IEEE Transactions on Biomedical Engineering* 52(4):630–638.

Cornforth, D., H.F. Jelinek, and M. Tarvainen. 2015. A comparison of nonlinear measures for the detection of cardiac autonomic neuropathy from heart rate variability. *Entropy* 17(3):1425–1440.

Cysarz, D., H. Bettermann, and P. van Leeuwen. 2000. Entropies of short binary sequences in heart period dynamics. *American Journal of Physiology, Heart and Circulation Physiology* 278(6): H2163–2172.

de Bruin, M.L, T.P. van Staa, S.V. Belitser, H.G.M. Leufkens, and A.W. Hoes. 2005. Predicting cardiac arrhythmias and sudden cardiac death in diabetic users of proarrhythmic drugs. *Diabetes Care* 28(2):440–442.

de Bruyne, M.C., J.A. Kors, A.W. Hoes, P. Klootwijk, J.M. Dekker, A. Hofman, J.H. van Bemmel, and D.E. Grobbee. 1999. Both decreased and increased heart rate variability on the standard 10-second electrocardiogram predict cardiac mortality in the elderly. *American Journal of Epidemiology* 150(12):1282–1288.

Dekker, J.M., R.S. Crow, A.R. Folsom, P.J. Hannan, D. Liao, C.A. Swenne, and E.G. Schouten. 2000. Low heart rate variability in a 2-minute rhythm strip predicts risk of coronary heart disease and mortality from several causes: The ARIC study. *Circulation* 102(11):1239–1244.

Friedman, G.D., A.L. Klatsky, and A.B. Siegelaub. 1975. Predictors of sudden cardiac death. *Circulation* 52(6 Suppl):III164–69.

Gao, J., B.M. Gurbaxani, J. Hu, K.J. Heilman, V.A. Emauele, G.F. Lewis, M. Davila, E.R. Unger, and J.-M.S. Lin. 2013. Multiscale analysis of heart rate variability in nonstationary environments. *Frontiers in Physiology* 4. doi: 10.3389/fphys.2013.00119.

Goldberger, A.L., and J.B. West. 1987. Application of nonlinear dynamics to clinical cardiology. In *Persectives in Biological Dynamics and Theoretical Medicine*, edited by S. Koslow, A. Mandell and M. Shlesinger, 195–213. New York, NY: The New York Academy of Sciences.

Grant, C.C., D.C.J. van Rensburg, N. Strydom, and M. Viljoen. 2011. Importance of tachogram length and period of recording during noninvasive investigation of the autonomic nervous system. *Annals of Noninvasive Electrocardiology* 16(2):131–139. doi: 10.1111/j.1542-474X.2011.00422.x.

Ho, Y.-L, C. Lin, Y.-H. Lin, and M.-T. Lo. 2011. The prognostic value of non-linear analysis of heart rate variability in patients with congestive heart failure—A pilot study of multiscale entropy. *PLoS One* 6(4):e18699. doi: 10.1371/journal.pone.0018699.

Hu, J., J. Gao, W-W. Tung, and Y. Cao. 2010. Multiscale analysis of heart rate variability: A comparison of different complexity measures. *Annals of Biomedical Engineering* 38(3):854–864.

Huikuri, H.V., J.M. Tapanainen, K. Lindgren, P. Raatikainen, T.H. Mäkikallio, K.E. Juhani Airaksinen, and R.J. Myerburg. 2003. Prediction of sudden cardiac death after myocardial infarction in the beta-blocking era. *Journal of the American College of Cardiology* 42(4):652–628.

Javorka, M., Z. Trunkvalterova, I. Tonhajzerova, Z. Lazarova, J. Javorkova, K. Javorka. 2008. Recurrences in heart rate dynamics are changed in patients with diabetes mellitus. *Clinical Physiology and Functional Imaging* 28(5):326–331.

Jelinek, H.F., T. Alothman, D.J. Cornforth, K. Khalaf, and A. Khandoker. 2014. Effect of biosignal pre-processing and recording length on clinical decision making for cardiac autonomic neuropathy. ESGCO 2014, Trento, Italy, pp. 3–4

Kamen, P.W., and A.M. Tonkin. 1995. Application of the Poincare plot to heart rate variability: A new measure of functional status in heart failure. *Australian and New Zealand Journal of Medicine* 25(1):18–26.

Karlsson, M., R. Hornsten, A. Rydberg, and U. Wiklund. 2012. Automatic filtering of outliers in RR intervals before analysis of heart rate variability in Holter recordings: A comparison with carefully edited data. *Biomedical Engineering Online* 11(2), doi: 10.1186/1475-925X-11-2.

Karmakar, C.K., A. Khandoker, J. Gubbi, and M. Palaniswami. 2009. Complex correlation measure: A novel desciptor for Poincaré plot. *BioMedical Engineering OnLine* 8(17), http://www.biomedical-engineering-online.com/content/8/1/17.

Kautzner, J., and A.J. Camm. 1997. Clinical relevance of heart rate variability. *Clinical Cardiology* 20(2):162–168.

Kemp, A.H., D.S. Quintana, K.L. Felmingham, S. Matthews, and H.F. Jelinek. 2012. Heart rate variability in unmedicated depressed patients without comorbid cardiovascular disease. *Plos One* 7(2):e30777. doi: 10.1371/journal.pone.0030777.

Kim, K.K., J.S. Kim, Y.G. Lim, and K.S. Park. 2009. The effect of missing RR-interval data on heart rate variability analysis in the frequency domain. *Physiological Measurement* 30(10):1039–1050. doi: 10.1088/0967-3334/30/10/005.

Kleiger, R.E., J.P. Miller, J.T. Bigger Jr, and A.J. Moss. 1987. Decreased heart rate variability and its association with increased mortality after acute myocardial infarction. *American Journal of Cardiology* 59(4):256–262.

Kleiger, R.E., P.K. Stein, M.S. Bosner, and J.N. Rottman. 1992. Time domain measurements of heart rate variability. *Cardiology Clinics* 10(3):487–498.

Kong, M.H., G.C. Fonarow, E.D. Peterson, A.B. Curtis, A.F. Hernandez, G.D. Sanders, K.L. Thomas, D.L. Hayes, and S.M. Al-Khatib. 2011. Systematic review of the incidence of sudden cardiac death in the United States. *Journal of the American College of Cardiology* 57(7):794–801. doi: 10.1016/j.jacc.2010.09.064.

Kuusela, T.A., T.J. Kaila, and M. Kahonen. 2003. Fine structure of the low-frequency spectra of heart rate and blood pressure. *BMC Physiology* 3(1):11.

Lane, R.E., M.R. Cowie, and A.W.C. Chow. 2005. Prediction and prevention of sudden cardiac death in heart failure. *Heart* 91:674–680. doi: 10.1136/hrt.2003.025254.

Lempel, A., and J. Ziv. 1976. On the complexity of finite sequences. *IEEE Transactions on Information Theory* 22(1):75–81.

Lerma, C., O. Infante, H. Perez-Grovas, and M.V. Jose. 2003. Poincare plot indexes of heart rate variability capture dynamic adaptations after haemodialysis in chronic renal failure patients. *Clinical Physiology and Functional Imaging* 23(2):72–80.

Liu, P.Y., W.C. Tsai, L.J. Lin, Y.H. Li, T.H. Chao, L.M. Tsai, and J.H. Chen. 2003. Time domain heart rate variability as a predictor of long-term prognosis after acute myocardial infarction. *Journal of the Formosan Medical Association* 102(7):474–479.

Lombardi, F. 2000. Chaos theory, heart rate variability, and arrhythmic mortality. *Circulation* 101(1):8–10.

Lombardi, F., T.H. Makikallio, R.J. Myerburg, and H.V. Huikuri. 2001. Sudden cardiac death: Role of heart rate variability to identify patients at risk. *Cardiovascular Research* 50(2):210–217. doi: S0008636301002218 [pii].

Mäkikallio, T.H., P. Barthel, R. Schneider, A. Bauer, J.M. Tapanainen, M.P. Tulppo, G. Schmidt, and H.V. Huikuri. 2005. Prediction of sudden cardiac death after acute myocardial infarction: Role of Holter monitoring in the modern treatment era. *European Heart Journal* 26(8):762–769.

Mäkikallio, T.H., H. Huikuri, U. Hintze, J. Videbæk, R.D. Mitrani, A. Castellanos, R.J. Myerburg, and M. Møller. 2001. Fractal analysis and time- and frequency-domain measures of heart rate variability as predictors of mortality in patients with heart failure. *American Journal of Cardiology* 87:178–182.

Marzbanrad, F., H.F. Jelinek, E. Ng, M. Tamayo, E. Hambly, C. McLachlan, S. Matthews, S. Palaniswami, and A.H. Khandoker. 2013. The effect of automated preprocessing of RR interval tachogram on discrimination capability of heart rate variability parameters. Zaragoza, Spain: Computing in Cardiology.

Moody, G.B. 1993. Spectral analysis of heart rate without resampling. In *Computers in Cardiology*, edited by A. Murray, pp. 715–718. London, UK, Washington: IEEE Computer Society Press.

Myerburg, R.J. 2001. Sudden cardiac death: Exploring the limits of our knowledge. *Journal of Cardiovascular Electrophysiology* 12(3):369–381. doi: 10.1046/j.1540-8167.2001.00369.x.

Odemuyiwa, O., M. Malik, T. Farrell, Y. Bashir, J. Poloniecki, and A.J. Camm. 1991. A comparison of the predicitive characteristics of HRV index and left ventricular ejection fraction for all-cause mortality, arrhythmic events and sudden cardiac death after acute myocardial infarction. *American Journal of Cardiology* 68:434–439.

Pacheco, J.R., D.T. Román, and H.T. Cruz. 2012. Distinguishing stationary/nonstationary scaling processes using wavelet Tsallis q-entropy. *Mathematical Problems in Engineering*:867042. doi: 10.1155/2012/867042.

Palazzolo, J.A., F.G. Estafanous, and P.A. Murray. 1998. Entropy measures of heart rate variation in conscious dogs. *American Journal of Physiology—Heart and Circulatory Physiology* 274(4):H1099–H1105.

Pan, J., and W.J. Tompkins. 1985. A real-time QRS detection algorithm. *IEEE Transactions in Biomedical Engineering* 32(3):230–236.

Peng, C.K., S. Havlin, H.E. Stanley, and A.L. Goldberger. 1995. Quantification of scaling exponents and crossover phenomena in nonstationary heartbeat time series. *Chaos* 5(1):82–87. doi: 10.1063/1.166141.

Perkiömä, J. 2011. Heart rate variability and nonlinear dynamics in risk stratification. *Frontiers in Physiology* 2. doi: 10.3389/fphys.2011.00081.

Pincus, S.M. 1991. Approximate entropy as a measure of system complexity. *Proceedings of the National Acadamy of Science U S A* 88(6):2297–2301.

Porges, S.W. 2007. The polyvagal theory. *Biological Psychiatry* 74(2):116–143.

Porta, A., S. Guzzetti, R. Furlan, T. Gnecchi-Ruscone, N. Montano, and A. Malliani. 2007. Complexity and nonlinearity in short-term heart period variability: Comparison of methods based on local nonlinear prediction. *IEEE Transactions on Biomedical Engineering* 54(1):94–106. doi: 10.1109/tbme.2006.883789.

Reed, M.J., C.E. Robertson, and P.S. Addison. 2005. Heart rate variability measurements and the prediction of ventricular arrhythmias. *Quarterly Journal of Medicine* 98(2):87–95. doi: 10.1093/qjmed/hci018.

Richman, J.S., and J.R. Moorman. 2000. Physiological time-series analysis using approximate entropy and sample entropy. *American Journal of Physiology—Heart and Circulatory Physiology* 278(6):H2039–H2049.

Sabir, I.N, G.D.K. Matthews, and C.L.-H. Huang. 2013. Sudden arrhythmic death: From basic science to clinical practice. *Frontier in Physiology* 4:339. doi: 10.3389/fphys.2013.00339.

Sapoznikov, D., M.H. Luria, Y. Mahler, and M.S. Gotsman. 1992. Computer processing of artifact and arrhythmias in heart rate variability analysis. *Computer Methods and Programs in Biomedicine* 39(1–2):75–84.

Saul, J.P., P. Albrecht, R.D. Berger, and R.J. Cohen. 1988. Analysis of long term heart rate variability: Methods, 1/f scaling and implications. *Computers in Cardiology* 14:419–422.

Schroeder, E.B., E.A. Whitsel, G.W. Evans, R.J. Prineas, L.E. Chambless, and G. Heiss. 2004. Repeatability of heart rate variability measures. *Journal of Electrocardiology* 37(3):163–172.

Singer, D.H., G.J. Martin, N. Magid, J.S. Weiss, J.W. Schaad, R. Kehoe, T. Zheutlin, D.J. Fintel, A.M. Hsieh, and M. Lesch. 1988. Low heart rate variability and sudden cardiac death. *Journal of Electrocardiology* 21 Suppl:S46–S55.

Singh, D., K. Vinod, and S.C. Saxena. 2004. Sampling frequency of the RR interval time series for spectral analysis of heart rate variability. *Journal of Medical Engineering and Technology* 28(6): 263–72. doi: 10.1080/03091900410001662350.

Sinnreich, R, J. Kark, D. Sapoznikov, and M. Luria. 1998. Five minute recordings of heart rate variability for population studies: Repeatability and age-sex characteristics. *Heart* 80(2):156–163.

Skinner, J.E., D.N. Weiss, J.M. Anchin, Z. Turianikova, I. Tonhajzerova, J. Javorkova, K. Javorka, M. Baumert, and M. Javorka. 2011. Nonlinear PD2i heart rate complexity algorithm detects autonomic neuropathy in patients with type 1 diabetes mellitus. *Clinical Neurophysiology* 122(7):1457–1462.

Smith, A.-L., H. Owen, and K.J. Reynolds. 2013. Heart rate variability indices for very short-term (30 beat) analysis. Part 1: Survey and toolbox. *Journal of Clinical Monitoring and Computing* 27(5): 569–576. doi: 10.1007/s10877-013-9471-4.

Stanley, H.E., L.A. Amaral, A.L. Goldberger, S. Havlin, P. Ch. Ivanov, and C.K. Peng. 1999. Statistical physics and physiology: Monofractal and multifractal approaches. *Physics A* 270:309–324.

Stein, P.K., M.S. Bosner, R.E. Kleiger, and B.M. Conger. 1994. Heart rate variability: A measure of cardiac autonomic tone. *American Heart Journal* 127(5):1376–1381.

Stein, P.K., P.P. Domitrovich, H.V. Huikuri, and R.E. Kleiger. 2005. Traditional and nonlinear heart rate variability are each independendly associated with mortality after myocardial infarction. *Journal of Cardiovascular Electrophysiology* 16(1):13–20.

Storck, N., M. Ericson, L. Lindblad, and M. Jensen-Urstad. 2001. Automatic computerized analysis of heart rate variability with digital filtering of ectopic beats. *Clinical Physiology* 21(1):15–24.

Struzik, Z.R., and J. Hayano. 2006. Spectral analysis of HRV without resampling. http://www.physionet.org/physiotools/lomb/lomb/html.

Teich, M.C., S.B. Lowen, B.M. Jost, and K. Vibe-Rheymer, eds. 2001. *Heart Rate Variability: Measures and Models*. Edited by M. Akay. Vol. II, *Nonlinear Biomedical Signal Processing, Dynamic Analysis and Modeling*. New York, NY: IEEE Press.

TFESC. 1996. Special report: Heart rate variability standards of measurement, physiological interpretation, and clinical use. *Circulation* 93(5):1043–1065.

Thayer, J.F., S.S. Yamamoto, and J.F. Brosschot. 2010. The relationship of autonomic imbalance, heart rate variability and cardiovascular disease risk factors. *Internatonal Journal of Cardiology* 141(2):122–131. doi: 10.1016/j.ijcard.2009.09.543.

Thuraisingham, R.A. 2006. Preprocessing RR interval time series for heart rate variability analysis and estimates of standard deviation of RR intervals. *Computer Methods and Programs in Biomedicine* 83(1):78–82. doi: 10.1016/j.cmpb.2006.05.002.

Thuraisingham, R., and G. Gottwald. 2006. On multiscale entropy analysis for physiological data. *Physica A* 366:323–332. doi: citeulike-article-id:2316796, 10.1016/j.physa.2005.10.008.

Tulppo, M.P., T.H. Mäkikallio, T.E.S. Takala, and T. Seppänen. 1996. Quantitative beat-to-beat analysis of heart rate dynamics during exercise. *American Journal of Physiology—Heart and Circulatory Physiology* 271:H244–H252.

Umetani, K., D.H. Singer, R. McCraty, and M. Atkinson 1998. Twenty-four hour time domain heart rate variability and heart rate: Relations to age and gender over nine decades. *Journal of the American College of Cardiology* 31(3):593–601.

Voss, A., R. Schroeder, S. Truebner, M. Goernig, H.R. Figulla, and A. Schirdewan. 2007. Comparison of nonlinear methods symbolic dynamics, detrended fluctuation, and Poincaré plot analysis in risk stratification in patients with dilated cardiomyopathy. *Chaos: An Interdisciplinary Journal of Nonlinear Science* 17(1):015120. doi: http://dx.doi.org/10.1063/1.2404633.

Wessel, N., A. Voss, H. Malberg, C. Ziehmann, H.U. Voss, A. Schirdewan, U. Meyerfeldt, and J. Kurths. 2000. Nonlinear analysis of complex phenomena in cardiological data. *Herzschrittmacher Therapie und Elektrophysiologie* 11:159–173.

Żebrowski, J.J., W. Popławska, R. Baranowski, and T. Buchner. 1999. Measuring the complexity of non-stationarity of non-linear interpretations of selected physiological processes. *ACTA Physica Polonica B* 30(8):2547–2570.

2

Historical Development of HRV Analysis

Andreas Voss

CONTENTS

Heart rate variability (HRV) is an expression of the immense complex interplay (Voss et al. 2009) of various biological systems and subsystems (Figure 2.1). Heart rate (HR) is strongly modulated by the combined effects of the sympathetic and parasympathetic nervous systems that are effecting heartbeat generation in the sinoatrial node. Therefore, measurement of changes in HR over time (HRV) provides information about physiological and/or impaired autonomic functioning. In a healthy subject, these variations are strongly correlated with central activity, breathing, circadian rhythm, vasomotion, and exercise (Hainsworth 2004).

In healthy subjects, the sinoatrial node located at the posterior wall of the right atrium initiates each beat of the heart. Due to the unstable membrane potential of the myocytes located in this region, action potentials are generated periodically at a fairly constant fre-

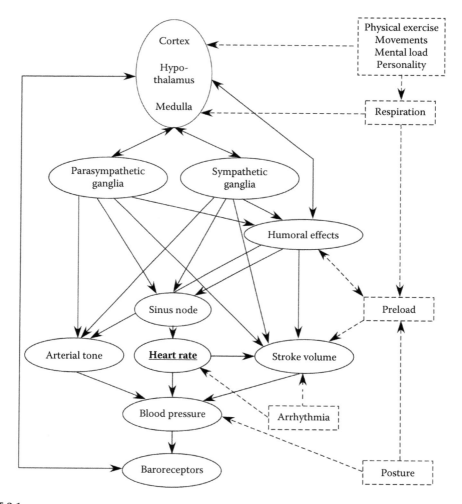

FIGURE 2.1
Simplified scheme of regulation of heart rate as an interplay of various biological systems and subsystems. (Courtesy of *Philos Transact A Math Phys Eng Sci.*) (From Voss, A. et al., *Philos Trans A Math Phys Eng Sci*, 367 (1887), 277–96, 2009.)

quency. This relatively constant frequency generated by the autorhythmicity of the sinoa-trial node is modulated by many factors that add variability to the HR signal at different frequencies (Stauss 2003; Task Force 1996) and over different scales (Cerutti et al. 2009).

Various studies (Ashkenazi et al. 1993; Busjahn et al. 1998; Voss et al. 1996a) suggest that there is a genetic component in HR generation and HRV, in addition to family envi-

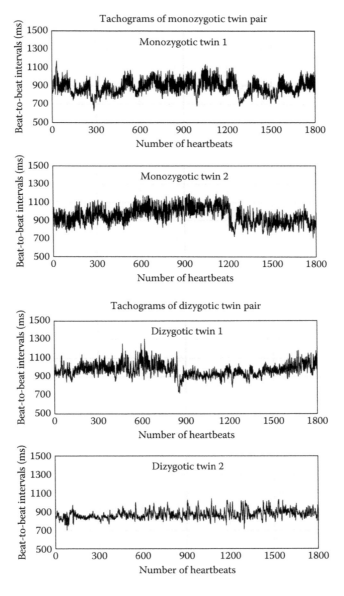

FIGURE 2.2
Genetic influences on heart rate variability (HRV). Monozygotic twins (top) show more similar tachograms than dizygotic twins (bottom). The reason for this is that monozygotic twins are genetically nearly identical while dizygotic twins are no more genetically similar than any other set of siblings.

ronmental influences (Figure 2.2). Further on, there are partly considerably influences of gender and age on short-term and long-term HRV (Murata et al. 1992; Ryan et al. 1994; Voss et al. 2015; Boettger et al. 2010).

The measurement of HRV from the electrocardiogram (ECG) or pulse curve is a bedside or an ambulant, noninvasive, low-cost, and simple to perform method, requiring standard medical equipment and dedicated software. The latter reflects the physiological or impaired balance of autonomic nervous system (ANS) regulation based on dedicated HR oscillations. Parasympathetic (vagal) activation corresponding to rapid dynamic control through acetylcholine targeting muscarinic receptors (high frequencies of the power spectrum) and sympathetic innervations have slower interaction via the β-adrenergic receptors. However, the autonomic regulation on the ventricular repolarization is not limited to the sinus nodal periodicity; there is a direct impact of the autonomic regulation on the cardiac cell of the ventricles (Couderc 2009).

From an electrophysiological standpoint, the P-to-P (PP) intervals reflect the variability of sinus node activity (Figure 2.3). However, reliable detection of P-waves is more difficult than QRS complex detection (dominant R peak) for several reasons, for example, low amplitudes, low signal-to-noise ratio, amplitude and morphological variability, and others. Nevertheless, RR intervals also reveal information about sinus node activity with sufficient accuracy because the spontaneous fluctuations of the PR interval are mostly lower than 2–4 ms (Esperer 1992).

Excluding arrhythmic events and artifacts from the RR-interval time series, we obtain the normal-to-normal (NN)-time series representing sinus node activity. The RR- or NN-interval time series plotted over time or beats are called tachograms.

HRV is a measure of variations in the HR over time (beats). Figure 2.4 shows the variation of the HR in a healthy subject and in patients with different impairments of the autonomic regulation.

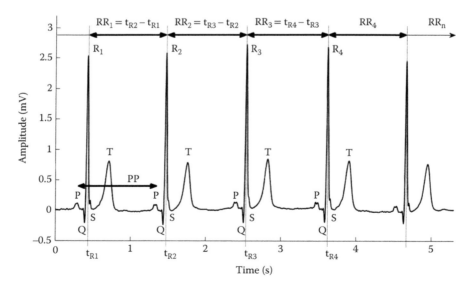

FIGURE 2.3
ECG with typical peaks and RR intervals.

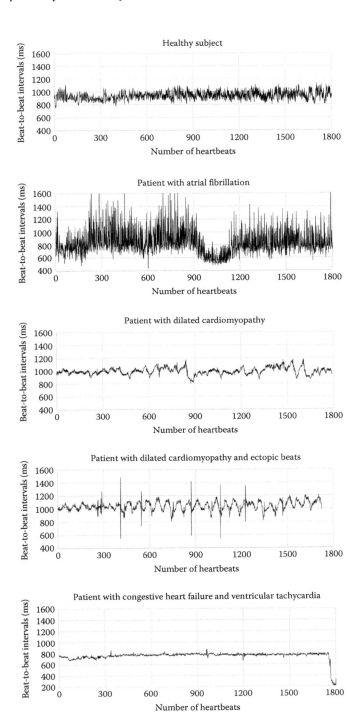

FIGURE 2.4
Tachograms from a healthy subject and patients with different heart diseases. With the exception of atrial fibrillation, all other heart diseases exhibit a reduced HRV. Atrial fibrillation generates an increased HRV caused by the lost coordination between the P-wave and R-peak.

2.1 History of HRV

Oscillations of the blood pressure and HR (pulse) have been known for a very long time. In the following review, some of the milestones in HR (pulse) detection and analysis are discussed.

Papyrun Eburs, an Egyptian papyrus (Figure 2.5) from about 1552 BCE, is the oldest preserved medical document. The papyrus contains chapters on different diseases and it

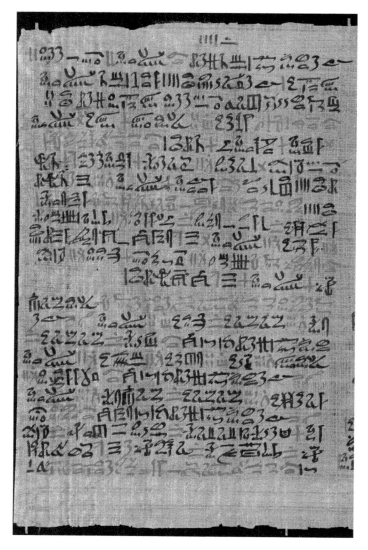

FIGURE 2.5

Papyrus Ebers, Kol.44, Universitätsbibliothek Leipzig (Courtesy of Reinhold Scholl). This page lists several possibilities to treat heart diseases. Unfortunately, the original pages related to pulse analysis got lost over the postwar years.

also includes a surprisingly accurate description of the circulatory system, noting the existence of blood vessels throughout the body and the heart's function as a center of the blood supply (Enersen 2015). In this context, the heart pulse and changes of the heart pulse are already mentioned. The Egyptians regarded the pulse as the voice of the heart and attempts to understand that voice led to an extensive pulse lore (Van Praagh and Van Praagh 1983).

Herophilos of Chalcedon (fourth century BCE) is an outstanding representative of ancient medicine. He is rightly counted as the father of anatomy. He was interested in different branches of medicine. Herophilos also found that the pulse is the result of the contractions and expansions of the arteries. However, he could not exactly explain where the pressure (pneuma) came from and suggested that "pneuma in the arteries could come from any proximate source." He did not see the direct connection between pulse and the heart (von Staden 1989).

Rufus of Ephesus, a famous ancient physician, lived approximately from 80 to 150 CE. He was the first to describe the relation between heart and pulse. He proposed (Bujalkova 2011) that the heart—as the origin of warmth, life, and pulsation—consists of the head, the bottom, and the heart cavities. The thicker left chamber is arterial, while the thinner right chamber, which is wider than the left one, is venous. Along both sides of the heart–head, he described wing-shaped free cavities which move synchronously with the pulsation of the heart—the so-called "heart ears."

Claudius Galen (Galen of Pergamon, about 129–200) and his scholarly teachings defined the practice of medicine in Western Europe for 1500 years. Galen was also an expert on the pulse; many consider him to be the originator of pulse diagnosis. He wrote at least 18 books on the pulse including at least eight treatises that described using pulse for diagnosis and predicting the prognosis of disease (Billman 2011). He stated that the power of pulsation has its origin in the heart itself and further that the fact that the heart, removed from the thorax, can be seen to move for a considerable time is a definite indication that it does not need nerves to perform its own function. Although Galen did not discuss the mechanism of the heart's automatic activity, he concluded that the pulsative faculty of the heart has its source in its own substance (Fye 1987). One of his more famous observations was that a woman's pulse sped up when she heard the name of her lover (Fullerton and Silverman 2009).

Stephen Hales (1677–1761) was the first to report that the beat-to-beat interval (BBI) and arterial pressure level varied during the respiratory cycle (Billman 2011).

Later on, in the eighteenth century, Albrecht von Haller's (1708–1777) observations on the heartbeat were his most significant contribution to cardiovascular physiology. He confirmed that the heart continues to beat despite the lack of any connection to the nervous system. Based on these experiments, he proposed that the heart muscle had intrinsic irritability that was stimulated by blood flowing over the organ's walls (Fye 1995). He also noticed that the beat of a healthy heart is not absolutely regular (Stys and Stys 1998).

Since its description by Carl Ludwig (1816–1895) in 1847 the mechanism of respiratory sinus arrhythmia (RSA) has been the subject of considerable research interest (Galletly and Larsen 1998). RSA is the variation in heartbeat interval with respiration.

This was followed in 1865 by Traube and in 1876 by Mayer, who published their results about periodical vasomotion and periodical blood pressure variations; these variabilities are known in the modern physiology (Esperer 1992).

In 1882, physiologist Augustus Desiré Waller recorded an ECG from his dog Jimmy and, later in 1887, for the first time (published), an ECG recording from a human (AlGhatrif and Lindsay 2012) using a capillary electrometer (Alexander Muirhead, an electrical engineer and pioneer of telegraphy, may have recorded a human ECG earlier in 1870 but this is controversial).

Dr. Willem Einthoven (1860–1927), a Dutch physiologist inspired by the work of Waller, refined the capillary electrometer even further and finally developed, in 1901, a new string galvanometer with very high sensitivity, which he used in his electrocardiograph (AlGhatrif and Lindsay 2012). This was the basis for future developments that made electrocardiography available for clinical use. In 1924, Einthoven was awarded the Nobel Prize in Physiology or Medicine for the invention of the electrocardiograph.

In 1935, Matthes performed the first pulse oximetry (PO) at the human ear (Matthes and Hauss 1938), the basis of a simpler method to record HR than the ECG.

In 1936, Anrep, Pascual, and Rössler proposed that the HR sinus arrhythmia is caused by the regulation of cardiac vagal outflow involving the same neuronal processes that generate the respiratory rhythm and reside within the brainstem (Garcia et al. 2013). This was more or less the introduction of interaction analyses in the investigation of couplings within the ANS.

The first device for ambulatory electrocardiography monitoring was developed in 1947 by Norman Holter (1914–1983). To become convinced of the usefulness of the ambulatory ECG in the late fifties, Holter conducted research on 200 patients in Great Falls (Gawłowska 2009). The experiment was successful in revealing some cases of exertional angina. This opened the possibility of investigating long-term HRV under normal circumstances and was at the same time the beginning of telemetry.

Hon and Lee (1963, 1965) noticed that fetal distress was accompanied by the changes in beat-to-beat variation of the fetal heart, even before there was detectable change in HR. This study was one of the very first applications of HRV analysis in clinical use.

Beginning in the early 1970s, several groups (Hyndman et al. 1971; Sayers 1973; Chess et al. 1975; Penaz et al. 1978; Akselrod et al. 1981) applied power spectral analysis to investigate the physiological basis for the individual frequency components that compose the periodic variations in HR (Billman 2011). Power spectral density (PSD) analysis performed using the fast Fourier transform (FFT) of RR-interval series or autoregressive (AR) methods reveal mainly three spectral components. In humans, these components are the high frequency (HF), the low frequency (LF), and the very low frequency (VLF) components. Most research concentrates on the LF and HF components due to the length of recording required for correct VLF analysis.

New developments following FFT or AR modeling are due to most of the biomedical signals recorded being nonlinear, nonstationary, and non-Gaussian in nature and therefore, it can be more advantageous to analyze them with higher order statistics/spectra compared to the use of second-order correlations and power spectra (Chua et al. 2010).

Although HRV was well recognized as a physiological phenomenon in the ensuing centuries, it was only widely appreciated in the 1960s and 1970s that a decrease in HRV accompanied autonomic failure and that this loss of HRV could be used as a measure of impaired autonomic function (Freeman and Chapleau 2013).

In 1978, Wolf et al. was the first to show that patients after a myocardial infarction (MI) with a reduced HRV had increased mortality. This was confirmed by Myers et al. (1986) who showed that HRV was reduced in cardiac patients known to be at increased risk of sudden cardiac death (SCD), when compared to those who were not at increased risk. These differences were greatest in power spectral methods. Then Kleiger et al. (1987) found that in patients recovering from MIs, those with the smallest HRV (standard deviation of RR intervals) had the greatest risk of dying suddenly. This finding set the basis for the use of HRV in post-acute myocardial infarction (AMI) risk stratification where it still holds its place as a tool of established practical value. Numerous studies have since supported the notion that decreased vagal activity, as indexed by HRV, predicts mortality in high risk as well as low risk populations.

During the 1980s, personal and bedside computers were available worldwide to measure and analyze HRV with simpler and more mobile computer-based techniques (Smith and Smith 1981). This offered much more distributed computational power and led to an exponential increase of studies that related to the analysis of HRV in the various fields of biology and medicine. In 1977, we counted about 160 Pubmed HRV references; this increased from 897 in 1987 to 3730 in 1997 and in 2015, we counted more than 17,500.

As a consequence of the outcomes from several studies, it became evident relatively early that autonomic regulation cannot be sufficiently characterized by calculating only a single index from the HRV (Cerutti et al. 2009). Therefore, combinations of indices only from HRV analysis or combinations of indices from HRV analysis and indices either from other biological signals (Guzzetti et al. 1991; Voss et al. 1996b) and/or medical parameters (Pedretti et al. 1993; Schmidt et al. 1996) were investigated in a multivariate approach.

One objective of coupling analyses was to characterize in more detail the behavior of known interactions such as baroreflex and RSA to get information about their physiological and pathophysiological developments. However, beneath these prominent autonomically mediated coupling mechanisms, there were many more such couplings within the ANS expected because of the very complex structure of HR generation (see Figure 2.1). One of the first approaches to obtain more information about the interplay of systems underlying autonomous regulation was introduced by Aarimaa et al. (1988); they investigated the interaction of HR and respiration in newborn babies by using the frequency cross-spectral densities of HRV and an impedance respirogram (Aarimaa et al. 1988). An overview of various available coupling analysis methods is provided in Schulz et al. (2013). Some prominent methods are described in the following methods section.

Beginning with the introduction of chaos theory to many different research fields, it was found that methods derived from nonlinear dynamics (NLD) provide new insights into the HRV changes under various physiological and pathophysiological conditions. They provide additional prognostic information and complement traditional time- and frequency-domain analyses of HRV (Voss et al. 2009).

Pioneering work was performed by the group of Glass (Guevara et al. 1981; Glass 1988) who introduced nonlinear approaches into heart rhythm analysis. Period-doubling bifurcations, in which the period of a regular oscillation doubles, were predicted theoretically and observed experimentally in the heart cells of embryonic chickens. Form, qualitative change, oscillation, stability, and other important biological notions found inherent expression in the new mathematical approach of NLD (Garfinkel 1983); Ritzenberg et al. (1984) were the first to provide evidence of nonlinear behavior in the ECG with the arterial blood pressure traces of a dog that had been injected with noradrenaline. The first approaches of HRV analyses based on nonlinear fractal dynamics were performed by Goldberger and West (1987). It was suggested that self-similar (fractal) scaling may underlie the 1/f-like spectra (Kobayashi and Musha 1982) as seen in multiple systems (e.g., interbeat interval variability and daily neutrophil fluctuations). They proposed that this fractal scale invariance may provide a mechanism for the "constrained randomness" underlying physiological variability and adaptability. Especially in the 1990s and later, various different NLD approaches were developed. Some of the most prominent ones are described in more detail in the methods section. To prove the ability of these methods, it is necessary to check the data for nonlinearity. One of the tests for nonlinearity is the surrogate data test. The method of using surrogate data in nonlinear time series analysis was introduced by Theiler et al. (1992).

In 1996—as a milestone in the history of HRV analysis—an international task force consisting of members from the European Society of Cardiology and the North American Society for Pacing and Electrophysiology published a report about standards of measurement, physiological interpretation, and clinical use of HRV (Task Force 1996).

After usable PO monitoring devices were available for reasonable prices in the mid-90s, they became standard equipment in clinical monitoring. A regular PO monitoring device continuously displays the arterial oxygen saturation value, SpO_2, and the current HR (pulse rate), averaged over some time interval. This inspired some researchers to assess the reliability of the detected PR and sometimes a photoplethysmographic (PPG)-derived breathing rate, both of which are also very interesting in telecare or when monitoring outpatients. However, pulse rate variability as an estimate of HRV has proved to be sufficiently accurate only for healthy (and mostly younger) subjects at rest (Schafer and Vagedes 2013).

A selection of further important methods, discoveries, developments, and applications are briefly discussed in Sections 2.2 through 2.5

2.2 Methods of HRV Analysis Based on Sinus Rhythm

In the following, we discuss some of the most prominent applied HRV analysis approaches that have shown clinical relevance without claiming that the presented selection of approaches is complete. These HRV approaches are further summarized in Table 2.1(Continued), with emphasis on their main properties regarding short- and long-term analyses, requirement of stationarity of the HR time series, and main output indices as well as recommendations and limitations for their application.

2.2.1 Linear Methods—Time Domain

HRV analyses in the time domain evaluate variability by determining the variations of normal-to-normal RR intervals (NN intervals) over a period of time. Here, a huge amount of statistical and geometrical indices can be directly determined from the NN intervals or can be derived from the differences between NN intervals. These indices involve mean, standard deviation, counting of the samples above or below a certain threshold, and other statistical measures that are based on the distribution of the data and not their order (Bravi et al. 2011). The most commonly used statistical and geometrical time-domain indices are as follows (Task Force 1996):

- meanNN: the mean value of NN intervals
- SDNN: the standard deviation of all NN intervals as a measure of global variability
- SDANN: the standard deviation of the averages of NN intervals in all 5-minute segments, which estimates the long-term components of HRV
- RMSSD: the square root of the mean squared differences of successive NN intervals, which estimates the short-term components of HRV

TABLE 2.1

Heart Rate Variability Analysis Approaches and Their Main Properties

Variability Approach	Domain	Recommendation and Limitations	Main Indices	Short Term	Long Term	Stationarity
Statistical representation	Time	NN intervals are required; sensitive to artifacts, ectopic beats, and noise	meanNN, SDNN, SDANN, RMSSD, SDNN index, SDSD, NN50, pNN50, HTI, TINN	X	X	X
Frequency representation	Frequency	Periodicity and NN intervals are required, sensitive to artifacts, ectopic beats, and noise*	Total power, ULF, VLF, LF, HF, LF/HF, LFn, HFn	X	X	X*
Power-law correlation	Nonlinear	Periodicity and large data sets are required; patient movement (slow frequency components) and artifacts influence spectral components	Scaling exponent β	–	X	X
Detrended fluctuation analysis	Nonlinear	At least 8000 data points and NN intervals are needed; monofractal method; sensitive to artifacts, ectopic beats, and noise; correlation with frequency domain indices	Scaling exponent α1 (short-term), scaling exponent α2 (long-term)	–	X	–
Multifractal analysis	Nonlinear	Require many local and theoretically infinite exponents to fully characterize their scaling properties	$D(h)$ with local exponent h	X	X	–
Symbolic dynamic	Nonlinear	Detailed information is lost but the more general dynamic behavior can be analyzed; outliers (ectopic beats, noise) influence symbol strings	Shannon and Rényi entropies, forbidden words, wpsum02, wpsum13, phvar, plvar, 0V, 1V, 2LV, 2UV, 0V%, 1V%, 2LV%, 2UV%	X	X	–
Correlation dimension	Nonlinear	The ability to determine the dimension depends on the number of data points; criterion to determine CD: $N > ^{(D/2)}$	CD	–	X	X
Lyapunov exponent/finite-time growth rates	Nonlinear	Requires large amounts of data; long computing times; system must remain stable; relatively difficult to implement	λ, λ_K	X	X	X

*For time-frequency approaches, stationarity is not required

(Continued)

TABLE 2.1 (Continued)

Heart Rate Variability Analysis Approaches and Their Main Properties

Variability Approach	Domain	Recommendation and Limitations	Main Indices	Short Term	Long Term	Stationarity
Poincaré plot	Nonlinear	SD1, SD2 dependent on other time-domain measures (SDANN, SDSD)	SD1, SD2, SD1/SD2	X	X	X
Recurrence plot	Nonlinear	Dependent on ε (threshold distance) and embedding dimension (10–20, not higher)	Isolated points, diagonal lines, horizontal/vertical lines	X	X	–
Approximate entropy	Nonlinear	Noise–free data are required; inherent bias exists by ApEn calculation because count self-matches and suggests more similarity than is present; dependency on the record length and is uniformly lower than expected for short records; lacks relative consistency; evaluate regularity on the shortest scale (one) only and ignore other scales; outliers (missed beat detections, artifacts) may affect the entropy values	ApEn	X	–	X
Sample entropy	Nonlinear	Time irreversibility is required; SampEn for higher pattern length values requires a substantially increased number of data points (beats); evaluate regularity on the shortest scale (one) only and ignore other scales; outliers (missed beat detections, artifacts) may affect the entropy values	SampEn	X	–	X
Multiscale entropy	Nonlinear	Time irreversibility is required; outliers (missed beat detections, artifacts) may affect the entropy values; as the number of data points decreases, the consistency of MSE results is progressively lost	MSE	X	X	X
Compression entropy	Nonlinear	Dependent on sample rate, the window length, and the lookahead buffer size; implementation has to consider integer numbers	H_{CE}	X	X	–

- SDNN index: the mean of the standard deviations of all NN intervals for all 5-minute segments
- SDSD: the standard deviation of differences between successive NN intervals
- NN50: the number of successive NN intervals differing by more than 50 ms from the preceding interval
- pNN50: NN50 divided by the total number of all NN intervals
- HTI: the HRV triangular index, which estimates overall HRV by determining the ratio of the total number of NN intervals to the number of NN intervals in the modal bin (128 Hz is the standard)
- TINN: the triangular interpolation of the NN interval histogram, created by determining the baseline width of the minimum square difference triangular interpolation of the highest peak of the histogram of all NN intervals.

2.2.2 Linear Methods—Frequency Domain

HR fluctuations, which reflect modulation of sinus node activity by autonomic and other homeostatic mechanisms, can be quantified and displayed using frequency-domain analysis. Frequency-domain measures use spectral analysis of a sequence of RR intervals and provide information on how power (variance) is distributed as a function of frequency or as a function of time and frequency. The introduction of power spectral analysis in HRV analysis provided a useful noninvasive technique for analyzing the autonomic mechanisms that control HR (Akselrod et al. 1981). Spectral analysis of the resting HR commonly produces several prominent peaks (Sayers 1973). Several animal and human experiments with pharmacological blockade of the ANS (Freeman 2006) have shown that the sympathetic and parasympathetic nervous systems mediate HR fluctuations in different frequency bands (Akselrod et al. 1981; Pagani et al. 1986).

Power spectrum analysis enables a quantitative representation of the contributing frequencies to an underlying biosignal. Thereby, these frequencies are classified as VLF (≤ 0.04 Hz), LF (0.04–0.15 Hz), and HF (0.15–0.4 Hz) for short-term recordings. For long-term recordings (24 hours), the VLF band can be further subdivided into the VLF (0.003–0.04 Hz) and the ultralow frequency (ULF; ≤ 0.003 Hz) bands. The ULF band may represent the circadian rhythm, the VLF band is possibly affected by temperature regulation and humoral systems, the LF band is sensitive to changes in cardiac sympathetic and parasympathetic nerve activity, and the HF band is synchronized to the respiratory rhythm and is primarily modulated by cardiac parasympathetic innervation (Stauss 2003; Valentini and Parati 2009). In addition, the components of higher frequencies (greater than 0.15 Hz) reflect oscillations of HR mediated by respiration via the RSA. The HF peak is also known to represent the respiratory frequency and is driven by the vagus nerve as indicated by the strong respiratory pattern of cardiac vagal motoneurons in the nucleus ambiguous (Rentero et al. 2002). In addition to the frequency bands, the total power (TP) of the spectrum (area under the curve) can be estimated as the variance of the NN interval segments (5 minutes, 24 hours) under investigation. The LF and HF power can also be represented in normalized units as LFn = LF/(LF + HF) and HFn = HF/(LF + HF).

As discussed above, many studies have presumed that LF power, especially if adjusted for HF power, TP, or respiration, provides an index of cardiac sympathetic "tone" and that the ratio of LF/HF power indicates "sympathovagal balance." However, recently, Goldstein et al. (2011) hypothesized that with or without adjustment for HF power, TP, or respiration, LF power seems to provide an index not of cardiac sympathetic tone but of baroreflex function! Manipulations and drugs that change LF power or LF/HF may do so not by affecting cardiac autonomic outflows directly but by affecting modulation of those outflows by baroreflexes.

For spectral analyses, the PSD function can be calculated either by parametric (AR models: Blackman–Tuckey's method, Welch's method, Burg's method, and Yule–Walker's method) and nonparametric (FFT) approaches or at least by applying the Lomb periodogram (a method to find periodicities in unevenly spaced data). Here, the Lomb method seems to be superior for PSD estimation of the HR spectrum than the FFT or AR models (Laguna et al. 1998).

To overcome the limitation of stationarity for estimating the power spectrum, several time-frequency approaches were introduced: the short-time Fourier transform (STFT), the Wigner–Ville transform (WVT), and the wavelet transform (WT).

2.2.3 Nonlinear Dynamics

Linear time and frequency-domain measures are often not sufficient to quantify the complex dynamics of HR generation. Therefore, various efforts have been made to apply nonlinear techniques (especially from NLD) to analyze HRV (Voss et al. 2009). These methods differ from the traditional time- and frequency-domain HRV analyses because they quantify the signal properties instead of assessing the magnitude of the HRV. They assess the self-affinity of heartbeat fluctuations over multiple time scales (fractal measures); the regularity/irregularity or randomness of heartbeat fluctuations (entropy measures); the coarse-grained dynamics of HR fluctuations based on symbols (symbolic dynamics); and the heartbeat dynamics based on a simplified phase-space embedding (Voss et al. 2009).

2.2.3.1 Power Law (Scaling Exponent β)

The frequency dependence of the power spectrum of heartbeat fluctuations was first reported in 1982 by Kobayashi and Musha in a normal young man. They found when plotting the power spectrum and frequency, f, of these RR intervals on a log–log graph (bilogarithmic scale), the plot can be described by a straight line with a slope equal to -1. In a log–log plot, the power law slope between 10^{-2} and 10^{-4} Hz is linear with a negative slope and reflects the degree to which the structure of the RR interval time series is self-similar over a scale of minutes to hours (Kleiger et al. 2005). The so-called $1/f$ relationship means that the power decreased approximately as a reciprocal of the underlying frequency, f. The slope of the regression line is also referred to as the scaling exponent, β, and provides an index for the long-term scaling characteristics.

2.2.3.2 Detrended Fluctuation Analysis (Fractal Scaling Exponent α1 and α2)

This method is based on a modified random walk analysis and was introduced and applied to physiologic time series by Peng et al. (1995). It quantifies the presence or absence of fractal correlation properties in nonstationary time series. The detrended fluctuation analysis (DFA) is based on the computation of the fractal scaling exponent α1 for short-term fractal scaling properties (calculated for the range $n = 4–16$ heartbeats) and the fractal scaling exponent α2 of long-term fractal scaling properties (calculated for the range $n = 16–64$ heartbeats; Peng et al. 1995). DFA offers clinicians the advantage of a means to investigate long-range correlations within a biological signal due to the intrinsic properties of the system producing the signal, rather than external stimuli unrelated to the "health" of the system (Seely and Macklem 2004).

2.2.3.3 Multifractal Analysis

Monofractal measures (DFA) assume that the same scaling properties are presented throughout an entire time series (Seely and Macklem 2004). The multifractal DFA (MDFA), introduced by Kantelhardt et al. (2002), is an alternative approach for the multifractal characterization of nonstationary time series based on a generalization of the monofractal DFA. Furthermore, Ivanov et al. (1999) demonstrated that the multifractal time series (biological dynamical system) require a large number of local scaling exponents to fully characterize their scaling properties. Multifractality in heartbeat dynamics indicates that the nonlinear control mechanisms involve coupled cascades of feedback loops in a system operating far from equilibrium (Goldberger et al. 2002). Thus, the multifractal method may add diagnostic power to contemporary analytic methods of the heartbeat (and other physiological) time-series analysis. The multifractality of heartbeat time series also enables us to quantify the greater complexity of the healthy dynamics compared to those of pathological conditions. Ivanov et al. (1999) found a loss of multifractality for a life-threatening condition, congestive heart failure (CHF), and that the healthy heartbeat is even more complex than previously suspected.

2.2.3.4 Symbolic Dynamics

Kurths and Voss introduced symbolic dynamics into HRV analysis (Kurths et al. 1995; Voss et al. 1996b) by developing special optimized measures for the analysis of HR dynamics. The application of symbolic dynamics has been proven to be sufficient for the investigation of complex systems and describes dynamic aspects within time series (Voss et al. 1996b). The concept of symbolic dynamics is based on a coarse-graining of the dynamics of the original HR time series applying a defined number of symbols. To classify dynamic changes within the NN interval time series, the NN intervals are first transformed into a symbol sequence with symbols from a given alphabet $A = \{0, 1, 2, 3\}$. Thus, 64 different word types using three successive symbols from the alphabet to characterize symbol strings are obtained. The resulting histogram contains the distribution of each single word within a word sequence. Based on the probability distribution of each word type, several indices can be calculated: the Shannon and Renyi entropy of the word distribution, a complexity measure; the number of seldom ($p < 0.001$) or never occurring word types referred to as forbidden words; wpsum02, the relative portion of words consisting only of the symbols "0" and "2" (measure for decreased HRV); wpsum13, the relative portion of words consisting only of the symbols "1" and "3" (measure for increased HRV); wsdvar, the standard deviation of a word sequence; phvarX, the portion of high-variability patterns in the NN interval time series >X ms; and plvarX, the portion of low-variability patterns in the NN interval time series <X ms.

Porta et al. (2001) introduced short-term symbolic dynamics (SSD) by fulfilling the needs of short-term analysis. Here, the short-term HR time series consisting of approximately 300 NN intervals can be analyzed. Thereby, the HR time series (NN interval) is transformed into a symbol sequence with the alphabet $A = \{0, 1, 2, 3, 4, 5\}$ based on six equally distributed class ranges and patterns of length 3 are constructed. These patterns are then sorted into four families. These are patterns with zero variation (0V), patterns with one variation (1V), patterns with two like variations (2LV), and patterns with two unlike variations (2UV). To obtain more detailed information about the dynamics of HR, some new pattern families can also be introduced (Heitmann et al. 2011; Schulz et al. 2010): ramp/ASC (three successive symbols form an ascending ramp), decline/DESC (three successive symbols form a descending ramp), PEAK (second symbol is larger than the other two symbols forming a peak), and VAL (second symbol is smaller than the other two symbols forming a valley). A further extension of the classical symbolic dynamic approach represents the segmented SSD. The segmented SSD was introduced in order to describe nonlinear aspects within long-term RR time series by applying a 24-hour segmentation algorithm in an enhanced way (Voss et al. 2010b; Schulz et al. 2014).

2.2.3.5 Correlation Dimension

Correlation dimension (CD) analysis of the heartbeat time series is based on the algorithm of Grassberger and Procaccia (1983). The CD can be thought of as a measure of the number of independent variables needed to describe the total system in phase space (Bogaert et al. 2001). It can be used to quantify the complexity of a dynamic system or a HR time series. In the presence of chaos, an attractor in phase space characterizes the dynamics of the system and its complexity can be quantified in terms of the properties of the attractor (Beckers et al. 2006). Low values of CD indicate that the complexity of the system is lost and that sympathetic and vagal stimulation are necessary to create complex dynamical systems of HR variations (Bogaert et al. 2001). Kanters et al. (1996) claimed that the CD of HRV signals is mostly due to linear correlations between the RR intervals. In general, CD values are decreased in cardiac diseases in comparison to healthy subjects. Hence, the algorithm of Grassberger and Procaccia (1983) is only applicable for the long-term time series and an increasing interest to overcome this limitation is under way.

Raab and Kurths (2001) introduced the method of large-scale dimension densities (LASDID) that allows the analysis of very short data sets for higher dimensional spatio-temporal systems and low-dimensional systems. Thus, it is possible to calculate the LASDID for short time series and obtain an overview of the changes in the dimension density in long time series (24 hours) (Raab et al. 2006a,b).

2.2.3.6 Lyapunov Exponent λ/Finite-Time Growth Rates λ_k

The Lyapunov exponent (λ) is a quantitative nonlinear measure to characterize a dynamical system and it quantifies the sensitivity of a system to initial conditions. A positive λ indicates a sensitive dependence on initial conditions and is considered the most relevant index of the presence of chaos in data (Eckmann and Ruelle 1985). The Lyapunov exponent determines the amount of instability or predictability of the system. A fully deterministic system will have a zero λ since it is fully predictable, whereas a random system will have large positive λ indicating no predictability (Yeragani et al. 2004). In practice, there are two algorithms available to estimate λ. The algorithm proposed by Wolf et al. (1978) is limited because of the required large data sets, stationarity, and long computing time. The method proposed by Rosenstein et al. (1993) overcomes these limitations and may be superior for the application to small cardiovascular data sets. In healthy individuals, the HRV of sinus rhythm has characteristics of chaos-like determinism, with a positive λ (Hagerman et al. 1996). The Lyapunov exponent reflects the "overall" properties of the instantaneous HR regulating system, which is why one cannot deduce from this measure-specific individual changes in the regulating system. A decrease in λ of the HR time series has been attributed to a decreased cardiac vagal function (Hagerman et al. 1996; Zwiener et al. 1996). In general, the Lyapunov exponent of HR time series is lower in diseased patients in comparison to healthy subjects.

Another approach derived from the concept of Lyapunov exponents to analyze the short-term predictability in RR intervals is suggested by Wessel et al. (2000); the method of finite-time growth rates λ_k. For HR time series, λ_k can be interpreted as an index of regularity. The smaller λ_k is the larger is the number of epochs with regular or predictable short-term dynamics in the HRV time series indicating a loss of short-term variability (Meyerfeldt et al. 2002).

2.2.3.7 Poincaré Plot Analysis

Poincaré plot analysis (PPA) represents a nonlinear quantitative technique of phase-space characterization, whereby the shape of the plot can be categorized into functional classes, as suggested by Kamen et al. (1996). PPA allows the calculation of HR dynamics with trends (Kamen et al. 1996; Weiss et al. 1994). The Poincaré plots are the two-dimensional graphical representation (scatter plots) of each NN interval or in the time series plotted against the subsequent NN interval. PPA provides a visual and quantitative analysis of NN interval sequences. Babloyantz and Destexhe (1988) qualitatively and quantitatively analyzed ECGs with Poincaré sections in 1988. Thereby, the shape of the plot that is assumed to be influenced by changes in the vagal and sympathetic modulation. The plots provide detailed beat-to-beat information on the behavior of the heart (Kamen et al. 1996). Typically, PPA shows an elongated cloud of points oriented along the line of identity. Only for graphical illustration, an ellipse characterizing the shape of the cloud of points can be drawn in the plot where the center of the ellipse is the mean NN value. In general, three indices are calculated from the Poincaré plots: the standard deviation of the instantaneous NN-interval variability (minor axis of the ellipse—SD1), the standard deviation of the long-term NN-interval variability (major axis of the ellipse—SD2), and the axes ratio (SD1/SD2) (Brennan et al. 2002; Kamen and Tonkin 1995). Analysis of Poincaré plots revealed increased randomness in beat-to-beat HR behavior demonstrated by an increase in the ratio between short-term and long-term HRV, suggesting that more random short-term HR behavior may be associated with a complicated clinical course (Laitio et al. 2000). This measure has not been used extensively for risk stratification and has proven useful for detecting preprocessing problems that significantly influence the calculation of HRV variables (Kleiger et al. 2005).

A further extension of the PPA is the segmented Poincaré plot analysis (SPPA), which was introduced by Voss et al. (2010a) as a nonlinear approach of phase-space characterization for the nonlinear quantification of NN time series based on the traditional PPA. Here, the cloud of points is rotated 45° clockwise around the main focus of the plot. The cloud of points is segmented into 12×12 equal rectangles whose size depends on the standard deviations SD1 (height) and SD2 (width) of the NN time series of the Poincaré plot. The number of points within each rectangle, related to the total number of points (*N*), was counted to obtain the single probabilities p_{ij} (row number: $i = 1 - 12$, column number: $j = 1 - 12$). Based on these single probabilities, the individual probability of each row (SPPA$_{r\_i}$) and each column (SPPA$_{c\_j}$) can be calculated by summation of the related single probabilities.

2.2.3.8 Recurrence Plots

Eckmann et al. (1987) introduced the method of recurrence plots (RPs) to visualize the recurrences of a trajectory (dynamical system) in its phase space. RPs are used to obtain information on nonstationary and aperiodicity of HR time series. The RPs can be quantified by four main features: isolated points (reflecting stochasticity in the signal), diagonal lines (index of determinism), and horizontal/vertical lines (reflecting local stationarity in the signal) (Bravi et al. 2011). The combination of these elements creates large-scale and small-scale patterns from which is possible to compute several features, mainly based on the count of the number of points within each element (Bravi et al. 2011). For the quantification of RP, Zbilut and Webber (1992) have provided the recurrence quantification analysis (RQA) tool, where different indices derived from RP are defined as recurrence point density, diagonal segments and paling in the RP, recurrence rate, determinism, average length of diagonal structures, entropy, and trend (Wessel et al. 2001).

The most important structures for RQA are diagonal and vertical lines. Diagonals reflect the repetitive occurrence of similar sequences of states in the system dynamics and express the similarity of system behavior in two distinct time sequences. Verticals result from a persistence of one state during some time interval (Javorka et al. 2009; Marwan et al. 2002, 2007).

2.2.3.9 Approximate Entropy/Sample Entropy

The approximate entropy (ApEn) represents a simple index for the overall "complexity" and "predictability" of time series (Pincus 1991). ApEn can be used to determine the degree of irregularity or disorder within a HR time series, measuring the underlying complexity of the system producing the dynamics. ApEn compares runs of patterns in time series; if similar patterns in a HR time series are found, ApEn estimates the logarithmic likelihood that the next intervals after each of the patterns will differ (i.e., the similarity of the patterns is more coincidence and lacks predictive value) (Ho et al. 1997). Two input parameters, m, the length of compared patterns and r, which defines the criterion of similarity, have to be fixed prior to the computation of ApEn. ApEn has revealed good statistically validity for $m = 2$ and $r = 15\%$ of the standard deviation of the HR time series. If a time series has more regularity and less complexity, the value of ApEn will be small. On the other hand, if a time series has more irregularity and complexity the value of ApEn will be higher. Pincus and Goldberger (1994) suggested that the reduction in entropy during pathology represents the system decoupling from external inputs or a reduction in the influence of these inputs.

The term "sample entropy" (SampEn) was introduced by Richman and Moorman (2000) as an improvement over the ApEn, acting as a simple index for the overall complexity and predictability of a time series (Pincus 1991). SampEn reflects the conditional probability that two sequences of m consecutive data points, which are similar to each other (within given tolerance r), will remain similar when one consecutive point is included, where self-matches are not included in calculating the probability. Changes in SampEn were interpreted in terms of the altered ANS control of either the atrial or the ventricular myocardium (or both) during discrete physiological states.

2.2.3.10 Multiscale Entropy

Entropy-based measures like ApEn and SampEn only evaluate regularity on one scale, the shortest one, and ignore other scales. Costa et al. (2002) introduced a new method called multiscale entropy analysis (MSE). Applying this method, multiple time scales were used to measure system complexity because the time series that are derived from the complex biological systems are likely to present structures on multiple spatiotemporal scales. The main advantage of MSE over other analysis methods is its ability to measure complexity according to the concept of complexity defined as "a meaningful structural richness" (Costa et al. 2005). MSE is based on consecutive coarse-grained time series determined by a scale factor τ. These coarse-grained time series for scale τ are obtained by taking the arithmetic mean of τ neighboring original values without overlapping. For scale 1, the coarse-grained time series is simply the original time series representing classical SampEn. MSE demonstrates that healthy dynamics are the most complex dynamics. Under pathologic conditions, MSE reveals a decrease in system complexity. Costa et al. (2002) found that the pathologic dynamics associated with either increased regularity/decreased variability or with increased variability due to loss of correlation properties are both characterized by a reduction in complexity. MSE seems to provide useful insights into the control mechanisms underlying physiologic dynamics over different scales (Costa et al. 2005). In the case of HR interval time series, it was suggested to extract the slopes of the MSE curve over the scales from $\tau = 1$ to 5 and from $\tau = 6$ to 20 (Costa et al. 2005; Bravi et al. 2011).

2.2.3.11 Compression Entropy

An approach to describe the entropy of a text was introduced in the framework of algorithmic information theory. Here, the entropy (Kolmogorov–Chaitin complexity) of a given text is defined as the smallest algorithm that is capable of generating the text (Li and Vitányi 1997). Although it is theoretically impossible to develop such algorithm data, compression techniques might be a sufficient approximation. Ziv and Lempel (1977) introduced a universal algorithm for lossless data compression (LZ77) using string-matching on a sliding window. Today, this algorithm is widely used and implemented in compression utilities such as GIF image compression and WinZip®. This algorithm can be applied in a modified way for analysis of HR time series (Baumert et al. 2004, 2005). Here, the compression entropy H_{CE} of heartbeat time series is affected by the sample rate, the window length, and the lookahead buffer size. H_{CE} indicates to what extent data from HR time series can be compressed using the detection of repetitive sequences. Reduced short-term fluctuations of HRV result in increased compression. It seems that entropy reduction reflects a change in sympathetic/parasympathetic HR control, probably an increase of the sympathetic influence and reduced vagal tone (Baumert et al. 2005). Assuming that the compressibility of a HR time series is a measure of its nonlinear complexity, the complexity of HR in patients is reduced and, therefore, H_{CE} decreases with increasing risk (Truebner et al. 2006).

2.2.3.11.1 Coupling Analyses of the Cardiovascular and Cardiorespiratory System

The analysis of the relationships within and between dynamic systems has become more and more a topic of great interest in different fields of science, for example, economics, physics, and life sciences. Especially in the medical field, the understanding of driver-response relationships between regulatory systems and within subsystems is of growing interest. In particular, the focus has recently moved toward the assessment of the strength of the relations and the directionality of couplings as two major aspects of investigations for a more detailed understanding of physiological regulatory mechanisms (Schulz et al. 2013; Porta and Faes 2013). Thereby, the cardiovascular and cardiorespiratory systems are characterized by a complex interplay of several linear and nonlinear subsystems. For the analyses of the cardiovascular and cardiorespiratory regulatory systems as well as the quantification of their interactions, a variety of linear as well as nonlinear uni-, bi-, and multivariate approaches have been proposed. The most applied approaches used to assess direct and indirect couplings can be grouped using traditional domain classification: Granger causality (GC), nonlinear prediction, entropy, symbolization, and phase synchronization. Commonly applied linear approaches include cross-correlation analysis in the time domain and cross-spectral power density or coherence analysis in the frequency domain, both of which are used to investigate the interrelationships between two time series. However, linear approaches are insufficient to quantify nonlinear structures and the complexity of the interplay of physiological (sub) systems is why nonlinear time series analysis seem to be often more suited to capture complex interactions between different time series.

These coupling approaches are partly based on the notion of GC, implying that if one time series has a causal influence on a second time series the knowledge of the past of the first time series is useful to predict future values of the second time series (Granger 1969; Wiener 1956). In biomedical applications, evaluation of causality is commonly performed by looking for directional dependencies within a set of multiple time series measured in the physiological system under investigation (Faes and Nollo 2010). There exist different concepts to assess GC—linear and nonlinear approaches.

Linear approaches based on parametric multivariate autoregressive models (MAR) and favoring the time and frequency domain. Starting in 1982, in the time domain, the linear GC (Geweke 1982), the causal transfer function (Faes et al. 2004), and, in 2012, the F-test and the Wald test (Bassani et al. 2012), as well as approaches based on predictability improvement and partial process decompositions (Porta et al. 2012), became of importance. The causal transfer function between closed loop interacting signals was proposed by Faes et al. (2004) and was validated in the field of cardiovascular and cardiorespiratory variability. Thereby, two time series x and y were described by a bivariate AR model, and the causal transfer function from x to y was estimated after imposing causality by setting to zero and then the model coefficients representative of the reverse effects from y to x.

In the frequency domain, these approaches targeting to the oscillatory nature of physiological variables and the peculiarity of specific control mechanisms of working in accordance to well defined time scales (Porta and Faes 2013). In this domain, partial directed coherence (PDC; Baccala and Sameshima 2001) and enhanced versions of this (e.g., normalized short time partial directed coherence [NSTPDC]) (Adochiei et al. 2013) are the most famous ones. These approaches are based on a fitted AR model and can detect direct and indirect causal information transfer since they measure exclusively direct effects between time series in multivariate dynamic systems. NSTPDC was introduced in 2013 for nonstationary signals to evaluate dynamic coupling changes and to detect the level and direction of couplings in multivariate- and complex dynamic systems.

Coupling approaches that are based on entropies have in common that they analyze a putative information transfer between time series. The concept of entropy addresses the uncertainty or predictability of a time series and was first introduced by Shannon in 1948 to quantify the information content within a time series. Here, the concept of mutual information analysis (MUI) was first introduced by Pompe in 1993 and can be applied to detect and quantify nondirectional linear and nonlinear interdependencies within one time series (univariate) or between different (bi- and multivariate) time series. MUI measures the information that x and y share in units called "bits" because of the application of log2 (Hoyer et al. 2002). Later on, Porta et al. (1999) introduced the cross-conditional entropy (CEx/y) based on the conditional entropy as a modification of the Shannon entropy. CEx/y quantifies the degree of coupling between two normalized time series (x, y) and represents a measure of the complexity of x with respect to y. In 2000, Schreiber introduced an information theoretical approach—the transfer entropy (TE) (Schreiber 2000) that is able to distinguish between driving and responding elements, to detect asymmetries in the interaction and to quantify the extent to which the dynamics of one process influences the conditioned transition probabilities of another. TE measures causality by a prediction improvement approach and extends the concept of Shannon entropy by taking into account the probabilities of transitions rather than static probabilities.

In 1998, Schaefer et al. used the concept of phase synchronization of chaotic oscillators (Schäfer et al. 1998) to analyze irregular nonstationary and noisy bivariate time series, applying the cardiorespiratory synchrogram, which is able to detect different synchronous states (n:m) and the transitions between the two time series (HR, respiration), and to distinguish between different periods of synchronization using their instantaneous phases. Here, the term "phase synchronization" is used to denote the state when a relation only between the phases (Φ1, Φ2) of interacting signals sets in, but the amplitudes remain chaotic and nearly uncorrelated (Pikovsky et al. 2001). Later on, in 2001, Rosenblum et al. proposed an approach also based on phase synchronization to detect and quantify the direction of the coupling of two time series by examining directly the oscillation phases. In 2010, Voss et al. (2010a) introduced the SPPA approach as a nonlinear approach of phase-space characterization for the nonlinear quantification of NN time series based on the traditional PPA. Thereby, the cloud of points is segmented into 12×12 equal rectangles whose size depends on the standard deviations SD1 (height) and SD2 (width) of the NN time series of the Poincaré plot. For the quantification single probabilities (pij) within each rectangle, the number of points within every rectangle is counted and normalized by the total number of all points. Based on these single probabilities, all row (i) and column (j) probabilities are calculated by summation of the related single probabilities. This approach was further enhanced for bi and multivariate coupling analyses using two-dimensional segmented Poincaré plot analysis (2DSPPA; Schulz et al. 2014; Seeck et al. 2013) and three-dimensional segmented Poincaré plot analysis (3DSPPA; Fischer and Voss 2014).

Coupling approaches that are based on symbolization enable a coarse-grain quantitative assessment of short-term dynamics of time series through the direct analysis of successive signal amplitudes that are based on discrete states (symbols). In 2002, Baumert et al. proposed the joint symbolic dynamics (JSD) approach that is based on the analysis of bivariate dynamic processes by means of symbols. Here, two time series were transformed in symbol sequences of different words. Therefore, a bivariate sample vector X of two time series (x, y) is transformed into a bivariate symbol vector S where n is beat-to-beat values using a given alphabet A = $\{0, 1\}$. JSD considers short-term beat-to-beat changes by allowing the assessment of overall short-term cardiovascular and cardiorespiratory couplings (CRCs). This approach was further enhanced in 2013 by Schulz et al. who introduced a new high-resolution version of JSD (HRJSD) that is characterized by three symbols which are formed on the basis of a threshold ($1 \neq 0$) for symbol transformation and which clusters the coupling behavior into eight word-type families for the quantification of cardiovascular and CRC patterns (Schulz et al. 2015). This circumvented the problems encountered by the classical JSD to distinguish between decreases and steady state as well as between small and large changes of autonomic regulation due to $l = 0$ and A = $\{0, 1\}$. JSD approaches have the main advantages that they are not sensitive to nonstationary time series and are capable of capturing nonlinear bivariate couplings by a simple procedure.

In summary, linear and nonlinear coupling approaches that are used to quantify direct or indirect interactions provide new insights into alterations of the cardiovascular and cardiorespiratory system and lead to an improved knowledge of the interacting regulatory mechanisms under different physiological and pathophysiological conditions. These approaches represent promising tools for detecting information flows in a multivariate sense. They also might be able to provide additional prognostic information in the medical field and might overcome or at least complement other traditional univariate analysis techniques.

2.3 Methods of HRV Analysis Not Based on Sinus Rhythm

2.3.1 Heart Rate Turbulence

Since the description of an early acceleration and late deceleration in HR following ventricular premature beats, called "heart rate turbulence" (HRT) (Schmidt et al. 1999), considerable progress has been made in the understanding of physiological mechanisms underlying this regulatory process (Voss et al. 2004). HRT characterizes short-term fluctuations in sinus cycle length that follow spontaneous ventricular premature complexes (VPCs) (Schmidt et al. 1999). The response to an endogenous disturbance of the HR–blood pressure sequence provides unique insights into regulation phenomena. In contrast to alternative methods that use exogenous stimuli as the baroreflex stimulation with phenylephrine, the HRT method enables a quantification and characterization of blood pressure regulation mechanisms caused by intrinsic triggers (Voss et al. 2004).

In normal subjects, the sinus rate briefly accelerates initially and subsequently decelerates compared with the pre-VPC rate, before returning to baseline. A similar pattern can also be induced by pacing, either by programmed ventricular stimulation or by an implanted device such as a cardiac defibrillator (Bauer et al. 2008).

The physiological mechanisms involved in HRT (the initiation of a short-term blood pressure regulation via the baroreflex) offers not only an explanation of why this method is particular suitable for risk stratification after MI but also gives new insights into different consequences of arrhythmias on cardiac mortality (Voss et al. 2004).

HRV, HRT, and baroreflex sensitivity, like many other physiological phenomena, reflect complex interactions between cells, tissues, and organs. The Task Force on Sudden Cardiac Death of the European Society of Cardiology recently recommended a risk stratification strategy that combines a marker of structural damage (such as left ventricular ejection fraction [LVEF]) with markers of autonomic imbalance (Papaioannou 2007).

2.4 Applications of HRV Analysis

Since the pioneering studies of the 1970s and 1980s, the field has rapidly expanded. Time and frequency and NLD techniques have been used to quantify HRV in various diseases and under various physiological conditions. Some of the most important application fields are as follows:

- Heart disease
- Monitoring and anesthesia
- Hypertension
- Sleep disorders
- Diseases of the central nervous system and brain damage
- Fetal and neonatal development and pregnancy
- Autonomic neuropathies and diabetes
- Mental stress, fatigue, and concentration
- Mind-body exercises

- Sports and physical activity
- Physiological influences on HRV
- Sepsis, inflammations, organ diseases, genetics, wellness, and so on

Some of these fields are discussed in more detail in the following sections. However, because of the amount of available publications and findings, the provided information must be incomplete and only a few references were selected.

2.4.1 Heart Disease

Heart failure is a clinical syndrome, with diagnosis based on a combination of typical signs and symptoms together with appropriate clinical tests (Krum and Abraham 2009). Considerable advances have been made in management of heart failure over the past few decades. Nevertheless, heart failure remains a major public health issue, with high prevalence and poor outcomes. Enhanced diagnostic precision coupled with early intervention could lessen the burden of disease. HRV has been proposed as an additional diagnostic tool as low HRV also increases the relative risk of death from cardiovascular diseases (Dekker et al. 2000) and increases the risk for SCD (Goldberger et al. 1984).

Reports from the original Framingham Heart Study cohort and the Framingham Offspring Study indicate that reduced HRV (decreased vagal tone or increased sympathetic tone) predicts not only increased risk for all-cause mortality but also deaths from coronary heart disease and CHF (Tsuji et al. 1996; Rubin et al. 2010).

Impaired autonomic activity has been shown to be an independent predictor of mortality after MI. Early decreases in HRV were shown (Stapelberg et al. 2012) to occur following MI and were then linked prognostically to mortality risk (Kleiger et al. 1987, 2005; Malik et al. 1990; Farrell et al. 1991; Casolo et al. 1992; Bigger et al. 1996; Voss et al. 1998; Camm et al. 2004; Huikuri and Stein 2013). It was found that within 2 months following MI, there is a significant recovery of HRV, which has been linked to the reestablishment of autonomic cardiac control (Lombardi et al. 1987). After 12 months, there is further significant recovery but HRV remains reduced compared to non-MI sufferers (Schwartz et al. 1988; Bigger et al. 1991). Over periods greater than 1 year, several studies demonstrated that HRV remains lowered post-MI and is associated with an increased risk of death (Bigger et al. 1992). The relative risk of mortality after MI is significantly higher in patients with decreased HRV (Kleiger et al. 1987; Bigger et al. 1988), regardless of time since AMI.

Certain abnormalities of autonomic function in the setting of structural cardiovascular disease have been associated with an adverse prognosis, including various markers of autonomic activity that have received increased attention as methods for identifying patients at risk for sudden death. As such both the sympathetic and the parasympathetic limbs can be characterized by tonic levels of activity, which are modulated by, and respond reflexively to, physiological changes (Lahiri et al. 2008).

In the Defibrillator in Acute Myocardial Infarction Trial (DINAMIT), HRV was used as a risk indicator and stratifying entry criterion but was not successful (Hohnloser et al. 2004).

An improvement in cardiac performance from cardiac resynchronization therapy (CRT) positively alters the autonomic control of HR and beta-blocker therapy seems to potentiate autonomic improvement combined with CRT (Gardini et al. 2010). Therefore, HRV might be a useful parameter for identifying patients who respond to CRT and who may require additional interventions (Xhyheri et al. 2012).

Research has also concentrated on attempts to predict the timing of the onset of fatal ventricular tachyarrhythmias (VTA; Wessel et al. 2000). However, the evidence of the value of HRV in predicting VTAs is less clear (Reed et al. 2005).

For a long time risk stratification in patients with dilated cardiomyopathy (DCM) seemed to be not or less successful (Grimm et al. 2003; Goldberger et al. 2014). However, the application of blood pressure variability (BPV; Voss et al. 2012b) and later the introduction of SPPA (Voss et al. 2010a, 2012a) led to a remarkable improved risk stratification in these patients.

Most cardiovascular drugs that improve morbidity and mortality, including beta-blockers, angiotensin converting enzyme (ACE) inhibitors, and statins, also increase HRV. Metoprolol, quinapril, captopril, enalapril, and atorvastatin have been shown (Bilchick and Berger 2006) in separate studies to increase HRV. The clinically observed increase in HRV with beta-blockers is likely related to the concomitant beneficial effects on the parasympathetic nervous system and renin–angiotensin–aldosterone axis. Importantly, beta-blockers may diminish the predictive value of HRV after MI, at least for sudden death (Huikuri et al. 2003).

Although several studies have reported on the clinical and prognostic value of HRV analysis in the assessment of patients with cardiovascular diseases, this technique has not yet been fully incorporated into routine clinical practice (Xhyheri et al. 2012).

2.4.2 Monitoring and Anesthesia

ANS dysfunction may complicate the perioperative course in the surgical patient undergoing anesthesia, increasing morbidity and mortality, and, therefore, it should be considered as an additional risk factor during pre- and postoperative evaluation (Bauernschmitt et al. 2004; Mazzeo et al. 2011). Furthermore, ANS dysfunction may complicate the clinical course of the critically ill patients admitted to intensive care units, in the case of trauma, sepsis, neurologic disorders, and cardiovascular diseases, and its occurrence adversely affects the outcome. In the care of these patients, the assessment of autonomic function may provide useful information concerning pathophysiology, risk stratification, early prognosis prediction, and treatment strategies. Given the role of ANS in the maintenance of systemic homeostasis, anesthesiologists, critical care specialists, and surgeons should recognize as critical the evaluation of ANS function.

2.4.3 Hypertension

One of the most important risk factors for cardiovascular diseases is hypertension. This association has been found in various studies. Autonomic dysfunction has been demonstrated before hypertension is established as well as in its early stages (Singh et al. 1998). Patients with hypertension exhibit increased LF power and reduced circadian patterns (Guzzetti et al. 1991). Langewitz et al. (1994) found decreased HF power and also a loss of circadian rhythm. The Framingham Heart Study (Singh et al. 1998) is one of the major studies which found reduced HRV in men and women with systemic hypertension and that LF power of HRV was associated with new onset hypertension in men.

The findings from large, epidemiological studies also provide strong evidence that vagal tone, as measured by HRV, is lower in subjects with hypertension than in normotensives even after adjustment for a range of covariates. Importantly, these studies suggest that decreases in vagal tone may precede the development of this critical risk factor for cardiovascular disease (Thayer et al. 2010). Analyzing HRV and other related parameters may be useful at enhancing our knowledge of the underlying pathophysiology, which in turn may improve therapeutic approaches for the subsets of hypertensive patients with signs of autonomic dysfunction (Carthy 2014).

2.4.4 Sleep Disorders

HRV has been applied to understand autonomic changes during different sleep stages. It has also been applied to understand the effect of sleep-disordered breathing (SDB), periodic limb movements, and insomnia both during sleep and during wakefulness. HRV has been successfully used to screen people for possible referral to a sleep laboratory. It has also been used to monitor the effects of continuous positive airway pressure (CPAP) therapy as part of sleep apnea treatment (Stein and Pu 2012).

Sleep is not just the absence of wakefulness but a regulated process with an important restorative function. Based on electroencephalographic recordings and characteristic patterns and waveforms one can distinguish wakefulness and five sleep stages grouped into light sleep, deep sleep, and rapid-eye-movement (REM) sleep. In order to explore the functions of sleep and sleep stages, Penzel et al. (2003) investigated the dynamics of sleep stages over the night and of HRV during the different sleep stages. Sleep is a complex biological phenomenon regulated by different biological pathways. Sleep stages and intermediate wake states have different distributions of their duration and this allowed Penzel et al. to create a model for the temporal sequence of sleep stages and wake states, showing that the sympathetic tone is strongly influenced by the sleep stages. Cardiovascular autonomic control plays a key role, varying among the transition to different sleep stages. In addition, the sleep-autonomic link has to be considered bidirectional (Tobaldini et al. 2013); in fact, autonomic changes can importantly alter sleep regulation and, on the other side, sleep disturbances can profoundly alter the physiological cardiac autonomic modulation. Nowadays, an increasing prevalence of sleep disorders such as SDB and neurological sleep-related disturbances have been described. The assessment of autonomic cardiovascular control using classical linear (Burr 2007) and, more recently, nonlinear (Migliorini et al. 2011) analysis of HRV has been widely used as a noninvasive tool to provide important information on autonomic changes in physiological and pathological sleep.

2.4.5 Diseases of the Central Nervous System and Brain Damage

It was reported by Lowensohn et al. in 1937 that normal cyclic changes in HR are reduced in the presence of severe brain damage (Lowensohn et al. 1977). Variability decreases rapidly if intracranial pressure rises and the rate of return of variability reflects the subsequent state of neuronal function, even when intracranial pressure has been restored to normal. They suggested that HRV may reflect the functional state of the central nervous system. However, these findings did not consider the influence of mean HR and of the respiratory pattern (Jennett 1977).

Low HRV has been observed in schizophrenic patients (Jindal et al. 2005; Bär et al. 2005). The mechanisms by which the vagal activity is suppressed in schizophrenia are obscure (Koponen et al. 2008), but disturbances in the corticosubcortical circuits modulating the ANS have been suggested by Bär et al. (2005). Previous studies have also suggested a role for the amygdala, insula, prefrontal cortex, and temporal lobes in cerebrogenic cardiovascular disturbances and sudden death (Williams et al. 2004).

Low HRV has also been found in association with the use of tricyclic antidepressants, clozapine, and thioridazine (Silke et al. 2002; Bär et al. 2008). Thus, the dysfunction of the cardioregulatory system may also be associated with functional and medication-related mechanisms rather than structural changes (Koponen et al. 2008).

Depressive patients frequently complain of symptoms of ANS dysfunction, such as dry mouth, diarrhea, and insomnia. These clinical observations propose the assumption of altered autonomic function in these patients. In contrast to these clinical assumptions, inconsistent results have been found in the studies of HRV in depressive patients (Voss et al. 2008; Stapelberg et al. 2012; Bär et al. 2004; Kemp et al. 2012).

2.4.6 Fetal and Neonatal Development and Pregnancy

Well-defined periods of active (AS) and quiet sleep (QS) are detected (Curzi-Dascalova 1995) as early as 27 weeks gestational age (w GA). Beyond 35 w GA, the amount of indeterminate sleep is reduced to <10% and, up to the normal term, sleep is marked by the prevalence of AS. AS differs from QS by faster respiratory rate and HR, more central respiratory pauses, lower amplitude of HF HRV (parasympathetico-dependent), and higher amplitude of LF HRV (sympathetico-dependent). In artificially ventilated infants, breathing is more dependent on the ventilator in QS than in AS. When they reach term, compared with normal full-term newborns, infants with intrauterine growth retardation or prematurity do not show significant differences of sleep structure, but present faster heart and respiratory rates, more respiratory pauses, and less HRV in both AS and QS; however, sleep-states-related cardiorespiratory modulations appear similar.

Pregnancy is discussed in more detail in Section 2.5.2.

The first postnatal period for preterm infants is characterized by periods of AS and QS states, with intermediate undetermined sleep phases. Preterm newborns have an immature ANS regulating brain and metabolic activity, HR, respiration, blood pressure, and body temperature. Porges and Furman (2011) showed that newborns initially use primitive brainstem–visceral circuits via ingestive behaviors as the primary mechanism to regulate physiological state (bodily functions). However, in addition to progressive maturation, cortical regulation of the brainstem develops during the first year of life (Longin et al. 2006). In QS, a decrease of HRV accompanied by less chaotic HR fluctuations has been investigated by applying linear and nonlinear methods in healthy full-term and preterm neonates with comorbidities (Doyle et al. 2009). Reulecke et al. (2012) found that CRC is not yet completely developed in very preterm neonates with 26–31 w GA. Significantly different regulation patterns in bivariate oscillations of HR and respiration during AS and QS can be recognized. On the one hand, these patterns were characterized by predominant monotonous regulating sequences originating from respiration independently from HR time series in AS, and to a minor degree in QS, and on the other hand by some prominent HR regulation sequences in QS independent of respiratory regulation.

2.4.7 Autonomic Neuropathies and Diabetes

Autonomic dysfunction has been related to a wide range of diabetic complications and to progression of the disease. Wheeler and Watkins (1973) documented the reduction or loss of beat-to-beat HRV of diabetics with autonomic neuropathy and demonstrated that the HRV was "abolished" by atropine but "unaltered" by sympathetic blockade. These authors hypothesized that the loss of HRV associated with diabetic autonomic neuropathy was due to vagal cardiac denervation (Freeman and Chapleau 2013).

Autonomic dysfunction has been related to a wide range of diabetic complications and to progression of the disease. Early detection of subclinical autonomic impairment through

HRV measurements in diabetic individuals may be important for risk stratification and subsequent therapeutic management, including pharmacologic and lifestyle interventions (Singh et al. 2000; Liao et al. 2002; Astrup et al. 2006; Xhyheri et al. 2012).

Diabetic subjects show parasympathetic impairment as assessed by frequency-domain measures, shifted toward the LF side and decline of the time-domain measures, namely SDNN, RMSDD, NN50 count, and pNN50. Autonomic dysfunction is associated with both an inadequate metabolic control of the disease and occurrence of diabetic neuropathy (Vinik et al. 2003). Further on, in disease progression, diabetic patients with autonomic dysfunction have a poor cardiovascular prognosis (8-year mortality up to 23%; Rathmann et al. 1993).

The results from the Diabetes Control and Complications Trial in patients with type 1 diabetes show that intensive glycemic control can prevent HRV imbalance, slowing the deterioration of autonomic dysfunction over time (Diabetes Control and Complications Trial Research Group 1993).

The prospective association between autonomic dysfunction, indexed by high HR and low HRV, and the development of diabetes was examined by Carnethon et al. in 8185 middle-aged men and women from the Atherosclerosis Risk in Communities (ARIC) Study (Carnethon et al. 2003). During the 8-year follow-up period, 1063 persons developed type 2 diabetes. Compared to those in the highest quartile of LF power, those in the lowest quartile had a 1.2-fold greater risk of developing diabetes after adjustment for age, race, gender, study center, education, alcohol use, smoking, heart disease, physical activity, and body mass index (BMI). Those with HR in the highest quartile had 1.6 greater risk of diabetes than those in the lowest HR quartile with similar results for analyses restricted to those with normal fasting glucose (Thayer and Sternberg 2006). Thus, early identification of cardiovascular autonomic neuropathy permits timely initiation of therapy (Xhyheri et al. 2012). Recently, it was found that in the general population aged 55–74 years, the prevalence of autonomic nervous dysfunction is increased not only in individuals with diabetes, but also in those with different degrees of glucose intolerance. It is associated with mortality and modifiable cardiovascular risk factors that may be used to screen for diminished HRV in clinical practice (Ziegler et al. 2015).

2.4.8 Mental Stress, Fatigue, and Concentration

Mental stress is reported to enhance sympathetic activity, alter sympathovagal balance, and reduce total HRV power (Malliani et al. 1991). Stress response is associated with increased energy expenditure (Tyagi et al. 2014) along with associated changes in HR, breath rate, and blood pressure. Psychosocial factors such as stressful life events, general stress, hostility, depression, and anxiety are also emerging as risk factors for cardiovascular diseases (Thayer and Sternberg 2006; Valentini and Parati 2009). Decreased HRV has been associated with several psychosocial conditions and states. Among them, work stress as a further psychosocial factor is strongly associated with HRV (Thayer et al. 2010). Several studies implicate altered ANS function and decreased parasympathetic activity as a possible mediator in this link. Low HRV is consistent with the cardiac symptoms of panic anxiety as well as with its psychological expressions in poor attentional control and emotion regulation, and behavioral inflexibility (Friedman and Thayer 1998). Similar reductions in HRV have been found in depression (Thayer et al. 1998), generalized anxiety disorder (Thayer et al. 1996; Kemp et al. 2014), and posttraumatic stress disorder (Cohen et al. 1999).

2.4.9 Mind and Body Exercises

Mind–body interventions tend to facilitate autonomic flexibility, enhance self-regulation, and induce relaxation that is characterized by parasympathetic dominance (Taylor et al. 2010) and increased HRV (Takahashi et al. 2005).

Yoga practitioners are reported to have lower HR, breath rate, blood pressure (Bharshankar et al. 2003), higher HRV (Muralikrishnan et al. 2012), and greater metabolic variability compared to nonyoga practitioners and metabolic syndrome patients with reduced oxygen requirements during resting conditions and more rapid poststress recovery (Tyagi et al. 2014). Regular yoga practitioners were also found to have higher vagal tone at all baseline states and higher variance to autonomic and metabolic measures during all active interventions with greater autonomic reactivity to, and recovery from, mental arithmetic stress.

The analysis of the circadian patterns of cardiophysiological parameters before and after eurhythmy therapy showed significant improvements in HRV in terms of greater day–night contrast caused by an increase of vagal activity and calmer and more complex HRV patterns during sleep (Seifert et al. 2013).

2.4.10 Sports and Physical Activity

The ANS is mainly involved in regulating the resting HR and the transient HR changes accompanying physical activity and after physical activity (Borresen and Lambert 2008).

In recent years, time- and frequency-domain indices and NLD indices of HRV has also gained increasing interest in sports and training sciences. In these fields, HRV is currently used for the noninvasive assessment of autonomic changes associated with short-term and long-term endurance exercise training in both leisure sports activity and high-performance training. Furthermore, HRV is being investigated as a diagnostic marker of overreaching and overtraining. A large body of evidence shows that, in healthy subjects and cardiovascular patients of all ages, regular aerobic training usually results in a significant improvement of overall as well as instantaneous HRV (Hottenrott et al. 2006). These changes, which are accompanied by significant reductions in HR both at rest and during submaximal exercise, reflect an increase in autonomic efferent activity and a shift in favor of enhanced vagal modulation of the cardiac rhythm. Regular aerobic training of moderate volume and intensity over a minimum period of 3 months seems to be necessary to ensure these effects, which might be associated with a prognostic benefit regarding overall mortality.

Regular physical activity affects HR at rest and at submaximal exercise intensity, as well as during the recovery after exercise (Borresen and Lambert 2008). From rest through increasing intensities of exercise, HR shows a gradual increase up to a peak value. Several studies using pharmacologic blockade have shown that such increase is primarily due to parasympathetic withdrawal, whereas at greater workloads, more pronounced increases of HR result from the combination of parasympathetic withdrawal and sympathetic activation, although even at very high-intensity exercise, there is never a total parasympathetic withdrawal (Valentini and Parati 2009). Regular physical activity training at submaximal exercise elicits a reduction of HR at rest (Wilmore et al. 2001; Smith et al. 1989) and at submaximal exercise, whereas maximum HR slightly decreases or remains unchanged with chronic training (Borresen and Lambert 2008). A number of studies with heterogeneous protocols in terms of follow-up duration, frequency, and duration of exercise sessions suggest that regular endurance training, besides increasing exercise tolerance and endurance, decreases resting HR (Valentini and Parati 2009). A decrease in intrinsic rhythmicity, a more predominant parasympathetic activity, and a slight decrease in the sympathetic contribution (Smith et al. 1989) have been suggested to mediate such change. Although many reports agree in demonstrating a decrease in HR at submaximal load (Wilmore et al. 2001; Skinner et al. 2003), most of the evidence suggests that maximal HR shows a negligible change with regular endurance training.

2.4.11 Physiological Influences on HRV

The dynamical fluctuations of biological signals provide a unique window to investigate the underlying mechanism of the biological systems in health and disease. However, before characterizing and interpreting impaired (pathophysiological) autonomic regulation due to an impaired HRV, the physiological basis must be known.

2.4.11.1 *Influences of Age, Gender, and Ethnicity*

It has been shown that the HRV strongly depends on age and gender. HRV reduces with aging and women up to the menopause exhibit higher vagal and reduced sympathetic activity compared to men (Ryan et al. 1994; Voss et al. 2015).

Choi et al. (2006) showed that three short-term HRV indices (HF, LF power, and LF/HF) were significantly related to age in Caucasian Americans but not in African Americans. The effect of age, ethnicity, and the age-by-ethnicity interaction on HF and LF power was significant, even after controlling for gender, BMI, and blood pressure. They concluded that young African Americans manifested a pattern of HRV response similarly to older Caucasian Americans. These results suggest that young African American individuals might show signs of premature aging in their ANS.

2.4.11.2 *Influences of Lifestyle*

Smokers exhibit increased sympathetic and reduced vagal activity as measured by HRV analysis leading to reduced HRV. One of the mechanisms by which smoking impairs the cardiovascular function is its effect on ANS control (Hayano et al. 1990; Niedermaier et al. 1993). Altered cardiac autonomic function, assessed by decrements in HRV, is associated with acute exposure to environmental tobacco smoke (ETS) and may be part of the pathophysiologic mechanisms linking ETS exposure and increased cardiac vulnerability (Pope et al. 2001). In addition, it was shown that the vagal modulation of the heart was blunted in heavy smokers, particularly during a parasympathetic maneuver (Rajendra Acharya et al. 2006).

HRV reduces with the acute ingestion of alcohol, suggesting sympathetic activation and/or parasympathetic withdrawal. Malpas et al. (1991) and Rajendra Acharya et al. (2006) have demonstrated vagal neuropathy in men with chronic alcohol dependence using 24-hour HRV analysis. Many additional lifestyle factors and behaviors influence HRV such as drugs, diet, sleep, and fitness, but these are not discussed here.

2.5 Time Course of HRV Analysis in Two Different Fields

2.5.1 HRV in Patients with DCM

Cardiomyopathy diseases are characterized by modifications of the heart muscle accompanied by abnormal findings of chamber size and wall thickness and/or an inadequate heart blood pumping function. The most common type of cardiomyopathy is DCM, which is defined by a left and/or right ventricular dilatation and dysfunction in the absence of coronary artery disease, hypertension, valvular disease, or congenital heart disease (Elliott et al. 2008). DCM is characterized by left ventricular dilation that is associated with systolic dysfunction. Diastolic dysfunction and impaired right ventricular function can develop (Jefferies and Towbin 2010). In the United States, the estimated incidence of DCM is 5–8 cases/100,000 population per year and the prevalence is 36 cases/100,000 population (Cooper 2005). Based on extrapolations, the global incidence of DCM is approximately 50 million new cases per year (Lassner et al. 2014). Furthermore, in the United States, for heart failure patients of age less than 60 years, 45% of the heart transplantations result from the consequences of DCM (Cooper 2005). Alone in the United States, the cost burden of caring for patients with DCM per year is $4–10 billion (Digiorgi et al. 2005; O'Connell and Bristow 1994) and until now only limited success in health care has been achieved. Therefore, in recent years, increased efforts have been made to investigate the causes and the progression of DCM, to optimize the treatment of DCM patients, and for early detection of patients at a high risk for a SCD contributing to the finding of an optimal timing for either prophylactic defibrillator implantation or, at worst, a cardiac transplantation (Voss et al. 2013).

HRV analysis in the field of DCM research began in the 1990s, mostly applying linear time, and frequency-domain HRV analysis. Recent studies of nonlinear HRV have become of great interest for DCM since linear HRV analysis revealed insufficient results in risk prediction of cardiac events.

In contrast to linear HRV indices providing only a small contribution to risk stratification in DCM (Grimm et al. 2003, 2005), nonlinear HRV analyses (Voss et al. 2007) and methods for analyzing BPV (Voss et al. 2012b) have shown new insights into the changed cardiovascular variability especially in DCM patients at high risk for a cardiac event compared to low risk patients. Nonlinear indices quantifying the structure and/or complexity of heartbeat time series and thus providing additional independent prognostic information in DCM will probably lead to improved risk prediction in DCM patients when combined with linear HRV indices, clinical parameters, or biochemical markers. Furthermore, an interesting approach to achieve improvements in the diagnosis of DCM and risk prediction in DCM is the combination of HRV analysis methods with methods investigating several other biosignals such as blood pressure, pulse wave, and respiration. Here, one obtains information about interactions, couplings, and synchronizations between these different regulatory systems.

The chronological order of HRV analysis in DCM below presents the most significant research results received until now (without a guarantee of completeness).

In 1991, the spectral analysis technique of HRV was applied to obtain a more detailed characterization of the changed autonomic profile in DCM (Binkley et al. 1991). This was achieved by comparing the power density spectra (Welch method, duration of RR-interval time series = 4 minutes) of 10 patients with idiopathic DCM (six males and four females, age = 49 ± 11 years) and 15 healthy males (age = 29 ± 7 years) at baseline and in response to pharmacologic interventions stimulating the sympathetic drive and reducing the parasympathetic tone. A parasympathetic withdrawal in DCM patients compared to healthy subjects was demonstrated, characterized by a considerably reduced HF band ($p < 0.05$) and high to LF areas ($p < 0.01$). Furthermore, parasympathetic withdrawal was demonstrated as an integral component of the autonomic imbalance characteristic in DCM, which can be detected noninvasively by the spectral analysis of HRV.

In 1993, researchers investigated possible mechanical influences leading to a reduced HRV in 20 DCM patients (Mbaissouroum et al. 1993). This was achieved by correlation of echocardiographic Doppler measures of the left ventricular function and sometime domain indices (MeanNN, RMSSD, pNN50, SDNN, and SDANN). The authors found a strong correlation between the left ventricular filling time and SDNN ($r = 81\%$) and SDANN ($r = 79\%$), respectively. Thus, they suggested a shortened left ventricular filling time in DCM as one important factor for the reduction of the HRV in DCM patients that usually have a higher HR than the healthy subjects. Because of the additional independent means of HRV indices, they proposed to also apply HRV indices for the assessment of DCM patients in addition to standard hemodynamic and imaging approaches.

In 1996, Fei et al. investigated long-term HRV (24-hour Holter ECG) in 41 patients with CHF secondary to idiopathic DCM performing a treadmill exercise test (Fei et al. 1996). From the frequency domain, the TP ($p = 0.009$) and LF ($p = 0.003$), but not the HF component of HRV were significantly lower in DCM patients ($n = 10$) with chronotropic incompetence compared with those without chronotropic incompetence. SDNN but not MeanNN from time-domain analysis was also significantly lower in DCM patients with chronotropic incompetence ($p = 0.030$). The authors assumed that decreased HRV in patients with CHF who have chronotropic incompetence could be explained by a relation between chronotropic incompetence and an abnormal autonomic influence on the heart in these patients. Also in 1996, Ponikowski et al. demonstrated the use of depressed time and frequency HRV indices calculated from 24-hour ambulatory ECGs for risk stratification of ventricular tachycardia and cardiac death (Ponikowski et al. 1996). The authors investigated 50 patients with moderate to severe CHF ($n = 12$ caused by idiopathic DCM and 38 caused by ischemic heart disease [IHD], 45 males and 5 females, age $= 59 \pm 9$ years, New York Heart Association [NYHA] II-III). Applying multiple regression analysis, decreased HF power was the only independent predictor of the presence of ventricular tachycardia independently of LVEF and MeanNN. Performing a univariate Cox analysis, lower SDNN, SDANN, SD, LFn, and HFn values ($p < 0.01$) were found to have the potential as independent predictors of cardiac death in patients who subsequently died. The Kaplan–Meier survival analysis revealed that SDNN and SDANN dichotomized at median values were the best predictors of mortality. In 1997, Ponikowski et al. confirmed these results in a study investigating a larger group of patients with moderate to severe CHF (90 males, 12 females, mean age 58 years, NYHA class II to IV) including CHF due to idiopathic DCM in 24 patients and IHD in 78 patients (Ponikowski et al. 1997). In multivariate analysis, they obtained SDNN, SDANN, and LF as independent predictors of survival (83 survivors and 19 deaths during a 20-month follow-up). In 1996, Hoffmann et al. performing also 24-hour HRV analysis, found that "neither time- nor frequency-domain indices of HRV differed significantly between idiopathic DCM patients with ($n = 10$) and without ($n = 61$) subsequent major arrhythmic events" (including sustained ventricular tachycardia, ventricular fibrillation, and SCD) (Hoffmann et al. 1996). They found only a trend toward lower SDANN ($p = 0.06$) and lower pNN50 ($p = 0.08$) in patients with major arrhythmic events indicating a tendency toward attenuated parasympathetic activity in these DCM patients compared to arrhythmia-free DCM patients.

In 1997, Szabó et al. demonstrated the suitability of a decreased SDNN and pNN50 index (from 24-hour ECG time series) reflecting an impaired vagal tone to predict an increased risk of a cardiac death and death due to progressive pump failure (Szabo et al. 1997). They investigated 159 patients from which 16 patients died due to SCD and 14 due to progressive pump failure during a follow-up of 23 months. In the same year, Fauchier et al. found that the patients with idiopathic DCM ($n = 93$), even those without CHF, had significantly decreased 24-hour time-domain indices (MeanNN, SDNN RMSSD) compared to healthy subjects ($n = 63$), which was related to left ventricular dysfunction and not to ventricular arrhythmias (Fauchier et al. 1997). The use of multivariate regression analysis determined an increased left ventricular end-diastolic diameter ($p = 0.0001$), a reduced SDNN ($p = 0.02$), and an increased pulmonary capillary wedge pressure ($p = 0.04$) as predictors of cardiac death ($n = 12$) or heart transplantation ($n = 8$).

In 1997, Yi et al. demonstrated that a SDNN value <50 ms (24-hour recording) was suitable to identify ($p = 0.0004$) patients with idiopathic DCM who were at increased risk of developing a progressive heart failure ($n = 28$) from a group of 64 DCM patients including also patients who remained clinically stable ($n = 36$) during a follow-up of 2 years (Yi et al. 1997). Also in 1997, Mortara et al. found that in stable CHF (87 patients without nonsustained ventricular tachycardia [NSVT] and 55 patients with presence of NSVT) the assessment of arterial baroreflex function, but not HRV frequency-domain analysis (LF, HF, and LF/HF), allows the identification of patients at high risk of NSVT (Mortara et al. 1997). Hoffmann et al. (2000) found a higher NYHA index, lower LVEF, increased LVEDD (all $p < 0.05$), and only slightly lower SDNN value ($p = 0.08$) in DCM patients with NSVT on Holter ($n = 42$) compared to patients without NSVT ($n = 95$) (Hoffmann et al. 2000). RMSSD and pNN50, reflecting primarily tonic vagal activity, and BRS, reflecting predominantly reflex vagal activity, were not different in patients with and without NSVT.

In 1998, Menz et al. compared baroreceptor sensitivity (BRS, phenylephrine method) and 24-hour time-domain HRV (SDNN, SDANN, and pNN50) as measures of cardiac autonomic tone in patients with coronary artery disease (CAD, $n = 49$) and idiopathic DCM ($n = 130$) (Menz et al. 1998). Only in a subgroup of patients with an LVEF $\leq 30\%$ did they find significant lower HRV indices ($p < 0.05$), but there was an unchanged BRS in patients with CAD compared to patients with idiopathic DCM. CAD and idiopathic DCM patients with an LVEF $\leq 30\%$ showed comparable alterations in cardiac autonomic tone. In the same year, Grimm et al. demonstrated preliminary results of the prospective Marburg Cardiomyopathy Study (MACAS, 24-hour Holter ECG recordings) based on 159 patients with idiopathic DCM (40 females, 119 males, age = 49 ± 12 years, LVEF = $32 \pm 10\%$) (Grimm et al. 1998). They reported that patients with a depressed LVEF <30% ($n = 54$) were characterized ($p < 0.05$) by a higher occurrence of left bundle branch blocks, NSVT, and T-wave alternans and by a decreased SDNN and BRS in comparison to patients with a preserved LVEF $\geq 30\%$ ($n = 76$).

In 1999, Fauchier et al. performed a study to evaluate the prognostic value of 24-hour time and frequency-domain HRV analysis for sudden death, resuscitated ventricular fibrillation, or sustained ventricular tachycardia in 116 patients with idiopathic DCM (91 males, age = 51 ± 12 years, LVEF = $34 \pm 12\%$; Fauchier et al. 1999). Using multivariate analysis, they could demonstrate that only a decreased SDNN index ($p = 0.02$, optimal cut-off level 100 ms) and ventricular tachycardia during the ECG recording ($p = 0.02$) predicted sudden death and/or arrhythmic events ($n = 16$ patients within a mean follow-up of 53 ± 39 months). Also in 1999, Jansson et al. investigated the treatment effects of captopril (ACE inhibitor) and metoprolol (selective beta-adrenergic receptor blocker) on the long-term HRV in 38 DCM patients (29 males, 9 females) with mild to moderate symptoms of heart failure. After 6 months of therapy, captopril treatment increased TP and LF in the frequency domain but there were no changes of time-domain indices found. Metoprolol treatment increased both time- and frequency-domain indices of HRV. They concluded that both drugs might have additive effects that are of prognostic importance in DCM patients. In 1999 and 2002, Malberg et al. showed that DCM patients ($n = 27$) were characterized by a 40%–50% lower number of systolic blood pressure/BBI fluctuations ($p < 0.05$) and a significantly lower BRS ($p < 0.05$) compared to healthy subjects ($n = 27$), which was confirmed for the first time using the short-term (30 minutes) linear dual sequence method (DSM;

Malberg et al. 1999, 2002). Additionally, they determined a parameter set of six indices of HRV, BPV, and DSM that classified 96% of DCM patients and healthy subjects correctly. In contrast to the standard baroreflex sequence method achieving 76% accuracy in classifying DCM patients, the DSM method achieved an improved accuracy of 84%. Bonaduce et al. (1999) demonstrated that LF/PF and pNN50 from 24-hour HRV analysis but not indices from the Poincaré plot had an independent and incremental prognostic value for CHF caused by CAD ($n = 57$) and idiopathic DCM ($n = 40$); this seemed useful in risk stratification of patients at high risk of cardiac death (32 patients during a 39 ± 18 months follow-up; Bonaduce et al. 1999).

Galinier et al. (2000) obtained IHD, cardiothoracic ratio $\geq 60\%$, and SDNN <67 ms as independent predictors for all-cause mortality ($n = 55$ patients during a 22 ± 18 months follow-up) in a DCM patient group ($n = 190$, age $= 61 \pm 12$ years; Galinier et al. 2000). For prediction of SCD ($n = 21$), IHD and from the frequency domain at daytime (10:00 h–19:00 h) lnLF power <3.3 were found to be independent predictors. In the same year, Lanza et al. found an association between LF/HF ratio <1.2 and cardiac death ($p < 0.03$), arrhythmic events ($p < 0.004$), and total cardiac events ($p < 0.002$) investigating 24-hour Holter recordings of 56 patients with idiopathic DCM (age $= 49 \pm 16$ years; Lanza et al. 2000). Using a multivariate Cox analysis, a LF/HF ratio <1.2 was the only independent predictor of arrhythmic events ($p < 0.02$) and the most powerful predictor of total cardiac events ($p < 0.009$).

In 2001, Malfatto et al. first investigated the correlation between an autonomic unbalance present in CHF and the ethology of the disease in 21 patients with ischemic heart failure and 21 with idiopathic DCM (Malfatto et al. 2001). In patients with ischemic heart failure, a greater sympathetic activation at rest under spontaneous breathing was found (higher LF and LF/HF, lower HF, $p < 0.05$) compared to patients with idiopathic DCM.

Mahon et al. found a significantly reduced ($p = 0.01$) short-term scaling component $\alpha 1$ (DFA on 24-hour Holter recordings) in both DCM patients ($n = 24$) and in asymptomatic relatives of DCM patients ($n = 22$) who have a left ventricular enlargement compared to healthy controls ($n = 14$) (Mahon et al. 2002). Furthermore, the time-domain index SDNN, the HRV triangular index and the frequency-domain indices ULF and VLF were markedly lower ($p < 0.05$) in DCM patients than in relatives or healthy controls. Also in 2002, Schumann et al. (2002) found a parameter set consisting of two short-term indices, LF/TP from linear frequency-domain and WPSUM13 from nonlinear symbolic dynamics, which was applicable for the early detection of several heart diseases (CAD: 30 males, 4 females, age $= 62 \pm 11$ years; DCM: 41 males, 9 females, age $= 52 \pm 10$ years; and MI: 42 males, 8 females, age $= 58 \pm 9$ years). For classification between the different heart diseases, a parameter set consisting of 24-hour long-term linear time-domain indices (meanNN, SDANN) and both a short- and a long-term Shannon entropy index of the AR spectrum were optimally suited.

In the following year, Hohenloser et al. determined only the microvolt-level T-wave alternans and BRS as significant univariate predictors of ventricular tachyarrhythmic events ($p < 0.035$ and $p < 0.015$, respectively) in 137 DCM patients (18 patients with ventricular tachyarrhythmic events during the 18-month follow-up) but not HRV indices from the time domain (meanNN and SDNN; Hohnloser et al. 2003).

In 2003, Minamihaba et al. investigated 24-hour ambulatory electrocardiography recordings from 32 IHD patients and 29 DCM patients presenting the ability of the HRV triangular index and SDNN to be indicators of disease severity in myocardial dysfunction, while MeanNN and LF/HF did not have such ability (Minamihaba et al. 2003). In the same year, Grimm et al. prospectively found in 343 patients with idiopathic DCM from the MACAS study that a reduced LVEF and a lack of beta-blocker use are important arrhythmia risk predictors, whereas signal-averaged ECG, BRS, HRV, and T-wave alternans do not seem to be helpful for arrhythmia risk stratification (46 patients during a 52 ± 21-month follow-up had sustained ventricular tachycardia, ventricular fibrillation, or sudden death; Grimm et al. 2003, 2005).

Following this work, Carvajal et al. reported on the ability of CD analysis to discriminate between 55 DCM patients (45 males, age = 52 ± 10 years) and 55 healthy controls (39 males, age = 50 ± 10 years). CD values were significantly lower ($p < 0.01$ for lag values ≥ 5) in DCM than in controls (Carvajal et al. 2005). In contrast to healthy subjects, in DCM patients, no differences were found between CD values during day and night. Also in 2005, Anastasiou-Nana et al. investigated the prognostic value of iodine-123-metaiodobenzylguanidine myocardial uptake and HRV in 52 DCM patients (age = 56 ± 12 years of age) from which 14 patients died during a 2-year follow-up (Anastasiou-Nana et al. 2005). They found similar time- and frequency-domain variables in survivors and nonsurvivors. A univariate Cox regression analysis indicated HF to be a predictor for sudden death ($p = 0.041$) but not a predictor for all-cause mortality.

In 2006, Rashba et al. demonstrated results from the Defibrillators in Nonischemic Cardiomyopathy Treatment Evaluation (DEFINITE; 274 participants, 200 males, age = 59 ± 12 years) trial showing that a preserved 24-hour HRV (SDNN >113 ms) was an indicator of an excellent prognosis in DCM patients during a 3-year follow-up (Rashba et al. 2006). Patients with preserved HRV may not benefit from prophylactic ICD placement.

Palacios et al. (2007) were the first to evaluate the prognostic value of nonlinear autonomic information flow (AIF) measures in patients with idiopathic DCM compared to linear standard HRV measures (Palacios et al. 2007). From AIF, most of the indices were determined to be suitable in discrimination between healthy subjects ($n = 12$, age = 42 ± 15 years of age) and DCM patients ($n = 32$, age = 48 ± 11 years of age), but from the frequency domain only lnLF was suitable. For the prognosis of DCM patients, the linear indices SDNN, HFn, LFn, and VLF, and the nonlinear AIF index PD(dHF) reflecting the HF band information flow could significantly discriminate 10 high-risk patients after aborted SCD from 22 low-risk patients without SCD after a 3-year follow-up.

In 2008, Klingenheben et al. found only a blunted BRS as a predictor of arrhythmic events (15 patients during a 22 ± 17-month follow-up) in 24-hour Holter recordings of 114 DCM patients ("Frankfurt DCM database"), whereas HRV and HRT achieved no predictive power for detection of arrhythmic events (Klingenheben et al. 2008).

In the following year, Valencia et al. tried to improve the risk stratification for cardiac death ($n = 26$) and SCD ($n = 12$) in 194 male patients with idiopathic DCM from the MUSIC2 database (Muerte Subita en Insuficiencia Cardiac; 3-year follow-up) using an entropy rate methodology (Valencia et al. 2009). Left atrium size enlargement, decreased linear HRV indices SDNN, and LFn during daytime and lower entropy rates during day- and nighttime were found to be independent predictors of an increased risk of death reflecting a lower HRV and an increase in regularity of the short-term HRV in high-risk DCM patients. A linear combination of entropy rate and SDNN determined during the daytime resulted in a specificity of 95% (85%) and sensitivity of 83% (81%) in discrimination between low-risk DCM patients and high-risk DCM patients at high risk for SCD (cardiac death).

Voss et al. first applied the SPPA in 2010 to assess its prognostic value for discriminating between idiopathic DCM patients at high risk ($n = 14$, age = 51 ± 15 years) and low-risk ($n = 77$, age = 52 ± 9 years) for SCD (Voss et al. 2010a). Two nonlinear column indices from SPPA (column 5 and column 8) demonstrated its suitability for a significant discrimination ($p < 0.002$) between the low- and high-risk DCM patients (Figure 2.6) whereas the linear short-term indices SD1, SD2, and SD1/SD2 from Poincaré analysis were comparable in

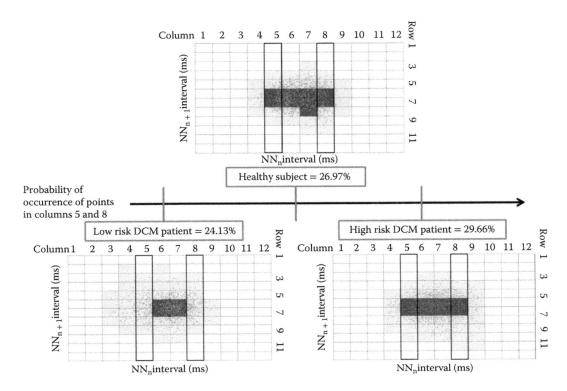

FIGURE 2.6
Results of segmented Poincaré plot analysis (SPPA) of a healthy subject (top), a low risk dilated cardiomyopathy (DCM) patient (bottom, left) and a high risk DCM patient (bottom, right); the probability of occurrence of points calculated from columns 5 and 8 is presented for each subject on the number line (center); light gray rectangles: probability of occurrence <5%, dark gray: probability of occurrence >5%.

both risk groups. In addition, indices from the lagged SPPA, applied by Voss et al. (2012a), obtained significant differences between low and high-risk DCM patients ($p = 0.00002$; sensitivity = 86%; specificity = 71%; Voss et al. 2012a). The use of multivariate statistics led to a sensitivity of 93%, specificity of 86%, and an area under the curve of 92% discriminating low and high risk. Considering the same low- and high-risk DCM patient groups, Voss et al. (2012b) demonstrated that BPV analysis also seems be useful for risk stratification of sudden death in patients with idiopathic DCM (Voss et al. 2012b). They found a significantly changed dynamics of blood pressure regulation (increased BPV) in high-risk patients. One BPV index from the nonlinear symbolic dynamics revealed especially significant univariate differences ($p < 0.001$; sensitivity: 86%; specificity 78%).

In 2013, Valencia et al. applied nonlinear HRV analysis methods (conditional entropy, refined multiscale entropy [RMSE], DFA, and linear time and frequency HRV analysis to the beat-to-beat series), for single and multiscale complexity analysis of HRV in 212 ischemic DCM patients (MUSIC2 database; Valencia et al. 2013). Beside an increase of NT-proBNP, NYHA, and left atrial size and a reduced LVEF, decreased nonlinear conditional entropy during nighttime ($p < 0.05$) was found in patients with a high risk for a SCD ($n = 13$) or a cardiac death ($n = 30$) in general compared to low-risk patients. Additionally ($p < 0.05$), decreased SDNN, LF/HF, and LFn during daytime, decreased short-term scaling exponent α1 from DFA during daytime, decreased nonlinear SampEn, and increased long-term scaling exponent from DFA during both day- and nighttime in patients at high risk for a cardiac death in general were reported.

In 2014, Goldberger et al. performed a meta-analysis taking into account 45 studies with 6088 patients (77% were male, age $= 53 \pm 15$ years, LVEF $= 31 \pm 11\%$) to estimate the performance of 12 commonly reported risk stratification tests as predictors of arrhythmic events in patients with nonischemic DCM (Goldberger et al. 2014). For meta-analysis, they extracted raw event rates and used mixed effects methodology in combination with a trim-and-fill method to estimate the influence of missing studies on the results. The highest odds ratio was determined for fragmented QRS and T-wave alternans (odds ratios: 6.73 and 4.66, 95% confidence intervals: 3.85–11.76 and 2.55–8.53, respectively). HRT and BRS were not suited for the prediction of arrhythmic outcomes. They suggested that the most probably combinations of risk stratification tests would be required to optimize risk stratification in nonischemic DCM. However, from HRV, only the index SDNN was considered! Also in 2014, Pezawas et al. investigated 60 DCM patients (median age = 57 years) and 30 healthy subjects (median age = 59 years) at multiple time points (initial assessment, assessment after 3 years and after a median follow-up of 7 years) applying the following methods: pharmacological BRS testing, standard time- and frequency-domain HRV analysis (SDNN, LF, and HF), exercise microvolt T-wave alternans and signal-averaged ECG, and corrected QT-time (Pezawas et al. 2014). Performing single time point analysis, microvolt T-wave alternans, BRS, and SDNN at initial testing added significant information regarding cardiac death observed in 21 patients. In the multiple time points analysis, only the microvolt T-wave alternans revealed additional information ($p < 0.001$) on resuscitated cardiac arrest ($n = 7$) or arrhythmic death ($n = 10$).

Valencia et al. (2015) investigated the suitability of the nonlinear symbolic dynamics analysis of RR and QT cardiac series for the differentiation between 44 ischemic DCM patients (26 males, age $= 46 \pm 17$ years) and 64 healthy subjects (39 males, age $= 50 \pm 15$ years) from the Intercity Digital ECG Alliance (IDEAL) database (Valencia et al. 2015). From the time-domain parameters a significantly decreased SDNN and increased MeanQT and MeanQTc during day- and nighttime and the whole 24-hour period were observed in the DCM group compared to the healthy group ($p < 0.01$). Both LFn and LF/HF from the frequency domain were significantly reduced ($p < 0.01$) in DCM patients but only during daytime or the whole 24-hour period. From symbolic dynamics, an increased occurrence rate of patterns without variations (0V%) and a reduced occurrence rate of patterns with one and two variation(s) (1V% and 2V%) were especially suitable indices for the detection of DCM patients ($p < 0.0005$, accuracy >80%). In the same year, Bas et al. investigated the suitability of the phase-rectified signal averaging (PRSA) method applied on 24-hour-ECG recordings for improved risk prediction in 42 idiopathic DCM patients from the IDEAL database (Bas et al. 2015). Acceleration and deceleration indices from the PRSA method demonstrated the capacity to significantly discriminate ($p < 0.001$) healthy subjects from DCM patients and high-risk from low-risk patients on a higher level than traditional temporal and spectral measures, reflecting more regularity of the ANS in high-risk DCM patients. Fischer et al. (2015) could significantly separate 56 low-risk (46 males, age $= 55 \pm 10$ years) and 13 high-risk (10 males, age $= 54 \pm 11$ years) DCM patients having an increased risk of SCD with indices from BPV and QT variability but not with indices from time- and frequency-domain HRV analysis (MeanNN, SDNN, RMSSD, LF, HF, and LF/HF) (Fischer et al. 2015). They found that QTV analysis in a multivariate approach has the ability for improved risk stratification in DCM patients with an increased risk of SCD. With a parameter set consisting of one diastolic BPV index (Shannon from symbolic dynamics) and one QT variability index (QTVlog), a sensitivity of 92.3% and specificity of 89.3% for discrimination between high and low risk DCM patients was achieved. With a parameter set consisting of two indices from the ECG analysis (indices from SPPA and QT variability), a sensitivity of 92.3% and specificity of 80.4% for risk discrimination was obtained.

In summary, studies about HRV analysis in DCM clearly present a reduced HRV and increased regularity in beat-to-beat time series both in DCM patients compared to healthy subjects and in DCM high-risk patients compared to DCM low-risk patients. However, in the literature, there exists a large discrepancy about the prognostic value of linear time- and frequency-domain HRV indices for risk identification in DCM patients. Several studies report on decreased linear HRV indices (SDNN, SDANN, RMSSD, pNN50, LF, HF, and LF/HF) in DCM patients with a high risk for arrhythmia events and cardiac death but other studies disprove the suitability of linear HRV indices for risk stratification. In all likelihood, differences in recording and analysis conditions including the length of the analyzed NN time series, methods, patient selection (inclusion and exclusion criteria), measurement conditions, follow-up duration, and study end-point definitions could be responsible for different results.

From nonlinear HRV analysis, especially entropy measures (entropy rate, conditional entropy, SampEn, and AIF), SSD indices and Poincaré plot indices (from SPPA and lagged SPPA) were found to be useful for risk stratification in DCM. Improvements in diagnosing DCM and in risk stratification were obtained by performing multivariate analysis and combining nonlinear methods in HRV analysis with analysis of further cardiovascular signals, for instance, blood pressure.

In general, HRV analysis, particularly in the nonlinear domain, seems to be a promising tool for risk assessment in DCM patients, and should be further investigated in large cohort studies.

2.5.2 HRV in Women Suffering from Preeclampsia

Hypertensive disorders during pregnancy are a leading cause of preterm birth, maternal and fetal morbidity, and mortality; 6%–8% of all pregnant women are affected (NHBPEP 2000). Among them preeclampsia (PE) is the most severe one. Fetal growth restriction and PE together affect around 10%–15% of all pregnancies worldwide (Cottrell and Sibley 2015). There are currently no therapies available to treat these pregnancy disorders. In addition, PE is linked to an increased risk for cardiovascular events, death, and stroke in women later in life. Therefore, PE is a considerable risk factor for long-term health in women (Amaral et al. 2015).

Early identification of pregnancy-induced hypertension (PIH) could facilitate treatment to avoid severe complications. The identification of specific ANS impairments characterized by changed HRV (and BPV) could help to detect at an early stage the high-risk patients in the group of women with PE.

The National High Blood Pressure Education Program Working Group on High Blood Pressure in Pregnancy classifies hypertension in pregnancy to one of four conditions: (1) chronic hypertension (CH), (2) gestational or PIH, (3) CH with superimposed PE, and (4) PE.

CH is defined as a blood pressure of more than 140/90 mmHg on two measurements before the 20th week of gestation or persisting beyond 12 weeks after delivery. PIH describes the development of hypertension after 20 weeks of gestation without proteinuria whereas PE is a multisystem disorder characterized by hypertension in combination with proteinuria in the second half of pregnancy (Zamorski and Green 2001; NHBPEP 2000; Leeman and Fontaine 2008). Although the etiology of PE is not yet fully understood, it is well established that PE is accompanied by low circulating blood volume and an increase in peripheral vascular resistance (Roberts and Redman 1993; Borghi et al. 2011). It is associated with disturbed placental development followed by endothelial dysfunction and can result in severe complications for the mother such as cerebral hemorrhage, lung edema, or liver hemorrhage and rupture. For the fetus, intrauterine growth restriction and preterm birth are possible consequences leading to a high risk of infant mortality or morbidity (VanWijk et al. 2000; NHBPEP 2000).

The first applications of HRV on fetal ECGs were found by Hon and Lee (1965) investigating fetal distress alterations in BBIs before HR changed. The application of HRV analysis in women suffering from hypertensive disorders and especially from PE started mostly in the middle of the 1990s.

In 1994, Eneroth-Grimfors et al. computed the variability in HR, blood pressure, and breathing movements in 12 healthy pregnant women, 13 preeclamptic women, and 10 non-pregnant controls using an AR spectral analysis algorithm (Eneroth-Grimfors et al. 1994). HRV was quantitated as the area under the spectral curve and a t-test was performed on logarithmic values. Women with PE were characterized by a significantly reduced HF peak compared to healthy pregnant ($p = 0.03$) and nonpregnant ($p = 0.02$) women. The present results indicate that PE is associated with decreased vagal control of the heart.

Ekholm et al. (1997) studied noninvasive electrocardiographic signals and arterial blood pressure from 14 women with PIH and 16 women with uncomplicated pregnancies of similar duration while breathing (1) with normal tidal volume at a frequency of 15 breaths per minute and (2) breathing tidal volume as deeply as possible at a frequency of six breaths per minute (Ekholm et al. 1997). For analysis of HR and systolic BPV, the AR model of spectral analysis was calculated. HR and systolic BPV were significantly increased in women with PIH compared to normotensive pregnant women (HF component of HRV [$p = 0.02$] while the women were breathing with a normal tidal volume).

In the following year, Eneroth et al. evaluated HRV applying time- and frequency-domain measures of 24-hour Holter ECG (Eneroth and Storck 1998). They investigated three groups of patients (15 preeclamptic, 15 women hospitalized due to other complications, and 15 healthy pregnant women) in the 28th–33rd weeks of gestation. Preeclamptic women had significantly longer NN intervals during the daytime compared to the other groups. Frequency-domain measures did not differ between the groups. Interestingly, the power of the maternal HR spectrum was clearly depressed, which affects the results. Nearly at the same time, Greenwood et al. performed standard microneurography to quantify single impulses of action potentials, together with processed multiunit bursts from fibers innervating the leg muscles, investigating vascular vasoconstrictive properties, HR, and finger arterial blood pressure at rest and their responses to standard isometric hand-grip exercise and cold pressor tests (Greenwood et al. 1998). Therefore, 13 patients with PIH and 11 healthy pregnant women were analyzed; PIH had higher levels of finger arterial blood pressure, more than 3 times the amount of single impulses of action potentials (per min and per 100 cardiac beats) and twofold the amount of multi-unit bursts. In the same year, Lewinsky et al. recorded 512 consecutive BBI maternal ECGs of 11 nonpregnant, 25 healthy pregnant, and 15 preeclamptic women in the rest left-lateral and supine positions and applied power spectral analysis to determine the relationship of sympathetic and parasympathetic tone as well as RSA to HRV (Lewinsky and Riskin-Mashiah 1998). As one result, healthy and preeclamptic women showed a significant decrease in RSA and an increase in sympathetic tone compared with nonpregnant women. Furthermore, only preeclamptic women shifting from the left lateral to the supine position demonstrated a marked increase in power within the VLF (0.04–0.15 Hz) range. In conclusion, PE is characterized by sympathetic overactivity and mediated by an increase in sympathetic nervous tone.

In 1999, Eneroth et al. analyzed the maternal power spectrum with an AR algorithm (LF peak—attributed to sympathetic tone, HF peak power (0.15–0.40 Hz)—reflecting vagal tone) of 24-hour Holter ECGs investigating 15 nonpregnant and preeclamptic women in the 32nd–36th weeks of gestation and 3–6 months postpartum, respectively (Eneroth et al. 1999). The power spectrum of maternal HRV did not differ between preeclamptic and nonpregnant women. However, the amplitude of all components became significantly higher after delivery compared to those during pregnancy except for the HF component in preeclamptic women, but the HF component was significantly lower in preeclamptic than in nonpregnant women ($p = 0.03$). In conclusion, Eneroth et al. indicated impaired vagal modulation even in the nonpregnant women, unlike those who had a normotensive pregnancy. In the same year, Ursem et al. applied 12 seconds of Doppler flow velocity waveform recordings from the umbilical artery at 10–20 weeks of gestation in 12 nulliparous women who subsequently developed PIH and gestational age-matched healthy nulliparous pregnant women, determining absolute values and beat-to-beat variability in fetal HR, peak systolic velocity, and time-averaged velocity (Ursem et al. 1999). In the results only variability in peak systolic velocity and time-averaged velocity were decreased in women who subsequently developed PIH. Therefore, the authors propose that the variability of the umbilical artery flow velocity is associated with the mechanical changes in the vascular bed of women who later develop PIH.

Yang et al. (2000) evaluated the changes of HRV in 17 nonpregnant, 17 healthy pregnant, and 11 preeclamptic women applying frequency-domain analysis of short-term from stationary BBI measuring to evaluate the total variance, LF, HF, ratio of LF to HF (LF/HF), and LF in normalized units (LF%; Yang et al. 2000). After that, the natural logarithm transformation was applied to variance, LF, HF, and LF/HF for the adjustment of the skewness of distribution. They found higher LF/HF and LF%, but lower RR value and HF in the healthy pregnant group compared to the nonpregnant group as well as lower HF, but higher LF/HF in the preeclamptic compared to all other groups. In conclusion, it was suggested that a healthy pregnancy is associated with a facilitation of sympathetic regulation and an attenuation of parasympathetic influence of HR, enhanced in preeclamptic pregnancy.

One year later, Greenwood et al. compared peripheral sympathetic discharge, its vasoconstrictor effect, and its baroreceptor control during pregnancy and postpartum in 21 healthy pregnant, 21 nonpregnant women, and 18 women suffering from PIH by muscle sympathetic nerve activity (MSNA) assessed from multiunit discharges and from single units with defined vasoconstrictor properties (s-MSNA; Greenwood et al. 2001). The s-MSNA in healthy pregnancies (38+/−6.6 impulses/100 beats) was greater ($p < 0.05$) than in nonpregnant women (19+/−1.8 impulses/100 beats) despite similar age and body weight, but less than in PIH women ($p < 0.001$) (146+/−23.5 impulses/100 beats), whereby MSNA followed a similar trend. Cardiac baroreceptor reflex sensitivity (BRS) was impaired in healthy pregnant and PIH women relative to nonpregnant women. After delivery, sympathetic activity decreased to values similar to those obtained in nonpregnant women with an increase in BRS. Furthermore, sympathetic output decreased in healthy pregnant women despite an insignificant change in blood pressure.

In 2004, Faber et al. also recorded continuous HR and blood pressure in 80 healthy pregnant women, 19 women with CH, 18 with PIH, and 44 with PE assessed by time- and frequency-domain analysis, NLD, and BRS (Faber et al. 2004). One result of their study was the markedly altered BPV in all three hypertensive groups compared to healthy pregnancies, especially in PE patients. Although the increase in PE patients did not lead to elevated spontaneous baroreflex events, BPV changed in CH and PIH paralleled by alterations in baroreflex parameters. The HRV is unaltered in CH and PE, but significantly impaired in PIH. Faber et al. concluded that the parameters of the HRV, BPV, and BRS differ between various hypertensive pregnancy disorders. Thus, distinct clinical manifestations of hypertension in pregnancy have different pathophysiological, regulatory, and compensatory mechanisms. In the same year, Rang et al. recorded the continuous HR and blood pressure by Portapres (TNO, Amsterdam, The Netherlands) during orthostatic stress, during rest in a supine and sitting position, and during paced breathing for periods of 1 minute at breathing frequencies of 6, 10, and 15 breaths/min (Rang et al. 2004). They applied HRV analysis for 21 pregnant woman with (multigravid) and without (primigravid) a history of PE, before pregnancy and at 6, 8, 12, 16, 20, and 32 weeks of gestation as well as 15 weeks after delivery with a classification after delivery as healthy pregnancy or PE (eight women). In this study, the spectral analysis was applied by analyzing baroreflex gain HRV and BPV as well as the phase angle between both the signals at LF (approximately 0.1 Hz) and HF (respiratory rate). Summarizing, women suffering from PE showed a significantly higher mean arterial pressure before and during pregnancy ($p = 0.001$), a significantly larger initial blood pressure drop to orthostatic stress before and in the first half of pregnancy ($p = 0.002$), and a significantly larger negative phase difference during supine rest at LF from 8 weeks onward ($p = 0.003$). These findings are compatible with increased resting sympathetic activity and decreased circulating volume, already present before and early in pregnancy.

The difference of instability and frequency-domain variability in HRs among healthy fetuses, preeclamptic fetuses, and fetuses affected by PE and growth restriction was investigated through of the antepartum fetal HRs by Yum et al. (2004). Very short-term intermittency (C1alpha) and the spectral powers were calculated to evaluate the instability and frequency-domain variability, respectively. The preeclamptic fetuses showed abnormally high C1alpha and LF as well as HF. The fetuses affected by PE and growth restriction showed even higher C1alpha and abnormally reduced LF than that of the preeclamptic fetuses. Conclusively, preeclamptic fetuses and fetuses affected by severe PE and growth restriction showed a greater abnormal instability and an abnormally reduced variability at LF range when compared to the HRs.

In 2005, Walther et al. recorded 30 minutes continuous blood pressure (Portapres signals, 200 Hz) under resting conditions from 16 pregnant women with CH (mean age: 30 years; range: 25–33 years) and 35 healthy pregnant women (mean age: 28 years; range: 24–30 years) starting at the 20th week of pregnancy every 4th week until delivery (Walther et al. 2005). As one result, the CH group had significantly increased blood pressure compared to healthy pregnant women (140 mmHg [132]–[148] vs. 111 mmHg [105]–[132]; $p < 0.001$) and an increased HR was found in both groups during the second half of pregnancy. Consequently, decreased HRV was distinctively presented in the CON group. Furthermore, both groups indicated increasing LF/HF related to a decrease in HF and a significant increase in LFn (LF power in normalized units), but no significant difference in HRV. In the contrast, VLF increased exclusively in woman suffering from CON.

Baier et al. (2006) applied discrete hidden Markov models (HMMs) to classify pregnancy disorders by recording RR and systolic blood pressure time series from 15 women with PIH, 34 with PE, and 41 healthy pregnant women beyond the 30th gestational week (Baier et al. 2006). The observation sequence was analyzed by symbolic dynamics.

HMMs were found to be sufficient to characterize different BPV with five to ten hidden states and HRV using 15 hidden states. PE and PIH revealed different pathophysiological autonomous regulation. In the same year, Voss et al. recorded high-resolution ECGs and noninvasive continuous blood pressure signals simultaneously for 30 minutes to analyze HRV, BPV, and BRS (Voss et al. 2006). Thirty-two healthy pregnant women (age 28 years, range 24–31 years), 16 women with abnormal uterine perfusion and normal outcome (AP–NO, age 29 years, range 28–33 years), and 19 women with abnormal uterine perfusion and pathologic (e.g., PIH or PE) outcome (AP–PO, age 26 years, range 25–30 years) were monitored every fourth week from the 20th week of pregnancy until delivery. The healthy pregnant women presented pregnancy-induced adaptation of cardiovascular control; in the course of gestation, BPV was increased while parameters of HRV and BRS were reduced. However, no changes during the second half of pregnancy could be observed in pregnancies with abnormal perfusion. Additionally, variability parameters were significantly altered in women with abnormal perfusion compared with healthy pregnant women, more pronounced in AP–PO compared with AP–NO. Abnormal uterine perfusion, independently of the pregnancy outcome, had a significant impact on maternal cardiovascular control. In the same year, Walther et al. recorded 30 minutes of noninvasive continuous blood pressure recordings to extract time series of systolic blood pressure (SBP) as well as diastolic blood pressure (DBP) values for the further analysis of HRV, BPV, and BRS (Walther et al. 2005). The data from 102 pregnancies with different uterine perfusions (pulsatility index >1.45: $n = 17$; bilateral notch: $n = 11$; pulsatility index and bilateral notch: $n = 30$; normal uterine Doppler: $n = 44$) were investigated to predict the PE ($n = 16$). The authors identified a combination of two variability indices (HF of DBP, VLF/TP of HRV) and one index from extend baroreflex sensitivity analysis, the number of tachycardic baroreflex events (Malberg et al. 2007), to predict PE several weeks before clinical manifestation with a sensitivity of 87.5%, a specificity of 83.7%, and a positive predictive accuracy (PPA) of 50.0%. While combining these results with Doppler investigations of uterine arteries, PPA increased to 71.4% (with a sensitivity of 93.7% and a specificity of 85.7%).

Baumert et al. investigated the monthly recorded ECGs from 32 healthy pregnant women with normal outcome, 32 pregnant women with abnormal perfusion (15 women with normal outcome and 17 women with developed PE or PIH), and 10 healthy nonpregnant women as controls (CON), starting from the 20th week of gestation until 3 days postpartum (Baumert et al. 2010). The objective of this study was to quantify longitudinal changes in ventricular repolarization during pregnancy. The QT(c) interval was unaltered in healthy pregnant women compared to CON, but the QT interval–HR hysteresis lag was shorter and the QT interval–HR regression residual was higher. Significantly smaller QT interval–HR regression residuals and a trend toward shorter QT(c) intervals could be found in pregnancies with abnormal uterine perfusion compared with healthy pregnant women. In conclusion, pregnancy has a significant effect on ventricular repolarization, whereby pregnancies with abnormal uterine perfusion and subsequent pathological outcomes have equal ventricular repolarization that precedes clinical symptoms. In the same year, Riedl et al. investigated the couplings between respiration, SBP and DBP, and HR from the data of 13 healthy pregnant women and 10 women suffering from PE applying nonlinear additive AR models with external input for a model-based coupling analysis following the idea of GC (Riedl et al. 2010). As the main result, they found that the coupling structure among HR, SBP, DBP, and respiration for healthy and preeclamptic women is the same and reliable. However, a significant increased respiratory influence on DBP could be found for preeclamptic women ($p = 0.003$) and the nonlinear respiratory influence on the HR is significantly different between the two groups

($p = 0.002$). Interestingly, the influence of SBP on HR is not selected, which indicates that the BRS estimation strongly demands the consideration of causal relationships between HR, blood pressure, and respiration. Finally, their results point to a potential role of respiration for understanding the pathogenesis of PE. Stutzman et al. (2010) studied the effects of an exercise program in normal weight and overweight/obese pregnant women on blood pressure and cardiac autonomic function determined by HRV and BRS (Stutzman et al. 2010). Twenty-two healthy pregnant women were recruited at 20 w GA (normal weight, $n = 10$; overweight/obese, $n = 12$) and assigned to either an exercise (walking) group or control (nonwalking) group, randomly. Women in the walking groups participated in a 16-week, low-intensity walking program and blood pressure, HRV and BRS were measured at rest and during exercise at the beginning (20 w GA) and end (36 w GA) of the walking program. One result indicated that women in the control groups (especially overweight women) showed changes in blood pressure, HRV, and BRS compared to the nonwalking group. Overweight women in the control group revealed an increased resting SBP of 10 mmHg and DBP of 7 mmHg. In addition, the authors found a declined HRV in the control group, but not in the walking group and a reduction in BRS and NN interval at rest in all groups except the walking normal weight group.

In the same year, Voss et al. (2010c) investigated alterations in cardiovascular regulations, applying the JDS method and revealing nonlinear interactions/couplings between two time series. Therefore, they investigated continuous, noninvasive 30-minute blood pressure and ECG from 20 healthy pregnant women before and after the 25th week of gestation as well as nine women with CH, nine with PIH, and 17 suffering from PE. It was shown that couplings in the cardiovascular regulation system were changed considerably between the first and the second part of gestation in healthy pregnancy. Further on, significant changes of these couplings led to a significant differentiation between healthy pregnancy and PE and between the CH or PIH and PE.

Seeck et al. investigated the differences in women suffering from PE with various other hypertensive pregnancy disorders (mean age 28.2 years, range 19–38 years, standard deviation 5.2 years) by applying the SPPA for the first time (Seeck et al. 2011). Continuous blood pressure was recorded for 30 minutes from 69 pregnant women with hypertensive disorders (29 with PE, 18 with CH, and 22 with PIH). The SPPA method as well as the traditional PPA method found highly significant differences ($p < 0.001$) between PE and other hypertensive disorders analyzing the DBP, but only the SPPA method revealed highly significant differences regarding the SBP. With SPPA they could increase the power of discrimination between chronic and gestational hypertension and PE to an area under the receiver operating characteristic (ROC) curve of 0.85 (versus 0.69 without using SPPA). In the same year, Tejera et al. applied an artificial neural network for the classification of women with healthy, hypertensive, and preeclamptic pregnancies in different gestational ages using maternal HRV indices composed by time intervals between consecutive NN heartbeats (Tejera et al. 2011). Considering also maternal history and blood pressure they obtained for PE a discrimination sensitivity of about 80% and a specificity of 85%–90%. Later on, they performed a comparative analysis of BPV and HRV complexity during pregnancy, applying a mixed unbalanced model for longitudinal statistical analysis as well as conventional spectral analysis, Lempel–Ziv complexity (see compression entropy), SampEn, approximated entropy, and DFA (Tejera et al. 2012a). In this study, they recorded 563 short (10 minute) ECGs from 217 pregnant women (135 healthy, 55 hypertensive, and 27 preeclamptic women) in several gestational ages in the sitting position. They reported significant differences between the hypertensive and healthy pregnant women with important considerations related to pregnancy adaptability and progression as well as the relationship of complexity and blood pressure with factors such as maternal age, familial history of diabetes, or hypertension. In a further study, they explored the correlations between HRV indices (complexity and spectral variables, calculated from short-term EGCs) and biochemical markers during the third trimester of the same healthy, hypertensive, and preeclamptic pregnancies (Tejera et al. 2012b). They found positive relations of complexity indices with hemoglobin concentration in the pathologic group and uric acid blood levels. The LF was negatively correlated with uric acid and creatinine concentration but positively correlated with platelet levels.

In 2013, Ramirez Avila et al. applied recurrence-based methods (RQA and the novel epsilon-recurrence networks) to distinguish pregnancies that develop life-threatening PE prior to the manifestation of the disease in the second trimester (Ramirez Avila et al. 2013). Therefore, they investigated HRV and systolic and diastolic BPV. They examined the coupling structures in the phase space, considering certain indices, for example, recurrence rate, determinism, laminarity, trapping time, and longest diagonal and vertical lines. The result of a quadratic discriminant analysis classified healthy pregnancies and upcoming preeclamptic patients with a sensitivity of 91.7% and a specificity of 45.8% in the case of RQA and 91.7% and 68% when using epsilon-recurrence networks, respectively.

In 2014, Voss et al. applied the bivariate segmented Poincaré plot analysis (BSPPA) to data of 35 pregnant women suffering from CH, PIH, and PE, investigating 30 minutes of noninvasive SBP and BBIs to quantify their couplings. They revealed significant different couplings between CH, PIH, and PE indicating that cardiovascular regulation can be considerably altered depending on the type of hypertensive disorder. An optimal multivariate set to distinguish best between CH and PE was estimated (sensitivity of 100%, specificity of 77.8%, and AUC of 90.8%) consisting of two BSPPA indices. In the same year, Fischer and Voss introduced the new 3DSPPAs, investigating 30 minutes of BBIs, respiration phase (RESP), noninvasive SBP, and DBP from 10 healthy nonpregnant women, 66 healthy pregnant women, and 56 hypertensive pregnant women (CH, PIH, and PE; Fischer and Voss 2014). SPPA3 discriminated the best between PIH and PE concerning coupling analysis of two or three different systems (BBI, DBP, RESP and BBI, SBP, DBP) reaching an accuracy of up to 82.9% (Figure 2.7). This could be increased to an accuracy of up to 91.2% by applying multivariate analysis differentiating between all pregnant women and PE.

Walther et al. (2014) recorded high-resolution ECG and noninvasive continuous blood pressure monitoring from 14 healthy pregnant women and 13 women with PE within 4 days before and 4 days after delivery and compared this to the values of 14 nonpregnant women. Blood pressure remained elevated 4 days postpartum, but markers for arterial stiffness normalized in women suffering from PE. However, none of the HRV and BRS parameters, altered due to either pregnancy or disease, returned back to normal levels 96 hours after the delivery, suggesting that 4 days after the delivery, the maternal cardiovascular system is still strongly affected by pregnancy independent of the health status.

The recently introduced new laboratory test, Elecsys (Roche, Penzberg, Germany), analyzes the angiogenic and antiangiogenic factors soluble fms-like tyrosine kinase (sFlt-1) and placental growth factor (PIGF) and their ratio (sFlt-1/PIGF to assess PE (Verlohren et al. 2010). Maternal serum concentrations of sFlt-1 and PIGF significantly separated healthy women and women with PE. The best performance was obtained in the identification of early-onset PE (area under the ROC of 0.97).

Pregnant women with suspected PE require intensive monitoring or hospitalization. The prediction of PE using Elecsys is successful starting from a gestational age of greater than 20 weeks. A combination of this test together with HRV and/or BPV analysis could

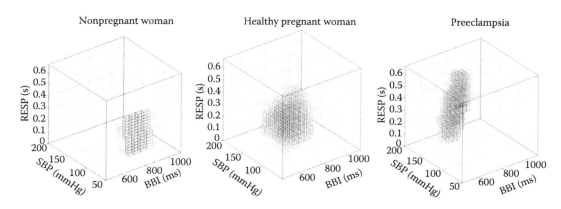

FIGURE 2.7
Three-dimensional segmented Poincaré plot analysis (SPPA3) shows the coupling between the three signals BBI, SBP, and RESP from a healthy nonpregnant woman (left), healthy pregnant woman (middle), and a woman suffering from preeclampsia (right). BBI, beat-to-beat intervals; RESP, respiratory rate; SBP, systolic blood pressure.

probably lead to an earlier prediction. Further on, HRV is known to be a risk stratifier in various heart diseases. Therefore, HRV and BPV analyses could be applied to determine the individual risk for the future development of cardiovascular diseases in PE women.

2.6 Outlook

The neuronal control of breathing and HR are closely linked, functionally as well as anatomically. CRC is strongly related to the occurrence of RSA. RSA is characterized by an HR increase during inspiration and a decrease during expiration and is dependent on both the frequency and the depth of respiration. Respiratory-mediated HRV is the most widely used index of cardiac parasympathetic function. The beat-to-beat variability of HR is predominantly mediated by the vagus nerve. The amplitude of the beat-to-beat variation with respiration is the most commonly used measure (Freeman 2006). Many disease states are present with cardiorespiratory instabilities and dysautonomia. Such cardiorespiratory dysautonomias include apnea of prematurity, sudden infant death syndrome (SIDS), obstructive sleep apnea, familial dysautonomia, and Rett syndrome (Garcia et al. 2013).

Cardiovascular homeostasis is maintained by input from baroreceptors in the carotid sinus and aortic arch (the "high pressure baroreceptors") and cardiopulmonary volume receptors in the atria, great veins, and ventricles (the "low pressure baroreceptors"). An increase in blood pressure inhibits efferent sympathetic outflow to the heart and peripheral vasculature and promotes efferent parasympathetic activity to the heart. This leads to a decrease in HR, systemic vascular resistance, and blood pressure. In contrast, a fall in blood pressure leads to an increase in HR and blood pressure (Fritsch et al. 1986; Andresen 1984).

The most specific classification domains of variability such as the time domain, the frequency domain, and the generalized nonlinear domain are still valid since the introduction of the task force. The task force itself was originally created to provide guidelines. With the help of these guidelines, medical science made considerable progress in discovery of physiological interrelations of autonomic regulation and its impairment. However, nowadays, these guidelines are (at least partly) out of date (Bravi et al. 2011). For instance, they recommended that equipment designed to analyze the HRV include the three specific statistical measures, plus one specific geometrical measure (Bravi et al. 2011). Several suggested methods (e.g., the power law approach) could not be proven to contribute to medical-oriented HRV analyses. The HF band, for instance, is limited to 0.4 Hz, leading in cases of elevated breathing rates (e.g., in patients with DCM or in schizophrenic patients) to miscalculations. Most of the positive validated methods from NLD were developed during the last 15–20 years and, therefore, are not included in the task force. Even though recently an updated paper was published (Sassi et al. 2015) several of these restrictions remained.

A new classification system is therefore needed to create new guidelines, one that is capable of giving a place to the increased number of techniques that currently are not classified but have been proved in representative studies to be effective in disease identification and assessment of health risk.

Although various studies have reported on the clinical and prognostic value of HRV analysis in the assessment of patients with different diseases, in most cases, this technique has not been fully established in medical practice. The reasons for this are manifold, leading to different or partly opposite results of HRV analyses for specific disease processes. Among the most important ones are as follows:

- Specific differences in the patient groups (inclusion and exclusion criteria, medication, comorbidities, risk factors, reference groups, etc.)
- Different length of the investigated time intervals
- Poor signal quality (increases the error in the precision of QRS complex detection)
- Dependency on signal preprocessing techniques (sampling frequency, applied filter technique, etc.)
- Recording conditions, as daytime (dependency on circadian rhythm), same/changing investigators (subjective influences), activity (lying in bed, ambulant, exercise), position (sitting, laying), and so on
- Same indices calculated with different methods (e.g., spectral indices as LFn, HFn from Fourier transform or from AR methods)
- Too low number of enrolled patients
- Univariate versus multivariate analyses
- Mostly retrospective studies, missing prospective and randomized studies

The analysis of causal and noncausal relationships within and between dynamic systems has become more and more a topic of great interest in different fields of science, for example, economics, physics, and life sciences. Especially in the medical field, the understanding of driver–response relationships between the regulatory systems and within subsystems is of growing interest. In particular, the focus has recently moved toward the assessment of the strength of the relations and the directionality of couplings as two major aspects of investigations for a more detailed understanding of physiological regulatory mechanisms and physiological networks (Schulz et al. 2013; Schulz and Voss 2014; Bashan et al. 2012).

The cardiovascular and cardiorespiratory systems are characterized by a complex interplay of several linear and nonlinear subsystems. For the analyses of the cardiovascular (Fischer and Voss 2014) and cardiorespiratory regulatory systems (Garcia et al. 2013) as well as the quantification of their interactions, a variety of linear as well as nonlinear uni-, bi-, and multivariate approaches have been proposed. However, linear approaches are insufficient to quantify nonlinear structures and the complexity of physiological (sub)systems' interplay suggests that nonlinear time series analysis may be often more suited to capture complex interactions between different time series (Schulz et al. 2013; Schulz and Voss 2014).

For the investigation of these systems, bivariate approaches are commonly applied. However, it can be assumed that the application of multivariate approaches (e.g., 3DSP-PAs (Fischer and Voss 2014), partial transfer entropy (pTE; Vakorin et al. 2009), nonuniform multivariate embedding (Faes et al. 2012), and PDC (Baccala and Sameshima 2001) will be increasingly used instead of bivariate ones since they improve the characterization of causal or noncausal interrelationships. Thereby, the assessment of these couplings and their causality can be performed by applying either linear or nonlinear time series analysis approaches. While nonlinear methods study complex signal interactions, linear methods favor the frequency-domain representation of biological signals (characterization of connectivity between specific oscillatory components). The application of linear and nonlinear approaches used to quantify direct or indirect as well as causal or noncausal relationships might provide new insights into alterations of the cardiovascular and cardiorespiratory system and possibly will lead to improved knowledge of the interacting regulatory mechanisms under different physiological and pathophysiological conditions. These approaches represent promising tools for detecting information flows in a multivariate sense. They also might be able to provide additional prognostic information in the medical field and might overcome or at least complement other traditional univariate analysis techniques (Schulz et al. 2013).

While HRV is a very simple and noninvasive method for recording data, the data itself, and its meaning, remain at least partly difficult to interpret. More research is needed to clarify further the interpretation of HRV; such research is promising in terms of better understanding both diseases and also their treatments.

References

Aarimaa, T., R. Oja, K. Antila, and I. Valimaki. 1988. Interaction of heart rate and respiration in newborn babies. *Pediatr Res* 24 (6):745–50. doi: 10.1203/00006450-198812000-00019.

Adochiei, F., S. Schulz, I. Edu, H. Costin, and A. Voss. 2013. A new normalised short time PDC for dynamic coupling analyses. *Biomed Tech (Berl)* Sep 7. doi: 10.1515/bmt-2013-4167.

Akselrod, S., D. Gordon, F. A. Ubel, D. C. Shannon, A. C. Berger, and R. J. Cohen. 1981. Power spectrum analysis of heart rate fluctuation: A quantitative probe of beat-to-beat cardiovascular control. *Science* 213 (4504):220–2.

AlGhatrif, M., and J. Lindsay. 2012. A brief review: History to understand fundamentals of electrocardiography. *J Community Hosp Intern Med Perspect* 2 (1). doi: 10.3402/jchimp.v2i1.14383.

Amaral, L. M., M. W. Cunningham, Jr., D. C. Cornelius, and B. LaMarca. 2015. Preeclampsia: Long-term consequences for vascular health. *Vasc Health Risk Manag* 11:403–15. doi: 10.2147/VHRM.S64798.

Anastasiou-Nana, M. I., J. V. Terrovitis, T. Athanasoulis, L. Karaloizos, A. Geramoutsos, L. Pappa, E. P. Tsagalou, S. Efentakis, and J. N. Nanas. 2005. Prognostic value of iodine-123-metaiodobenzylguanidine myocardial uptake and heart rate variability in chronic congestive heart failure secondary to ischemic or idiopathic dilated cardiomyopathy. *Am J Cardiol* 96 (3):427–31. doi: 10.1016/j.amjcard.2005.03.093.

Andresen, M. C. 1984. Short- and long-term determinants of baroreceptor function in aged normotensive and spontaneously hypertensive rats. *Circ Res* 54 (6):750–9.

Ashkenazi, I. E., A. Reinberg, A. Bicakova-Rocher, and A. Ticher. 1993. The genetic background of individual variations of circadian-rhythm periods in healthy human adults. *Am J Hum Genet* 52 (6):1250–9.

Astrup, A. S., L. Tarnow, P. Rossing, B. V. Hansen, J. Hilsted, and H. H. Parving. 2006. Cardiac autonomic neuropathy predicts cardiovascular morbidity and mortality in type 1 diabetic patients with diabetic nephropathy. *Diabetes Care* 29 (2):334–9.

Babloyantz, A., and A. Destexhe. 1988. Is the normal heart a periodic oscillator? *Biol Cybern* 58 (3): 203–11.

Baccala, L. A., and K. Sameshima. 2001. Partial directed coherence: A new concept in neural structure determination. *Biol Cybern* 84 (6):463–74.

Baier, V., M. Baumert, P. Caminal, M. Vallverdu, R. Faber, and A. Voss. 2006. Hidden Markov models based on symbolic dynamics for statistical modeling of cardiovascular control in hypertensive pregnancy disorders. *IEEE Trans Biomed Eng* 53 (1):140–3. doi: 10.1109/TBME.2005.859812.

Bär, K. J., W. Greiner, T. Jochum, M. Friedrich, G. Wagner, and H. Sauer. 2004. The influence of major depression and its treatment on heart rate variability and pupillary light reflex parameters. *J Affect Disord* 82 (2):245–52. doi: 10.1016/j.jad.2003.12.016.

Bär, K. J., M. Koschke, S. Berger, S. Schulz, M. Tancer, A. Voss, and V. K. Yeragani. 2008. Influence of olanzapine on QT variability and complexity measures of heart rate in patients with schizophrenia. *J Clin Psychopharmacol* 28 (6):694–8. doi: 10.1097/JCP.0b013e31818a6d25.

Bär, K. J., A. Letzsch, T. Jochum, G. Wagner, W. Greiner, and H. Sauer. 2005. Loss of efferent vagal activity in acute schizophrenia. *J Psychiatr Res* 39 (5):519–27. doi: 10.1016/j.jpsychires. 2004.12.007.

Bas, R., M. Vallverdu, J. F. Valencia, A. Voss, A. B. de Luna, and P. Caminal. 2015. Evaluation of acceleration and deceleration cardiac processes using phase-rectified signal averaging in healthy and idiopathic dilated cardiomyopathy subjects. *Med Eng Phys* 37 (2):195–202. doi: 10.1016/j.medengphy.2014.12.001.

Bashan, A., R. P. Bartsch, J. W. Kantelhardt, S. Havlin, and PCh Ivanov. 2012. Network physiology reveals relations between network topology and physiological function. *Nat Commun* 3:702. doi: 10.1038/ncomms1705.

Bassani, T., V. Magagnin, S. Guzzetti, G. Baselli, G. Citerio, and A. Porta. 2012. Testing the involvement of baroreflex during general anesthesia through Granger causality approach. *Comput Biol Med* 42 (3):306–12. doi: 10.1016/j.compbiomed.2011.03.005.

Bauer, A., M. Malik, G. Schmidt, P. Barthel, H. Bonnemeier, I. Cygankiewicz, P. Guzik, F. Lombardi, A. Muller, A. Oto, et al. 2008. Heart rate turbulence: Standards of measurement, physiological interpretation, and clinical use: International Society for Holter and Noninvasive Electrophysiology Consensus. *J Am Coll Cardiol* 52 (17):1353–65. doi: 10.1016/j.jacc.2008.07.041.

Bauernschmitt, R., H. Malberg, N. Wessel, B. Kopp, E. U. Schirmbeck, and R. Lange. 2004. Impairment of cardiovascular autonomic control in patients early after cardiac surgery. *Eur J Cardiothorac Surg* 25 (3):320–6. doi: 10.1016/j.ejcts.2003.12.019.

Baumert, M., V. Baier, J. Haueisen, N. Wessel, U. Meyerfeldt, A. Schirdewan, and A. Voss. 2004. Forecasting of life threatening arrhythmias using the compression entropy of heart rate. *Methods Inf Med* 43 (2):202–6. doi: 10.1267/METH04020202.

Baumert, M., V. Baier, A. Voss, L. Brechtel, and J. Haueisen. 2005. Estimating the complexity of heart rate fluctuations—An approach based on compression entropy. *Fluct Noise Lett* 5 (4):L557–L563. doi: 10.1142/S0219477505003026.

Baumert, M., A. Seeck, R. Faber, E. Nalivaiko, and A. Voss. 2010. Longitudinal changes in QT interval variability and rate adaptation in pregnancies with normal and abnormal uterine perfusion. *Hypertens Res* 33 (6):555–60. doi: 10.1038/hr.2010.30.

Baumert, M., T. Walther, J. Hopfe, H. Stepan, R. Faber, and A. Voss. 2002. Joint symbolic dynamic analysis of beat-to-beat interactions of heart rate and systolic blood pressure in normal pregnancy. *Med Biol Eng Comput* 40 (2):241–5.

Beckers, F., B. Verheyden, and A. E. Aubert. 2006. Aging and nonlinear heart rate control in a healthy population. *Am J Physiol Heart Circ Physiol* 290 (6):H2560–70. doi: 10.1152/ajpheart.00903. 2005.

Bharshankar, J. R., R. N. Bharshankar, V. N. Deshpande, S. B. Kaore, and G. B. Gosavi. 2003. Effect of yoga on cardiovascular system in subjects above 40 years. *Indian J Physiol Pharmacol* 47 (2):202–6.

Bigger, J. T., Jr., J. L. Fleiss, L. M. Rolnitzky, R. C. Steinman, and W. J. Schneider. 1991. Time course of recovery of heart period variability after myocardial infarction. *J Am Coll Cardiol* 18 (7):1643–9.

Bigger, J. T., Jr., J. L. Fleiss, R. C. Steinman, L. M. Rolnitzky, R. E. Kleiger, and J. N. Rottman. 1992. Frequency domain measures of heart period variability and mortality after myocardial infarction. *Circulation* 85 (1):164–71.

Bigger, J. T., Jr., R. E. Kleiger, J. L. Fleiss, L. M. Rolnitzky, R. C. Steinman, and J. P. Miller. 1988. Components of heart rate variability measured during healing of acute myocardial infarction. *Am J Cardiol* 61 (4):208–15.

Bigger, J. T., Jr., R. C. Steinman, L. M. Rolnitzky, J. L. Fleiss, P. Albrecht, and R. J. Cohen. 1996. Power law behavior of RR-interval variability in healthy middle-aged persons, patients with recent acute myocardial infarction, and patients with heart transplants. *Circulation* 93 (12):2142–51.

Bilchick, K. C., and R. D. Berger. 2006. Heart rate variability. *J Cardiovasc Electrophysiol* 17 (6):691–4. doi: 10.1111/j.1540-8167.2006.00501.x.

Billman, G. E. 2011. Heart rate variability—A historical perspective. *Front Physiol* 2:86. doi: 10.3389/fphys.2011.00086.

Binkley, P. F., E. Nunziata, G. J. Haas, S. D. Nelson, and R. J. Cody. 1991. Parasympathetic withdrawal is an integral component of autonomic imbalance in congestive heart failure: Demonstration in human subjects and verification in a paced canine model of ventricular failure. *J Am Coll Cardiol* 18 (2):464–72.

Boettger, M. K., S. Schulz, S. Berger, M. Tancer, V. K. Yeragani, A. Voss, and K. J. Bar. 2010. Influence of age on linear and nonlinear measures of autonomic cardiovascular modulation. *Ann Noninvasive Electrocardiol* 15 (2):165–74. doi: 10.1111/j.1542-474X.2010.00358.x.

Bogaert, C., F. Beckers, D. Ramaekers, and A. E. Aubert. 2001. Analysis of heart rate variability with correlation dimension method in a normal population and in heart transplant patients. *Auton Neurosci* 90 (1–2):142–7. doi: 10.1016/S1566-0702(01)00280-6.

Bonaduce, D., M. Petretta, F. Marciano, M. L. Vicario, C. Apicella, M. A. Rao, E. Nicolai, and M. Volpe. 1999. Independent and incremental prognostic value of heart rate variability in patients with chronic heart failure. *Am Heart J* 138 (2 Pt 1):273–84.

Borghi, C., A. F. Cicero, D. D. Esposti, V. Immordino, S. Bacchelli, N. Rizzo, F. Santi, and E. Ambrosioni. 2011. Hemodynamic and neurohumoral profile in patients with different types of hypertension in pregnancy. *Intern Emerg Med* 6 (3):227–34. doi: 10.1007/s11739-010-0483-5.

Borresen, J., and M. I. Lambert. 2008. Autonomic control of heart rate during and after exercise: Measurements and implications for monitoring training status. *Sports Med* 38 (8):633–46.

Bravi, A., A. Longtin, and A. J. Seely. 2011. Review and classification of variability analysis techniques with clinical applications. *Biomed Eng Online* 10:90. doi: 10.1186/1475-925X-10-90.

Brennan, M., M. Palaniswami, and P. Kamen. 2002. Poincare plot interpretation using a physiological model of HRV based on a network of oscillators. *Am J Physiol Heart Circ Physiol* 283 (5):H1873–86. doi: 10.1152/ajpheart.00405.2000.

Bujalkova, M. 2011. Rufus of Ephesus and his contribution to the development of anatomical nomenclature. *Acta Med Hist Adriat* 9 (1):89–100.

Burr, R. L. 2007. Interpretation of normalized spectral heart rate variability indices in sleep research: A critical review. *Sleep* 30 (7):913–9.

Busjahn, A., A. Voss, H. Knoblauch, M. Knoblauch, E. Jeschke, N. Wessel, J. Bohlender, J. McCarron, H. D. Faulhaber, H. Schuster, R. Dietz, and F. C. Luft. 1998. Angiotensin-converting enzyme and angiotensinogen gene polymorphisms and heart rate variability in twins. *Am J Cardiol* 81 (6):755–60.

Camm, A. J., C. M. Pratt, P. J. Schwartz, H. R. Al-Khalidi, M. J. Spyt, M. J. Holroyde, R. Karam, E. H. Sonnenblick, J. M. Brum, and Investigators AzimiLide post Infarct surVival Evaluation.

2004. Mortality in patients after a recent myocardial infarction: A randomized, placebo-controlled trial of azimilide using heart rate variability for risk stratification. *Circulation* 109 (8):990–6. doi: 10.1161/01.CIR.0000117090.01718.2A.

Carnethon, M. R., S. H. Golden, A. R. Folsom, W. Haskell, and D. Liao. 2003. Prospective investigation of autonomic nervous system function and the development of type 2 diabetes: The Atherosclerosis Risk in Communities Study, 1987–1998. *Circulation* 107 (17):2190–5. doi: 10.1161/01.CIR.0000066324.74807.95.

Carthy, E. R. 2014. Autonomic dysfunction in essential hypertension: A systematic review. *Ann Med Surg (Lond)* 3 (1):2–7. doi: 10.1016/j.amsu.2013.11.002.

Carvajal, R., N. Wessel, M. Vallverdu, P. Caminal, and A. Voss. 2005. Correlation dimension analysis of heart rate variability in patients with dilated cardiomyopathy. *Comput Methods Programs Biomed* 78 (2):133–40. doi: 10.1016/j.cmpb.2005.01.004.

Casolo, G. C., P. Stroder, C. Signorini, F. Calzolari, M. Zucchini, E. Balli, A. Sulla, and S. Lazzerini. 1992. Heart rate variability during the acute phase of myocardial infarction. *Circulation* 85 (6):2073–9.

Cerutti, S., D. Hoyer, and A. Voss. 2009. Multiscale, multiorgan and multivariate complexity analyses of cardiovascular regulation. *Philos Trans A Math Phys Eng Sci* 367 (1892):1337–58. doi: 10.1098/rsta.2008.0267.

Chess, G. F., R. M. Tam, and F. R. Calaresu. 1975. Influence of cardiac neural inputs on rhythmic variations of heart period in the cat. *Am J Physiol* 228 (3):775–80.

Choi, J. B., S. Hong, R. Nelesen, W. A. Bardwell, L. Natarajan, C. Schubert, and J. E. Dimsdale. 2006. Age and ethnicity differences in short-term heart-rate variability. *Psychosom Med* 68 (3):421–6. doi: 10.1097/01.psy.0000221378.09239.6a.

Chua, K. C., V. Chandran, U. R. Acharya, and C. M. Lim. 2010. Application of higher order statistics/spectra in biomedical signals–A review. *Med Eng Phys* 32 (7):679–89. doi: 10.1016/j.medengphy.2010.04.009.

Cohen, H., M. A. Matar, Z. Kaplan, and M. Kotler. 1999. Power spectral analysis of heart rate variability in psychiatry. *Psychother Psychosom* 68 (2):59–66.

Cooper, L. T., Jr. 2005. The natural history and role of immunoadsorption in dilated cardiomyopathy. *J Clin Apher* 20 (4):256–60. doi: 10.1002/jca.20045.

Costa, M., A. L. Goldberger, and C. K. Peng. 2002. Multiscale entropy analysis of complex physiologic time series. *Phys Rev Lett* 89 (6):068102.

Costa, M., A. L. Goldberger, and C. K. Peng. 2005. Multiscale entropy analysis of biological signals. *Phys Rev E Stat Nonlin Soft Matter Phys* 71 (2 Pt 1):021906.

Cottrell, E. C., and C. P. Sibley. 2015. From pre-clinical studies to clinical trials: Generation of novel therapies for pregnancy complications. *Int J Mol Sci* 16 (6):12907–12924. doi: 10.3390/ijms160612907.

Couderc, J. P. 2009. Cardiac regulation and electrocardiographic factors contributing to the measurement of repolarization variability. *J Electrocardiol* 42 (6):494–9. doi: 10.1016/j.jelectrocard.2009.06.019.

Curzi-Dascalova, L. 1995. Development of the sleep and autonomic nervous system control in premature and full-term newborn infants. *Arch Pediatr* 2 (3):255–62.

Dekker, J. M., R. S. Crow, A. R. Folsom, P. J. Hannan, D. Liao, C. A. Swenne, and E. G. Schouten. 2000. Low heart rate variability in a 2-minute rhythm strip predicts risk of coronary heart disease and mortality from several causes: The ARIC Study. Atherosclerosis Risk in Communities. *Circulation* 102 (11):1239–44.

Diabetes Control and Complications Trial Research Group. 1993. The effect of intensive treatment of diabetes on the development and progression of long-term complications in insulin-dependent diabetes mellitus. *N Engl J Med* 329 (14):977–86. doi: 10.1056/NEJM199309303291401.

Digiorgi, P. L., M. S. Reel, B. Thornton, E. Burton, Y. Naka, and M. C. Oz. 2005. Heart transplant and left ventricular assist device costs. *J Heart Lung Transplant* 24 (2):200–4. doi: 10.1016/j.healun.2003.11.397.

Doyle, O. M., I. Korotchikova, G. Lightbody, W. Marnane, D. Kerins, and G. B. Boylan. 2009. Heart rate variability during sleep in healthy term newborns in the early postnatal period. *Physiol Meas* 30 (8):847–60. doi: 10.1088/0967-3334/30/8/009.

Eckmann, J. P., and D. Ruelle. 1985. Ergodic theory of chaos and strange attractors. *Rev Mod Phys* 57 (3):617–56.

Eckmann, J. P., S. O. Kamphorst, and D. Ruelle. 1987. Recurrence plots of dynamical systems. *Europhys Lett* (4):973–7.

Ekholm, E. M., K. U. Tahvanainen, and T. Metsala. 1997. Heart rate and blood pressure variabilities are increased in pregnancy-induced hypertension. *Am J Obstet Gynecol* 177 (5):1208–12.

Elliott, P., B. Andersson, E. Arbustini, Z. Bilinska, F. Cecchi, P. Charron, O. Dubourg, U. Kuhl, B. Maisch, W. J. McKenna, L. Monserrat, et al. 2008. Classification of the cardiomyopathies: A position statement from the European Society Of Cardiology Working Group on Myocardial and Pericardial Diseases. *Eur Heart J* 29 (2):270–6. doi: 10.1093/eurheartj/ehm342.

Eneroth-Grimfors, E., M. Westgren, M. Ericson, C. Ihrman-Sandahl, and L. E. Lindblad. 1994. Autonomic cardiovascular control in normal and pre-eclamptic pregnancy. *Acta Obstet Gynecol Scand* 73 (9):680–4.

Eneroth, E., and N. Storck. 1998. Preeclampsia and maternal heart rate variability. *Gynecol Obstet Invest* 45 (3):170–3.

Eneroth, E., M. Westgren, M. Ericsson, L. E. Lindblad, and N. Storck. 1999. 24-hour ECG frequency-domain measures in preeclamptic and healthy pregnant women during and after pregnancy. *Hypertens Pregnancy* 18 (1):1–9.

Enersen, O. D. 2015. Ebers' papyrus. Whonamedit? http://www.whonamedit.com/synd.cfm/443.html.

Esperer, H. D. 1992. Die Herzfrequenzvariabilität, ein neuer Parameter für die nichtinvasive Risikostratifizierung nach Myokardinfarkt und arrhythmogener Synkope. Gegenwärtiger Stand und Perspektiven. *Herzschr. Elektrophys.* 3:1–16.

Faber, R., M. Baumert, H. Stepan, N. Wessel, A. Voss, and T. Walther. 2004. Baroreflex sensitivity, heart rate, and blood pressure variability in hypertensive pregnancy disorders. *J Hum Hypertens* 18 (10):707–12. doi: 10.1038/sj.jhh.1001730.

Faes, L., and G. Nollo. 2010. Extended causal modeling to assess Partial Directed Coherence in multiple time series with significant instantaneous interactions. *Biol Cybern* 103 (5):387–400. doi: 10.1007/s00422-010-0406-6.

Faes, L., G. Nollo, and A. Porta. 2012. Non-uniform multivariate embedding to assess the information transfer in cardiovascular and cardiorespiratory variability series. *Comput Biol Med* 42 (3):290–7. doi: 10.1016/j.compbiomed.2011.02.007.

Faes, L., A. Porta, R. Cucino, S. Cerutti, R. Antolini, and G. Nollo. 2004. Causal transfer function analysis to describe closed loop interactions between cardiovascular and cardiorespiratory variability signals. *Biol Cybern* 90 (6):390–9. doi: 10.1007/s00422-004-0488-0.

Farrell, T. G., Y. Bashir, T. Cripps, M. Malik, J. Poloniecki, E. D. Bennett, D. E. Ward, and A. J. Camm. 1991. Risk stratification for arrhythmic events in postinfarction patients based on heart rate variability, ambulatory electrocardiographic variables and the signal-averaged electrocardiogram. *J Am Coll Cardiol* 18 (3):687–97.

Fauchier, L., D. Babuty, P. Cosnay, M. L. Autret, and J. P. Fauchier. 1997. Heart rate variability in idiopathic dilated cardiomyopathy: Characteristics and prognostic value. *J Am Coll Cardiol* 30 (4):1009–14.

Fauchier, L., D. Babuty, P. Cosnay, and J. P. Fauchier. 1999. Prognostic value of heart rate variability for sudden death and major arrhythmic events in patients with idiopathic dilated cardiomyopathy. *J Am Coll Cardiol* 33 (5):1203–7.

Fei, L., P. J. Keeling, N. Sadoul, X. Copie, M. Malik, W. J. McKenna, and A. J. Camm. 1996. Decreased heart rate variability in patients with congestive heart failure and chronotropic incompetence. *Pacing Clin Electrophysiol* 19 (4 Pt 1):477–83.

Fischer, C., A. Seeck, R. Schroeder, M. Goernig, A. Schirdewan, H. R. Figulla, M. Baumert, and A. Voss. 2015. QT variability improves risk stratification in patients with dilated cardiomyopathy. *Physiol Meas* 36 (4):699–713. doi: 10.1088/0967-3334/36/4/699.

Fischer, C., and A. Voss. 2014. Three-dimensional segmented poincare plot analyses SPPA3 investigates cardiovascular and cardiorespiratory couplings in hypertensive pregnancy disorders. *Front Bioeng Biotechnol* 2:51. doi: 10.3389/fbioe.2014.00051.

Freeman, R. 2006. Assessment of cardiovascular autonomic function. *Clin Neurophysiol* 117 (4):716–30. doi: 10.1016/j.clinph.2005.09.027.

Freeman, R., and M. W. Chapleau. 2013. Testing the autonomic nervous system. *Handb Clin Neurol* 115:115–36. doi: 10.1016/B978-0-444-52902-2.00007-2.

Friedman, B. H., and J. F. Thayer. 1998. Anxiety and autonomic flexibility: A cardiovascular approach. *Biol Psychol* 49 (3):303–23.

Fritsch, J. M., D. L. Eckberg, L. D. Graves, and B. G. Wallin. 1986. Arterial pressure ramps provoke linear increases of heart period in humans. *Am J Physiol* 251 (6 Pt 2):R1086–90.

Fullerton, J. B., and M. E. Silverman. 2009. Claudius Galen of Pergamum: Authority of medieval medicine. *Clin Cardiol* 32 (11):E82–3. doi: 10.1002/clc.20388.

Fye, W. B. 1987. The origin of the heart beat: A tale of frogs, jellyfish, and turtles. *Circulation* 76 (3): 493–500.

Fye, W. B. 1995. Albrecht von Haller. *Clin Cardiol* 18 (5):291–2.

Galinier, M., A. Pathak, J. Fourcade, C. Androdias, D. Curnier, S. Varnous, S. Boveda, P. Massabuau, M. Fauvel, J. M. Senard, and J. P. Bounhoure. 2000. Depressed low frequency power of heart rate variability as an independent predictor of sudden death in chronic heart failure. *Eur Heart J* 21 (6):475–82. doi: 10.1053/euhj.1999.1875.

Galletly, D. C., and P. D. Larsen. 1998. Relationship between cardioventilatory coupling and respiratory sinus arrhythmia. *Br J Anaesth* 80 (2):164–8.

Garcia, A. J., 3rd, J. E. Koschnitzky, T. Dashevskiy, and J. M. Ramirez. 2013. Cardiorespiratory coupling in health and disease. *Auton Neurosci* 175 (1–2):26–37. doi: 10.1016/j.autneu.2013.02.006.

Gardini, A., P. Lupo, E. Zanelli, S. Bisetti, and R. Cappato. 2010. Diagnostic capabilities of devices for cardiac resynchronization therapy. *J Cardiovasc Med (Hagerstown)* 11 (3):186–9. doi: 10.2459/JCM.0b013e3283303036.

Garfinkel, A. 1983. A mathematics for physiology. *Am J Physiol* 245 (4):R455–66.

Gawłowska, J., and Wranicz, J.K. 2009. Norman J. "Jeff" Holter (1914–1983). *Cardiol J* 16 (4):386–387.

Geweke, J. 1982. Measurement of linear dependence and feedback between multiple time series. *J Am Statist Ass* 77 (378):304–313.

Glass, L., and Mackey, M. C. 1988. *From Clocks to Chaos: The Rhythms of Life.* Princeton, NJ: Princeton University Press.

Goldberger, A. L., L. A. Amaral, J. M. Hausdorff, PCh Ivanov, C. K. Peng, and H. E. Stanley. 2002. Fractal dynamics in physiology: Alterations with disease and aging. *Proc Natl Acad Sci U S A* 99 Suppl 1:2466–72. doi: 10.1073/pnas.012579499.

Goldberger, A. L., L. J. Findley, M. R. Blackburn, and A. J. Mandell. 1984. Nonlinear dynamics in heart failure: Implications of long-wavelength cardiopulmonary oscillations. *Am Heart J* 107 (3):612–5.

Goldberger, A. L., and B. J. West. 1987. Applications of nonlinear dynamics to clinical cardiology. *Ann N Y Acad Sci* 504:195–213.

Goldberger, J. J., H. Subacius, T. Patel, R. Cunnane, and A. H. Kadish. 2014. Sudden cardiac death risk stratification in patients with nonischemic dilated cardiomyopathy. *J Am Coll Cardiol* 63 (18):1879–89. doi: 10.1016/j.jacc.2013.12.021.

Goldstein, D. S., O. Bentho, M. Y. Park, and Y. Sharabi. 2011. Low-frequency power of heart rate variability is not a measure of cardiac sympathetic tone but may be a measure of modulation of cardiac autonomic outflows by baroreflexes. *Exp Physiol* 96 (12):1255–61. doi: 10.1113/expphysiol.2010.056259.

Granger, C. W. J. 1969. Investigating causal relations by econometric models and cross-spectral methods. *Econometrica* 37 (3):424–438.

Grassberger, P., and I. Procaccia. 1983. Measuring the strangeness of strange attractors. *Physica D* 9:189–208.

Greenwood, J. P., E. M. Scott, J. B. Stoker, J. J. Walker, and D. A. Mary. 2001. Sympathetic neural mechanisms in normal and hypertensive pregnancy in humans. *Circulation* 104 (18):2200–4.

Greenwood, J. P., J. B. Stoker, J. J. Walker, and D. A. Mary. 1998. Sympathetic nerve discharge in normal pregnancy and pregnancy-induced hypertension. *J Hypertens* 16 (5):617–24.

Grimm, W., M. Christ, J. Bach, H. H. Muller, and B. Maisch. 2003. Noninvasive arrhythmia risk stratification in idiopathic dilated cardiomyopathy: Results of the Marburg Cardiomyopathy Study. *Circulation* 108 (23):2883–91. doi: 10.1161/01.CIR.0000100721.52503.85.

Grimm, W., M. Christ, J. Sharkova, and B. Maisch. 2005. Arrhythmia risk prediction in idiopathic dilated cardiomyopathy based on heart rate variability and baroreflex sensitivity. *Pacing Clin Electrophysiol* 28 Suppl 1:S202–6. doi: 10.1111/j.1540-8159.2005.00033.x.

Grimm, W., C. Glaveris, J. Hoffmann, V. Menz, N. Mey, S. Born, and B. Maisch. 1998. Noninvasive arrhythmia risk stratification in idiopathic dilated cardiomyopathy: Design and first results of the Marburg Cardiomyopathy Study. *Pacing Clin Electrophysiol* 21 (11 Pt 2):2551–6.

Guevara, M. R., L. Glass, and A. Shrier. 1981. Phase locking, period-doubling bifurcations, and irregular dynamics in periodically stimulated cardiac cells. *Science* 214 (4527):1350–3.

Guzzetti, S., S. Dassi, M. Pecis, R. Casati, A. M. Masu, P. Longoni, M. Tinelli, S. Cerutti, M. Pagani, and A. Malliani. 1991. Altered pattern of circadian neural control of heart period in mild hypertension. *J Hypertens* 9 (9):831–8.

Hagerman, I., M. Berglund, M. Lorin, J. Nowak, and C. Sylvén. 1996. Chaos-related deterministic regulation of heart rate variability in time- and frequency domains: Effects of autonomic blockade and exercise. *Cardiovasc Res* 31:410–8.

Hainsworth, R. 2004. Physiological background of heart rate variability. In *Dynamic Electrocardiology*, edited by Camm A.J. Malik M., 3–12. New York, NY: Blackwell Futura.

Hayano, J., M. Yamada, Y. Sakakibara, T. Fujinami, K. Yokoyama, Y. Watanabe, and K. Takata. 1990. Short- and long-term effects of cigarette smoking on heart rate variability. *Am J Cardiol* 65 (1): 84–8.

Heitmann, A., T. Huebner, R. Schroeder, S. Perz, and A. Voss. 2011. Multivariate short-term heart rate variability: A pre-diagnostic tool for screening heart disease. *Med Biol Eng Comput* 49 (1):41–50. doi: 10.1007/s11517-010-0719-6.

Ho, K. K., G. B. Moody, C. K. Peng, J. E. Mietus, M. G. Larson, D. Levy, and A. L. Goldberger. 1997. Predicting survival in heart failure case and control subjects by use of fully automated methods for deriving nonlinear and conventional indices of heart rate dynamics. *Circulation* 96 (3):842–8.

Hoffmann, J., W. Grimm, V. Menz, U. Knop, and B. Maisch. 1996. Heart rate variability and major arrhythmic events in patients with idiopathic dilated cardiomyopathy. *Pacing Clin Electrophysiol* 19 (11 Pt 2):1841–4.

Hoffmann, J., W. Grimm, V. Menz, and B. Maisch. 2000. Cardiac autonomic tone and its relation to nonsustained ventricular tachyarrhythmias in idiopathic dilated cardiomyopathy. *Clin Cardiol* 23 (2):103–8.

Hohnloser, S. H., T. Klingenheben, D. Bloomfield, O. Dabbous, and R. J. Cohen. 2003. Usefulness of microvolt T-wave alternans for prediction of ventricular tachyarrhythmic events in patients with dilated cardiomyopathy: Results from a prospective observational study. *J Am Coll Cardiol* 41 (12):2220–4.

Hohnloser, S. H., K. H. Kuck, P. Dorian, R. S. Roberts, J. R. Hampton, R. Hatala, E. Fain, M. Gent, S. J. Connolly, and Dinamit Investigators. 2004. Prophylactic use of an implantable cardioverter-defibrillator after acute myocardial infarction. *N Engl J Med* 351 (24):2481–8. doi: 10.1056/NEJMoa041489.

Hon, E. H., and S. T. Lee. 1963. Electronic evaluation of the fetal heart rate. III. Patterns preceding fetal death, further observations. *Am J Obstet Gynecol* 87:814–26.

Hon, E. H., and S. T. Lee. 1965. The fetal electrocardiogram. 3. Display techniques. *Am J Obstet Gynecol* 91:56–60.

Hottenrott, K., O. Hoos, and H. D. Esperer. 2006. Heart rate variability and physical exercise. Current status. *Herz* 31 (6):544–52. doi: 10.1007/s00059-006-2855-1.

Hoyer, D., U. Leder, H. Hoyer, B. Pompe, M. Sommer, and U. Zwiener. 2002. Mutual information and phase dependencies: Measures of reduced nonlinear cardiorespiratory interactions after myocardial infarction. *Med Eng Phys* 24 (1):33–43. doi: S1350453301001205 [pii].

Huikuri, H. V., and P. K. Stein. 2013. Heart rate variability in risk stratification of cardiac patients. *Prog Cardiovasc Dis* 56 (2):153–9. doi: 10.1016/j.pcad.2013.07.003.

Huikuri, H. V., J. M. Tapanainen, K. Lindgren, P. Raatikainen, T. H. Makikallio, K. E. Juhani Airaksinen, and R. J. Myerburg. 2003. Prediction of sudden cardiac death after myocardial infarction in the beta-blocking era. *J Am Coll Cardiol* 42 (4):652–8.

Hyndman, B. W., R. I. Kitney, and B. M. Sayers. 1971. Spontaneous rhythms in physiological control systems. *Nature* 233 (5318):339–41.

Ivanov, P. C., L. A. Amaral, A. L. Goldberger, S. Havlin, M. G. Rosenblum, Z. R. Struzik, and H. E. Stanley. 1999. Multifractality in human heartbeat dynamics. *Nature* 399 (6735):461–5. doi: 10.1038/20924.

Jansson, K., I. Hagerman, R. Ostlund, K. E. Karlberg, E. Nylander, O. Nyquist, and U. Dahlstrom. 1999. The effects of metoprolol and captopril on heart rate variability in patients with idiopathic dilated cardiomyopathy. *Clin Cardiol* 22 (6):397–402.

Javorka, M., Z. Turianikova, I. Tonhajzerova, K. Javorka, and M. Baumert. 2009. The effect of orthostasis on recurrence quantification analysis of heart rate and blood pressure dynamics. *Physiol Meas* 30 (1):29.

Jefferies, J. L., and J. A. Towbin. 2010. Dilated cardiomyopathy. *Lancet* 375 (9716):752–62. doi: 10.1016/S0140-6736(09)62023-7.

Jennett, S. 1977. Heart-rate variability in brain-damaged adults. *Lancet* 1 (8016):860.

Jindal, R., E. M. MacKenzie, G. B. Baker, and V. K. Yeragani. 2005. Cardiac risk and schizophrenia. *J Psychiatry Neurosci* 30 (6):393–5.

Kamen, P. W., H. Krum, and A. M. Tonkin. 1996. Poincare plot of heart rate variability allows quantitative display of parasympathetic nervous activity in humans. *Clin Sci (Lond)* 91 (2):201–8.

Kamen, P. W., and A. M. Tonkin. 1995. Application of the Poincare plot to heart rate variability: A new measure of functional status in heart failure. *Aust N Z J Med* 25 (1):18–26.

Kantelhardt, J., S. Zschiegner, E. Koscielnybunde, S. Havlin, A. Bunde, and H Stanley. 2002. Multifractal detrended fluctuation analysis of nonstationary time series. *Physica A* 316:87–114.

Kanters, J. K., M. V. Hojgaard, E. Agner, and N. H. Holstein-Rathlou. 1996. Short- and long-term variations in non-linear dynamics of heart rate variability. *Cardiovasc Res* 31 (3):400–9.

Kemp, A. H., A. R. Brunoni, I. S. Santos, M. A. Nunes, E. M. Dantas, R. Carvalho de Figueiredo, A. C. Pereira, A. L. Ribeiro, J. G. Mill, R. V. Andreao, J. F. Thayer, I. M. Bensenor, and P. A. Lotufo. 2014. Effects of depression, anxiety, comorbidity, and antidepressants on resting-state heart rate and its variability: An ELSA-Brasil cohort baseline study. *Am J Psychiatry* 171 (12):1328–34. doi: 10.1176/appi.ajp.2014.13121605.

Kemp, A. H., D. S. Quintana, K. L. Felmingham, S. Matthews, and H. F. Jelinek. 2012. Depression, comorbid anxiety disorders, and heart rate variability in physically healthy, unmedicated patients: Implications for cardiovascular risk. *PLOS ONE* 7 (2):e30777. doi: 10.1371/journal.pone.0030777.

Kleiger, R. E., J. P. Miller, J. T. Bigger, Jr., and A. J. Moss. 1987. Decreased heart rate variability and its association with increased mortality after acute myocardial infarction. *Am J Cardiol* 59 (4):256–62. doi: 0002-9149(87)90795-8 [pii].

Kleiger, R. E., P. K. Stein, and J. T. Bigger, Jr. 2005. Heart rate variability: Measurement and clinical utility. *Ann Noninvasive Electrocardiol* 10 (1):88–101. doi: 10.1111/j.1542-474X.2005.10101.x.

Klingenheben, T., P. Ptaszynski, and S. H. Hohnloser. 2008. Heart rate turbulence and other autonomic risk markers for arrhythmia risk stratification in dilated cardiomyopathy. *J Electrocardiol* 41 (4):306–11. doi: 10.1016/j.jelectrocard.2007.10.004.

Kobayashi, M., and T. Musha. 1982. 1/f fluctuation of heartbeat period. *IEEE Trans Biomed Eng* 29 (6):456–7. doi: 10.1109/TBME.1982.324972.

Koponen, H., A. Alaraisanen, K. Saari, O. Pelkonen, H. Huikuri, M. J. Raatikainen, M. Savolainen, and M. Isohanni. 2008. Schizophrenia and sudden cardiac death: A review. *Nord J Psychiatry* 62 (5):342–5. doi: 901960942 [pii]10.1080/08039480801959323.

Krum, H., and W. T. Abraham. 2009. Heart failure. *Lancet* 373 (9667):941–55. doi: 10.1016/S0140-6736(09)60236-1.

Kurths, J., A. Voss, P. Saparin, A. Witt, H. J. Kleiner, and N. Wessel. 1995. Quantitative analysis of heart rate variability. *Chaos* 5 (1):88–94. doi: 10.1063/1.166090.

Laguna, P., G. B. Moody, and R. G. Mark. 1998. Power spectral density of unevenly sampled data by least-square analysis: Performance and application to heart rate signals. *IEEE Trans Biomed Eng* 45 (6):698–715. doi: 10.1109/10.678605.

Lahiri, M. K., P. J. Kannankeril, and J. J. Goldberger. 2008. Assessment of autonomic function in cardiovascular disease: Physiological basis and prognostic implications. *J Am Coll Cardiol* 51 (18):1725–33. doi: 10.1016/j.jacc.2008.01.038.

Laitio, T. T., H. V. Huikuri, E. S. Kentala, T. H. Makikallio, J. R. Jalonen, H. Helenius, K. Sariola-Heinonen, S. Yli-Mayry, and H. Scheinin. 2000. Correlation properties and complexity of peri-operative RR-interval dynamics in coronary artery bypass surgery patients. *Anesthesiology* 93 (1):69–80.

Langewitz, W., H. Ruddel, and H. Schachinger. 1994. Reduced parasympathetic cardiac control in patients with hypertension at rest and under mental stress. *Am Heart J* 127 (1):122–8.

Lanza, G. A., M. G. Bendini, A. Intini, G. De Martino, M. Galeazzi, V. Guido, and A. Sestito. 2000. Prognostic role of heart rate variability in patients with idiopathic dilated cardiomyopathy. *Ital Heart J* 1 (1):56–63.

Lassner, D., M. Rohde, C. Sabine Siegismund, U. Kühl, U. Michael Gross, F. Escher, C. Tschöpe, and H. P. Schultheiss. 2014. Myocarditis—Personalized medicine by expanded endomyocardial biopsy diagnostics. *WJCD* 04 (06):325–340. doi: 10.4236/wjcd.2014.46042.

Leeman, L., and P. Fontaine. 2008. Hypertensive disorders of pregnancy. *Am Fam Physician* 78 (1): 93–100.

Lewinsky, R. M., and S. Riskin-Mashiah. 1998. Autonomic imbalance in preeclampsia: Evidence for increased sympathetic tone in response to the supine-pressor test. *Obstet Gynecol* 91 (6):935–9.

Li, M., and Paul M.B. Vitányi. 1997. *An Introduction to Kolmogorov Complexity and Its Applications*. New York, NY: Springer Publishing Company, Incorporated.

Liao, D., M. Carnethon, G. W. Evans, W. E. Cascio, and G. Heiss. 2002. Lower heart rate variability is associated with the development of coronary heart disease in individuals with diabetes: The atherosclerosis risk in communities (ARIC) study. *Diabetes* 51 (12):3524–31.

Lombardi, F., G. Sandrone, S. Pernpruner, R. Sala, M. Garimoldi, S. Cerutti, G. Baselli, M. Pagani, and A. Malliani. 1987. Heart rate variability as an index of sympathovagal interaction after acute myocardial infarction. *Am J Cardiol* 60 (16):1239–45.

Longin, E., T. Gerstner, T. Schaible, T. Lenz, and S. Konig. 2006. Maturation of the autonomic nervous system: Differences in heart rate variability in premature vs. term infants. *J Perinat Med* 34 (4):303–8. doi: 10.1515/JPM.2006.058.

Lowensohn, R. I., M. Weiss, and E. H. Hon. 1977. Heart-rate variability in brain-damaged adults. *Lancet* 1 (8012):626–8.

Mahon, N. G., A. E. Hedman, M. Padula, Y. Gang, I. Savelieva, J. E. Waktare, M. M. Malik, H. V. Huikuri, and W. J. McKenna. 2002. Fractal correlation properties of R-R interval dynamics in asymptomatic relatives of patients with dilated cardiomyopathy. *Eur J Heart Fail* 4 (2):151–8.

Malberg, H., R. Bauernschmitt, A. Voss, T. Walther, R. Faber, H. Stepan, and N. Wessel. 2007. Analysis of cardiovascular oscillations: A new approach to the early prediction of pre-eclampsia. *Chaos* 17 (1):015113. doi: 10.1063/1.2711660.

Malberg, H., N. Wessel, A. Hasart, K. J. Osterziel, and A. Voss. 2002. Advanced analysis of spontaneous baroreflex sensitivity, blood pressure and heart rate variability in patients with dilated cardiomyopathy. *Clin Sci (Lond)* 102 (4):465–73.

Malberg, H., N. Wessel, A. Schirdewan, K. J. Osterziel, and A. Voss. 1999. Dual sequence method for analysis of spontaneous baroreceptor reflex sensitivity in patients with dilated cardiomyopathy. *Z Kardiol* 88 (5):331–7.

Malfatto, G., G. Branzi, S. Gritti, L. Sala, R. Bragato, G. B. Perego, G. Leonetti, and M. Facchini. 2001. Different baseline sympathovagal balance and cardiac autonomic responsiveness in ischemic and non-ischemic congestive heart failure. *Eur J Heart Fail* 3 (2):197–202.

Malik, M., T. Farrell, and A. J. Camm. 1990. Circadian rhythm of heart rate variability after acute myocardial infarction and its influence on the prognostic value of heart rate variability. *Am J Cardiol* 66 (15):1049–54.

Malliani, A., M. Pagani, F. Lombardi, and S. Cerutti. 1991. Cardiovascular neural regulation explored in the frequency domain. *Circulation* 84 (2):482–92.

Malpas, S. C., E. A. Whiteside, and T. J. Maling. 1991. Heart rate variability and cardiac autonomic function in men with chronic alcohol dependence. *Br Heart J* 65 (2):84–8.

Marwan, N., N. Wessel, U. Meyerfeldt, A. Schirdewan, and J. Kurths. 2002. Recurrence-plot-based measures of complexity and their application to heart-rate-variability data. *Phys Rev E Stat Nonlin Soft Matter Phys* 66 (2 Pt 2):026702.

Marwan, N., M. Carmen Romano, M. Thiel, and J. Kurths. 2007. Recurrence plots for the analysis of complex systems. *Physics Rep* 438 (5–6):237–329. doi: http://dx.doi.org/10.1016/j.physrep. 2006.11.001.

Matthes, K., and W. Hauss. 1938. Lichtelektrische Plethysmogramme. *Klinische Wochenschrift* 17 (35):1211–213.

Mazzeo, A. T., E. La Monaca, R. Di Leo, G. Vita, and L. B. Santamaria. 2011. Heart rate variability: A diagnostic and prognostic tool in anesthesia and intensive care. *Acta Anaesthesiol Scand* 55 (7):797–811. doi: 10.1111/j.1399-6576.2011.02466.x.

Mbaissouroum, M., C. O'Sullivan, S. J. Brecker, H. B. Xiao, and D. G. Gibson. 1993. Shortened left ventricular filling time in dilated cardiomyopathy: Additional effects on heart rate variability? *Br Heart J* 69 (4):327–31.

Menz, V., W. Grimm, J. Hoffmann, S. Born, C. Schmidt, and B. Maisch. 1998. Baroreflex sensitivity and heart rate variability in coronary disease compared to dilated cardiomyopathy. *Pacing Clin Electrophysiol* 21 (11 Pt 2):2416–9.

Meyerfeldt, U., N. Wessel, H. Schutt, D. Selbig, A. Schumann, A. Voss, J. Kurths, C. Ziehmann, R. Dietz, and A. Schirdewan. 2002. Heart rate variability before the onset of ventricular tachycardia: Differences between slow and fast arrhythmias. *Int J Cardiol* 84 (2–3):141–51. doi: S0167527302001390 [pii].

Migliorini, M., M. O. Mendez, and A. M. Bianchi. 2011. Study of heart rate variability in bipolar disorder: Linear and non-linear parameters during sleep. *Front Neuroeng* 4:22. doi: 10.3389/fneng.2011.00022.

Minamihaba, O., M. Yamaki, H. Tomoike, and I. Kubota. 2003. Severity in myocardial dysfunction contributed to long-term fluctuation of heart rate, rather than short-term fluctuations. *Ann Noninvasive Electrocardiol* 8 (2):132–8.

Mortara, A., M. T. La Rovere, G. D. Pinna, P. Parziale, R. Maestri, S. Capomolla, C. Opasich, F. Cobelli, and L. Tavazzi. 1997. Depressed arterial baroreflex sensitivity and not reduced heart rate variability identifies patients with chronic heart failure and nonsustained ventricular tachycardia: The effect of high ventricular filling pressure. *Am Heart J* 134 (5 Pt 1):879–88.

Muralikrishnan, K., B. Balakrishnan, K. Balasubramanian, and F. Visnegarawla. 2012. Measurement of the effect of Isha Yoga on cardiac autonomic nervous system using short-term heart rate variability. *J Ayurveda Integr Med* 3 (2):91–6. doi: 10.4103/0975-9476.96528.

Murata, K., P. J. Landrigan, and S. Araki. 1992. Effects of age, heart rate, gender, tobacco and alcohol ingestion on R-R interval variability in human ECG. *J Auton Nerv Syst* 37 (3):199–206.

Myers, G. A., G. J. Martin, N. M. Magid, P. S. Barnett, J. W. Schaad, J. S. Weiss, M. Lesch, and D. H. Singer. 1986. Power spectral analysis of heart rate variability in sudden cardiac death: Comparison to other methods. *IEEE Trans Biomed Eng* 33 (12):1149–56. doi: 10.1109/TBME.1986. 325694.

NHBPEP. 2000. Report of the National High Blood Pressure Education Program Working Group on High Blood Pressure in Pregnancy. *Am J Obstet Gynecol* 183 (1):S1–S22.

Niedermaier, O. N., M. L. Smith, L. A. Beightol, Z. Zukowska-Grojec, D. S. Goldstein, and D. L. Eckberg. 1993. Influence of cigarette smoking on human autonomic function. *Circulation* 88 (2):562–71.

O'Connell, J. B., and M. R. Bristow. 1994. Economic impact of heart failure in the United States: Time for a different approach. *J Heart Lung Transplant* 13 (4):S107–12.

Pagani, M., F. Lombardi, S. Guzzetti, O. Rimoldi, R. Furlan, P. Pizzinelli, G. Sandrone, G. Malfatto, S. Dell'Orto, E. Piccaluga, M. Turieland, G. Baselli, S. Cerutti, and A. Malliani. 1986. Power spectral analysis of heart rate and arterial pressure variabilities as a marker of sympatho-vagal interaction in man and conscious dog. *Circ Res* 59 (2):178–93.

Palacios, M., H. Friedrich, C. Gotze, M. Vallverdu, A. B. de Luna, P. Caminal, and D. Hoyer. 2007. Changes of autonomic information flow due to idiopathic dilated cardiomyopathy. *Physiol Meas* 28 (6):677–88. doi: 10.1088/0967-3334/28/6/006.

Papaioannou, V. E. 2007. Heart rate variability, baroreflex function and heart rate turbulence: Possible origin and implications. *Hellenic J Cardiol* 48 (5):278–89.

Pedretti, R., M. D. Etro, A. Laporta, S. Sarzi Braga, and B. Caru. 1993. Prediction of late arrhythmic events after acute myocardial infarction from combined use of noninvasive prognostic variables and inducibility of sustained monomorphic ventricular tachycardia. *Am J Cardiol* 71 (13):1131–41.

Penaz, J., N. Honzikova, and B. Fiser. 1978. Spectral analysis of resting variability of some circulatory parameters in man. *Physiol Bohemoslov* 27 (4):349–57.

Peng, C. K., S. Havlin, H. E. Stanley, and A. L. Goldberger. 1995. Quantification of scaling exponents and crossover phenomena in nonstationary heartbeat time series. *Chaos* 5 (1):82–7. doi: 10.1063/1.166141.

Penzel, T., J. W. Kantelhardt, C. C. Lo, K. Voigt, and C. Vogelmeier. 2003. Dynamics of heart rate and sleep stages in normals and patients with sleep apnea. *Neuropsychopharmacology* 28 (Suppl 1):S48–53. doi: 10.1038/sj.npp.1300146.

Pezawas, T., A. Diedrich, R. Winker, D. Robertson, B. Richter, L. Wang, D. W. Byrne, and H. Schmidinger. 2014. Multiple autonomic and repolarization investigation of sudden cardiac death in dilated cardiomyopathy and controls. *Circ Arrhythm Electrophysiol* 7 (6):1101–8. doi: 10.1161/CIRCEP.114.001745.

Pikovsky, A., M. Rosenblum, and J. Kurths. 2001. *Synchronization: A Universal Concept in Nonlinear Science*. Cambridge: Cambridge University Press.

Pincus, S. M. 1991. Approximate entropy as a measure of system complexity. *Proc Natl Acad Sci U S A* 88 (6):2297–301.

Pincus, S. M., and A. L. Goldberger. 1994. Physiological time-series analysis: What does regularity quantify? *Am J Physiol* 266 (4 Pt 2):H1643–56.

Pompe, B. 1993. Measuring statistical dependencies in a time series. *J. Stat. Phys.* 73(3):587–610.

Ponikowski, P., S. D. Anker, A. Amadi, T. P. Chua, E. Cerquetani, D. Ondusova, C. O'Sullivan, S. Adamopoulos, M. Piepoli, and A. J. Coats. 1996. Heart rhythms, ventricular arrhythmias, and death in chronic heart failure. *J Card Fail* 2 (3):177–83.

Ponikowski, P., S. D. Anker, T. P. Chua, R. Szelemej, M. Piepoli, S. Adamopoulos, K. Webb-Peploe, D. Harrington, W. Banasiak, K. Wrabec, and A. J. Coats. 1997. Depressed heart rate variability as an independent predictor of death in chronic congestive heart failure secondary to ischemic or idiopathic dilated cardiomyopathy. *Am J Cardiol* 79 (12):1645–50.

Pope, C. A., 3rd, D. J. Eatough, D. R. Gold, Y. Pang, K. R. Nielsen, P. Nath, R. L. Verrier, and R. E. Kanner. 2001. Acute exposure to environmental tobacco smoke and heart rate variability. *Environ Health Perspect* 109 (7):711–6.

Porges, S. W., and S. A. Furman. 2011. The early development of the autonomic nervous system provides a neural platform for social behavior: A polyvagal perspective. *Infant Child Dev* 20 (1): 106–118. doi: 10.1002/icd.688.

Porta, A., G. Baselli, F. Lombardi, N. Montano, A. Malliani, and S. Cerutti. 1999. Conditional entropy approach for the evaluation of the coupling strength. *Biol Cybern* 81 (2):119–29.

Porta, A., T. Bassani, V. Bari, G. D. Pinna, R. Maestri, and S. Guzzetti. 2012. Accounting for respiration is necessary to reliably infer Granger causality from cardiovascular variability series. *IEEE Trans Biomed Eng* 59 (3):832–41. doi: 10.1109/TBME.2011.2180379.

Porta, A., and L. Faes. 2013. Assessing causality in brain dynamics and cardiovascular control. *Philos Trans A Math Phys Eng Sci* 371 (1997):20120517. doi: 10.1098/rsta.2012.0517.

Porta, A., S. Guzzetti, N. Montano, R. Furlan, M. Pagani, A. Malliani, and S. Cerutti. 2001. Entropy, entropy rate, and pattern classification as tools to typify complexity in short heart period variability series. *IEEE Trans Biomed Eng* 48 (11):1282–91. doi: 10.1109/10.959324.

Raab, C., and J. Kurths. 2001. Estimation of large-scale dimension densities. *Phys Rev E Stat Nonlin Soft Matter Phys* 64 (1 Pt 2):016216.

Raab, C., J. Kurths, A. Schirdewan, and N. Wessel. 2006a. Normalized correlation dimension for heart rate variability analysis. *Biomed Tech (Berl)* 51 (4):229–32. doi: 10.1515/BMT.2006.043.

Raab, C., N. Wessel, A. Schirdewan, and J. Kurths. 2006b. Large-scale dimension densities for heart rate variability analysis. *Phys Rev E Stat Nonlin Soft Matter Phys* 73 (4 Pt 1):041907.

Rajendra Acharya, U., K. P. Joseph, N. Kannathal, C. M. Lim, and J. S. Suri. 2006. Heart rate variability: A review. *Med Biol Eng Comput* 44 (12):1031–51. doi: 10.1007/s11517-006-0119-0.

Ramirez Avila, G. M., A. Gapelyuk, N. Marwan, H. Stepan, J. Kurths, T. Walther, and N. Wessel. 2013. Classifying healthy women and preeclamptic patients from cardiovascular data using recurrence and complex network methods. *Auton Neurosci* 178 (1–2):103–10. doi: 10.1016/j.autneu.2013.05.003.

Rang, S., H. Wolf, G. A. van Montfrans, and J. M. Karemaker. 2004. Serial assessment of cardiovascular control shows early signs of developing pre-eclampsia. *J Hypertens* 22 (2):369–76.

Rashba, E. J., N. A. Estes, P. Wang, A. Schaechter, A. Howard, W. Zareba, J. P. Couderc, J. Perkiomaki, J. Levine, and A. Kadish. 2006. Preserved heart rate variability identifies low-risk patients with nonischemic dilated cardiomyopathy: Results from the DEFINITE trial. *Heart Rhythm* 3 (3):281–6. doi: 10.1016/j.hrthm.2005.11.028.

Rathmann, W., D. Ziegler, M. Jahnke, B. Haastert, and F. A. Gries. 1993. Mortality in diabetic patients with cardiovascular autonomic neuropathy. *Diabet Med* 10 (9):820–4.

Reed, M. J., C. E. Robertson, and P. S. Addison. 2005. Heart rate variability measurements and the prediction of ventricular arrhythmias. *QJM* 98 (2):87–95. doi: 10.1093/qjmed/hci018.

Rentero, N., A. Cividjian, D. Trevaks, J. M. Pequignot, L. Quintin, and R. M. McAllen. 2002. Activity patterns of cardiac vagal motoneurons in rat nucleus ambiguus. *Am J Physiol Regul Integr Comp Physiol* 283 (6):R1327–34. doi: 10.1152/ajpregu.00271.2002.

Reulecke, S., S. Schulz, and A. Voss. 2012. Autonomic regulation during quiet and active sleep states in very preterm neonates. *Front Physiol* 3:61. doi: 10.3389/fphys.2012.00061.

Richman, J. S., and J. R. Moorman. 2000. Physiological time-series analysis using approximate entropy and sample entropy. *Am J Physiol Heart Circ Physiol* 278 (6):H2039–49.

Riedl, M., A. Suhrbier, H. Stepan, J. Kurths, and N. Wessel. 2010. Short-term couplings of the cardiovascular system in pregnant women suffering from pre-eclampsia. *Philos Trans A Math Phys Eng Sci* 368 (1918):2237–50. doi: 10.1098/rsta.2010.0029.

Ritzenberg, A. L., D. R. Adam, and R. J. Cohen. 1984. Period multupling-evidence for nonlinear behaviour of the canine heart. *Nature* 307 (5947):159–61.

Roberts, J. M., and C. W. Redman. 1993. Pre-eclampsia: More than pregnancy-induced hypertension. *Lancet* 341 (8858):1447–51.

Rosenblum, M., A. Pikovsky, C. Schäfer, P. A. Tass, and J. Kurths. 2001. *Phase synchronization: From theory to data analysis, Handbook of Biological Physics.* Vol. 4. Amsterdam: Elsevier Science.

Rosenstein, M. T., J. J. Collins, and C. J. De Luca. 1993. A practical method for calculating largest Lyapunov exponents from small data sets. *Phys. D* 65 (1–2):117–134. doi: 10.1016/0167-2789(93)90009-p.

Rubin, M. F., S. M. Brunelli, and R. R. Townsend. 2010. Variability–The drama of the circulation. *J Clin Hypertens (Greenwich)* 12 (4):284–7. doi: 10.1111/j.1751-7176.2009.00262.x.

Ryan, S. M., A. L. Goldberger, S. M. Pincus, J. Mietus, and L. A. Lipsitz. 1994. Gender- and age-related differences in heart rate dynamics: Are women more complex than men? *J Am Coll Cardiol* 24 (7):1700–7. doi: 0735-1097(94)90177-5 [pii].

Sassi, R., S. Cerutti, F. Lombardi, M. Malik, H. V. Huikuri, C. K. Peng, G. Schmidt, Y. Yamamoto, Reviewers Document, B. Gorenek, et al. 2015. Advances in heart rate variability signal analysis:

Joint position statement by the e-Cardiology ESC Working Group and the European Heart Rhythm Association co-endorsed by the Asia Pacific Heart Rhythm Society. *Europace.* doi: 10.1093/europace/euv015.

Sayers, B. M. 1973. Analysis of heart rate variability. *Ergonomics* 16 (1):17–32. doi: 10.1080/00140137308924479.

Schafer, A., and J. Vagedes. 2013. How accurate is pulse rate variability as an estimate of heart rate variability? A review on studies comparing photoplethysmographic technology with an electrocardiogram. *Int J Cardiol* 166 (1):15–29. doi: 10.1016/j.ijcard.2012.03.119.

Schäfer, C., M. G. Rosenblum, J. Kurths, and H. H. Abel. 1998. Heartbeat synchronized with ventilation. *Nature* 392 (6673):239–40. doi: 10.1038/32567.

Schmidt, G., M. Malik, P. Barthel, R. Schneider, K. Ulm, L. Rolnitzky, A. J. Camm, J. T. Bigger, Jr., and A. Schomig. 1999. Heart-rate turbulence after ventricular premature beats as a predictor of mortality after acute myocardial infarction. *Lancet* 353 (9162):1390–6. doi: 10.1016/S0140-6736(98)08428-1.

Schmidt, G., G. E. Morfill, P. Barthel, M. Hadamitzky, H. Kreuzberg, V. Demmel, R. Schneider, K. Ulm, and A. Schomig. 1996. Variability of ventricular premature complexes and mortality risk. *Pacing Clin Electrophysiol* 19 (6):976–80.

Schreiber, T. 2000. Measuring information transfer. *Phys Rev Lett* 85 (2):461–4.

Schulz, S., F. C. Adochiei, I. R. Edu, R. Schroeder, H. Costin, K. J. Bar, and A. Voss. 2013. Cardiovascular and cardiorespiratory coupling analyses: A review. *Philos Trans A Math Phys Eng Sci* 371 (1997):20120191. doi: 10.1098/rsta.2012.0191.

Schulz, S., J. Haueisen, K. J. Bar, and V. Andreas. 2015. High-resolution joint symbolic analysis to enhance classification of the cardiorespiratory system in patients with schizophrenia and their relatives. *Philos Trans A Math Phys Eng Sci* 373 (2034). doi: 10.1098/rsta.2014.0098.

Schulz, S., M. Koschke, K. J. Bär, and A. Voss. 2010. The altered complexity of cardiovascular regulation in depressed patients. *Physiol Meas* 31 (3):303–21. doi: 10.1088/0967-3334/31/3/003.

Schulz, S., J. Ritter, K. Oertel, K. Witt, K. J. Bär, O. Guntinas-Lichius, and A. Voss. 2014. Altered autonomic regulation as a cardiovascular risk marker for patients with sudden sensorineural hearing loss. *Otol Neurotol* 35 (10):1720–9. doi: 10.1097/MAO.0000000000000622.

Schulz, S., and A. Voss. 2014. Cardiovascular and cardiorespiratory coupling analysis—State of the art and future perspectives. Cardiovascular Oscillations (ESGCO), 2014 8th Conference of the European Study Group on, Trento, 25–28 May 2014.

Schumann, A., N. Wessel, A. Schirdewan, K. J. Osterziel, and A. Voss. 2002. Potential of feature selection methods in heart rate variability analysis for the classification of different cardiovascular diseases. *Stat Med* 21 (15):2225–42. doi: 10.1002/sim.979.

Schwartz, P. J., A. Zaza, M. Pala, E. Locati, G. Beria, and A. Zanchetti. 1988. Baroreflex sensitivity and its evolution during the first year after myocardial infarction. *J Am Coll Cardiol* 12 (3):629–36.

Seeck, A., M. Baumert, C. Fischer, A. Khandoker, R. Faber, and A. Voss. 2011. Advanced Poincare plot analysis differentiates between hypertensive pregnancy disorders. *Physiol Meas* 32 (10):1611–22. doi: 10.1088/0967-3334/32/10/009.

Seeck, A., W. Rademacher, C. Fischer, J. Haueisen, R. Surber, and A. Voss. 2013. Prediction of atrial fibrillation recurrence after cardioversion-interaction analysis of cardiac autonomic regulation. *Med Eng Phys* 35 (3):376–82. doi: 10.1016/j.medengphy.2012.06.002.

Seely, A. J., and P. T. Macklem. 2004. Complex systems and the technology of variability analysis. *Crit Care* 8 (6):R367–84. doi: 10.1186/cc2948.

Seifert, G., J. L. Kanitz, K. Pretzer, G. Henze, K. Witt, S. Reulecke, and A. Voss. 2013. Improvement of circadian rhythm of heart rate variability by eurythmy therapy training. *Evid Based Complement Alternat Med* 2013:564340. doi: 10.1155/2013/564340.

Shannon, C. E. 1948. *A Mathematical Theory of Communication.* New York, NY: American Telephone and Telegraph Company.

Silke, B., C. Campbell, and D. J. King. 2002. The potential cardiotoxicity of antipsychotic drugs as assessed by heart rate variability. *J Psychopharmacol* 16 (4):355–60.

Singh, J. P., M. G. Larson, C. J. O'Donnell, P. F. Wilson, H. Tsuji, D. M. Lloyd-Jones, and D. Levy. 2000. Association of hyperglycemia with reduced heart rate variability (The Framingham Heart Study). *Am J Cardiol* 86 (3):309–12.

Singh, J. P., M. G. Larson, H. Tsuji, J. C. Evans, C. J. O'Donnell, and D. Levy. 1998. Reduced heart rate variability and new-onset hypertension: Insights into pathogenesis of hypertension: The Framingham Heart Study. *Hypertension* 32 (2):293–7.

Skinner, J. S., S. E. Gaskill, T. Rankinen, A. S. Leon, D. C. Rao, J. H. Wilmore, and C. Bouchard. 2003. Heart rate versus %VO2max: Age, sex, race, initial fitness, and training response–HERITAGE. *Med Sci Sports Exerc* 35 (11):1908–13. doi: 10.1249/01.MSS.0000093607.57995.E3.

Smith, M. L., D. L. Hudson, H. M. Graitzer, and P. B. Raven. 1989. Exercise training bradycardia: The role of autonomic balance. *Med Sci Sports Exerc* 21 (1):40–4.

Smith, S. E., and S. A. Smith. 1981. Heart rate variability in healthy subjects measured with a bedside computer-based technique. *Clin Sci (Lond)* 61 (4):379–83.

Stapelberg, N. J., I. Hamilton-Craig, D. L. Neumann, D. H. Shum, and H. McConnell. 2012. Mind and heart: Heart rate variability in major depressive disorder and coronary heart disease—A review and recommendations. *Aust N Z J Psychiatry* 46 (10):946–57. doi: 10.1177/0004867412444624.

Stauss, H. M. 2003. Heart rate variability. *Am J Physiol Regul Integr Comp Physiol* 285 (5):R927–31. doi: 10.1152/ajpregu.00452.2003.

Stein, P. K., and Y. Pu. 2012. Heart rate variability, sleep and sleep disorders. *Sleep Med Rev* 16 (1):47–66. doi: 10.1016/j.smrv.2011.02.005.

Stutzman, S. S., C. A. Brown, S. M. Hains, M. Godwin, G. N. Smith, J. L. Parlow, and B. S. Kisilevsky. 2010. The effects of exercise conditioning in normal and overweight pregnant women on blood pressure and heart rate variability. *Biol Res Nurs* 12 (2):137–48. doi: 10.1177/1099800410375979.

Stys, A., and T. Stys. 1998. Current clinical applications of heart rate variability. *Clin Cardiol* 21 (10):719–24.

Szabo, B. M., D. J. van Veldhuisen, N. van der Veer, J. Brouwer, P. A. De Graeff, and H. J. Crijns. 1997. Prognostic value of heart rate variability in chronic congestive heart failure secondary to idiopathic or ischemic dilated cardiomyopathy. *Am J Cardiol* 79 (7):978–80.

Takahashi, T., T. Murata, T. Hamada, M. Omori, H. Kosaka, M. Kikuchi, H. Yoshida, and Y. Wada. 2005. Changes in EEG and autonomic nervous activity during meditation and their association with personality traits. *Int J Psychophysiol* 55 (2):199–207. doi: 10.1016/j.ijpsycho.2004.07.004.

Task Force. 1996. Heart rate variability: Standards of measurement, physiological interpretation and clinical use. Task Force of the European Society of Cardiology and the North American Society of Pacing and Electrophysiology. *Circulation* 93 (5):1043–65.

Taylor, A. G., L. E. Goehler, D. I. Galper, K. E. Innes, and C. Bourguignon. 2010. Top-down and bottom-up mechanisms in mind-body medicine: Development of an integrative framework for psychophysiological research. *Explore (NY)* 6 (1):29–41. doi: 10.1016/j.explore.2009.10.004.

Tejera, E., M. J. Areias, A. I. Rodrigues, J. M. Nieto-Villar, and I. Rebelo. 2012a. Blood pressure and heart rate variability complexity analysis in pregnant women with hypertension. *Hypertens Pregnancy* 31 (1):91–106. doi: 10.3109/10641955.2010.544801.

Tejera, E., M. J. Areias, A. I. Rodrigues, A. Ramoa, J. M. Nieto-Villar, and I. Rebelo. 2012b. Relationship between heart rate variability indexes and common biochemical markers in normal and hypertensive third trimester pregnancy. *Hypertens Pregnancy* 31 (1):59–69. doi: 10.3109/10641955.2010.544802.

Tejera, E., M. Jose Areias, A. Rodrigues, A. Ramoa, J. Manuel Nieto-Villar, and I. Rebelo. 2011. Artificial neural network for normal, hypertensive, and preeclamptic pregnancy classification using maternal heart rate variability indexes. *J Matern Fetal Neonatal Med* 24 (9):1147–51. doi: 10.3109/14767058.2010.545916.

Thayer, J. F., B. H. Friedman, and T. D. Borkovec. 1996. Autonomic characteristics of generalized anxiety disorder and worry. *Biol Psychiatry* 39 (4):255–66. doi: 10.1016/0006-3223(95)00136-0.

Thayer, J. F., M. Smith, L. A. Rossy, J. J. Sollers, and B. H. Friedman. 1998. Heart period variability and depressive symptoms: Gender differences. *Biol Psychiatry* 44 (4):304–6.

Thayer, J. F., and E. Sternberg. 2006. Beyond heart rate variability: Vagal regulation of allostatic systems. *Ann N Y Acad Sci* 1088:361–72. doi: 10.1196/annals.1366.014.

Thayer, J. F., S. S. Yamamoto, and J. F. Brosschot. 2010. The relationship of autonomic imbalance, heart rate variability and cardiovascular disease risk factors. *Int J Cardiol* 141 (2):122–31. doi: 10.1016/j.ijcard.2009.09.543.

Theiler, J., S. Eubank, A. Longtin, B. Galdrikian, and J. Doyne Farmer. 1992. Testing for nonlinearity in time series: The method of surrogate data. *Phys D* 58 (1–4):77–94. doi: 10.1016/0167-2789(92)90102-s.

Tobaldini, E., L. Nobili, S. Strada, K. R. Casali, A. Braghiroli, and N. Montano. 2013. Heart rate variability in normal and pathological sleep. *Front Physiol* 4:294. doi: 10.3389/fphys.2013.00294.

Truebner, S., I. Cygankiewicz, R. Schroeder, M. Baumert, M. Vallverdu, P. Caminal, R. Vazquez, A. Bayes de Luna, and A. Voss. 2006. Compression entropy contributes to risk stratification in patients with cardiomyopathy. *Biomed Tech (Berl)* 51 (2):77–82. doi: 10.1515/BMT.2006.014.

Tsuji, H., M. G. Larson, F. J. Venditti, Jr., E. S. Manders, J. C. Evans, C. L. Feldman, and D. Levy. 1996. Impact of reduced heart rate variability on risk for cardiac events. The Framingham Heart Study. *Circulation* 94 (11):2850–5.

Tyagi, A., M. Cohen, J. Reece, and S. Telles. 2014. An explorative study of metabolic responses to mental stress and yoga practices in yoga practitioners, non-yoga practitioners and individuals with metabolic syndrome. *BMC Complement Altern Med* 14:445. doi: 10.1186/1472-6882-14-445.

Ursem, N. T., E. B. Clark, B. B. Keller, W. C. Hop, and J. W. Wladimiroff. 1999. Do heart rate and velocity variability derived from umbilical artery velocity waveforms change prior to clinical pregnancy-induced hypertension? *Ultrasound Obstet Gynecol* 14 (4):244–9. doi: 10.1046/j.1469-0705.1999.14040244.x.

Vakorin, V. A., O. A. Krakovska, and A. R. McIntosh. 2009. Confounding effects of indirect connections on causality estimation. *J Neurosci Methods* 184 (1):152–60. doi: 10.1016/j.jneumeth.2009.07.014.

Valencia, J. F., M. Vallverdu, A. Porta, A. Voss, R. Schroeder, R. Vazquez, A. Bayes de Luna, and P. Caminal. 2013. Ischemic risk stratification by means of multivariate analysis of the heart rate variability. *Physiol Meas* 34 (3):325–38. doi: 10.1088/0967-3334/34/3/325.

Valencia, J. F., M. Vallverdu, I. Rivero, A. Voss, A. B. de Luna, A. Porta, and P. Caminal. 2015. Symbolic dynamics to discriminate healthy and ischaemic dilated cardiomyopathy populations: An application to the variability of heart period and QT interval. *Philos Trans A Math Phys Eng Sci* 373 (2034). doi: 10.1098/rsta.2014.0092.

Valencia, J. F., M. Vallverdu, R. Schroeder, A. Voss, R. Vazquez, A. Bayes de Luna, and P. Caminal. 2009. Complexity of the short-term heart-rate variability. *IEEE Eng Med Biol Mag* 28 (6):72–8. doi: 10.1109/MEMB.2009.934621.

Valentini, M., and G. Parati. 2009. Variables influencing heart rate. *Prog Cardiovasc Dis* 52 (1):11–9. doi: 10.1016/j.pcad.2009.05.004.

Van Praagh, R., and S. Van Praagh. 1983. Aristotle's "triventricular" heart and the relevant early history of the cardiovascular system. *Chest* 84 (4):462–8.

VanWijk, M. J., K. Kublickiene, K. Boer, and E. VanBavel. 2000. Vascular function in preeclampsia. *Cardiovasc Res* 47 (1):38–48.

Verlohren, S., A. Galindo, D. Schlembach, H. Zeisler, I. Herraiz, M. G. Moertl, J. Pape, J. W. Dudenhausen, B. Denk, and H. Stepan. 2010. An automated method for the determination of the sFlt-1/PlGF ratio in the assessment of preeclampsia. *Am J Obstet Gynecol* 202 (2):161 e1–161 e11. doi: 10.1016/j.ajog.2009.09.016.

Vinik, A. I., R. E. Maser, B. D. Mitchell, and R. Freeman. 2003. Diabetic autonomic neuropathy. *Diabetes Care* 26 (5):1553–79.

von Staden, H. 1989. *Herophilus: The Art of Medicine in Early Alexandria*. Cambridge: Cambridge University Press.

Voss, A., V. Baier, A. Schirdewan, and U. Leder. 2004. Physiological hypotheses on heart rate turbulence. In *Dynamic Electrocardiography*, M. Malik and A. J. Camm (eds.), 203–210. Oxford, UK: Blackwell Publishing.

Voss, A., M. Baumert, V. Baier, H. Stepan, T. Walther, and R. Faber. 2006. Autonomic cardiovascular control in pregnancies with abnormal uterine perfusion. *Am J Hypertens* 19 (3):306–12. doi: 10.1016/j.amjhyper.2005.08.008.

Voss, A., A. Busjahn, N. Wessel, R. Schurath, H. D. Faulhaber, F. C. Luft, and R. Dietz. 1996a. Familial and genetic influences on heart rate variability. *J Electrocardiol* 29 Suppl:154–60.

Voss, A., C. Fischer, and R. Schroeder. 2014. Coupling of heart rate and systolic blood pressure in hypertensive pregnancy. *Methods Inf Med* 53 (4):286–90. doi: 10.3414/ME13-02-0045.

Voss, A., C. Fischer, R. Schroeder, H. R. Figulla, and M. Goernig. 2010a. Segmented Poincare plot analysis for risk stratification in patients with dilated cardiomyopathy. *Methods Inf Med* 49 (5):511–5. doi: 10.3414/ME09-02-0050.

Voss, A., C. Fischer, R. Schroeder, H. R. Figulla, and M. Goernig. 2012a. Lagged segmented Poincare plot analysis for risk stratification in patients with dilated cardiomyopathy. *Med Biol Eng Comput* 50 (7):727–36. doi: 10.1007/s11517-012-0925-5.

Voss, A., M. Goernig, R. Schroeder, S. Truebner, A. Schirdewan, and H. R. Figulla. 2012b. Blood pressure variability as sign of autonomic imbalance in patients with idiopathic dilated cardiomyopathy. *Pacing Clin Electrophysiol* 35 (4):471–9. doi: 10.1111/j.1540-8159.2011.03312.x.

Voss, A., K. Hnatkova, N. Wessel, J. Kurths, A. Sander, A. Schirdewan, A. J. Camm, and M. Malik. 1998. Multiparametric analysis of heart rate variability used for risk stratification among survivors of acute myocardial infarction. *Pacing Clin Electrophysiol* 21 (1 Pt 2):186–92.

Voss, A., J. Kurths, H. J. Kleiner, A. Witt, N. Wessel, P. Saparin, K. J. Osterziel, R. Schurath, and R. Dietz. 1996b. The application of methods of non-linear dynamics for the improved and predictive recognition of patients threatened by sudden cardiac death. *Cardiovasc Res* 31 (3):419–33. doi: 0008636396000089 [pii].

Voss, A., R. Schroeder, P. Caminal, M. Vallverdú, H. Brunel, I. Cygankiewicz, R. Vázquez, and A. Bayés de Luna. 2010b. Segmented symbolic dynamics for risk stratification in patients with ischemic heart failure. *Cardiovas Eng Tech* 1 (4):290–298. doi: 10.1007/s13239-010-0025-3.

Voss, A., R. Schroeder, A. Heitmann, A. Peters, and S. Perz. 2015. Short-term heart rate variability–Influence of gender and age in healthy subjects. *PLOS ONE* 10 (3):e0118308. doi: 10.1371/journal.pone.0118308.

Voss, A., R. Schroeder, S. Truebner, M. Goernig, H. R. Figulla, and A. Schirdewan. 2007. Comparison of nonlinear methods symbolic dynamics, detrended fluctuation, and Poincare plot analysis in risk stratification in patients with dilated cardiomyopathy. *Chaos* 17 (1):015120. doi: 10.1063/1.2404633.

Voss, A., R. Schroeder, M. Vallverdu, S. Schulz, I. Cygankiewicz, R. Vazquez, A. Bayes de Luna, and P. Caminal. 2013. Short-term vs. long-term heart rate variability in ischemic cardiomyopathy risk stratification. *Front Physiol* 4:364. doi: 10.3389/fphys.2013.00364.

Voss, A., S. Schulz, M. Koschke, and K. J. Bar. 2008. Linear and nonlinear analysis of autonomic regulation in depressed patients. *Conf Proc IEEE Eng Med Biol Soc* 2008:2653–6. doi: 10.1109/IEMBS.2008.4649747.

Voss, A., S. Schulz, R. Schroeder, M. Baumert, and P. Caminal. 2009. Methods derived from nonlinear dynamics for analysing heart rate variability. *Philos Trans A Math Phys Eng Sci* 367 (1887):277–96. doi: 10.1098/rsta.2008.0232.

Voss, A., A. Seeck, and M. Baumert. 2010c. Altered interactions of heart rate and blood pressure during normal and abnormal pregnancy. *Conf Proc IEEE Eng Med Biol Soc* 2010:1695–8. doi: 10.1109/IEMBS.2010.5626838.

Walther, T., A. Voss, M. Baumert, S. Truebner, H. Till, H. Stepan, N. Wessel, and R. Faber. 2014. Cardiovascular variability before and after delivery: Recovery from arterial stiffness in women with preeclampsia 4 days post partum. *Hypertens Pregnancy* 33 (1):1–14. doi: 10.3109/10641955.2013.821481.

Walther, T., N. Wessel, M. Baumert, A. Voss, H. Stepan, and R. Faber. 2005. Longitudinal analysis of heart rate variability in chronic hypertensive pregnancy. *Hypertens Res* 28(2):113–8

Weiss, J. N., A. Garfinkel, M. L. Spano, and W. L. Ditto. 1994. Chaos and chaos control in biology. *J Clin Invest* 93 (4):1355–60. doi: 10.1172/JCI117111.

Wessel, N., N. Marwan, U. Meyerfeldt, A. Schirdewan, and J. Kurths. 2001. Recurrence quantification analysis to characterise the heart rate variability before the onset of ventricular tachycardia. In *Medical Data Analysis*, edited by Jose Crespo, Victor Maojo and Fernando Martin, 295–301. Heidelberg: Springer Berlin Heidelberg.

Wessel, N., C. Ziehmann, J. Kurths, U. Meyerfeldt, A. Schirdewan, and A. Voss. 2000. Short-term forecasting of life-threatening cardiac arrhythmias based on symbolic dynamics and finite-time growth rates. *Phys Rev E Stat Phys Plasmas Fluids Relat Interdisc Topics* 61 (1):733–9.

Wheeler, T., and P. J. Watkins. 1973. Cardiac denervation in diabetes. *Br Med J* 4 (5892):584–6.

Wiener, N. 1956. The theory of prediction. In *Modern Mathematics for Engineers*, edited by Beckenbach, E.F, vol. series 1. New York, NY: McGraw-Hill.

Williams, L. M., P. Das, A. W. Harris, B. B. Liddell, M. J. Brammer, G. Olivieri, D. Skerrett, M. L. Phillips, A. S. David, A. Peduto, and E. Gordon. 2004. Dysregulation of arousal and amygdala-prefrontal systems in paranoid schizophrenia. *Am J Psychiatry* 161 (3):480–9.

Wilmore, J. H., P. R. Stanforth, J. Gagnon, T. Rice, S. Mandel, A. S. Leon, D. C. Rao, J. S. Skinner, and C. Bouchard. 2001. Heart rate and blood pressure changes with endurance training: The HERITAGE Family Study. *Med Sci Sports Exerc* 33 (1):107–16.

Wolf, M. M., G. A. Varigos, D. Hunt, and J. G. Sloman. 1978. Sinus arrhythmia in acute myocardial infarction. *Med J Aust* 2 (2):52–3.

Xhyheri, B., O. Manfrini, M. Mazzolini, C. Pizzi, and R. Bugiardini. 2012. Heart rate variability today. *Prog Cardiovasc Dis* 55 (3):321–31. doi: 10.1016/j.pcad.2012.09.001.

Yang, C. C., T. C. Chao, T. B. Kuo, C. S. Yin, and H. I. Chen. 2000. Preeclamptic pregnancy is associated with increased sympathetic and decreased parasympathetic control of HR. *Am J Physiol Heart Circ Physiol* 278 (4):H1269–73.

Yeragani, V. K., R. K. A. Radhakrishna, K. R. Ramakrishnan, and S. H. Srinivasan. 2004. Measures of LLE of heart rate in different frequency bands: A possible measure of relative vagal and sympathetic activity. *Nonlinear Anal-Real* 5 (3):441–462. doi: 10.1016/j.nonrwa.2003.07.002.

Yi, G., J. H. Goldman, P. J. Keeling, M. Reardon, W. J. McKenna, and M. Malik. 1997. Heart rate variability in idiopathic dilated cardiomyopathy: Relation to disease severity and prognosis. *Heart* 77 (2):108–14.

Yum, M. K., C. R. Kim, E. Y. Park, and J. H. Kim. 2004. Instability and frequency-domain variability of heart rates in fetuses with or without growth restriction affected by severe preeclampsia. *Physiol Meas* 25 (5):1105–13.

Zamorski, M. A., and L. A. Green. 2001. NHBPEP report on high blood pressure in pregnancy: A summary for family physicians. *Am Fam Physician* 64 (2):263–70, 216.

Zbilut, J.P., and C.L. Webber. 1992. Embeddings and delays as derived from quantification of recurrence plots. *Phys Lett A* (171):199–203.

Ziegler, D., A. Voss, W. Rathmann, A. Strom, S. Perz, M. Roden, A. Peters, C. Meisinger, and Kora Study Group. 2015. Increased prevalence of cardiac autonomic dysfunction at different degrees of glucose intolerance in the general population: The KORA S4 survey. *Diabetologia* 58 (5):1118–28. doi: 10.1007/s00125-015-3534-7.

Ziv, J., and A. Lempel. 1977. Universal algorithm for sequential data compression. *IEEE Trans Inf Ther* 23:337–343. doi: 10.1109.

Zwiener, U., D. Hoyer, R. Bauer, B. Luthke, B. Walter, K. Schmidt, S. Hallmeyer, B. Kratzsch, and M. Eiselt. 1996. Deterministic–chaotic and periodic properties of heart rate and arterial pressure fluctuations and their mediation in piglets. *Cardiovasc Res* 31 (3):455–65.

3

A Descriptive Approach to Signal Processing

Dragana Bajić, Goran Dimić, Tatjana Lončar-Turukalo, Branislav Milovanović, and Nina Japundžić-Žigon

CONTENTS

3.1 Introduction

Digital signal processing is a tool that is used not only in classic engineering but also in a range of multidisciplinary applications. To understand the benefits that a particular signal processing method offers, the researchers must be aware of the theory underlying the method, as well as the limitations thereof.

At first glance, there is a wide range of excellent introductory books, primers, and tutorials on signal processing. Unfortunately, many such texts assume that the reader is familiar with mathematics and stochastic processes theory at university level and sometimes with fundamentals of communications theory. The reader should be fluent in mathematical terms, theorems, and lemmas in order to benefit from such material. On the one hand, signal processing penetrates all aspects of contemporary life, but on the other, a would-be consumer of the benefits that signal processing offers may find this material challenging.

The aim of this chapter is to describe the introductory topics of signal processing using no mathematical terms and no mathematical expression. Another important issue is to show that signal processing is not a magic wand that gives a solution at a single sweep. Signal processing has its limitations and wielding the powerful tools it offers requires carefulness and understanding. A correct approach is based on interdisciplinary teamwork.

This chapter is not intended for signal processing experts, who might find the descriptive approach without the mathematical strictness too simplified. It is intended for the absolute beginners who do not wish to study mathematics in order to understand, for example, what power spectrum density estimation really means.

3.2 From Analog to Digital: A Necessary Prerequisite for Signal Processing

A classical electrocardiograph (ECG) is an *analog* signal. It is continuous in time, meaning that it is defined at any instant in time. It is also continuous in space, meaning that its amplitude can assume any possible value. The resolution of analog signals is infinitesimally small and such signals appear in a continuous manner, just like the sinusoidal signal presented in Figure 3.1a.

On the other hand, most computers are digital machines that do not have an infinitesimally small resolution. Digital computers are fundamentally based on discrete or discontinuous numbers and cannot process a signal that is continuous in time or continuous in amplitude. An analog signal needs to be converted into *digital* form to become fit for computer input and for subsequent processing. For this reason, almost every research paper on cardiovascular signal analysis contains a statement similar to the following: "The arterial blood pressure signal was digitized at 1000 Hz and transmitted to the computer equipped with the corresponding receiver." This statement describes the process of conversion from a continuous analog biomedical signal into a digital representation of that signal. This process is achieved by an analog-to-digital (A/D) conversion performed in the electronic circuits of the computer or in some attached electronic device, in order to provide a sequence of numbers that is readable and treatable by the computer.

The A/D conversion consists of two processes:

- Sampling (to make a signal discrete in time)
- Quantization (to make a signal discrete in space)

The final output of an A/D convertor is a stream of numbers expressed as *binary digits (bits)*, which only consist of two symbols—zero and one. For example, the number "35" could be represented as "00100011," although there are several alternate representations.

3.2.1 The Sampling Theorem

While analog signals are appropriate for ECG signals written on millimeter paper, digitalization offers many possibilities to all aspects of medical data analysis, from electronic wristbands that record sleep patterns to the most sophisticated diagnostic devices.

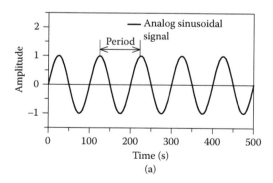
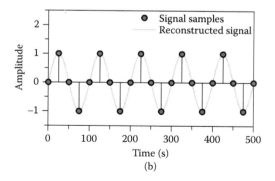

FIGURE 3.1

(a) Analog sinusoidal signal. (b) Discrete signal samples (light gray dots) and the signal reconstructed from the samples (gray line, the same as the original signal).

The concept of digital medical data relies upon findings published in a historic paper by Claude Shannon, an American mathematician and cryptographer, in 1949: "Communication in the presence of noise" (Shannon 1949). Shannon proved that a signal, under some constraints, can be represented by a series of its discrete samples. So the sinusoidal signal from Figure 3.1a can be represented by a series of its amplitudes (samples) shown in Figure 3.1b. From these samples, a likeness of the original signal can be reconstructed. The fidelity of that reconstruction depends upon the quality of the digitization process. In the example above, the "blood pressure signal was digitized at 1000 Hz." This rate of 1000 Hz indicates that the signal was sampled 1000 times per second, which is appropriate for the blood pressure signal and would enable the original signal to be constructed with no loss of information. Shannon's theory is able to predict the sampling rate necessary to allow the signal to be perfectly reconstructed.

Before Shannon's work, there existed some abstract mathematical elaborations, as well as heuristic engineering trials, but without a clear application possibility. The only comparable achievement on sampling was "On the transmission capacity of the 'ether' and of cables in electrical communications" (Kotelnikov 1933). The paper was written and presented in Russian and its importance was recognized immediately. But, according to Lukatela (1979, 1982), the Soviet authorities locked the paper in, thus successfully removing it from the eyes of outer world. In spite of this obstacle, Kotelnikov's contribution was (much later) acknowledged and praised worldwide. In the year 2000, at age 92, Vladimir Aleksandovich Kotelnikov received the US IEEE Alexander Graham Bell Medal.

3.2.2 Quantization

The previous section treated sampling in time, but it is also necessary to perform quantization, since an analog signal can take any possible amplitude value, so it is still continuous in space and far from the required stream of zeros and ones.

This procedure—quantization—is illustrated in Figure 3.2. The upper panel (a) shows a continuous signal. Its time samples (dark gray dots) lie within the regions called

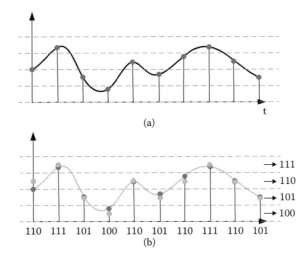

FIGURE 3.2
(a) Original signal and its samples (light gray dots). (b) Discrete amplitude values of the signal samples (red dots); discrete samples can get one out of four possible values, coded as 100, 101, 110, or 111.

quantization levels, bounded by light gray dashed borders. To each signal sample placed within the same quantization region, the same value is associated. It is shown by light gray dots in panel (b). Since there are four pairs of light gray dashed borders (four quantization levels), the light gray dots—that is, quantized samples—can assume only one out of four different values. The signal becomes double discrete: after the sampling made it discrete in time, the quantization made it discrete in space.

The A/D conversion is complete when the doubly discrete signal is coded, and there are many ways of doing this, which depend on the equipment being used. The four discrete amplitude levels shown in Figure 3.3 could be coded using the numbers +1, +2, +3, and +4. But it is more convenient to present them as binary numbers. In this example, the four amplitude levels are finally coded using three bits per sample and denoted 1 00, 1 01, 1 10, and 1 11 (the first "1" is the sign "+"). The original signal and its final form—a stream of binary digits (bits)—are presented in Figure 3.3, where black rectangles correspond to the ones and zeros.

Unfortunately, as Figure 3.2b shows, the dark gray dots (original samples) and light gray dots (quantized samples) do not overlap; the quantization procedure has induced errors, in the form of quantization noise. These errors are irreversible; they remain within the signal reconstructed from the quantized samples. The amount of error introduced depends on the number of quantization levels in the quantization process. The quantization levels define an important parameter—a resolution of the signal.

Intuitively, if the number of quantization levels increase, the region borders would be closer together, so the difference between the original signal sample and its quantized counterpart (the error) would be smaller and the signal resolution would increase. This is illustrated in Figure 3.4. The upper panel (a) presents the original signal quantized in two ways: with eight levels and with 64 levels. Both quantized signals are a staircase-shaped approximation of the original one, but the 64-level approximation looks much better. The "much better" appearance is justified in the lower panel that shows the quantization error, which is much lower for the 64-level case.

The theoretical measure that describes the relationship between the signal and the corresponding error induced by quantization is called signal-to-(quantization) noise ratio. If this ratio is large, then the signal is much stronger than the noise and the noise can be neglected. Biomedical signal acquisition systems are as a rule designed to keep the signal resolution sufficiently high, keeping the quantization error unnoticeable.

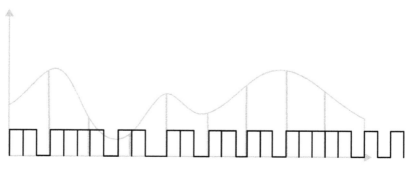

FIGURE 3.3
The original signal (gray line) and its digital counterpart—a binary stream of "ones" and "zeros."

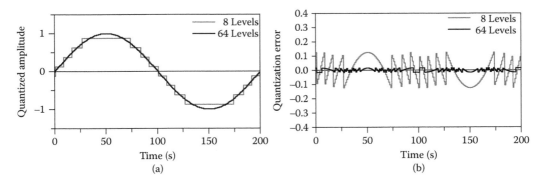

FIGURE 3.4

(a) A sinusoidal signal quantized using eight levels and 64 levels. (b) Error induced by quantization: error decreases and signal resolution increases if the number of levels increases.

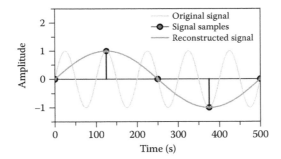

FIGURE 3.5

An outcome of the inadequate sampling frequency: the reconstructed signal differs from the original signal

3.2.3 Limits of Digitalization

To recap, A/D conversion consists of sampling and quantization. The latter procedure induces negligible errors, while the first one allows for perfect signal reconstruction if some constraints are satisfied. These constraints are an important issue. To illustrate the problem, consider an example presented in Figure 3.5. It presents the same sinusoidal signal as in Figure 3.1a, but with samples taken at wider intervals apart. The signal reconstructed from these samples is obviously wrong, but it does not mean that the sampling theorem does not work. It only means that it is not applied correctly. The sampling theorem acknowledges that any signal is made up of a range of frequencies, but can be completely determined by sampling at twice the rate of the highest frequency. Figure 3.1b illustrates this principle, as the sampling intervals, shown by the gray dots, occur at twice the frequency of the signal.

An example that illustrates the difference between signals with "quick" and "slow" changes is shown in Figure 3.6. It presents the heart rate recorded from two different species—from a healthy human in lying position and from a freely moving rat. The points in time when the samples are taken are marked with dashed lines. The sampling rate that is sufficient for a human signal fails to capture most of the changes in the faster signal recorded from a small animal. So, for small animals, the sampling instants should be more frequent.

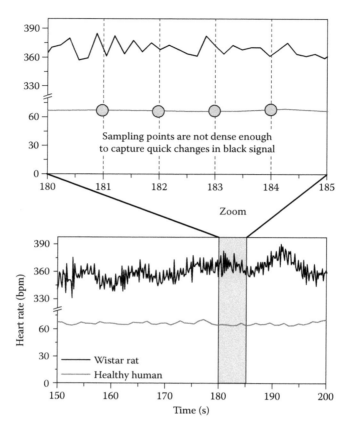

FIGURE 3.6
Signal with "quick" changes (black line) and "slow" changes (gray line); sampling epochs (vertical dashed lines) are not "dense" enough so most of the quick changes in the black signal are "missed."

Relying on the observations of "quick" and "slow" is not a precise method for assessment of the maximum frequency component of the signal, and therefore, to calculate the sampling rate required. A useful approach to achieve this is to describe the signal in the *frequency domain*.

3.3 Frequency Domain and Power Density Spectrum

While it is quite simple to observe the signal as it is recorded in time, as health care professionals have done since the first commercial ECG equipment appeared—a presentation of a signal in the frequency domain might appear quite abstract. One of the most well-known methods to achieve this is the Fourier transform. This is based on the theory that a signal can be represented as a sum of sine and cosine signals. A sine signal periodically repeats itself along the time axis, like the one shown in Figure 3.1a. It has the properties of amplitude, which refers to the vertical range of the signal, and frequency, which is the number of repetitions that occur during one second. If a period of a sine is equal to 0.1 seconds, than the sine repeats 10 times during a second and its frequency is 10 cycles per second or 10 Hz (*Hertz*). A cosine is the same as a sine, except that it is shifted in time. These sine and cosine components are known collectively as the spectrum of the signal.

A simple example is a decomposition of a rectangular signal. A perfect decomposition would have an infinite number of frequency components but only the first four are presented in Figure 3.7, upper panel. The first component has the largest amplitude and the lowest frequency. The subsequent components are smaller in amplitude but larger in frequency. The middle panel shows the successive summation of sine components. The more sine signals that are added, the better is the approximation of the rectangular signal. In the lower panel, each component is represented by a point with the same color as the ones in the top panel. The difference is that in the lower panel, the horizontal axis shows frequency and the vertical axis the amplitude of the spectral component. This is known as a frequency domain presentation. Such a graph can be used to determine which frequency

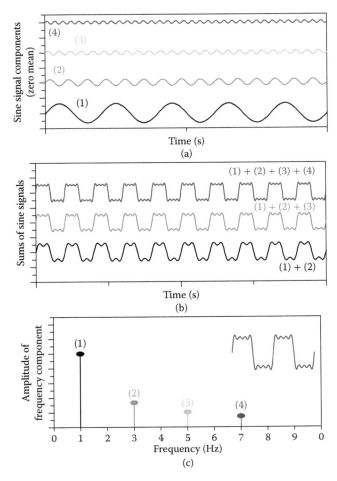

FIGURE 3.7
(a) Four sine components in time domain: from bottom to top their respective frequency is increasing. (b) Rectangular waveform approximated by summing the first two, three, and four sine components. (c) Sine components in the frequency domain.

components are significant: the higher ones have lower amplitudes and can be neglected. The fast changes in the signal are a consequence of high frequency components.

Observing Figure 3.7c, the highest significant frequency may be determined. The minimum sampling rate (i.e., sampling frequency) that must be used to reconstruct the original signal up to and including this frequency component is two times this frequency.

This analysis is possible if the signal can be decomposed into the sum of sine and cosine waveforms and obtain their ordinates in the frequency domain. However, the Fourier transform treats periodic signals of infinite duration: if the signals do not repeat over infinite time, this process is not strictly valid. Biomedical signals do not fit into this category so some tricks have to be applied. As an illustration of this problem, a spectrum of a sampled sine signal with a frequency of 1000 Hz and of finite duration is shown alongside its ideal theoretical counterpart in Figure 3.8. The gray dot shows the frequency ordinate obtained using a Fourier transform if the signal is periodic and infinite. If the signal is not infinite, the black figure centered around 1000 Hz is obtained, along with side lobes representing other frequencies that are introduced by the discontinuities of a finite signal. If the act of sampling is also taken into account, further reflections are obtained above and below 1000 Hz, shown by the additional mirror images of the central figure shown at left and right.

In order to present a finite aperiodic biomedical signal in the frequency domain, a mathematical technique is used to estimate its strength at different frequencies, to obtain an estimate of its power spectral density (PSD). This is a different but related process: the Fourier transform calculates the exact amplitude of a signal at an exact frequency, while from biomedical signals, an estimate is made to represent what is happening in the vicinity of a particular frequency.

It is important to stress that this is an estimate and not an exact process. Consequently, there exists a range of parametric and nonparametric methods, each one yielding estimates that are similar, but not exactly the same. The parameters taken from such estimates are also similar, but not exactly the same. There is no standard that would suggest which estimation method should be used, so researchers are free to choose one out of the numerous approved methods. The maximal frequency component that could be extracted from a signal is at a half of the sampling frequency. An illustrative example is presented in Figure 3.9, which shows the estimates of PSD of an animal (rat) heart rate signal. The estimates are evaluated using three usual methods: periodogram, Weltch,

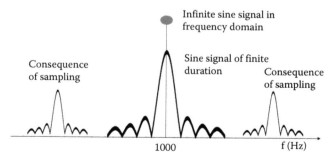

FIGURE 3.8
Sine signal in the frequency domain: gray dots indicate ideal sine signal; the finite sampled sine signal contains some other spectral components.

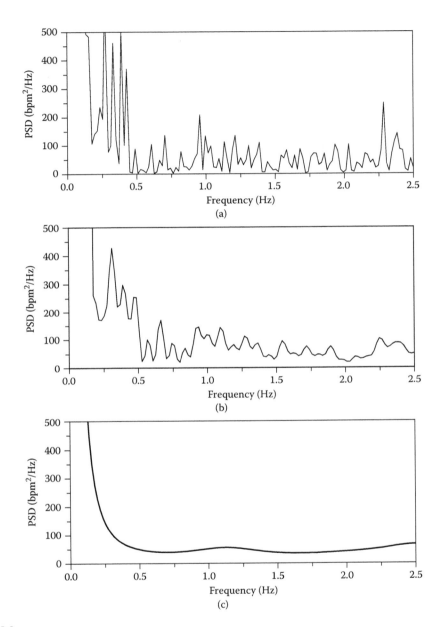

FIGURE 3.9
Alternative estimates of the power spectral density of a heart rate signal from Wistar rat. (a) Periodogram method. (b) Weltch method. (c) Burg method.

and Burg. Although the estimates obtained using different methods seems to be different, they all point out the frequency regions where most of the signal power is concentrated. All methods clearly show that the heart rate signal of a Wistar rat has increased power in the vicinities of 1 and 2.25 Hz. The estimates differ in smoothness, not in component estimation.

3.4 Stationary Signals

In addition to the fact that spectral components of a signal can only be estimated, there is another fact that must be considered: the estimation of PSD may have to be *stationary* for the entire length of the signal. Statistical theory defines the stationarity at many levels. But in practical applications, it is usually assumed that signals are *wide sense stationary* (WSS). One reason for such an assumption lies in a fact that *strict sense stationarity* is difficult, if not impossible, to prove.

WSS implies that statistical parameters, such as mean and variance, have to be stable, no matter at what point in the signal they are estimated. Since the estimation of statistical parameters is based on time averages, a test for stationarity checks whether the parts of signal are turbulent or not. For example, the heart rate signal shown in Figure 3.10 is not stationary in mean, since its partial mean values (time averages), taken at different places along the time axis, differ too much. It is possible to perform an informal test for stationarity by visually inspecting the graph of such a signal.

The stationarity is of particular importance in PSD estimation because, although the discussion so far has covered the detection of the fast-changing components of the signal, the slow components are also important. This is illustrated in Figure 3.11. The signal available is a sinusoidal signal that is gradually increasing because it is added to another sine signal of much lower frequency. The composite signal is obviously not stationary. Unfortunately, the signal is too short to deduce which one out of the two low-frequency sine signals is a cause of the increasing trend in the short signal from Figure 3.11. The only solution is to measure the signal over a longer time period, so that the spectrum estimation would give the correct result.

For this reason, the signals for estimation cannot be too short. Knowing this limitation, one must be careful not to make conclusions based on signals that are too short. On the other hand, if the signal is long, there are more chances that it would become nonstationary. This is usually a consequence of subject movement. It can be easily recognized and removed from the signal.

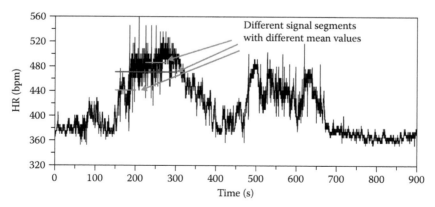

FIGURE 3.10
Nonstationary high-resolution signal of Wistar rat subjected to air-jet stress.

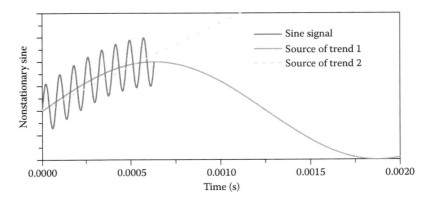

FIGURE 3.11
Nonstationary sine signal (dark gray line), too short to find out which one out of two low-frequency sine signals is a cause of the increasing trend.

3.5 Conclusion

This chapter provides an explanation of signal processing basic functions, without going into the mathematics of probability and random processes. However, just as a medical doctor can talk to a patient without highly sophisticated medical terms, anatomic names, and chemical formulae, signal processing features can be explained without the mathematical formulae, strict theorems, or lemmas. It is the hope that this text will contribute to interdisciplinary understanding of biosignal time series analysis. For the same reason, the literature list is quite small. For deeper insight into the problems, there are many books written for engineers, since they contain less mathematics and more application examples.

References and Further Readings

C. E. Shannon, Communication in the presence of noise, *Proceedings of the Institute of Radio Engineers*, vol. 37, no. 1, pp. 10–21, Jan. 1949. Reprint as classic paper in *Proceedings of the IEEE*, vol. 86, no. 2, (Feb. 1998).

V. A. Kotelnikov, On the transmission capacity of "ether" and wire in electrocommunications, (English translation), Izd. Red. Upr. Svyazzi RKKA (1933), Reprint in *Modern Sampling Theory: Mathematics and Applications*, Editors: J. J. Benedetto and P. J. S. G. Ferreira. Boston, MA: Birkhauser, 2000, ISBN 0-8176-4023-1.

G. Lukatela, *Statistical Communication Theory and Information Theory*. Belgrade: GK Publications, 1979, 1982.

A. Papoulis, *Probability, Random Variables, and Stochastic Processes*, 9th edition (1965, 1st edition). Tokyo: McGraw-Hill Kogakusha.

J. G. Proakis, D. G. Manolakis, *Digital Signal Processing: Principles, Algorithms and Applications*, 4th edition. Upper Saddle River, NJ: Pearson, Prentice Hall, 2007.

4

Linear and Nonlinear Parametric Models in Heart Rate Variability Analysis

Gaetano Valenza, Luca Citi, and Riccardo Barbieri

CONTENTS

4.1 Introducing Physiological Models of Cardiovascular Control and Related Parametric Formulation

In the last few decades, mathematical modeling and signal processing techniques have played an important role in the study of cardiovascular control physiology and heartbeat dynamics. An example application of these methodological approaches is given by the extensive number of studies on cardiovascular control dynamics mediated by the autonomic nervous system (ANS). This system is very often investigated through analysis of event series obtained by computing the time intervals between two consecutive R-waves as detected from the electrocardiogram (ECG), that is, the RR intervals. Because the heartbeat is controlled by the ANS, the RR series show preferred oscillations around their mean value, defined as heart rate variability (HRV) [1,2]. The parametric models discussed later in this chapter have been extensively used to characterize each RR interval value as dependent on a linear regression of its previous RR values, providing an effective formulation to explain these peculiar periodic oscillations.

4.1.1 ANS Control of the Heart Rate

The ANS comprises the sympathetic nervous system (SNS) and parasympathetic nervous system (PNS). In general, increased SNS activity (and/or diminished PNS tone) leads to an increase in heart rate (HR), whereas low SNS activity or high PNS activity causes HR to decrease. The two autonomic branches act synergically to modulate the heartbeat in order to maintain blood pressure at controlled levels, and HRV is the result of their balancing action. Several studies report on a significant relationship between ANS dynamics and cardiovascular mortality [1,2]. Consequently, a huge effort has been devoted to the analysis and modeling of HRV in order to provide effective and reliable quantifiers of ANS dynamics. Extensive description of the physiological mechanisms behind the generation of HR fluctuations can be found in Refs. [1–4]. The effect of these SNS–PNS interactions results in two main oscillatory components that are usually differentiated in the HRV spectral profile [1–4]: (a) the high-frequency (HF) band (0.15–0.40 Hz), which reflects effects of respiration on HR, also referred to as respiratory sinus arrhythmia (RSA); and (b) the low-frequency (LF) band (0.04–0.15 Hz), which represents oscillations related to regulation of blood pressure and vasomotor tone including the so-called 0.1 Hz fluctuation. The less studied very low-frequency (VLF) band (<0.04 Hz) is thought to relate, among other factors, to thermoregulation and kidney functioning. In this sense, linear analysis and parametric modeling aimed at identifying a limited number of oscillatory components represent a very efficient and parsimonious methodological tool. Nevertheless, the information behind heartbeat dynamics goes beyond the simplistic identification of linear components. Several nonlinear measures of HRV, in fact, such as Lyapunov exponents, $1/f$ slope, approximate entropy (ApEn), and detrended fluctuation analysis (DFA), have been widely used to uncover nonlinear fluctuations in HR that are not otherwise apparent [1,2,5]. Consequently, such measures provided important quantifiers of cardiovascular control dynamics, mediated by the ANS, and they have been found to be of prognostic value in aging and diseases [6–13]. Although the detailed physiology behind complex dynamics of heartbeat variations has not been completely clarified, nonlinear HRV dynamics may be partly explained by the various nonlinear neural interactions and integrations occurring at the neuron and receptor levels, and they underlie the complex output of the sinoatrial node in response to changing levels of efferent autonomic inputs [14]. It is thought that the complexity of healthy dynamics can be understood to be an essential part of their capability to adapt to a varying environment.

4.1.2 A Brief History of Linear and Nonlinear Parametric Models of Heartbeat Dynamics

HRV is the discrete time series that serves as a gold standard to evaluate autonomic functions in healthy subjects and in patients with different pathologies, which can or cannot be strictly related to the cardiovascular system. The first historical studies (from 1920) highlighting the emergence of HRV as a physiologically meaningful measure were focused on RSA. Since 1978, when Wolf et al. [15] described the relationship between decreased RR variability and mortality in postmyocardial infarction, several methodologies and measures have been proposed and are now described in the literature [1,2] ranging from simple descriptors to nonlinear models.

In 1973, Sayers first proposed a spectral analysis of HRV, although it was used to evaluate autonomic control on the cardiovascular dynamics since 1981 [16]. Since then, spectral analysis has been taken as a reference method for the identification and quantification of the principal oscillations that characterize HRV, especially during significant parasympathetic changes. Fourier-based techniques were initially pursued for HRV spectral analysis, maybe for their simplicity and widespread diffusion. However, a major limitation of this approach is related to poor spectral resolution, especially when short time frames are used [17].

Parametric modeling based on a simple linear regression on the past heartbeat event, instead, is able to achieve a better spectral resolution even for short frames of data [18] (although the model order and parameter estimation have to be optimized). As mentioned above, parametric modeling refers to a (proper) mathematical description of the physiological system under study. Such a mathematical description is characterized by a formula defined by parameters that have to be estimated and tuned by looking at observed physiological data. In the case of the linear autoregressive (AR) model of ANS dynamics through HRV data, parametrization means that the prediction of the next heartbeat is defined as an algebraic sum (i.e., positive and negative weighted sums) of past RR intervals. The first parametric estimates of HRV started being published in the early 1980s by Jarisch et al. [19], Brovelli et al. [20], Baselli et al. [21], Giddens et al. [22], Bartoli et al. [23], Kitney et al. [24], Pagani et al. [25], and Lombardi et al. [26]. In 2005, Barbieri et al. [27] proposed to embed such widely used parametric linear modeling within a point-process framework through which the RR interval series is seen as a binary stochastic (i.e, having a random probability distribution or pattern that may be analyzed statistically but may not be precisely predicted) series characterized by interevent probability functions. With this approach, the methodological knowledge gained so far was enriched with instantaneous estimates in the time and frequency domain, and goodness-of-fit measures (see details in Section 4.2.3).

Since the early 1990s, several studies suggesting the use of nonlinear autoregressive (NAR) models for heartbeat dynamics have been published [28–30]. In particular, NAR modeling has been used to determine whether chaotic determinism is present in a resting-state heartbeat time series through Lyapunov exponents [28], and to evaluate the degree of nonlinearity of HRV [29] and low-dimensional chaotic dynamics [30]. Of note, in 2002, the application of nonlinear autoregressive moving average (NARMA) models for heartbeat dynamics [31–33] was proposed. These NARMA models have been used to describe the closed loop between HR and baroreflex control [32] to predict the outcome of invasive cardiac electrophysiological studies through Lyapunov exponents [31] and to search the possible presence of determinism in HRV series [33]. As a clinical outcome, it has been shown that NAR model-based HRV analysis improves the assessment of several clinical conditions including dilated cardiomyopathy [34], obstructive sleep apnea syndrome with and without hypertension [35], and postural changes [36,37]. Recently, we built on this literature by embedding NAR modeling within a point-process framework [38–44]. In this case, a major methodological improvement was the use of the Laguerre expansion of the Wiener–Volterra AR terms in order to achieve a more effective system identification [38,40,45]. Of note, this method is ideal for modeling physiological systems because it accounts for the nonlinear and time-varying behavior of stochastic systems. The basic mathematical formulation related to all these pioneering studies is reported in the following sections.

Finally, it is worthwhile mentioning that a significant part of the parametric modeling proposed in the literature to assess cardiovascular functions involves multivariate modeling. As an example, multivariate parametric models were proposed to assess the relationship between arterial blood pressure, HR, and respiratory control [46–49]

In this chapter, we describe the use of linear and nonlinear parametric models whose definition is governed by stochastic mathematical functions with a finite number of parameters, which are able to provide a better spectral resolution on short frames of data. In the case of heartbeat dynamics, these models refer to autoregressive (AR) models. A general block scheme for the kinds of parametric modeling considered in this chapter is shown in Figure 4.1.

The RR interval series is seen as the output of an AR system (the cardiovascular system) which is controlled by the ANS. The regression can take into account linear and nonlinear combinations of the past events. In the case of nonlinear regression models, the Wiener–Volterra models can be considered. Finally, it is possible to perform the regression on the actual RR intervals or on its variations, that is, considering the derivative series. Once the model parameters are estimated, it is possible to extract several features of ANS dynamics through proper quantitative tools. In the next section, linear parametric models are described considering the standard and point-process formulation, followed by the related quantitative tools and feature extraction. The same logical flow is adopted for the description of the nonlinear parametric models. Concluding the chapter, exemplary appli-

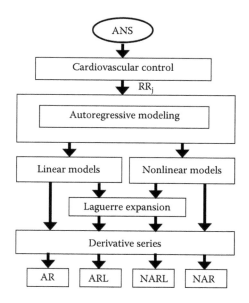

FIGURE 4.1
An overview of the linear and nonlinear parametric modeling described in detail in this chapter. ARL and NARL stand for linear and nonlinear autoregressive (AR) model with the Laguerre expansion of the kernel, respectively.

cations including HRV assessment through point-process nonlinear models during postural change protocols and after cardiac heart failure (CHF) are reported.

4.2 Linear Parametric Models

4.2.1 Preprocessing

Before estimating the RR interval series, a preprocessing step with the ECG signal is usually required. This step aims at increasing the signal-to-noise ratio (SNR) of the signal as well as extracting and subtracting the signal baseline. Removing such an oscillation, in fact, usually improves the performance of the algorithms for automatic wave detection. The baseline can be defined as a deviation from the ECG isoelectric line below approximately 0.5 Hz and is due to electrode movement artifacts, and respiration activity. Once the ECG is preprocessed, an R-wave (or more generally a QRS complex) detection algorithm should be used. This choice depends on the characteristics of the specific ECG signal (see reviews in Refs. [50,51]), for example, SNR, signal power, and ECG leads. Nevertheless, not all of the RR intervals obtained by the automatic QRS detection algorithm are correct. Any technical artifact (i.e., errors due to the R-peak detection algorithm) in the RR interval time series may interfere with the analysis of these signals. Therefore, an artifact correction algorithm is needed. In this case, a proper piecewise cubic spline interpolation method [52,53] can be adopted. Moreover, physiological artifacts could also be present in the RR series as ectopic beats and arrhythmic events. Therefore, checking by visual inspection for physiological artifacts should always be performed and only artifact-free sections must be included in further analysis. Next, a previously developed algorithm [54] based on the point process statistics (local likelihood) that is able to perform a real-time RR interval error detection and correction is also presented.

As a standard definition, the interval between two successive QRS complexes is defined as the RR interval (t_{R-R}) and the HR (beats per minute) is given as

$$HR = \frac{60}{t_{R-R}} \qquad (4.1)$$

As HR is a time series comprised of a sequence of nonuniform RR intervals, this signal should be further resampled at a certain frequency before performing further processing. Many studies report resampling rates between 2 and 4 Hz. Of note, a resampling rate of 7 Hz has been suggested in Refs. [55–57] as the most appropriate value. A popular heartbeat resampling algorithm is the one proposed by Berger et al. [58]. This algorithm is based on using an arbitrary frequency at which the HR samples will be evenly spaced in time and using a local time window defined at each HR sample point as the time interval extending from the previous sample to the next. Successively, the number of RR intervals (including fractions of them) that occur within this local window are counted. The value r_i of the HR at each sample point is taken to be $r_i = f_r - n_i/2$, where f_r was the sampling frequency of the resulting HR signal and n_i was the number of RR intervals falling into the local window centered at the *i*th sample point [58].

Note that interpolation is not mandatorily required to perform a parametric HRV analysis. It is possible, in fact, to consider the RR interval series as an intrinsically discrete stochastic series, or as a non-uniform discretization of a continuous signal.

4.2.2 The AR Model

Considering the heartbeat dynamics as a sequence of N samples $\{y(1), ..., y(n)\}$ representing a single realization of a discrete-time AR stochastic process, it is possible to write the following model:

$$y(n) = \sum_{k=1}^{p} a(k) y(n-k) + w(n) \qquad (4.2)$$

where n is the discrete-time index, $a(k)$ are AR coefficients, p is the model order, and $w(n)$ is a zero-mean white noise of variance equal to σ^2. Consequently, the AR(p) model is characterized by the AR parameters $\{a[1], a[2], ..., a[p], \sigma^2\}$. Equation 4.2 can also be expressed in the z-transform domain:

$$Y(z) = Y(z) \left(\sum_{k=1}^{p} a_k z^{-k} \right) + W(z) = H(z)W(z) \qquad (4.3)$$

where $Y(z)$ and $W(z)$ are the z-transform of $y(n)$ and $w(n)$, respectively, and

$$H(z) = \frac{1}{1 - \sum_{k=1}^{p} a_k z^{-k}} \qquad (4.4)$$

Several methods can be used to estimate the AR model parameters. A standard approach is a last square-based method, which estimates the a_k coefficients by minimizing the following cost function:

$$J_N = \sum_{n=1}^{N} \psi^{N-n} e_N(n)^2 \qquad (4.5)$$

where $e_N(n) = y(n) - \sum_{k=1}^{p} a(k) y(n-k)$ and $0 < \psi \leq 1$ is the forgetting factor.

Of note, as a step further, in order to take into account the nonstationarity of the RR interval series, the AR model estimation has been made time-varying [37,59–62] such that its parameters are estimated sample-by-sample through a recursive relationship $a(n+1, k) = F[a(n, k)]$ [59], with F standing for a linear or nonlinear function.

Concerning the model order, its estimation can be performed using Akaike's final prediction error, Akaike's information criterion [63], the Bayesian information criterion, Parzen's criterion of AR transfer function, and Riassen's minimum description length method [64]. However, it has been demonstrated that these criteria underestimate the actual model order [64], and it has been recommended that an order not less than $p = 16$ should be used for spectral analysis of short RR time series resampled at 4 Hz [64]. Suggestions concerning other practical issues using parametric modeling of heartbeat dynamics can be found in Refs. [65–67].

Of note, the abovementioned standard parametric modeling has been successful in a huge number of clinical applications including hemodialysis [68], presence of ectopic beats [69], and postural changes [70].

4.2.3 Point-Process Framework

The point-process framework primarily defines the probability of having a heartbeat event at each moment in time. Defining $t \in (0, T]$ as the observation interval and $0 \leq u_1 < \cdots < u_k < u_{k+1} < \cdots < u_K \leq T$ as the times of the events, it is possible to define $N(t) = \max\{k : u_k \leq t\}$

as the sample path of the associated counting process. Its differential, $dN(t)$, denotes a continuous-time indicator function, where $dN(t) = 1$ when there is an event (the ventricular contraction), or $dN(t) = 0$ otherwise. The left continuous sample path is defined as $\widetilde{N}(t) = \lim_{\tau \to t^-} N(\tau) = \max\{k : u_k < t\}$. Given the R-wave events $\{u_j\}_{j=1}^J$ detected from the ECG, $RR_j = u_j - u_{j-1} > 0$ denotes the jth RR interval. Assuming history dependence, the inverse Gaussian probability distribution of the waiting time $t - u_j$ until the next R-wave event is [27]

$$f(t|\mathcal{H}_t, \xi(t)) = \left[\frac{\xi_0(t)}{2\pi(t - u_j)^3}\right]^{\frac{1}{2}} \times \exp\{-\frac{1}{2}\frac{\xi_0(t)[t - u_j - \mu_{RR}(t, \mathcal{H}_t, \xi(t))]^2}{\mu_{RR}(t, \mathcal{H}_t, \xi(t))^2(t - u_j)}\} \qquad (4.6)$$

where $j = \widetilde{N}(t)$ is the index of the previous R-wave event before time t, $\mathcal{H}_t = (u_j, RR_j, RR_{j-1}, ..., RR_{j-M+1})$ is the history of events, $\xi(t)$ is the vector of the time-varing parameters, $\mu_{RR}(t, \mathcal{H}_t, \xi(t))$ is the first-moment statistic (mean) of the distribution, and $\xi_0(t) > 0$ is the shape parameter of the inverse Gaussian distribution. Since $f(t|\mathcal{H}_t, \xi(t))$ indicates the probability of having a beat at time t given that a previous beat has occurred at u_j, $\mu_{RR}(t, \mathcal{H}_t, \xi(t))$ can be interpreted as the expected waiting time until the next event occurs. The use of an inverse Gaussian distribution $f(t|\mathcal{H}_t, \xi(t))$, characterized at each moment in time, is motivated both physiologically (the integrate-and-fire initiating the cardiac contraction [27]) and by goodness-of-fit comparisons [71]. Here, the instantaneous mean $\mu_{RR}(t, \mathcal{H}_t, \xi(t))$ is expressed as a linear combination of present and past RR intervals:

$$\mu_{RR}(t, \mathcal{H}_t, \xi(t)) = \gamma_0 + \sum_{i=1}^{p} \gamma_1(i, t)\, RR_{\widetilde{N}(t)-i} \qquad (4.7)$$

It has been shown that performing the estimations on the derivative RR interval series improves model performance and the achievement of stationarity within the sliding time window W (usually $70 < W < 90$ seconds) [38–44,72–74]:

$$\mu_{RR}(t, \mathcal{H}_t, \xi(t)) = RR_{\widetilde{N}(t)} + \gamma_0 + \sum_{i=1}^{p} \gamma_1(i, t)\left(RR_{\widetilde{N}(t)-i} - RR_{\widetilde{N}(t)-i-1}\right) \qquad (4.8)$$

In both equations, the coefficients γ_0 and $\{\gamma_1(i)\}$ correspond to the time-varying zero- and first-order coefficients, respectively. Since $\mu_{RR}(t, \mathcal{H}_t, \xi(t))$ is defined in continuous time, it is possible to obtain an instantaneous RR mean estimate at a very fine timescale (with an arbitrarily small bin size Δ), which requires no interpolation between the arrival times of two beats. Given the proposed parametric model, all linear indices are defined as a time-varying function of the parameters $\xi(t) = [\xi_0(t), \gamma_0(t), \gamma_1(1, t), ..., \gamma_1(p, t)]$.

The unknown time-varying parameter vector $\xi(t)$ is estimated by means of a local maximum likelihood method [27,75,76]. Briefly, given a local observation interval $(t - l, t]$ of duration l, a subset $U_{m:n}$ of the R-wave events is considered. Specifically, $m = N(t - l) + 1$ and $n = N(t)$. At each time t, the unknown time-varying parameter vector $\xi(t)$ is found such that the following local log-likelihood is maximized:

$$L(\xi(t)\,|\,U_{m:n}) = \sum_{k=m+P-1}^{n-1} w(t - u_{k+1})\, \log[f(u_{k+1}\,|\,\mathcal{H}_{u_{k+1}}, \xi(t))] + \log \int_t^\infty f(\tau\,|\,\mathcal{H}_t, \xi(t))\, d\tau \qquad (4.9)$$

where $w(\tau) = e^{\varpi\tau}$ is an exponential weighting function for the local likelihood. In Equation 4.9, the latter term accounts for the next, not yet observed, RR interval (right censoring). A Newton–Raphson procedure is used to maximize the local log-likelihood in Equation 4.9 and compute the local maximum likelihood estimate of $\xi(t)$ [75]. Because there is significant overlap between adjacent local likelihood intervals, the Newton–Raphson procedure is started at t with the previous local maximum likelihood estimate at time $t - \Delta$, where Δ defines the time interval shift to compute the next parameter update.

The model goodness-of-fit is based on the Kolmogorov–Smirnov (KS) test and associated KS statistics (see details in [27,77]). Autocorrelation plots are considered to test the independence of the model-transformed intervals [27]. Once the order $\{p\}$ is determined, the initial model coefficients are estimated by the method of least squares [78]. In order to provide reliable results, just like other dynamical methods, these point-process-based processing techniques require an uninterrupted series of RR intervals, with a minimum recommended length of 60 seconds. Nevertheless, peak detection errors and ectopic beats often determine abrupt changes in the RR interval series that may result in substantial deviations of the HRV indices, especially in changes in the dynamics. In addition, they could potentially bias the statistical outcomes. Therefore, the actual heartbeat data can be preprocessed using a previously developed algorithm [54] based on the point-process statistics (local likelihood) that is able to perform real-time RR interval error detection and correction. Specifically, the algorithm assesses whether the actual observation is in agreement with the resulting model or if, instead, the alternative hypothesis of an erroneous beat is more likely.

4.2.4 Quantitative Tools and Feature Extraction

The abovementioned approaches based on linear parametric modeling allow for two levels of quantitative characterization of heartbeat dynamics: time-domain estimation and linear power spectrum estimation. Namely, given the RR interval series, estimates of mean RR, RR interval standard deviation, mean HR, and HR standard deviation can be extracted. Of note, using the point-process framework, instantaneous time-domain and frequency-domain estimates of heartbeat dynamics can be derived. In particular, the instantaneous time-domain characterization is based on the first- and the second-order moments of the underlying probability structure of heartbeat generation [27].

Although features defined in the time domain are simple and widely used, they are unable to discern between SNS and PNS activity (although RMSSD can be considered to reflect mainly PNS activity since it is computed as differences between successive beats). Frequency-domain analysis has been extensively pursued, contributing to the understanding of the autonomic background of RR interval fluctuations in the HR record. The linear power spectrum estimation, in fact, reveals the linear mechanisms governing the heartbeat dynamics in the frequency domain as regulated by the ANS.

Using a standard linear parametric AR model, the power spectral density (PSD) of $y(n)$ can be calculated as follows:

$$P_y(f) = \frac{\sigma^2 \Delta t}{|1 - \sum_{k=1}^{p} a_k z^{-k}|^2_{z=e^{j2\pi f \Delta t}}} \tag{4.10}$$

where Δt is the sampling rate of $y(n)$.

Using a point-process linear model, it is possible to compute the time-varying parametric (linear) autospectrum $P_y(f,t)$ given the time-varying parameter set $\xi(t)$ for the instantaneous RR interval mean $\mu_{RR}(t, \mathcal{H}_t, \xi(t))$. In order to facilitate the description of the spectral and bispectral estimation using point-process nonlinear models, Equation 4.10 can be rewritten as follows [79]:

$$Q(f, t) = S_{xx}(f, t)H_1(f, t)H_1(-f, t) \tag{4.11}$$

where $S_{xx}(f, t) = \sigma_{RR}^2$, and $H_1(f) = \Gamma_1'(f)^{-1}$ with $\Gamma_1'(f_1)$ standing for the Fourier transform of the extended AR kernel $\gamma_1'(i)$ defined as

$$\gamma_1'(i) = \begin{cases} 1, & \text{if } i = 0 \\ -\gamma_1(i) & \text{if } 1 \leq i \leq M \end{cases} \tag{4.12}$$

When performing the regression on the derivative RR interval series (see Equation 4.8), the time-varying parametric autospectrum of the RR intervals is given by multiplying its derivative spectrum $Q(f, t)$ in Equation 4.11 by the quantity $2(1 - \cos(\omega))$ [40,72].

Three main oscillatory components are usually differentiated in the HRV spectral profile [1,2]: the HF band (0.15–0.40 Hz), which reflects the effects of respiration on HR, historically also referred to as RSA; the LF band (0.04–0.15 Hz), which represents oscillations related to regulation of blood pressure and vasomotor tone; and the VLF band (<0.04 Hz), which is thought to relate, among other factors, to thermoregulation and kidney functioning. However, the VLF band is usually <0.04 Hz and is almost never considered as an ANS marker because it is related more to thermal regulation [80]. Broad evidence supports vagal origin of the HF component [1,2,81]. In contrast, the interpretation of the LF band is controversial. In fact, the current opinion on the fact that the LF power and LF/HF ratio are indices of sympathetic cardiac control and autonomic balance, respectively, is highly challenged and suggest that the HRV power spectrum, including its LF components, is mainly determined by the parasympathetic dynamics [81]. Moreover, the LF and HF power in normalized units (i.e., $LFnorm = LF/(LF + HF)$ and $HFnorm = HF/(LF + HF)$) are proposed to give more information about the sympathovagal balance [1].

Concerning the calculation of the abovementioned spectral features, by integrating Equation 4.10 (when considering standard linear AR models) and by integrating Equation 4.11 (when considering standard point-process linear AR models) in each frequency band, it is possible to compute the VLF, LF, and HF indices.

4.3 Nonlinear Parametric Models

In this section, nonlinear parametric models are formally defined and applied to exemplary nonlinear physiological dynamics such as heartbeat dynamics. Here, the prediction of the next heartbeat is defined as an algebraic sum of past RR intervals, including higher order combinations of such values. In our exemplary applications reported below, we focus on quadratic and cubic combinations.

4.3.1 NAR and NARMA Models

A NAR model can be expressed, in a general form, as follows:

$$y(k) = \mathbf{F}(y(k - 1), y(k - 2), ..., y(k - M)) + \epsilon(k) \tag{4.13}$$

where $y(k)$ is a time series, M is the maximum lags considered for the process, and $\epsilon(k)$ are independent, identically distributed Gaussian random variables, which account for uncertainties and possible unmodelled dynamics. This model can be can be written as a Taylor expansion:

$$y(k) = \gamma_0 + \sum_{i=1}^{M} \gamma_1(i)\, y(k-i) + \sum_{n=2}^{\infty} \sum_{i_1=1}^{M} \cdots \sum_{i_n=1}^{M} \gamma_n(i_1, \cdots, i_n) \prod_{j=1}^{n} y(k-i_j) + \epsilon(k) \qquad (4.14)$$

where the quadratic kernel $\gamma_2(i,j)$ is assumed to be symmetric. We also define the extended kernels $\gamma_1'(i)$ and $\gamma_2'(i,j)$ as

$$\gamma_1'(i) = \begin{cases} 1, & \text{if } i=0 \\ -\gamma_1(i) & \text{if } 1 \le i \le M \end{cases} \qquad (4.15)$$

$$\gamma_2'(i,j) = \begin{cases} 0, & \text{if } ij=0 \wedge i+j \le M \\ -\gamma_2(i,j) & \text{if } 1 \le i \le M \wedge 1 \le j \le M \end{cases}. \qquad (4.16)$$

The AR structure of Equation 4.14 allows for system identification with only exact knowledge on output data and with only a few assumptions on input data (noise assumptions).

NAR models can be seen as a special case of NARMA models, which can be expressed, in a general form, as follows:

$$y(k) = \mathbf{F}(y(k-1), y(k-2), ..., y(k-M_y), \epsilon(k), \epsilon(k-1), ..., \epsilon(k-M_e)) \qquad (4.17)$$

where $\epsilon(k)$ are independent, identically distributed Gaussian random variables, and M_y and M_e are the maximum lags considered for the process and noise terms, respectively. Consequently, an extended version of the NARMA model can be can be written as

$$y(k) = \gamma_0 + \sum_{i=1}^{M} \gamma_1(i)\, y(k-i) + \sum_{n=2}^{\infty} \sum_{i_1=1}^{M} \cdots \sum_{i_n=1}^{M} \gamma_n(i_1, ..., i_n) \prod_{j=1}^{n} y(k-i_j)$$

$$+ \sum_{i=1}^{M} \phi_1(i)\, \epsilon(k-i) + \sum_{n=2}^{\infty} \sum_{i_1=1}^{M} \cdots \sum_{i_n=1}^{M} \phi_n(i_1, ..., i_n) \prod_{j=1}^{n} \epsilon(k-i_j) \qquad (4.18)$$

4.3.2 Laguerre Expansion of the Input–Output Volterra Kernels

Let the jth-order discrete-time orthonormal Laguerre function be (see Figure 4.2)

$$\phi_j(k) = \alpha^{\frac{k-j}{2}} (1-\alpha)^{\frac{1}{2}} \sum_{i=0}^{j} (-1)^i \binom{k}{i} \binom{j}{i} \alpha^{j-i}(1-\alpha)^i, \ (k \ge 0)$$

where α is the discrete-time Laguerre parameter $(0 < \alpha < 1)$, which determines the rate of exponential asymptotic decline of these functions. Usually, the choice of the Laguerre parameter α is rather critical in achieving efficient expansions.

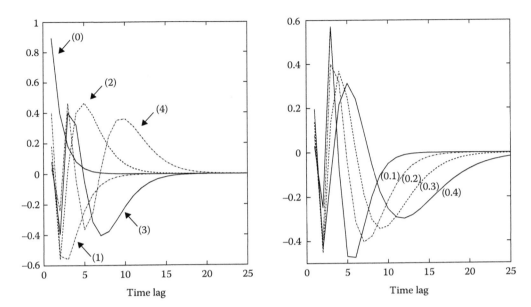

FIGURE 4.2
(Left) First four Laguerre functions for $\alpha = 0.2$ plotted over the first 25 lags. The order of each Laguerre basis is indicated under brackets. (Right) The third Laguerre functions for $\alpha = 0.1, 0.2, 0.3, 0.4$. The corresponding α value is indicated in parentheses.

Given the Laguerre function, $\phi_j(k)$, and the signal, $y(k)$, the jth-order Laguerre filter output is

$$l_j(k) = \sum_{i=0}^{\infty} \phi_j(i)\, y(k - i) \tag{4.19}$$

whose computation can be accelerated significantly by use of the following recursive relation [82]:

$$l_0(k) = \sqrt{\alpha}\, l_0(k-1) + \sqrt{1-\alpha}\, y(k-1) \tag{4.20}$$

$$l_j(k) = \sqrt{\alpha}\, l_j(k-1) + \sqrt{\alpha}\, l_{j-1}(k) + \tag{4.21}$$

$$\sqrt{\alpha}\, l_{j-1}(k-1),\; j \geq 1 \tag{4.22}$$

Using Laguerre expansion up to order P for the linear terms and up to order Q for the nonlinear ones, since the $\{\phi_i(t)\}$ form a complete orthonormal set in functional space $\mathcal{L}_2$, we can write [83]

$$\gamma_0 = g_0 \tag{4.23}$$

$$\gamma_1(i) = \sum_{m=0}^{P} g_1(m)\phi_m(i) \tag{4.24}$$

$$\gamma_2(i,j) = \sum_{m=0}^{Q} \sum_{n=0}^{m} g_2(m,n)\phi_m(i)\phi_n(j) \tag{4.25}$$

Here g_0, $g_1(m)$, and $g_2(m,n)$ are constant coefficients. As the expansion goes to zero as i and j go to infinity, the expansion can be truncated at delay M. Using Equations 4.19 and 4.23 through 4.25, it is possible to write

$$y(k) = g_0 + \sum_{i=0}^{P} g_1(i)\, l_i(k-1) + \sum_{i=0}^{Q} \sum_{j=0}^{i} g_2(i,j)\, l_i(k-1)\, l_j(k-1) + \epsilon(k) \qquad (4.26)$$

Equation 4.26 is the nonlinear autoregressive with Laguerre expansion (NARL) model. In this case, the number of parameters to estimate is $N = \{1\} + \{(P+1)\} + \{(Q+1)(Q+2)/2\}$. The AR order M of the NAR model corresponding to the NARL model depends on how fast the Laguerre functions decay to 0. It is also noteworthy that when $\alpha = 0$ the filter output becomes $l_j(k) = (-1)^j y(k-j)$ and the NARL model corresponds, apart from the sign, to the NAR model.

Quantitative tools of NAR or NARL modeling are defined through their equivalent input–output Wiener–Volterra models. The general scheme of such a quantitative characterization is shown in Figure 4.3.

The input–output model of a general NAR dynamical system can be written using a Wiener–Volterra [84] series as

$$y(k) = h_0 + \sum_{i=1}^{M} h_1(i)\, \epsilon(k-i) + \sum_{n=2}^{\infty} \sum_{i_1=1}^{M} \cdots \sum_{i_n=1}^{M} h_n(i_1, \ldots, i_n) \prod_{j=1}^{n} \epsilon(k-i_j) \qquad (4.27)$$

where the functions $h_n(\tau_1, \ldots, \tau_n)$ are the Volterra kernels, which represent the nonlinear dynamic system.

Just like for a linear AR model, there is an equivalent infinite-memory moving average model, in fact, a quadratic NAR (or NARL) model can be linked to an input–output Volterra model, driven by the same noise term. The transformation between Equations 4.14 and 4.27 can be performed in the frequency domain by using the following relationships [85] between the Fourier transforms of the Volterra kernels of order p, $H_p(f_1, \ldots, f_n)$, and the

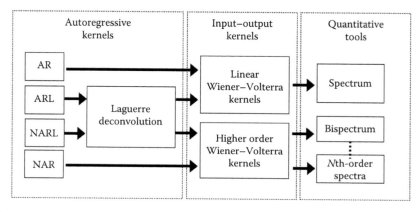

FIGURE 4.3
Block diagram of the point-process quantitative tools derivation.

Fourier transforms of the extended NAR terms, $\Gamma'_1(f_1)$ and $\Gamma'_2(f_1,f_2)$:

$$\sum_{k=mid(\rho)}^{\rho} \sum_{\sigma \in \sigma_\rho} H_k(f_{\sigma(1)}, \ldots, f_{\sigma(r)}, \omega_{\sigma(r+1)} + f_{\sigma(r+2)}, \ldots, f_{\sigma(\rho-1)} + f_{\sigma(\rho)}) \times \Gamma'_1(f_{\sigma(1)}) \cdots \Gamma'_1(f_{\sigma(r)})$$

$$\times \Gamma'_2(f_{\sigma(r+1)}, f_{\sigma(r+2)}) \cdots \Gamma'_2(f_{\sigma(\rho-1)}, f_{\sigma(\rho)}) = 0 \qquad (4.28)$$

where ρ is a given integer representing the kernel order, $mid(\rho) = \lceil \rho/2 \rceil$, $r = 2k - \rho$ and σ_ρ is the permutation set of N_ρ. Obviously, there is the need to truncate the series to a reasonable order for actual application. In this chapter, we model cardiovascular activity with a cubic input–output Volterra by means of the following relationships with the NARI:

$$H_1(f) = \frac{1}{\Gamma'_1(f)} \qquad (4.29)$$

$$H_2(f_1,f_2) = -\frac{\Gamma'_2(f_1,f_2)}{\Gamma'_1(f_1)\Gamma'_1(f_2)} H_1(f_1 + f_2) \qquad (4.30)$$

$$H_3(f_1,f_2,f_3) = -\frac{1}{6} \sum_{\sigma_3} \frac{\Gamma'_2\left(f_{\sigma_3(1)}, f_{\sigma_3(2)}\right)}{\Gamma'_1\left(f_{\sigma_3(1)}\right)\Gamma'_1\left(f_{\sigma_3(2)}\right)} \times H_2\left(f_{\sigma_3(1)} + f_{\sigma_3(2)}, f_{\sigma_3(3)}\right). \qquad (4.31)$$

Once the vector of the AR time-varing parameters $\xi(t)$ is estimated, it is possible to derive instantaneous quantitative tools such as the nth-order spectral representations.

4.3.3 Point-Process Framework

A nonlinear stochastic model embedded within a point-process framework is able to instantaneously assess the complex cardiovascular dynamics. Just like the previous formulation of point-process linear models, the core of the framework is the definition of the interbeat probability function to predict the waiting time of the next heartbeat, that is, the R-wave event, which in this case is a linear and nonlinear combination of the previous R-wave events. In particular, we describe the most performant model we developed so far which combines the inhomogeneous inverse Gaussian point-process framework previously defined in Refs. [27,86] with a novel AR structure linked to input–output definitions based on Laguerre expansions of the Volterra kernels [82,87–90]. This method employs the orthonormal basis of the discrete-time Laguerre functions to expand the kernels and reduces the number of unknown parameters that need be estimated. In order to define the related quantitative tools, we link a second-order NAR model with Laguerre expansion of kernels (hereinafter called NARL) to an equivalent infinite-order input–output Volterra model, which we then truncate at the third order. Therefore, NARL estimates allow for the instantaneous estimation of the high-order polyspectra [85], such as bispectrum and trispectrum [91,92].

Here, we propose a novel formulation based on the Laguerre expansions where the previous RR intervals are embedded, with the instantaneous RR mean defined as

$$\mu_{RR}(t, \mathcal{H}_t, \xi(t)) = RR_{\widetilde{N}(t)} + g_0(t) + \sum_{i=0}^{p} g_1(i,t)\, l_i(t^-) + \sum_{i=0}^{q} \sum_{j=0}^{q} g_2(i,j,t)\, l_i(t^-)\, l_j(t^-) \qquad (4.32)$$

where

$$l_i(t^-) = \sum_{n=1}^{\tilde{N}(t)} \phi_i(n) \left(RR_{\tilde{N}(t)-n} - RR_{\tilde{N}(t)-n-1} \right) \tag{4.33}$$

is the output of the Laguerre filters just before time t. The coefficients $g_0, \{g_1(i)\}$ and $\{g_2(i,j)\}$ correspond to the time-varying zero-, first-, and second-order NARL coefficients, respectively.

The corresponding NAR Wiener–Volterra model with degree of nonlinearity 2 and long-term memory [82] becomes

$$\mu_{RR}(t, \mathcal{H}_t, \xi(t)) = RR_{\tilde{N}(t)} + \gamma_0 + \sum_{i=1}^{\infty} \gamma_1(i, t) \, (RR_{\tilde{N}(t)-i} - RR_{\tilde{N}(t)-i-1})$$

$$+ \sum_{i=1}^{\infty} \sum_{j=1}^{\infty} \gamma_2(i, j, t) \, (RR_{\tilde{N}(t)-i} - RR_{\tilde{N}(t)-i-1}) \times (RR_{\tilde{N}(t)-j} - RR_{\tilde{N}(t)-j-1}) \tag{4.34}$$

Note that, even if there is a parallel in the degree of nonlinearities between the NAR and the NARL models (e.g., you can explicate the quadratic function of the previous observation RR intervals), the latter reflects a very different characterization.

4.3.4 Quantitative Tools and Feature Extraction

The abovementioned approaches based on nonlinear parametric modeling allow for three levels of quantitative characterization of heartbeat dynamics: time-domain estimation, linear power spectrum estimation, and higher order spectral (HOS) representation. Next, the parametric estimation of spectrum, bispectrum, and trispectrum is described in detail considering the point-process formulation as a reference model. It is straightforward, in fact, to consider the estimates from the standard nonlinear parametric formulation as a particular case of the point-process dynamical estimates occurring at $t = t^*$. Note that the bispectrum complements the linear dynamical information given by the spectrum by providing a quantification of the nonlinear interactions between the system frequencies. Through bispectral analysis, for instance, it is possible to obtain enhanced estimates of the parasympathetic dynamics (see the bispectral HH index) as well as estimates of the dynamical interaction between low frequencies and high frequencies (see the bispectral LH index).

To summarize, the necessary steps to estimate the quantitative tools from nonlinear models are as follows:

1. From $\gamma_n(...)$ find $\gamma'_n(...)$.
2. Compute the Fourier transforms $\Gamma'_n(...)$ of the kernels $\gamma'_n(...)$.
3. Compute the input–output Volterra kernels $H_k(...)$ from the $\Gamma'_n(...)$ of the AR model.
4. Estimate the nth-order spectra such as the instantaneous spectrum $Q(f, t)$ and bispectrum $\text{Bis}(f_1, f_2, t)$.

4.3.4.1 Dynamic Spectrum Estimation

The linear power spectrum estimation reveals the linear mechanisms governing the heartbeat dynamics in the frequency domain. In particular, given the input–output Volterra kernels of a NAR model for the instantaneous RR interval mean $\mu_{RR}(t, H_t, \xi(t))$, it is possible to compute the time-varying parametric (linear) autospectrum [79]:

$$Q(f, t) = S_{xx}(f, t)H_1(f, t)H_1(-f, t) - \frac{3}{2\pi} \int H_3(f, f_2, -f_2, t)S_{xx}(f_2, t)df_2 \qquad (4.35)$$

where $S_{xx}(f, t) = \sigma_{RR}^2$. The time-varying parametric autospectrum of the RR intervals is given by multiplying its derivative spectrum $Q(f, t)$ by the quantity $2(1 - \cos(\omega))$ [72]. Of note, estimates from standard parametric nonlinear models are defined by Equation 4.35 at a certain time as $t = t^*$. Just like described for linear modeling (see Section 4.2.4), by integrating Equation 4.35 in each frequency band, it is possible to compute the index within the VLF (VLF = 0.01–0.05 Hz), LF (LF = 0.05–0.15 Hz), and HF (HF = 0.15–0.5 Hz) ranges.

4.3.4.2 Bispectrum Estimation

The HOS representation allows for the consideration of statistics beyond the second order, and phase relations between frequency components otherwise suppressed [92,93]. HOS, also known as polyspectra, are spectral representations of higher order statistics, that is, moments and cumulants of third order and beyond. HOS can detect deviations from linearity, stationarity, or Gaussianity. Particular cases of HOS are the third-order spectrum (bispectrum) and the fourth-order spectrum (trispectrum) [93].

A general definition of the bispectrum is as follows:

$$B(f_1, f_2) = \iint_{t_1, t_2 = -\infty}^{+\infty} c_3(t_1, t_2) e^{-j(2\pi f_1 t_1 + 2\pi f_2 t_2)} dt_1 dt_2 \qquad (4.36)$$

with the condition

$$|\omega_1|, |\omega_2| \leq \pi \text{ for } \omega = 2\pi f$$

The $c_3(t_1, t_2)$ variable represents the third-order cumulant, which is defined as follows:

$$c_3(t_1, t_2) = E\{s(t_1)s(t_2)s(t_1 + t_2)\} \qquad (4.37)$$

where $s(t)$ is a square integrable stationary signal with zero mean. Thus, the bispectrum measures the correlation among three spectral peaks, ω_1, ω_2, and $(\omega_1 + \omega_2)$ and estimates the phase coupling.

Concerning the bispectral parametric estimation of nonlinear models, let $H_2(f_1, f_2, t)$ denote the Fourier transform of the second-order Volterra kernel coefficients. The analytical solution for the bispectrum of a nonlinear system response with stationary, zero-mean Gaussian input is [94]

$$\begin{aligned}
\text{Bis}(f_1, f_2, t) = \; &2H_2(f_1 + f_2, -f_2, t)H_1(-f_1 - f_2, t)H_1(f_2, t) \times S_{xx}(f_1 + f_2, t)S_{xx}(f_2, t) \\
&+ 2H_2(f_1 + f_2, -f_1, t) \times H_1(-f_1 - f_2, t)H_1(f_1, t)S_{xx}(f_1 + f_2, t)S_{xx}(f_1, t) \\
&+ 2H_2(-f_1, -f_2, t)H_1(f_1, t)H_1(f_2, t) \times S_{xx}(f_1, t)S_{xx}(f_2, t)
\end{aligned} \qquad (4.38)$$

Of note, an expression similar to Equation 4.38 was derived in the early work of Brillinger [95], and later in the appendix of Ref. [96].

Given the dynamical bispectrum $\text{Bis}(f_1, f_2, t)$, at each t, it is possible to estimate the bispectral features as described in detail in the following section.

4.3.4.3 Feature Extraction

Of note, it has been demonstrated that the bispectrum has several symmetry properties [97], which divide the (f_1, f_2) plane in symmetric zones. Therefore, the bispectrum of a real signal is uniquely defined by its values in the triangular region of computation, $0 \leq f_1 \leq f_2 \leq f_1 + f_2 \leq 1$, provided there is no bispectral aliasing [98–100]. Specifically introducing the bispectral parameter, $P(a)$, which is invariant to translation, DC level, amplification, and scale. It is defined as follows:

$$P(a) = \arctan \left(\frac{I_i(a)}{I_r(a)} \right) \tag{4.39}$$

where

$$I(a) = I_r(a) + jI_i(a) = \int_{f_1=0^+}^{\frac{1}{1+a}} B(f_1, af_1)df_1 \tag{4.40}$$

for $0 < a \leq 1$ and $j = \sqrt{-1}$ where a is the slope of the straight line on which the bispectrum is integrated.

Mean magnitude and phase entropy [101] are also calculated within the triangular region of computation. Mean magnitude is defined as

$$M_{\mathrm{mean}} = \frac{1}{L} \sum_{\Omega} |B(f_1, af_1)| \tag{4.41}$$

and phase entropy is

$$P_{e=} \sum_n p(\Psi_n)\log(p(\Psi_n)) \tag{4.42}$$

$$p(\Psi_n) = \frac{1}{L} \sum_{\Omega} 1 \left(\Phi \left(B(f_1, af_1) \right) \in \Psi_n \right) \tag{4.43}$$

$$\Psi_n = \{ \Phi | -\pi + 2\pi n/N \leq \phi \leq -\pi + 2\pi(n+1)/N \} \tag{4.44}$$

with $n = 0, 1, ..., N - 1$, where L is the number of points within the triangular region of computation, Φ refers to the phase angle of the bispectrum, Ω refers to the space of the defined triangular region of computation, and $1(.)$ is an indicator function, which is equal to 1 when the phase angle Φ is within the range of bin Ψ_n in Equation 4.44.

The mean magnitude of the bispectrum can be useful in discriminating between processes with similar power spectra but different third-order statistics. However, it is sensitive to amplitude changes.

The normalized bispectral entropy (P_1) is equal to

$$P_1 = - \sum_n p_n \log(p_n) \tag{4.45}$$

where

$$p_n = \frac{|B(f_1, af_1)|}{\sum_{\Omega} |B(f_1, af_1)|} \tag{4.46}$$

and Ω is the triangular region of computation.

The normalized bispectral squared entropy (P_2) is calculated as

$$P_2 = -\sum_n p_n \log(p_n) \tag{4.47}$$

where

$$p_n = \frac{|B(f_1, af_1)|^2}{\sum_\Omega |B(f_1, af_1)|^2} \tag{4.48}$$

and Ω is the triangular region of computation.

In addition, the sum of logarithmic amplitudes of the bispectrum can be computed as [102]

$$\text{Hbis}_1(t) = \sum_\Omega \log(|\text{Bis}(f_1, f_2, t)|) \tag{4.49}$$

As is well known, the sympathovagal linear effects on HRV are mainly characterized by the LF and HF spectral powers. Through bispectral analysis, it is possible to further evaluate the nonlinear sympathovagal interactions by integrating $|B(f_1, f_2)|$ in the appropriate frequency bands. Specifically, it is possible to evaluate

$$\text{LL}(t) = \int_{f_1=0^+}^{0.15} \int_{f_2=0^+}^{0.15} \text{Bis}(f_1, f_2, t) df_1 df_2 \tag{4.50}$$

$$\text{LH}(t) = \int_{f_1=0^+}^{0.15} \int_{f_2=0.15^+}^{0.4} \text{Bis}(f_1, f_2, t) df_1 df_2 \tag{4.51}$$

$$\text{HH}(t) = \int_{f_1=0.15^+}^{0.4} \int_{f_2=0.15^+}^{0.4} \text{Bis}(f_1, f_2, t) df_1 df_2 \tag{4.52}$$

4.3.4.4 Dynamic Trispectrum Estimation

Brillinger [103], Billings [84], Priestley [104], and others have demonstrated that there is a closed-form solution for homogeneous systems with Gaussian inputs. Thus, the transfer function of a m-order homogeneous system is estimated by the following relation:

$$H_m(f_1, \ldots, f_m) = \frac{S_{yx\ldots x}(-f_1, \cdots, -f_m)}{m! S_{xx}(f_1) \cdots S_{xx}(f_m)} \tag{4.53}$$

where the numerator is the $m + 1 - n$th order cross-polyspectrum between y and x. This result is a generalization of the classical result from the transfer function of a linear system resulting from $m = 1$. Therefore, the cross-trispectrum (Fourier transform of the third-order moment) can be estimated as

$$\mathcal{T}(f_1, f_2, f_3, t) \approx 3! S_{xx}(f_1, t) S_{xx}(f_2, t) S_{xx}(f_3, t) \times H_3(f_1, f_2, f_3, t) \qquad (4.54)$$

4.4 Exemplary Applications

In this section, we describe two exemplary applications of the above-described point-process NARL model on actual heartbeat data gathered from healthy subjects undergoing postural changes, and patients with severe CHF.

4.4.1 Postural Changes

In this study, we validate the point-process NARL as related to real physiological dynamics in a study of the RR interval time series recorded from 10 healthy subjects undergoing a tilt-table protocol (75° head-up tilt over 50 seconds); see further details in Refs. [27,105,106]. Briefly, each subject was first placed horizontally in a supine position, with restraints used to secure him/her at the waist, arms, and hands. The subject was then tilted from the horizontal to the vertical position and returned to the horizontal position. The study was conducted at the Massachusetts Institute of Technology (MIT), General Clinical Research Center (GCRC) and was approved by the MIT Institutional Review Board and the GCRC Scientific Advisory Committee. Of note, tilt-table recordings have been widely recommended for the study of both stationary and nonstationary HRV assessment [1,27,105,107,108]. A single-lead ECG was continuously recorded for each subject during the study, and the RR intervals were extracted using a curve length-based QRS detection algorithm [109].

To perform a proper model order selection, we integrated the KS and autocorrelation analysis by considering the AIC criterion (for comparison analysis exclusively) using the first 5-minute recordings of resting state. For the NARL model, we obtained $4 \leq P \leq 8$ as the optimal linear order and $3 \leq P \leq 4$ and $2 \leq Q \leq 3$ for the nonlinear model. One representative KS and autocorrelation plot is shown in Figure 4.4. For all the considered subjects, nearly all of the KS plots and more than 97% of the autocorrelation samples were within the 95% confidence bounds. The tracking results are shown in Figure 4.5.

We further applied an established time-domain method [110] to the RR time series in order to test the presence of nonlinearity in the heartbeat intervals. The outcomes from the nonlinearity test further validate that the nonlinear terms estimated by our goodness-of-fit procedures are not a result of an overfitting identification. Specifically, data coming from the tilt-table protocol is characterized by a relevant presence of nonlinearity and nonstationarity in the RR time series for all the considered subjects (see [40]).

We also evaluated the statistical differences between the supine and upright epochs before and after the slow transitions of the tilt-table protocol. The difference was expressed in terms of P-values from a nonparametric rank-sum test [111], under the null hypothesis that the medians of the two sample groups are equal. Given the rank-sum statistics, we also calculated the area under the receiver operating characteristic (ROC) curve [112], hereinafter area under the curve (AUC). The results from the tilt-table dataset are shown in

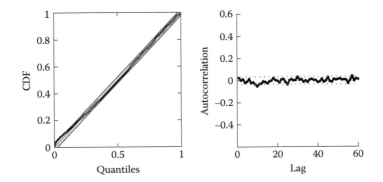

FIGURE 4.4
KS plot (left) and autocorrelation plot (right) from a representative subject of the tilt-table protocol using a point-process nonlinear model. The dashed lines in all plots indicate the 95% confidence bounds.

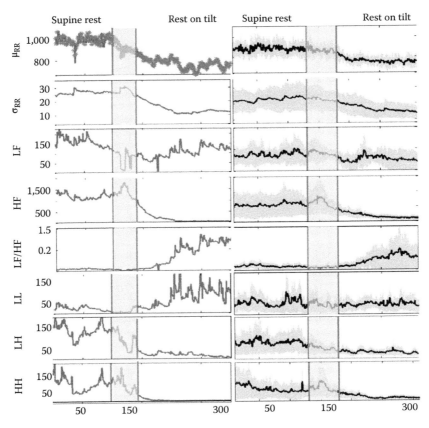

FIGURE 4.5
Instantaneous heartbeat statistics computed from a representative subject (N. 1, left column) and averaged along all 10 subjects of the tilt-table protocol (right column) using a NARL model. In the first panel, the estimated $\mu_{RR}(t)$ is superimposed on the recorded RR series. Below, the instantaneous heartbeat power spectra evaluated in low frequency (LF) and in high frequency (HF), the sympatho-vagal balance (LF/HF), and several bispectral statistics are reported. Given a considered feature X, plots on the right panels are expressed as $X = \text{Median}(X) \pm \text{MAD}(X)$.

Tables 4.1 and 4.2. We computed standard recommended time domain and morphological features such as the root mean square of successive differences of intervals (RMSSD), the percentage of successive differences of intervals which differ by more than 50 ms (pNN50% expressed as a percentage of the total number of heartbeats analyzed), and the triangular index (TINN) [1].

From our model linear coefficients, we computed the instantaneous RR standard deviation (a time-varying version of the SDNN [1]) as well the LF and the HF power and

TABLE 4.1

Standard and Instantaneous Measures of HRV: Results from the Tilt-Table Experimental Dataset.

Standard Time-Domain Measures of HRV				
Statistical Index	**Rest**	**Tilt**	***P* value**	**AUC**
RMSSD(ms)	32.1 ± 12.6	19.7 ± 4.5	<0.05	0.699
NN50(count)	31.0 ± 29.0	6.0 ± 5.5	<0.02	0.728
pNN50(%)	10.2 ± 9.5	1.74 ± 1.4	<0.02	0.728
HRV_tri_ind	8.03 ± 1.4	7.3 ± 1.6	>0.05	0.661
TINN (ms)	195.0 ± 70.0	150.0 ± 45.0	>0.05	0.641
σ_{RR}(ms)	21.3 ± 6.7	14.81 ± 4.7	<0.03	0.717
Instantaneous Standard Frequency-Domain Measures of HRV				
Statistical Index	**Rest**	**Tilt**	***P* value**	**AUC**
LF (ms^2)	373.4 ± 217.0	287.7 ± 135.9	>0.05	0.420
HF (ms^2)	242.4 ± 140.4	82.04 ± 61.1	<0.03	0.719
LF/HF (n.u.)	0.96 ± 0.57	2.30 ± 2.13	>0.05	0.632

P values are obtained by rank-sum test between the Rest and Tilt epochs. Values are expressed as $X = \text{Median}(X) \pm \text{MAD}(X)$.

TABLE 4.2

Instantaneous Higher Order Measures of HRV: Results from the Tilt-Table Experimental Dataset

Instantaneous Higher Order Measures of HRV				
Statistical Index	**Rest**	**Tilt**	**P value**	**AUC**
$\overline{P(a)}$	0.02 ± 0.45	-0.22 ± 0.72	>0.05	0.599
$\sigma_{P(a)}$	0.71 ± 0.19	0.36 ± 0.19	<0.02	0.739
$M_{\text{mean}}(10^3)$	67.4 ± 28.8	40.7 ± 21.4	<0.05	0.653
P_e	5.19 ± 0.08	5.33 ± 0.06	<0.05	0.747
P_1	8.81 ± 0.24	9.03 ± 0.27	>0.05	0.578
P_2	7.61 ± 0.42	7.83 ± 0.8	>0.05	0.554
$H\text{bis}_1(10^3)$	162.7 ± 6.4	153.0 ± 3.5	<0.02	0.742
LL(10^6)	163.9 ± 146.2	162.2 ± 135.4	>0.05	0.542
LH(10^6)	429.7 ± 229.8	183.2 ± 82.9	<0.02	0.743
HH(10^6)	974.5 ± 632.1	289 ± 194.5	<0.005	0.789

P values are obtained by rank-sum test between the Rest and Tilt epochs. Values are expressed as $X = \text{Median}(X) \pm \text{MAD}(X)$.

their ratio (i.e., sympato-vagal balance, LF/HF), whereas by estimating the dynamic bispectrum by the nonlinear coefficients (see Equation 4.38), we computed all the bispectral features defined in Section 4.3.4.3. All features were calculated instantaneously with a 5-ms temporal resolution. To average among the group, we considered the median values over the estimated instantaneous time series according to the protocol timeline. Values are expressed as median and its respective absolute deviation (i.e., for a feature X, $X = \text{Median}(X) \pm \text{MAD}(X)$, where $\text{MAD}(X) = \text{Median}(|X - \text{Median}(X)|)$). As a first outcome, we can observe that the values and the confidence intervals of all the linear features are quite similar among the different models, thus demonstrating that the inclusion of nonlinear terms in the model does not effect the linear part of the signal. Nevertheless, it is important to note that the NARL model provides the best overall results in terms of statistical difference between the rest and tilt conditions. This demonstrates that choosing the most proper model is important even in the computation of less complex measures, such as variance. Also note that all significant higher order indices show better P-value and AUC when compared with standard measures.

From a clinical point of view, our results suggest that linear AR parametric models clearly relate to the sympathovagal physiological model. In addition, a more comprehensive and reliable characterization of the ANS functions on cardiovascular control can be performed through nonlinear models and related estimates. Our results also demonstrate that time-varying models and related estimates are also needed to properly identify critical events in heartbeat dynamics. On the other hand, it is important to point out that, although nonlinear features derived by the nonlinear parametric model have proved very effective in characterizing autonomic dynamics, current knowledge on the nonlinear correlates does not relate to specific physiological processes, thus calling for more evolved nonlinear models that can go beyond the black box approach. A major achievement of linking nonlinear estimates to specific physiological mechanisms would be to obtain specific biomarkers allowing effective clinical stratifications in health and disease.

4.4.2 Cardiac Heart Failure

The second heartbeat dataset was retrieved from a public source: Physionet (http://www.physionet.org/) [113]. It consists of RR time series recorded from 14 CHF patients (from the *BIDMC–CHF* Database) and 16 healthy subjects (from the *MIT–BIH* Normal Sinus Rhythm Database: http://www.physionet.org/physiobank/database/nsrdb/). Each RR time series was artifact-free (upon human visual inspection and artifact rejection) and lasted about 50 minutes (small segments of the original over 20-hour recordings). These recordings have been taken as a landmark for studying complex heartbeat interval dynamics [6,7,10,114]. Of note, the NARL model gives the best fit results for 27 of the 30 subjects [40]. This is due to the capability of the Laguerre coefficients to intrinsically embed all the previous information (i.e., long-term memory). In addition, having less regressors improves the performance of the parameter identification. Using this data, we studied the difference between healthy and CHF subjects. The difference was expressed in terms of P-values from a nonparametric rank-sum test [111], under the null hypothesis that the medians of the two sample groups are equal. Given the rank-sum statistics, we also calculated the area under the ROC curve [112], hereinafter AUC. These longer recordings provide an ideal dataset for nonlinear and complex HRV analysis, as demonstrated by the large number of published outcomes [7,10,114]). Results are shown in Tables 4.3 and 4.4. Here, in addition to the standard measures considered for the first protocol we also computed several widely used nonlinear features such as the ApEn [115], the sample entropy (SampEn)

TABLE 4.3

Standard and Instantaneous Measures of HRV: Results from the Second Experimental Dataset

Standard Time-Domain and Nonlinear Measures of HRV				
	CHF ($n = 14$)	**Healthy ($n = 16$)**	**P value**	**AUC**
RMSSD	0.0121 ± 0.0036	0.0432 ± 0.0145	$>4e^{-4}$	0.888
NN50	13.5 ± 12.00	912.50 ± 633.00	$>3e^{-4}$	0.892
pNN50	0.2357 ± 0.2246	21.5406 ± 15.4908	$>1e^{-4}$	0.919
TINN	0.1575 ± 0.0650	0.2975 ± 0.0500	$>3e^{-4}$	0.892
ApEn	1.2130 ± 0.1032	1.2177 ± 0.1066	>0.05	0.495
SampEn	1.5670 ± 0.2690	1.4092 ± 0.1522	>0.05	0.633
DFA-α_1	0.8498 ± 0.2191	1.0820 ± 0.1467	>0.05	0.709
DFA-α_2	1.1552 ± 0.1335	0.9286 ± 0.0544	<0.05	0.736
σ_{RR}(ms)	8.31 ± 2.2	24.7 ± 7.0	$>5e^{-4}$	0.875
Instantaneous Standard Frequency-Domain Measures of HRV				
	CHF ($n = 14$)	**Healthy ($n = 16$)**	**P value**	**AUC**
LF(ms^2)	7.28 ± 6.1	316.0 ± 127.2	$>1.5e^{-5}$	0.973
HF(ms^2)	30.59 ± 21.0	606.1 ± 344.7	$>5e^{-4}$	0.879
LF/HF (n.u.)	0.08 ± 0.1	0.86 ± 0.7	>0.04	0.728

P values are obtained from the rank-sum test between the CHF and healthy subject groups. Values are expressed as $X = \text{Median}(X) \pm \text{MAD}(X)$.

TABLE 4.4

Instantaneous Higher Order Measures of HRV: Results from the CHF Experimental Dataset.

Instantaneous Higher Order Measures of HRV				
	CHF ($n = 14$)	**Healthy ($n = 16$)**	**P value**	**AUC**
$\overline{P(a)}$	-0.33 ± 0.29	-0.21 ± 0.3	>0.05	0.518
$\sigma_{P(a)}$	0.62 ± 0.22	0.48 ± 0.06	>0.05	0.312
$M_{\text{mean}}(10^3)$	16.65 ± 8.24	81.6 ± 57.9	$>2e^{-3}$	0.848
P_e	5.05 ± 0.14	5.26 ± 0.04	$>3e^{-3}$	0.830
P_1	9.25 ± 0.06	8.76 ± 0.42	$>5e^{-3}$	0.808
P_2	8.57 ± 0.20	7.34 ± 0.75	$>3e^{-3}$	0.821
$H\text{bis}_1(10^3)$	146.7 ± 7.06	166.5 ± 6.7	$>4e^{-4}$	0.853
LL(10^6)	8.6 ± 7.8	211.9 ± 134.0	$>2e^{-5}$	0.960
LH(10^6)	46.6 ± 34.0	549.6 ± 351.5	$>2e^{-4}$	0.911
HH(10^7)	19.2 ± 14.5	230.1 ± 190.9	$>7e^{-3}$	0.795

P values are obtained from the rank-sum test between the CHF and healthy subject groups. Values are expressed as $X = \text{Median}(X) \pm \text{MAD}(X)$.

[116], and the DFA [114]. Results show that, on average, the CHF patients show significantly lower σ_{RR}. However, σ_{RR} depends on linear estimates exclusively, leading to the need for complementary nonlinear measures. If we reasonably hypothesize that the NARL bispectral estimation allows for the evaluation of the interactions between the sympathetic

and parasympathetic systems, our results indicate that on average the CHF patients show lower interactions between the two peripheral nervous systems, evaluated by means of LL, LH, and HH. These findings are in agreement with the current literature whereby disorders in these interactions may lead to abnormalities (e.g., heart failure [117]). With respect to the considered standard morphological and nonlinear features, most of the NARL spectral and bispectral features show more significant results. Specifically, differently than what is found in the shorter tilt-table protocol, here the LF and the LL values related to slower autonomic influences (possibly sympathetic) show the most significant decrease, with the highest AUC among all other parameters. This relevant outcome may be possibly attributed to the capability of the Laguerre coefficients to better capture the slow dynamics (i.e., long-term memory) when longer data are available.

4.5 Final Remarks and Perspectives

In this chapter, a mathematical overview of parametric models used for HRV analysis is presented. These parametric models are usually based on AR relationships and are preferred over the nonparametric ones because of the high resolution in the frequency-domain analysis even with short time series (once the model parameters are estimated, reliable AR-based estimates can be obtained using only a few seconds of heartbeat dynamics). The model order and the parameter vector, however, need to be effectively estimated in order to obtain reliable features in the time and frequency domain. We split the chapter into two main logical parts, which are related to linear and nonlinear models. Each part includes the standard and point-process mathematical formulation, followed by the most common quantitative tools and feature extraction that can be applied.

As a general consideration, the parameter estimation of linear models is easier to perform with respect to nonlinear models. This is due to the higher number of parameters and higher sensitivity to the input signal amplitude variation that are intrinsic in the nonlinear formulation (because of the quadratic and cubic history dependence). Nevertheless, nonlinear models are able to provide the same quantitative tools as linear models (i.e., measures defined in the time and frequency domain), with additional estimates related to higher order statistics such as bispectrum and trispectrum. Last but not least, series of heartbeat dynamics can be seen as the output of the cardiovascular system, which is indeed a nonlinear system in normal conditions [14]. Of note, as described in Section 4.2.3, by performing the regression on the derivative series, the NARL model improves the achievement of stationarity [40,72] and consequently improves system identification. These statements are also confirmed by the experimental results reported in Section 4.4. The results from nonlinearity tests performed on actual RR interval series gathered on healthy subjects undergoing structured (postural changes) and unstructured activities, in fact, demonstrate that the RR interval series is indeed an output of a nonlinear system [40]. Moreover, such nonlinearity tends to be lost during pathological conditions such as severe CHF. Moreover, goodness-of-fit analyses through KS statistics and autocorrelation plots demonstrate that nonlinear models outperform the linear ones by achieving a better prediction of the next heartbeat event [40]. Of note, nonlinear models also allow the definition of other measures of complexity related to entropy [44,118,119] and Lyapunov exponents [41,73,120].

Concerning the difference between the standard (linear and nonlinear) and point-process implementation, it has been demonstrated how the latter approach outperforms the former one by significantly improving the prediction of the next heartbeat event [27]. Moreover, the point-process approach is exclusively able to provide goodness-of-fit measure as well as instantaneous estimates in the time and frequency domain, both relevant features required by an effective statistical signal processing tool.

4.6 Summary

One of the greatest advancements in applied mathematics has been its use in the functioning of biological and physiological systems. The nature and complexity of the modeling mathematical framework of choice spans from very high dimensional mathematical objects aimed at reproducing each single element participating in the biological/physiological system in question, to very simple (often black box) formulations aimed at characterizing the overall dynamics of selective features and variables of interest. Among these models, parametric models (as opposed to nonparametric models, which do not assume any basic structure of the system generating the experimental data) are defined by mathematical formulations derived by using a finite number of parameters associated with the physiological system dynamics under study. These parameters are usually collected together to form a single k-dimensional vector revealing the physiological dynamics under study. Once estimated, the model is fixed, and does not change to accommodate the complexity of the data, as can easily happen when using nonparametric models. Throughout a historical overview of the most relevant methodologies based on parametric models for HRV analysis, this chapter points out how parametric models have proven to be a fundamental methodological tool for the assessment of the ANS control of heartbeat dynamics.

The chapter further reports details on advanced probabilistic models for instantaneous HRV assessment. Specifically, we focus on one of the most recent advances in linear and nonlinear regressive models used for HRV analysis where point-process theory is exploited to characterize the probability of any heartbeat occurrence. As the interbeat probability function is defined at each moment in time, it is possible to obtain instantaneous estimates of heartbeat dynamics, opening new dramatic scenarios in understanding underlying physiological linear and nonlinear processes.

Finally, we report the most significant features that can be extracted from both linear and nonlinear parametric models and conclude the presentation with some exemplary applications, such as HRV assessment during postural change protocols and after CHF.

References

1. A. Camm, M. Malik, J. Bigger, et al., Heart rate variability: Standards of measurement, physiological interpretation, and clinical use, *Circulation*, vol. 93, no. 5, pp. 1043–1065, 1996.
2. U. R. Acharya, K. P. Joseph, N. Kannathal, et al., Heart rate variability: A review, *Medical and Biological Engineering and Computing*, vol. 44, no. 12, pp. 1031–1051, 2006.
3. H. M. Stauss, Heart rate variability, *American Journal of Physiology-Regulatory, Integrative and Comparative Physiology*, vol. 285, no. 5, pp. R927–R931, 2003.
4. G. G. Berntson, J. T. Bigger, D. L. Eckberg, et al., Heart rate variability: Origins, methods, and interpretive caveats, *Psychophysiology*, vol. 34, pp. 623–648, 1997.

5. N. Wessel, H. Malberg, R. Bauernschmitt, et al., Nonlinear methods of cardiovascular physics and their clinical applicability, *International Journal of Bifurcation and Chaos*, vol. 17, no. 10, pp. 3325–3371, 2007.

6. F. Atyabi, M. Livari, K. Kaviani, et al., Two statistical methods for resolving healthy individuals and those with congestive heart failure based on extended self-similarity and a recursive method, *Journal of Biological Physics*, vol. 32, no. 6, pp. 489–495, 2006.

7. L. Glass, Introduction to controversial topics in nonlinear science: Is the normal heart rate chaotic? *Chaos: An Interdisciplinary Journal of Nonlinear Science*, vol. 19, no. 2, 028501, 2009

8. L. Glass, Synchronization and rhythmic processes in physiology, *Nature*, vol. 410, no. 6825, pp. 277–284, 2001.

9. A. Goldberger, C. Peng, and L. Lipsitz, What is physiologic complexity and how does it change with aging and disease? *Neurobiology of Aging*, vol. 23, no. 1, pp. 23–26, 2002.

10. C. Poon and C. Merrill, Decrease of cardiac chaos in congestive heart failure, *Nature*, vol. 389, no. 6650, pp. 492–495, 1997.

11. M. P. Tulppo, A. M. Kiviniemi, A. J. Hautala, et al., Physiological background of the loss of fractal heart rate dynamics, *Circulation*, vol. 112, no. 3, pp. 314–319, 2005.

12. G. Wu, N. Arzeno, L. Shen, et al., Chaotic signatures of heart rate variability and its power spectrum in health, aging and heart failure, *PLOS ONE*, vol. 4, no. 2, p. e4323, 2009.

13. O. Stiedl and M. Meyer, Fractal dynamics in circadian cardiac time series of corticotropin-releasing factor receptor subtype-2 deficient mice, *Journal of Mathematical Biology*, vol. 47, no. 2, pp. 169–197, 2003.

14. K. Sunagawa, T. Kawada, and T. Nakahara, Dynamic nonlinear vago-sympathetic interaction in regulating heart rate, *Heart and Vessels*, vol. 13, no. 4, pp. 157–174, 1998.

15. M. Wolf, G. Varigos, D. Hunt, et al., Sinus arrhythmia in acute myocardial infarction, *The Medical Journal of Australia*, vol. 2, no. 2, pp. 52–53, 1978.

16. S. Akselrod, D. Gordon, F. A. Ubel, D. C. Shannon, A. Berger, and R. J. Cohen, Power spectrum analysis of heart rate fluctuation: A quantitative probe of beat-to-beat cardiovascular control, *Science*, vol. 213, no. 4504, pp. 220–222, 1981.

17. S. M. Kay and S. L. Marple Jr, Spectrum analysis—A modern perspective, *Proceedings of the IEEE*, vol. 69, no. 11, pp. 1380–1419, 1981.

18. L. Marple, Resolution of conventional Fourier, autoregressive, and special ARMA methods of spectrum analysis, in *Acoustics, Speech, and Signal Processing, IEEE International Conference on ICASSP'77.*, vol. 2. IEEE, 1977, pp. 74–77.

19. W. Jarisch and J. S. Detwiler, Statistical modeling of fetal heart rate variability, *IEEE Transactions on Biomedical Engineering*, no. 10, pp. 582–589, 1980.

20. M. Brovelli, G. Baselli, S. Cerutti, et al., Computerized analysis for an experimental validation of neurophysiological models of heart rate control, *Computers in Cardiology*, vol. 2, pp. 205–208, 1983.

21. G. Baselli, D. Bolis, S. Cerutti, et al., Autoregressive modeling and power spectral estimate of rr interval time series in arrhythmic patients, *Computers and Biomedical Research*, vol. 18, no. 6, pp. 510–530, 1985.

22. D. P. Giddens and R. I. Kitney, Neonatal heart rate variability and its relation to respiration, *Journal of Theoretical Biology*, vol. 113, no. 4, pp. 759–780, 1985.

23. F. Bartoli, G. Baselli, and S. Cerutti, AR identification and spectral estimate applied to the RR interval measurements, *International Journal of Bio-medical Computing*, vol. 16, no. 3, pp. 201–215, 1985.

24. R. Kitney, T. Fulton, A. McDonald, et al., Transient interactions between blood pressure, respiration and heart rate in man, *Journal of Biomedical Engineering*, vol. 7, no. 3, pp. 217–224, 1985.

25. M. Pagani, F. Lombardi, S. Guzzetti, et al., Power spectral analysis of heart rate and arterial pressure variabilities as a marker of sympatho-vagal interaction in man and conscious dog. *Circulation Research*, vol. 59, no. 2, pp. 178–193, 1986.

26. F. Lombardi, G. Sandrone, S. Pernpruner, et al., Heart rate variability as an index of sympathovagal interaction after acute myocardial infarction, *The American Journal of Cardiology*, vol. 60, no. 16, pp. 1239–1245, 1987.

27. R. Barbieri, E. Matten, A. Alabi, et al., A point process model of human heartbeat intervals: New definitions of heart rate and heart rate variability, *American Journal of Physiology-Heart and Circulatory Physiology*, vol. 288, no. 1, p. H424, 2005.

28. K. Chon, J. Kanters, N. Iyengar, et al., Detection of chaotic determinism in stochastic short time series, in *Engineering in Medicine and Biology Society, 1997. Proceedings of the 19th Annual International Conference of the IEEE*, vol. 1. IEEE, 1997, pp. 275–277.

29. C. Bian and X. Ning, Nonlinearity degree of short-term heart rate variability signal, *Chinese Science Bulletin*, vol. 49, no. 5, pp. 530–534, 2004.

30. M. Osaka, H. Kumagai, K. Sakata, et al., Low-order chaos in sympathetic nerve activity and scaling of heartbeat intervals, *Physical Review E*, vol. 67, no. 4, p. 041915, 2003.

31. A. A. Armoundas, K. Ju, N. Iyengar, et al., A stochastic nonlinear autoregressive algorithm reflects nonlinear dynamics of heart-rate fluctuations, *Annals of Biomedical Engineering*, vol. 30, no. 2, pp. 192–201, 2002.

32. H. Wang, K. Ju, and K. H. Chon, Closed-loop nonlinear system identification via the vector optimal parameter search algorithm: Application to heart rate baroreflex control, *Medical Engineering and Physics*, vol. 29, no. 4, pp. 505–515, 2007.

33. M. Gomes, A. Souza, H. Guimaraes, et al., Investigation of determinism in heart rate variability, *Chaos: An Interdisciplinary Journal of Nonlinear Science*, vol. 10, no. 2, pp. 398–410, 2000.

34. N. Wessel, H. Malberg, R. Bauernschmitt, et al., Nonlinear additive autoregressive model-based analysis of short-term heart rate variability, *Medical and Biological Engineering and Computing*, vol. 44, no. 4, pp. 321–330, 2006.

35. M. Riedl, A. Suhrbier, H. Malberg, et al., Modeling the cardiovascular system using a nonlinear additive autoregressive model with exogenous input, *Physical Review E*, vol. 78, no. 1, p. 011919, 2008.

36. L. Faes, H. Zhao, K. H. Chon, et al., Time-varying surrogate data to assess nonlinearity in nonstationary time series: Application to heart rate variability, *IEEE Transactions on Biomedical Engineering*, vol. 56, no. 3, pp. 685–695, 2009.

37. M. P. Tarvainen, S. D. Georgiadis, P. O. Ranta-aho, et al., Time-varying analysis of heart rate variability signals with a Kalman smoother algorithm, *Physiological Measurement*, vol. 27, no. 3, p. 225, 2006.

38. G. Valenza, L. Citi, R. Garcia, et al., Complexity variability assessment of nonlinear time-varying cardiovascular control. *Scientific reports*, 7, 2017.

39. G. Valenza, A. Greco, C. Gentili, et al., Combining electroencephalographic activity and instantaneous heart rate for assessing brain -heart dynamics during visual emotional elicitation in healthy subjects, *Phil. Trans. R. Soc. A, vol. 374, no. 2067*, 20150176, 2016.

40. G. Valenza, L. Citi, E. Scilingo, et al., Point-process nonlinear models with Laguerre and Volterra expansions: Instantaneous assessment of heartbeat dynamics, *IEEE Transactions on Signal Processing*, vol. 61, no. 11, pp. 2914–2926, 2013.

41. G. Valenza, L. Citi, and R. Barbieri, Instantaneous nonlinear assessment of complex cardiovascular dynamics by Laguerrevolterra point process models, in *Engineering in Medicine and Biology Society (EMBC), 2013 35th Annual International Conference of the IEEE*. IEEE, 2013, pp. 6131–6134.

42. G. Valenza, L. Citi, C. Gentili, et al., Characterization of depressive states in bipolar patients using wearable textile technology and instantaneous heart rate variability assessment, *IEEE Journal of Biomedical and Health Informatics*, 2015.

43. G. Valenza, L. Citi, A. Lanatá, et al., Revealing real-time emotional responses: A personalized assessment based on heartbeat dynamics, *Nature Scientific Reports*, vol. 4, no. 4998, pp. 1–13, 2014.

44. G. Valenza, L. Citi, E. P. Scilingo, et al., Inhomogeneous point-process entropy: An instantaneous measure of complexity in discrete systems, *Physical Review E*, vol. 89, no. 5, p. 052803, 2014.

45. V. Marmarelis, Modeling methology for nonlinear physiological systems, *Annals of Biomedical Engineering*, vol. 25, no. 2, pp. 239–251, 1997.

46. R. Barbieri, R. A. Waldmann, V. Di Virgilio, et al., Continuous quantification of baroreflex and respiratory control of heart rate by use of bivariate autoregressive techniques, *Annals of Noninvasive Electrocardiology*, vol. 1, no. 3, pp. 264–277, 1996.

47. R. Barbieri, G. Parati, and J. P. Saul, Closed versus open-loop assessment of heart rate baroreflex, *Engineering in Medicine and Biology Magazine, IEEE*, vol. 20, no. 2, pp. 33–42, 2001.

48. R. DeBoer, J. M. Karemaker, J. Strackee, et al., Hemodynamic fluctuations and baroreflex sensitivity in humans: A beat-to-beat model, *American Journal of Physiology*, vol. 253, no. 3 Pt 2, pp. H680–H689, 1987.

49. G. Baselli, S. Cerutti, S. Civardi, et al., Cardiovascular variability signals: Towards the identification of a closed-loop model of the neural control mechanisms, *IEEE Transactions on Biomedical Engineering*, vol. 35, no. 12, pp. 1033–1046, 1988.

50. B. Kohler, C. Hennig, and R. Orglmeister, The principals of software QRS detection, *IEEE Engineering in Medicine and Biology*, vol. 6, no. 1, pp. 42–57, 2002.

51. M. Elgendi, B. Eskofier, S. Dokos, et al., Revisiting QRS detection methodologies for portable, wearable, battery operated, and wireless ECG systems, *PLOS ONE*, vol. 9, no. 1, p. e84018, 2014.

52. N. Lippman, K. Stein, and B. Lerman, Nonlinear predictive interpolation. A new method for the correction of ectopic beats for heart rate variability analysis, *Journal of Electrocardiology*, vol. 26, p. 14, 1993.

53. N. Lippman, K. Stein, and B. Lerman, Comparison of methods for removal of ectopy in measurement of heart rate variability, *American Journal of Physiology Heart and Circulatory Physiology*, vol. 267, no. 1, p. H411, 1994.

54. L. Citi, E. Brown, and R. Barbieri, A real-time automated point process method for detection and correction of erroneous and ectopic heartbeats, *IEEE Transactions on Biomedical Engineering*, vol. 59, pp. 2828–2837, 2012.

55. G. D. Clifford and L. Tarassenko, Quantifying errors in spectral estimates of HRV due to beat replacement and resampling, *IEEE Transactions on Biomedical Engineering*, vol. 52, no. 4, pp. 630–638, 2005.

56. H. J. Jelinek, T. Alothman, D. J. Cornforth, et al., Effect of biosignal preprocessing and recording length on clinical decision making for cardiac autonomic neuropathy, in *Cardiovascular Oscillations (ESGCO), 2014 8th Conference of the European Study Group on*. IEEE, 2014, pp. 3–4.

57. D. Singh, K. Vinod, S. C. Saxena, et al., Effects of RR segment duration on HRV spectrum estimation, *Physiological Measurement*, vol. 25, no. 3, p. 721, 2004.

58. R. Berger, S. Akselrod, D. Gordon, et al., An efficient algorithm for spectral analysis of heart rate variability, *IEEE Transactions on Biomedical Engineering*, no. 9, pp. 900–904, 2007.

59. L. T. Mainardi, A. M. Bianchi, G. Baselli, et al., Pole-tracking algorithms for the extraction of time-variant heart rate variability spectral parameters, *IEEE Transactions on Biomedical Engineering*, vol. 42, no. 3, pp. 250–259, 1995.

60. L. T. Mainardi, On the quantification of heart rate variability spectral parameters using time–frequency and time-varying methods, *Philosophical Transactions of the Royal Society A: Mathematical, Physical and Engineering Sciences*, vol. 367, no. 1887, pp. 255–275, 2009.

61. M. Arnold, X. Milner, H. Witte, et al., Adaptive AR modeling of nonstationary time series by means of Kalman filtering, *IEEE Transactions on Biomedical Engineering*, vol. 45, no. 5, pp. 553–562, 1998.

62. J. McNames and M. Aboy, Statistical modeling of cardiovascular signals and parameter estimation based on the extended Kalman filter, *IEEE Transactions on Biomedical Engineering*, vol. 55, no. 1, pp. 119–129, 2008.

63. H. Akaike, Fitting autoregressive models for prediction, *Annals of the Institute of Statistical Mathematics*, vol. 21, no. 1, pp. 243–247, 1969.

64. A. Boardman, F. S. Schlindwein, A. P. Rocha, et al., A study on the optimum order of autoregressive models for heart rate variability, *Physiological Measurement*, vol. 23, no. 2, p. 325, 2002.

65. R. L. Burr and M. J. Cowan, Autoregressive spectral models of heart rate variability: Practical issues, *Journal of Electrocardiology*, vol. 25, pp. 224–233, 1992.
66. R. Takalo, H. Hytti, and H. Ihalainen, Tutorial on univariate autoregressive spectral analysis, *Journal of Clinical Monitoring and Computing*, vol. 19, no. 6, pp. 401–410, 2005.
67. P. B. Persson, Spectrum analysis of cardiovascular time series, *American Journal of Physiology-Regulatory, Integrative and Comparative Physiology*, vol. 273, no. 4, pp. R1201–R1210, 1997.
68. S. Cavalcanti, L. Chiari, S. Severi, et al., Parametric analysis of heart rate variability during hemodialysis, *International Journal of Bio-medical Computing*, vol. 42, no. 3, pp. 215–224, 1996.
69. J. Mateo and P. Laguna, Analysis of heart rate variability in the presence of ectopic beats using the heart timing signal, *IEEE Transactions on Biomedical Engineering*, vol. 50, no. 3, pp. 334–343, 2003.
70. F. Ng, S. Wong, P. Gomis, et al., Probabilistic assessment of autonomic nervous system fluctuations during tilt table tests, in *Engineering in Medicine and Biology Society, 2008. EMBS 2008. 30th Annual International Conference of the IEEE*. IEEE, 2008, pp. 4692–4695.
71. Z. Chen, E. Brown, and R. Barbieri, Assessment of autonomic control and respiratory sinus arrhythmia using point process models of human heart beat dynamics, *IEEE Transactions on Biomedical Engineering*, vol. 56, no. 7, pp. 1791–1802, 2009.
72. C. Granger and R. Joyeux, An introduction to long-memory time series models and fractional differencing, *Journal of Time Series Analysis*, vol. 1, no. 1, pp. 15–29, 1980.
73. L. Citi, G. Valenza, and R. Barbieri, Instantaneous estimation of high-order nonlinear heartbeat dynamics by lyapunov exponents, in *Engineering in Medicine and Biology Society (EMBC), 2012 Annual International Conference of the IEEE*. IEEE, 2012, pp. 13–16.
74. G. Valenza, L. Citi, and R. Barbieri, Estimation of instantaneous complex dynamics through Lyapunov exponents: A study on heartbeat dynamics. *PloS one*, vol. 9, no. 8, e105622, 2014.
75. C. Loader, *Local Regression and Likelihood*. Springer Verlag, New York, 1999.
76. R. Tibshirani and T. Hastie, Local likelihood estimation, *Journal of the American Statistical Association*, pp. 559–567, 1987.
77. E. Brown, R. Barbieri, U. Eden, et al., Likelihood methods for neural spike train data analysis, *Computational Neuroscience: A Comprehensive Approach*, pp. 253–286, 2003.
78. D. T. Westwick and R. E. Kearney, *Explicit Least-Squares Methods, In Identification of Nonlinear Physiological Systems*. John Wiley and Sons, Hoboken, NJ, 2003.
79. P. Koukoulas and N. Kalouptsidis, Nonlinear system identificationusing Gaussian inputs, *Signal Processing, IEEE Transactions on*, vol. 43, no. 8, pp. 1831–1841, 1995.
80. B. Sayers, Analysis of heart rate variability. *Ergonomics*, vol. 16, no. 1, p. 17, 1973.
81. G. A. Reyes del Paso, W. Langewitz, L. J. Mulder, et al., The utility of low frequency heart rate variability as an index of sympathetic cardiac tone: A review with emphasis on a reanalysis of previous studies, *Psychophysiology*, vol. 50, no. 5, pp. 477–487, 2013.
82. V. Marmarelis, Identification of nonlinear biological system using Laguerre expansions of kernels, *Annals of Biomedical Engineering*, vol. 21, pp. 573–589, 1993.
83. M. Schetzen, *The Volterra and Wiener Theories of Nonlinear Systems*, Wiley, Hoboken, NJ, 1980.
84. S. Billings, Identification of nonlinear system—A survey, *Proceedings of the IEEE*, vol. 127, pp. 272–285, 1980.
85. J. Le Caillec and R. Garello, Nonlinear system identification using autoregressive quadratic models, *Signal Processing*, vol. 81, no. 2, pp. 357–379, 2001.
86. R. Barbieri, M. Quirk, L. Frank, et al., Construction and analysis of non-Poisson stimulus-response models of neural spiking activity, *Journal of Neuroscience Methods*, vol. 105, no. 1, pp. 25–37, 2001.
87. M. Akay, *Nonlinear Biomedical Signal Processing Vol. II: Dynamic Analysis and Modeling*. Wiley-IEEE Press, Hoboken, NJ, 2000.
88. M. Korenberg and L. Paarmann, Orthogonal approaches to time-series analysis and system identification, *Signal Processing Magazine, IEEE*, vol. 8, no. 3, pp. 29–43, 1991.
89. M. Korenberg, Parallel cascade identification and kernel estimation for nonlinear systems, *Annals of Biomedical Engineering*, vol. 19, no. 4, pp. 429–455, 1991.

90. V. Marmarelis and T. Berger, General methodology for nonlinear modeling of neural systems with Poisson point-process inputs, *Mathematical Biosciences*, vol. 196, no. 1, pp. 1–13, 2005.

91. C. Nikias and J. Mendel, Signal processing with higher-order spectra, *Signal Processing Magazine, IEEE*, vol. 10, no. 3, pp. 10–37, 1993.

92. C. Nikias and A. Petropulu, Higher-order spectra analysis: A nonlinear signal processing framework, 1993.

93. C. Nikias and M. Raghuveer, Bispectrum estimation: A digital signal processing framework, *Proceedings of the IEEE*, vol. 75, no. 7, pp. 869–891, 1987.

94. J. Nichols, C. Olson, J. Michalowicz, et al., The bispectrum and bicoherence for quadratically nonlinear systems subject to non-Gaussian inputs, *IEEE Transactions on Signal Processing*, vol. 57, no. 10, pp. 3879–3890, 2009.

95. D. Brillinger, An introduction to polyspectra, *The Annals of Mathematical Statistics*, pp. 1351–1374, 1965.

96. J. Caillec and R. Garello, Asymptotic bias and variance of conventional bispectrum estimates for 2-D signals, *Multidimensional Systems and Signal Processing*, vol. 16, no. 1, pp. 49–84, 2005.

97. C. Nikias, *Higher-Order Spectral Analysis: A Nonlinear Signal Processing Framework*, Upper Saddle River, NJ: PTR Prentice-Hall, Inc., 1993.

98. D. R. Brillinger, M. Rosenblatt, and P. Petropulu, Computation and interpretation of kth order spectra, In *Spectral Analysis of Time Series*, B. Harris (Ed.), New York, NY: Wiley, pp. 189–232, 1967.

99. K. Chua, V. Chandran, U. Acharya, et al., Cardiac state diagnosis using higher order spectra of heart rate variability, *Journal of Medical Engineering and Technology*, vol. 32, no. 2, pp. 145–155, 2008.

100. A. Lanatá, G. Valenza, C. Mancuso, et al., Robust multiple cardiac arrhythmia detection through bispectrum analysis, *Expert Systems with Applications*, vol. 38, no. 6, pp. 6798–6804, 2011.

101. T. N. Chang and S. Sun, Blind detection of photomontage using higher order statistics, *IEEE International Symposium on Circuits and Systems (ISCAS)*, Vancouver, Canada, 2004.

102. S. Zhou, J. Gan, and F. Sepulveda, Classifying mental tasks based on features of higher-order statistics from EEG signals in brain-computer interface, *Information Sciences*, vol. 178, no. 6, pp. 1629–1640, 2008.

103. D. Brillinger, The identification of polynomial systems by means of higher order spectra* 1, *Journal of Sound and Vibration*, vol. 12, no. 3, pp. 301–313, 1970.

104. M. Priestley, *Spectral Analysis and Time Series*, Academic Press, Cambridge, MA, 1981.

105. T. Heldt, M. B. Oefinger, M. Hoshiyama, et al., Circulatory response to passive and active changes in posture, *Computers in Cardiology*, vol. 30, pp. 263–266, 2003.

106. T. Heldt, E. B. Shim, R. D. Kamm, et al., Computational modeling of cardiovascular response to orthostatic stress, *Journal of Applied Physiology (Bethesda, Md.: 1985)*, vol. 92, no. 3, pp. 1239–1254, Mar. 2002.

107. A. Porta, E. Tobaldini, S. Guzzetti, et al., Assessment of cardiac autonomic modulation during graded head-up tilt by symbolic analysis of heart rate variability, *American Journal of Physiology-Heart and Circulatory Physiology*, vol. 293, no. 1, pp. H702–H708, 2007.

108. K. Chon, T. Mullen, and R. Cohen, A dual-input nonlinear system analysis of autonomic modulation of heart rate, *IEEE Transactions on Biomedical Engineering*, vol. 43, no. 5, pp. 530–544, 1996.

109. W. Zong and G. Moody, WQRS-single-channel QRS detector based on length transform, *Physionet*. http://www.physionet.org/physiotools/1.htm, 2003.

110. A. Barnett and R. Wolff, A time-domain test for some types of nonlinearity, *IEEE Transactions on Signal Processing*, vol. 53, no. 1, pp. 26–33, 2005.

111. F. Wilcoxon, Individual comparisons by ranking methods, *Biometrics Bulletin*, vol. 1, no. 6, pp. 80–83, 1945.

112. S. Mason and N. Graham, Areas beneath the relative operating characteristics (ROC) and relative operating levels (ROL) curves: Statistical significance and interpretation, *Quarterly Journal of the Royal Meteorological Society*, vol. 128, no. 584, pp. 2145–2166, 2002.

113. A. Goldberger, L. Amaral, L. Glass, et al., PhysioBank, PhysioToolkit, and PhysioNet: Components of a new research resource for complex physiologic signals, *Circulation*, vol. 101, no. 23, p. e215, 2000.

114. C. Peng, S. Havlin, H. Stanley, et al., Quantification of scaling exponents and crossover phenomena in nonstationary heartbeat time series, *Chaos: An Interdisciplinary Journal of Nonlinear Science*, vol. 5, no. 1, p. 82, 1995.

115. Y. Fusheng, H. Bo, and T. Qingyu, Approximate entropy and its application in biosignal analysis, *Nonlinear Biomedical Signal Processing*, p. 72, 2000.

116. J. Richman and J. Moorman, Physiological time-series analysis using approximate entropy and sample entropy, *American Journal of Physiology-Heart and Circulatory Physiology*, vol. 278, no. 6, p. H2039, 2000.

117. P. Schwartz and G. De Ferrari, Sympathetic–parasympathetic interaction in health and disease: Abnormalities and relevance in heart failure, *Heart Failure Reviews*, pp. 1–7, 2010.

118. G. Valenza, M. Nardelli, G. Bertschy, et al., Mood states modulate complexity in heartbeat dynamics: A multiscale entropy analysis, *EPL (Europhysics Letters)*, vol. 107, no. 1, p. 18003, 2014.

119. A. Lanata, G. Valenza, M. Nardelli, et al., Complexity index from a personalized wearable monitoring system for assessing remission in mental health, *IEEE Journal of Biomedical and Health Informatics*, vol. 19, no. 1, pp. 132–139, 2015.

120. L. Citi, G. Valenza, P. Purdon, et al., Monitoring heartbeat nonlinear dynamics during general anesthesia by using the instantaneous dominant Lyapunov exponent, in *Engineering in Medicine and Biology Society (EMBC), 2012 Annual International Conference of the IEEE*. IEEE, 2012, pp. 3124–3127.

5

Assessing Complexity and Causality in Heart Period Variability through a Model-Free Data-Driven Multivariate Approach

Alberto Porta, Luca Faes, Giandomenico Nollo, Anielle C. M. Takahashi, and Aparecida M. Catai

CONTENTS

5.1 Introduction

Heart rate variability, that is, the spontaneous fluctuations of the inverse of heart period (HP) over time, is one of the most studied physiological time series. The key features of its success are: the relevance of the information encoded in it (Akselrod et al., 1981; Task Force of the European Society of Cardiology and the North American Society of Pacing and Electrophysiology, 1996), thus making more and more clinically relevant HP variability assessment; and the richness of the observed dynamics (Goldberger, 1996), thus prompting for the application of virtually any tool for signal processing to it. Most of the approaches applied to HP variability are model-based, being spectral analysis grounded on autoregressive modeling of the most frequently exploited one in univariate applications (Pagani et al., 1986). Model-based approaches are largely utilized in multivariate applications as well (Xiao et al., 2005; Porta et al., 2006, 2009) to describe the influences of determinants driving HP fluctuations through well-known physiological pathways. Among the determinants of HP variability, systolic arterial pressure (SAP) variability and respiration (RESP) play a relevant role by contributing directly to HP oscillations through the baroreflex (Baselli et al., 1994; Mullen et al., 1997; Porta et al., 2000b) and the coupling between respiratory centers and vagal outflow (Baselli et al., 1994; Triedman et al., 1995; Eckberg, 2003; Porta et al., 2012b), respectively. While the univariate model-based approach allows the description of the time course and frequency content of HP variability (Task Force of the European Society of Cardiology and the North American Society of Pacing and Electrophysiology, 1996), the multivariate model-based techniques permit the description of the relationship between HP variability and its determinants in terms of gain (Baselli et al., 1994; Patton et al., 1996), phase (Halamek et al., 2003; Porta et al., 2011), correlation (Porta et al., 2000b), degree of association along a given temporal direction (Porta et al., 2002; Nollo et al., 2005), and directionality of the interactions (Porta et al., 2012a, 2013b; Faes et al., 2013).

While the importance of model-based approaches is indubitable, model-free data-driven multivariate techniques are gaining more and more attention. This interest is motivated by the awareness that the description of the multivariate data set might be imprecise, and even incorrect, when the predefined model class does not match with the mechanism generating the recorded dynamics. Since, in physiological systems, the full description of the data–generating mechanism is more an exception than a rule, especially in integrated system physiology, the likelihood that the data-generating mechanism is perfectly described by a given model class is very low. In addition, even in the fortunate case of matching between a model class and data-generating mechanism, model parameters and their number should be estimated from noisy realizations, thus leading to discrepancies between the true parameters and the estimated ones and, consequently, between the dynamics generated by the model and by the original system (Soderstrom and Stoica, 1988). The waiver of making assumptions about the data-generating mechanism not only has contributed to an increase the appeal and popularity of model-free data-driven multivariate approaches but also has enlarged the possibility to describe time series dynamics without forcing them to fulfill to hypotheses that clearly do not hold in reality (e.g., linearity and/or Gaussian distributions).

The aim of this study is to emphasize the importance of model-free data-driven multivariate approaches in describing HP variability and cardiovascular control mechanisms responsible for inducing HP changes via modifications of different cardiovascular variables such as SAP and RESP. The goal was achieved through the application of a previously proposed model-free data-driven multivariate framework devised to assess complexity and causality over a multivariate set composed by several, simultaneously recorded, cardiovascular variability series (Porta et al., 2014). The approach was applied to assess: the complexity of the cardiac control, through the evaluation of the amount of irregularity of HP variability in a multivariate space accounting for HP, SAP, and RESP; and the degree of involvement of the cardiac baroreflex and cardiopulmonary pathway in governing cardiovascular interactions, through the evaluation of the strength of the causal link from SAP and RESP to HP variability. Modifications of complexity and causality during supine resting condition (REST) and during the orthostatic challenge resulting from active standing (STAND) were quantified as a function of age.

5.2 Methods

5.2.1 Estimating Complexity from HP Series via a Model-Free Data-Driven Multivariate Approach

We make reference to Porta et al. (2014) for the description of the model-free data-driven multivariate framework for the assessment of complexity of HP variability given the universe of knowledge $\Omega = \{HP,SAP,RESP\}$. Two approaches were considered (Porta et al., 2014). The first approach exploited a local predictability (LP) technique based on a k-nearest-neighbor approach (Farmer and Sidorowich, 1987; Abarbanel et al., 1994; Porta et al., 2007c). The HP complexity was estimated as the degree of HP unpredictability when past values of the same series and present and past samples of SAP and RESP were known. The degree of unpredictability was assessed as the degree of uncorrelation between the original and predicted signals (Porta et al., 2007c). It ranged from 0 to 1, where 0 indicated perfect predictability and null complexity, while 1 indicated null predictability and maximal complexity. The second approach computed the HP complexity as the residual HP uncertainty given past samples of the same series and present and past values of SAP and RESP. The residual HP uncertainty was quantified via conditional entropy (CE) estimated again via a k-nearest-neighbor approach (Porta et al., 2013a). The CE was divided by the Shannon entropy of HP series to obtain an index of complexity ranging again from 0 to 1, where 0 indicated perfect predictability and null complexity, while 1 indicated null predictability and maximal complexity (Porta et al., 2007a). The key feature of both LP and CE methods for the assessment of HP complexity was the construction of a multivariate nonuniform optimal embedding space where the dynamical interactions among HP, SAP, and RESP were unfolded and univocally described (Vlachos and Kugiumtzis, 2010; Faes et al., 2011; Porta et al., 2014). The embedding space was multivariate, nonuniform, and optimal because it could be formed by time-delayed components of different signals (here HP, SAP, and RESP); the time separation between adjacent components could be variable and the components were selected such a way to produce the maximal reduction of unpredictability or uncertainty in the case of LP and CE methods, respectively (Porta et al., 2014). The overall procedure was iterated until the minimum of HP unpredictability or uncertainty was reached (Porta et al., 2014) and the number of components at the minimum was labeled as $q_{HP^{LPo}}$ and $q_{HP^{CEo}}$, respectively. The degree of unpredictability and uncertainty at $q_{HP^{LPo}}$ and $q_{HP^{CEo}}$, respectively, was indicated as the normalized complexity index (NCI) and indicated as $NCI_{HP^{LP}}$ and $NCI_{HP^{CE}}$. Since the optimal embedding space could be formed by components of HP, SAP, and RESP, all these signals could contribute to $q_{HP^{LPo}}$. We indicated in the following with $q_{HP \to HP^{LPo}}$, $q_{SAP \to HP^{LPo}}$, and $q_{RESP \to HP^{LPo}}$ the number of components of HP, SAP, and RESP contributing to $q_{HP^{LPo}}$ with $q_{HP^{LPo}} = q_{HP \to HP^{LPo}} + q_{SAP \to HP^{LPo}} + q_{RESP \to HP^{LPo}}$. The relations $q_{HP \to HP^{LPo}} = 0$, $q_{SAP \to HP^{LPo}} = 0$, and $q_{RESP \to HP^{LPo}} = 0$, respectively, indicated that HP, SAP, or RESP did not influence the current value of HP. When $q_{HP \to HP^{LPo}} \neq 0$, $q_{SAP \to HP^{LPo}} \neq 0$, and $q_{RESP \to HP^{LPo}} \neq 0$, the minimal delay of past values of HP, SAP, and RESP on the current value of HP could be estimated, respectively. Similar decomposition of $q_{HP^{CEo}}$ could be obtained with $q_{HP^{CEo}} = q_{HP \to HP^{CEo}} + q_{SAP \to HP^{CEo}} + q_{RESP \to HP^{CEo}}$ and the minimal delay of interactions from HP, SAP, and RESP to HP could be estimated as well provided that $q_{HP \to HP^{CEo}} \neq 0$, $q_{SAP \to HP^{CEo}} \neq 0$, and $q_{RESP \to HP^{CEo}} \neq 0$, respectively.

5.2.2 Estimating Causality Indexes from SAP and RESP to HP a via a Model-Free Data-Driven Multivariate Approach

We make reference to Porta et al. (2014) for the description of the model-free data-driven multivariate framework for the assessment of causality indexes from SAP to HP along the cardiac baroreflex and from RESP to HP along the cardiopulmonary pathway given the universe of knowledge $\Omega = \{HP, SAP, RESP\}$. Two approaches were considered (Porta et al., 2014), based on the notion of Granger causality (Granger, 1980) and transfer entropy (Schreiber, 2000).

The first approach estimated the strength of the causal relation from a cause series to an effect one via a causality ratio (CR) quantifying the fractional decrement of the unpredictability of the assigned effect resulting from the inclusion of the presumed cause in the restricted set of signals that intentionally excluded the presumed cause (Granger, 1980). More specifically, if the presumed cause was SAP, the effect was HP and the reduced set was {HP, RESP}; the fractional decrement of the HP unpredictability due to the inclusion of SAP measured the strength of the causal relation from SAP to HP along the cardiac baroreflex (Porta et al., 2014). This index is indicated as $CR_{SAP \to HP^{LP}}$ in the following. If the presumed cause was RESP, the effect was HP and the restricted set was {HP, SAP}; the fractional decrement of the HP unpredictability due to the inclusion of RESP quantified the strength of the causal relation from RESP to HP along the cardiopulmonary pathway (Porta et al., 2014). This index is indicated as $CR_{RESP \to HP^{LP}}$ in the following. $CR_{SAP \to HP^{LP}} = 0$ and $CR_{RESP \to HP^{LP}} = 0$ indicated that the enlargement of the embedding space by including SAP and RESP respectively did not lead to the addition of any components of SAP and RESP, respectively, thus suggesting the absence of causality from SAP and RESP to HP. Conversely, $CR_{SAP \to HP^{LP}} < 0$ and $CR_{RESP \to HP^{LP}} < 0$ indicated that SAP and RESP, respectively, carried unique information about the future HP evolution that could not be derived from any signal in the restricted set, and according to the concept of Granger causality (Granger, 1980), it could be stated that SAP and RESP Granger-caused HP, respectively.

The second approach assessed the strength of the causal relation from a cause series to an effect one via a CR quantifying the fractional decrement of the information carried by the effect series resulting from the inclusion of the presumed cause in the restricted set of signals that deliberately excluded the presumed cause (Schreiber, 2000). In this case, the indexes measuring the strength of the casual relation from SAP and RESP to HP along the cardiac baroreflex and cardiopulmonary pathway respectively are labeled as $CR_{SAP \to HP^{CE}}$ and $CR_{RESP \to HP^{CE}}$ in the following. Analogously to the LP approach, $CR_{SAP \to HP^{CE}} = 0$ and $CR_{RESP \to HP^{CE}} = 0$ suggested the absence of causality from SAP and RESP to HP, while $CR_{SAP \to HP^{LP}} < 0$ and $CR_{RESP \to HP^{LP}} < 0$ indicated the presence of a causal relation from SAP and RESP to HP, respectively.

5.3 Experimental Protocol and Data Analysis

5.3.1 Experimental Protocol

We studied 100 nonsmoking healthy humans (54 males). The age of the subjects ranges from 21 to 70 years. The overall range of age was uniformly divided into five bins of size of 10 years. Table 5.1 summarizes the characteristics of the overall population and of any subgroup in the considered bins of age. The population was balanced in terms of gender to limit the influences of this confounding factor on the analysis (Barnett et al., 1999). All the subjects were apparently healthy, had no history, and no clinical evidence of any disease based on clinical and physical examinations, laboratory tests, standard electrocardiogram (ECG), and a maximum cardiopulmonary exercise test conducted by a physician. They were not taking any medication known to interfere with cardiovascular control. Smokers and habitual drinkers were excluded from this study. All subjects were evaluated in the afternoon. The experiments were carried out in a climatically controlled room (22–23° C) with relative air humidity at 40%–60%. Subjects were instructed not to consume caffeinated and alcoholic beverages as well as not to perform strenuous exercises on the day before the recording. They were also instructed to ingest a light meal at least 2 hours prior to the test.

TABLE 5.1

Characteristics of the Population

Age Bin (Years)	All Ages	21–30	31–40	41–50	51–60	61–70
Number of subjects	100 (54 M/46 F)	20 (10 M/10 F)	20 (11 M/9 F)	20 (10 M/10 F)	20 (10 M/10 F)	20 (13 M/7 F)
Age (years)	45 (21–70)	26	34	45	55	65
Weight (kg)	71 (43–100)	71	69	70	71	72
Height (cm)	167 (146–197)	168	168	167	169	164
BMI (kg · m^{-2})	25 (17.4–33.4)	23.9	24.8	25.4	25.1	26.7

M = male; F = female; BMI = body mass index. Values are given as median (1st quartile–3rd quartile).

On the day of the experiment, the subjects were interviewed and examined before the test to verify whether they were in good health and had a regular night of sleep. Prior to the recording, the volunteers were made familiar with the equipment and with the experimental procedure. During the entire protocol, the subjects breathed spontaneously but they were not allowed to talk. The study was performed according to the Declaration of Helsinki and it was approved by the Human Research Ethics Committee of the Federal University of São Carlos (protocol number 173/2011). A written informed consent was obtained from all subjects.

ECG (modified lead I), continuous plethysmographic arterial pressure (Finometer PRO, Finapress Medical System, The Netherlands), and respiratory movements via thoracic belt (Marazza, Monza, Italy) were digitalized using a commercial device (BioAmp Power Lab, AD Instruments, Australia). Signals were sampled at 400 Hz. The arterial pressure was measured from the middle finger of the left hand maintained at the level of heart by fixing the subject's arm to his/her thorax. All the experimental sessions of the protocol included two periods in the same order: (1) 15 minutes at REST and (2) 15 minutes during STAND. Before REST, we allowed 10 minutes for stabilization. The arterial pressure signal was cross-calibrated in each session using a measure provided by a sphygmomanometer at the onset of REST. The autocalibration procedure of the arterial pressure device was switched off after the first automatic calibration at the onset of the session. Analyses were performed after about 2 minutes from the start of each period.

5.3.2 Beat-to-Beat Variability Series Extraction and Index Calculation

After detecting the QRS complex on the ECG and locating the peak of the QRS complex using parabolic interpolation, HP was approximated as the temporal distance between two consecutive parabolic apexes. The maximum arterial pressure inside of the nth HP, HP(n), was taken as the nth SAP, SAP(n). The signal of the thoracic movements was downsampled once per cardiac beat at the occurrence of the first QRS peak delimiting HP(n), thus obtaining the nth RESP measure, RESP(n). The occurrences of QRS and SAP peaks were carefully checked to avoid erroneous detections or missed beats. After extracting the series HP $= \{$HP(n), $n = 1, \ldots, N\}$, SAP $= \{$SAP(n), $n = 1, \ldots, N\}$ and RESP $= \{$RESP(n), $n = 1, \ldots, N\}$, where n is the progressive cardiac beat counter and N is the total cardiac beat number, sequences of 256 consecutive measures were randomly selected inside REST and STAND periods, thus focusing on short-term cardiovascular regulatory mechanisms (Task Force of the European Society of Cardiology and the North American Society of Pacing and Electrophysiology, 1996). If evident nonstationarities, such as very slow drifting of the mean or sudden changes of the variance, were present despite the linear detrending, the random selection was carried out again. Traditional time domain parameters such as the mean and the variance of HP and SAP were calculated and indicated as μ_{HP}, μ_{SAP}, σ^2_{HP}, and σ^2_{SAP}. They were expressed in ms, mmHg, ms^2, and mmHg^2, respectively. RESP values were expressed in arbitrary units (a.u.). The possible immediate (i.e., within the same cardiac beat) effects of SAP and RESP on HP (Eckberg, 1976; Porta et al., 2012a) were accounted for by testing the presence of zero-lag interactions of SAP(n) and RESP(n) on HP(n). The number of nearest neighbors, k, was set to 30 for both LP and CE approaches (Porta et al., 2014). The maximal number of lagged components derived from each series and tested for the construction of the optimal embedding space was fixed to 10 and the maximal number of components forming the multivariate embedding space was fixed to 15. This choice imposed that

$q_{HP \to HP^{LPo}}$, $q_{SAP \to HP^{LPo}}$, $q_{RESP \to HP^{LPo}}$, $q_{HP \to HP^{CEo}}$, $q_{SAP \to HP^{CEo}}$, and $q_{RESP \to HP^{CEo}}$ ranged from 0 to 10, while $q_{HP^{LPo}}$ and $q_{HP^{CEo}}$ ranged from 0 to 15.

5.3.3 Statistical Analysis

After pooling together all the data regardless of age and the experimental condition (i.e., REST and STAND), we performed a paired *t*-test to check the significance of the difference between the optimal number of samples, q_{HP^o}, leading to the minimal unpredictability or uncertainty of the HP series assessed according to the LP and CE approaches, respectively. If the normality test (Kolmogorov–Smirnov test) was not fulfilled, the Wilcoxon signed rank test was utilized. After pooling together all the data regardless of age, the same test was exploited to evaluate the effect of the orthostatic challenge (i.e., STAND) on traditional parameters (i.e., μ_{HP}, σ^2_{HP}, μ_{SAP}, and σ^2_{SAP}) and, after having assigned the method (i.e., LP or CE), on NCI and CR. Two-way repeated measures analysis of variance (one factor repetition, Holm–Sidak test for multiple comparisons) was utilized to test the significance of the differences between the number of samples of HP, SAP, and RESP contributing to q_{HP^o} within the same method (i.e., LP and CE) and between methods within the same parameter. The $\chi 2$ test was utilized to test the effect of the experimental condition within the method (i.e., LP or CE) and the effect of the method within the experimental condition (i.e., REST or STAND) on the percentage of subjects with immediate influences from SAP and RESP to HP (McNemar's test). Linear regression analysis of μ_{HP}, σ^2_{HP}, μ_{SAP}, and σ^2_{SAP} on age was carried out. Pearson product-moment correlation coefficient was calculated. The same analysis was carried out to check the dependence of NCI and CR, as computed from LP and CE approaches, on age. Statistical analysis was carried out using a commercial statistical program (Sigmaplot, ver.11, Systat Software, San Jose, CA, USA). A $p < .05$ was always considered significant.

5.4 Results

5.4.1 Representative Examples of Complexity and Causality Analyses of HP Dynamics

Figure 5.1 shows a representative example of HP, SAP, and RESP series recorded at REST in a healthy young subject (age = 26 years) and in a healthy old individual (age = 70 years). This example shows a tendency of the HP series toward a reduction of HP variance, σ^2_{HP}, with age in the presence of an unchanged HP mean, μ_{HP}: μ_{HP} and σ^2_{HP} are 899 ms and 1758 ms^2, respectively in Figure 5.1a and 871 ms and 579 ms^2, respectively in Figure 5.1d. Conversely, SAP mean, μ_{SAP}, and variance, σ^2_{SAP}, tend to increase: μ_{SAP} and σ^2_{SAP} are 119 mmHg and 8 mmHg^2 in Figure 5.1b and 155 mmHg and 64 mmHg^2 in Figure 5.1e. In this example, $NCI_{HP^{LP}}$ and $NCI_{HP^{CE}}$ are 0.35 and 0.78, respectively, in the young subject and they are lower in the old individual (i.e., 0.19 and 0.68), thus indicating a reduction of complexity in terms of unpredictability and amount of information of the HP series. In the young subject, $CR_{SAP \to HP^{LP}}$ and $CR_{SAP \to HP^{CE}}$ are −0.03 and 0 and $CR_{RESP \to HP^{LP}}$ and $CR_{RESP \to HP^{CE}}$ are −0.59 and −0.19. In the old individual, $CR_{SAP \to HP^{LP}}$ and $CR_{SAP \to HP^{CE}}$ are equal to those derived from the young one. Conversely, in the old subject, $CR_{RESP \to HP^{LP}}$ and $CR_{RESP \to HP^{CE}}$ are less negative (−0.34 and −0.06).

Figure 5.2 shows a representative example of HP, SAP, and RESP series recorded during STAND in a healthy young subject (age = 30 years) and in a healthy old individual

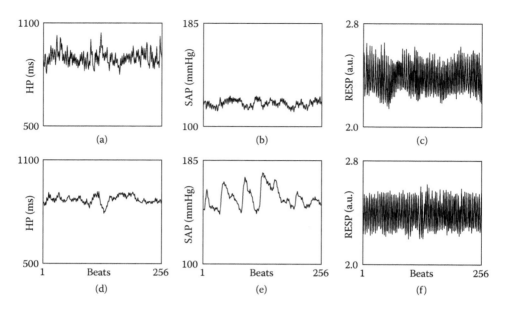

FIGURE 5.1
HP, SAP, and RESP series recorded at REST in a healthy young (age = 26 years) subject are shown in (a), (b), and (c), respectively, while those recorded in the same condition in a healthy old (age = 70 years) individual are depicted in (d), (e), and (f), respectively.

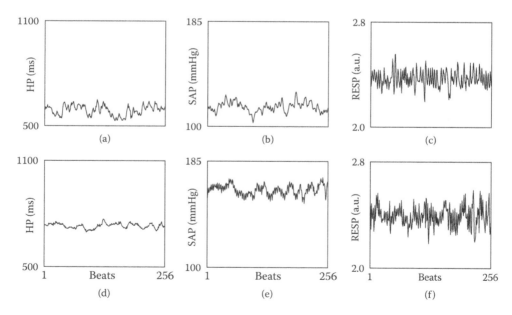

FIGURE 5.2
HP, SAP, and RESP series recorded during STAND in a healthy young (age = 30 years) subject are shown in (a), (b), and (c), respectively, while those recorded in the same condition in a healthy old (age = 70 years) individual are depicted in (d), (e), and (f), respectively.

(age = 70 years). This example shows a tendency toward an increase of μ_{HP} and to a decrease of σ^2_{HP} with age: μ_{HP} and σ^2_{HP} were 588 ms and 784 ms^2 in Figure 5.2a and 732 ms and 201 ms^2 in Figure 5.2d. μ_{SAP} exhibits a marked increase from 117 (Figure 5.2b) to 162 mmHg (Figure 5.2e), while σ^2_{SAP} is similar (i.e., 21 and 17 mmHg^2). In this example, $NCI_{HP^{LP}}$ is 0.13 in the young subject and higher in the old individual (i.e., 0.19), thus indicating an increase of complexity in terms of unpredictability of the HP series. $NCI_{HP^{CE}}$ is more balanced, 0.61 and 0.62 in the young and old subject, respectively. In the young subject, $CR_{SAP \to HP^{LP}}$, $CR_{SAP \to HP^{CE}}$, $CR_{RESP \to HP^{LP}}$, and $CR_{RESP \to HP^{CE}}$ are $-0.36, 0, 0$, and 0. In the old subject, $CR_{SAP \to HP^{LP}}$ becomes less negative (i.e., -0.09) and $CR_{SAP \to HP^{CE}}$, $CR_{RESP \to HP^{LP}}$ and $CR_{RESP \to HP^{CE}}$ are similar (i.e., 0, -0.02, and 0, respectively).

5.4.2 Optimal Number of Components and Zero-Lag Interactions

The bar graph in Figure 5.3 shows the mean (plus standard deviation) of the total number of components (i.e., the optimal embedding dimension), q_{HP^o}, leading to the smallest unpredictability of the HP series according to the LP technique, and to the minimal amount of information carried by the HP series according to CE. Values of q_{HP^o} were pooled together independently of the experimental condition (i.e., REST and STAND) and age. The LP and CE approaches had different levels of parsimoniousness: the number of components necessary to reduce the HP uncertainty to the minimum was significantly smaller than the one needed to decrease the unpredictability to the nadir (the median value of $q_{HP^{LPo}}$ and $q_{HP^{CEo}}$ was 4 and 2, respectively).

q_{HP^o} was decomposed into three terms, $q_{HP \to HP^o}$, $q_{SAP \to HP^o}$, and $q_{RESP \to HP^o}$, featuring the number of HP, SAP, and RESP samples contributing to the reduction of unpredictability and uncertainty of the HP series. Figure 5.4 reports the mean (plus standard deviation) of $q_{HP \to HP^o}$ (white bar), $q_{SAP \to HP^o}$ (gray bar), and $q_{RESP \to HP^o}$ (black bar) as a function of the method (i.e., LP and CE). Values of $q_{HP \to HP^o}$, $q_{SAP \to HP^o}$, and $q_{RESP \to HP^o}$ were pooled together regardless of the experimental condition (i.e., REST and STAND) and age. The LP approach led to values of $q_{HP \to HP^{LPo}}$ larger than $q_{SAP \to HP^{LPo}}$ and $q_{RESP \to HP^{LPo}}$, while $q_{SAP \to HP^{LPo}}$ and $q_{RESP \to HP^{LPo}}$ were similar. The CE technique clearly suggested a different importance of HP, SAP, and RESP in diminishing HP uncertainty. Indeed, $q_{HP \to HP^{CEo}}$ was the largest value and $q_{SAP \to HP^{CEo}}$ was the smallest one. The difference between $q_{HP^{LPo}}$

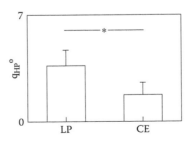

FIGURE 5.3
Bar graph shows mean plus standard deviation of the optimal total number of components, q_{HP^o}, leading to the smallest unpredictability of HP series according to the LP approach (i.e., $q_{HP^{LPo}}$) and to the minimal amount of information carried by HP series according to CE (i.e., $q_{HP^{CEo}}$). The values of q_{HP^o} were pooled together regardless of the experimental conditions (i.e., REST and STAND) and age. The symbol * indicates a significant difference with $p < .001$.

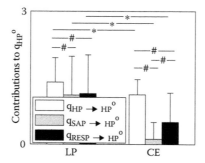

FIGURE 5.4
Grouped bar graph shows mean plus standard deviation of the number of HP ($q_{HP\rightarrow HP^o}$, white bar), SAP ($q_{SAP\rightarrow HP^o}$, gray bar), and RESP ($q_{RESP\rightarrow HP^o}$, black bar) samples contributing to the optimal number of components, q_{HP^o}, leading to the smallest unpredictability of HP series according to the LP approach (i.e., $q_{HP\rightarrow HP^{LPo}}$, $q_{SAP\rightarrow HP^{LPo}}$ and $q_{RESP\rightarrow HP^{LPo}}$) and to the minimal amount of information carried by HP series according to CE (i.e., $q_{HP\rightarrow HP^{CEo}}$, $q_{SAP\rightarrow HP^{CEo}}$, and $q_{RESP\rightarrow HP^{CEo}}$). The values of $q_{HP\rightarrow HP^o}$, $q_{SAP\rightarrow HP^o}$, and $q_{RESP\rightarrow HP^o}$ were pooled together regardless of the experimental condition (i.e., REST and STAND) and age. The symbol * indicates a significant difference with $p < .05$ within the same index while varying the method. The symbol # indicates a significant difference with $p < .05$ within the same method while varying the index.

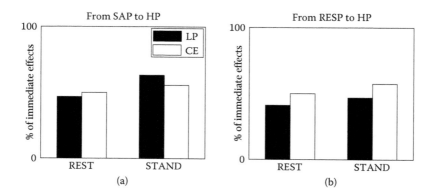

FIGURE 5.5
Grouped bar graphs show the percentage of subjects with immediate effects (i.e., zero-lag interactions) from SAP to HP (a) and from RESP to HP (b) as a function of the experimental condition (REST and STAND). The percentage was calculated by accounting solely for subjects with $q_{SAP\rightarrow HP^o} \neq 0$ and $q_{RESP\rightarrow HP^o} \neq 0$ in (a) and (b), respectively. Black bars represent the percentage of subjects with immediate effects assessed according to LP approach, while the white bars represent that computed according to CE. Subjects were pooled together independently of age. No significant difference was detected.

and $q_{HP^{CEo}}$, reported in Figure 5.3, was explained in Figure 5.4 in terms of a significant decline of $q_{HP\rightarrow HP^{CEo}}$, $q_{SAP\rightarrow HP^{CEo}}$, and $q_{RESP\rightarrow HP^{CEo}}$ compared to $q_{HP\rightarrow HP^{LPo}}$, $q_{SAP\rightarrow HP^{LPo}}$, and $q_{RESP\rightarrow HP^{LPo}}$, respectively.

Figure 5.5 shows the effect of the orthostatic stimulus on the percentage of subjects exhibiting immediate effects (i.e., zero-lag interactions) from SAP to HP (Figure 5.5a) and from RESP to HP (Figure 5.5b). Subjects were pooled together independently of age. Among subjects with $q_{SAP\rightarrow HP^o} \neq 0$ and $q_{RESP\rightarrow HP^o} \neq 0$, the percentage of subjects with immediate effects did not vary with the type of approach (i.e., LP or CE) and the experimental condition (i.e., REST or STAND).

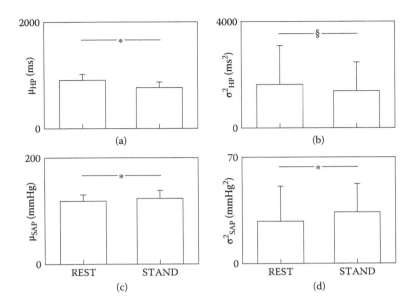

FIGURE 5.6
Bar graphs show mean plus standard deviation of HP mean, μ_{HP} (a), HP variance, σ^2_{HP} (b), SAP mean, μ_{SAP} (c), and SAP variance, σ^2_{SAP} (d) as a function of the experimental condition (i.e., REST and STAND). Values of μ_{HP}, σ^2_{HP}, μ_{SAP}, and σ^2_{SAP} were pooled together regardless of age. The symbols * and § indicate a significant difference with $p < .001$ and $p < .05$, respectively.

5.4.3 Effects of Orthostatic Challenge on HP Complexity and Causality Indexes

Figure 5.6 shows the bar graphs of μ_{HP}, σ^2_{HP}, μ_{SAP}, and σ^2_{SAP} (mean plus standard deviation) as a function of the experimental condition (i.e., REST and STAND). Values of μ_{HP}, σ^2_{HP}, μ_{SAP}, and σ^2_{SAP} were pooled together independently of age. STAND induced a significant decrease of μ_{HP} (Figure 5.6a) and σ^2_{HP} (Figure 5.6b) and a significant increase of μ_{SAP} (Figure 5.6c) and σ^2_{SAP} (Figure 5.6d).

Figure 5.7 reports the bar graphs of NCI_{HP} (mean plus standard deviation) as a function of the experimental condition (i.e., REST and STAND) estimated by the LP and CE approaches. Values of NCI_{HP} were pooled together independently of age. Both LP (Figure 5.7a) and CE (Figure 5.7b) techniques detected a significant decrease of NCI_{HP} during STAND, thus suggesting that the orthostatic challenge reduced unpredictability and uncertainty of the HP series.

Figure 5.8 reports the bar graphs of $CR_{SAP \to HP}$ and $CR_{RESP \to HP}$ (mean minus standard deviation) as a function of the experimental condition (i.e., REST and STAND) estimated by the LP and CE approaches. Values of $CR_{SAP \to HP}$ and $CR_{RESP \to HP}$ were pooled together independently of age. $CR_{SAP \to HP}{}^{LP}$ became significantly more negative during STAND (Figure 5.8a) and this trend revealed an augmentation of the strength of the causal link from SAP to HP. $CR_{SAP \to HP}{}^{CE}$ was unable to detect the same effect of STAND (Figure 5.8b). STAND affected $CR_{RESP \to HP}$ as well (Figure 5.8c and d). Indeed, $CR_{RESP \to HP}$ significantly moved toward 0, thus indicating a reduced strength of the causal link from RESP to HP. This finding was confirmed both by $CR_{RESP \to HP}{}^{LP}$ (Figure 5.8c) and $CR_{RESP \to HP}{}^{CE}$ (Figure 5.8d).

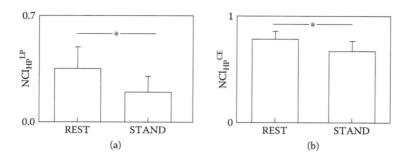

FIGURE 5.7

Bar graphs show mean plus standard deviation of NCI of the HP series, NCI_{HP}, in (a) and (b), as a function of the experimental condition (REST and STAND). The bar graph in (a) is relevant to indexes computed according to the LP approach, while the bar graph in (b) is relevant to those calculated according to CE. Values of NCI_{HP} were pooled together regardless of age. The symbol * indicates a significant difference with $p < .001$.

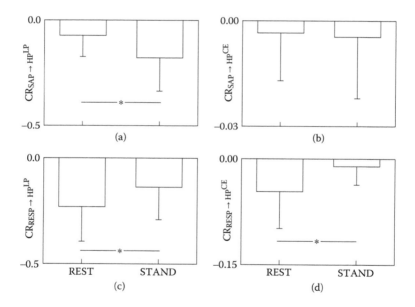

FIGURE 5.8

Bar graphs show mean minus standard deviation of CR from SAP to HP, $CR_{SAP \to HP}$, in (a) and (b), and of CR from RESP to HP, $CR_{RESP \to HP}$, in (c) and (d) as a function of the experimental condition (REST and STAND). The bar graphs in (a) and (c) are relevant to indexes computed according to the LP approach, while bar graphs (b) and (d) are relevant to those calculated according to CE. Values of $CR_{SAP \to HP}$ and $CR_{RESP \to HP}$ were pooled together regardless of age. The symbol * indicates a significant difference with $p < .001$.

5.4.4 Linear Regression Analysis on HP Complexity and Causality Indexes on Age

Table 5.2 reviews the results of linear regression analysis of time domain HP and SAP variability parameters on age at REST. While μ_{HP} was unrelated to age, σ^2_{HP}, μ_{SAP}, and σ^2_{SAP} were found significantly correlated with age. The correlation coefficient, r_P, was negative in the case of σ^2_{HP}, thus indicating that the magnitude of the HP variations progressively decreased with age and was positive in the case of μ_{SAP} and σ^2_{SAP}, thus evidencing that

TABLE 5.2

Linear Regression Analysis of Time-Domain HP and SAP Variability Parameters on Age at REST

	r_P	p	Significance
μ_{HP}	0.0418	6.80×10^{-1}	No
σ^2_{HP}	−0.391	5.77×10^{-5}	Yes
μ_{SAP}	0.243	1.48×10^{-2}	Yes
σ^2_{SAP}	0.403	3.22×10^{-5}	Yes

μ_{HP} = HP mean; σ^2_{HP} = HP variance; μ_{SAP} = SAP mean; σ^2_{SAP} = SAP variance; r_P = Pearson product-moment correlation coefficient; p = probability of type-I error; Yes/No = the variable is/is not significantly related to age with $p < .05$.

TABLE 5.3

Linear Regression Analysis of Time-Domain HP and SAP Variability Parameters on Age during STAND

	r_P	p	Significance
μ_{HP}	0.306	1.97×10^{-3}	Yes
σ^2_{HP}	−0.430	7.88×10^{-6}	Yes
μ_{SAP}	0.299	2.54×10^{-3}	Yes
σ^2_{SAP}	0.0104	9.18×10^{-1}	No

μ_{HP} = HP mean; σ^2_{HP} = HP variance; μ_{SAP} = SAP mean; σ^2_{SAP} = SAP variance; r_P = Pearson product-moment correlation coefficient; p = probability of type-I error; Yes/No = the variable is/is not significantly related to age with $p < .05$.

TABLE 5.4

Linear Regression Analysis of Model-Free Data-Driven Multivariate Indexes of HP Complexity on Age at REST

	r_P	p	Significance
$NCI_{HP^{LP}}$	−0.357	2.69×10^{-4}	Yes
$NCI_{HP^{CE}}$	−0.317	1.33×10^{-3}	Yes

$NCI_{HP^{LP}}$, $NCI_{HP^{CE}}$ = normalized complexity index of HP series derived from LP and CE approaches; r_P = Pearson product-moment correlation coefficient; p = probability of type-I error; Yes/No = the variable is/is not significantly related to age with $p < .05$.

both SAP and the magnitude of its changes increased with age. It is worth noting that p assessed over σ^2_{SAP} was three orders of magnitude larger than that relevant to μ_{SAP}.

Table 5.3 summarizes the results of linear regression analysis of time-domain HP and SAP parameters on age during STAND. Different from REST, μ_{HP} was significantly linearly correlated with age. r_P was positive, thus suggesting that orthostatic challenge induced a tachycardic response becoming less and less important with age. Similarly to REST, the progressive decrease of σ^2_{HP} and the gradual increase of μ_{SAP} were significant. During STAND no linear relation was detected between σ^2_{SAP} and age.

Table 5.4 reports the results of linear regression analysis of HP complexity parameters on age at REST. $NCI_{HP^{LP}}$ and $NCI_{HP^{CE}}$ were significantly linearly correlated with age. r_P was negative, thus suggesting a progressive loss of complexity of HP dynamics with age. Table 5.5 summarizes the results of linear regression analysis of HP complexity indexes on age during STAND. This table suggests a different behavior between HP complexity indexes assessed according to LP and CE techniques. Only $NCI_{HP^{LP}}$ was found significantly related to age (the type-I error probability of the linear relation of $NCI_{HP^{CE}}$ on age was close to the significance level). r_P of $NCI_{HP^{LP}}$ on age was positive, thus suggesting that HP variability during STAND became more and more unpredictable with age.

Table 5.6 reports the results of linear regression analysis of parameters assessing causality from SAP and RESP to HP on age at REST. Both $CR_{SAP \to HP^{LP}}$ and $CR_{SAP \to HP^{CE}}$ were unrelated to age. Conversely, both $CR_{RESP \to HP^{LP}}$ and $CR_{RESP \to HP^{CE}}$ progressively became less negative with age (r_P was positive), thus suggesting that aging reduced the strength of the causal link from RESP to HP. Table 5.7 summarizes the results of linear regression analysis of parameters assessing causality from SAP and RESP to HP on age during STAND. Causality analysis indicated another different behavior between the LP and CE approaches. Indeed, while $CR_{SAP \to HP^{LP}}$ was significantly linearly correlated with age, $CR_{SAP \to HP^{CE}}$ was unrelated to it. r_P of $CR_{SAP \to HP^{LP}}$ on age was positive, thus indicating that the strength of the causal link from SAP to HP became gradually weaker and weaker

TABLE 5.5

Linear Regression Analysis of Model-Free Data-Driven Multivariate Indexes of HP Complexity on Age during STAND

	r_P	p	Significance
$NCI_{HP^{LP}}$	0.244	1.42×10^{-2}	Yes
$NCI_{HP^{CE}}$	0.179	7.52×10^{-2}	No

$NCI_{HP^{LP}}$, $NCI_{HP^{CE}}$ = normalized complexity index of HP series derived from LP and CE approaches; r_P = Pearson product-moment correlation coefficient; p = probability of type-I error; Yes/No = the variable is/is not significantly related to age with $p < .05$.

TABLE 5.6

Linear Regression Analysis of Model-Free Data-Driven Multivariate Causality Indexes from SAP and RESP to HP on Age at REST

	r_P	p	Significance
$CR_{SAP \to HP^{LP}}$	-0.0677	5.03×10^{-1}	No
$CR_{SAP \to HP^{CE}}$	0.0203	8.41×10^{-1}	No
$CR_{RESP \to HP^{LP}}$	0.201	4.47×10^{-2}	Yes
$CR_{RESP \to HP^{CE}}$	0.380	9.47×10^{-5}	Yes

$CR_{SAP \to HP^{LP}}$, $CR_{SAP \to HP^{CE}}$ = causality ratio from SAP to HP series derived from LP and CE approaches; $CR_{RESP \to HP^{LP}}$, $CR_{RESP \to HP^{CE}}$ = causality ratio from RESP to HP series derived from LP and CE approaches; r_P = Pearson product-moment correlation coefficient; p = probability of type-I error; Yes/No = the variable is/is not significantly related to age with $p < .05$.

TABLE 5.7

Linear Regression Analysis of Model-Free Data-Driven Multivariate Causality Indexes from SAP and RESP to HP on Age during STAND

	r_P	p	Significance
$CR_{SAP \to HP}^{LP}$	0.326	9.51×10^{-4}	Yes
$CR_{SAP \to HP}^{CE}$	0.00152	9.88×10^{-1}	No
$CR_{RESP \to HP}^{LP}$	−0.149	1.40×10^{-1}	No
$CR_{RESP \to HP}^{CE}$	−0.182	7.00×10^{-2}	No

$CR_{SAP \to HP}^{LP}$, $CR_{SAP \to HP}^{CE}$ = causality ratio from SAP to HP series derived from LP and CE approaches; $CR_{RESP \to HP}^{LP}$, $CR_{RESP \to HP}^{CE}$ = causality ratio from RESP to HP series derived from LP and CE approaches; r_P = Pearson product-moment correlation coefficient; p = probability of type-I error; Yes/No = the variable is/is not significantly related to age with $p < .05$.

with age. The LP and CE approaches provided similar results in the case of causality from RESP to HP: indeed, both $CR_{RESP \to HP}^{LP}$ and $CR_{RESP \to HP}^{CE}$ were unrelated to age.

5.5 Discussion

5.5.1 Discussion of the Methodological Findings

The first part of the discussion is mainly devoted to methodological issues supporting the relevance of applying model-free data-driven multivariate techniques in studies carried out to elucidate mechanisms underpinning cardiovascular regulation and, more specifically, to quantify the complexity of the cardiac control and the strength of the causal relations among cardiovascular variables. In this section, a subsection is devoted to the comparison between two traditional approaches for the assessment of complexity and causality (i.e., LP and CE) in the context of the analysis of cardiovascular control. This comparison was allowed by the peculiar characteristic of the specific model-free data-driven multivariate framework adopted in this study (Porta et al., 2014).

5.5.1.1 On the Importance of Applying a Model-Free Data-Driven Multivariate Framework for the Evaluation of the Cardiovascular Control from Spontaneous Physiological Variations

The present study stresses the importance of applying a model-free data-driven multivariate approach for the characterization of HP variability and its dependence on variations of physiological variables different from HP such as SAP and RESP. Traditionally, parameters helpful to describe HP variability were computed via both model-free (Akselrod et al., 1981) and model-based (Pagani et al., 1986) univariate techniques. However, the univariate approach fails in accounting for possible influences of physiological variables over HP variability, thus providing a limited interpretation of the HP dynamics, preventing the understanding of the origin of HP changes and limiting the clinical application of HP variability indexes due to the lack of association to specific physiological mechanisms. In order to overcome these shortcomings, multivariate model-based approaches have been proposed (Baselli et al., 1994; Mullen et al., 1997; Xiao et al., 2005; Porta et al., 2006, 2009). These methods were found very helpful in providing a more complete picture of HP variability via the quantification of transfer functions linking fluctuations of cardiovascular variables to HP changes (Mullen et al., 1997; Xiao et al., 2005) and the decomposition of HP variability into the contributions attributable to specific physiological mechanisms (Porta et al., 2006, 2012b). However, these methods hypothesize that the interactions among variability series could be faithfully explained in terms of linear relations usually described by standard linear multivariate regression models (Baselli et al., 1994; Mullen et al., 1997; Xiao et al., 2005; Porta et al., 2006, 2009). Even though the hypothesis of linearity might hold in several experimental conditions and the small amount of HP changes, especially in pathological subjects, might allow the linearization of a nonlinear system about the mean values of the variables, linear dynamics or small variations cannot be considered ubiquitous features in HP variability studies. In addition, even if one of the two abovementioned prerequisites holds, the general structure of the adopted model class might lead to inefficient reproduction of the HP dynamics especially when the model order was kept low to avoid overparametrization. According to these considerations, model-free data-driven techniques should be favored in exploratory studies based on little information about the underlying system, while model-based approaches should be considered as a secondary option. Conversely, due to the usual superior computational efficiency of model-based approaches compared to model-free ones, model-based techniques should be privileged when more robust information about the system's behavior is provided. However, even in this case the application of a model-free data-driven multivariate approach should not be discarded because it can provide an additional check about the final conclusions of the analysis.

5.5.1.2 *Application of a Model-Free Data-Driven Multivariate Framework for the Evaluation of Complexity of HP Dynamics and the Causal Relations from SAP and RESP to HP Variability*

The model-free data-driven multivariate approach to the assessment of complexity of a time series and to the evaluation of the strength of the causal relations between two series while accounting for the confounding influences of signals different from the presumed cause and assigned effect proposed in Porta et al. (2014) was applied to HP, SAP, and RESP series recorded to quantify the influences of aging on cardiovascular regulation. The adopted approach is completely different from more traditional techniques for the assessment of complexity of HP variability and this difference is the consequence of its multivariate nature. Indeed, in the usual definition, complexity is evaluated according to the degree of irregularity of the HP dynamics computed solely on the basis of the past history of HP series via both LP (Sugihara et al., 1996; Porta et al., 2000a, 2007c) and CE (Pincus et al., 1993; Porta et al., 2000c, 2007b, 2013a; Richman and Moorman, 2000; Javorka et al., 2008). Conversely, complexity evaluation provided by the adopted approach is based on the past history of all the signals included in the multivariate universe of knowledge $\Omega = \{HP,SAP,RESP\}$. Therefore, while traditional indexes measure low complexity only in the presence of repetitive patterns in the designated effect signal (i.e., HP), with our definition, low complexity may also be encountered when complex dynamics of the effect signal are explained by the dynamics of the other signals included in Ω.

The exploitation of a multivariate universe of knowledge $\Omega = \{HP,SAP,RESP\}$ is particularly attractive in cardiovascular variability studies. Indeed, even though the vast majority of the applications assessing cardiovascular variability interactions are based on a bivariate universe of knowledge $\Omega = \{HP, SAP\}$, for example, in the case of the assessment of baroreflex sensitivity (Laude et al., 2004), it was demonstrated that RESP is a latent confounder for the HP-SAP variability interactions (Porta et al., 2012a; Bassani et al., 2013) due to contemporaneous RESP actions on both HP and SAP variability (Saul et al., 1991; Baselli et al., 1994). Therefore, conditioning for RESP is mandatory to correctly disambiguate the temporal directions of the interactions between HP and SAP, thus suggesting that the minimal set of cardiovascular variability series deserving attention to describe cardiovascular regulation is $\Omega = \{HP, SAP, RESP\}$. The importance of considering $\Omega = \{HP, SAP, RESP\}$ is dramatically evident in experimental conditions in which the RESP drive is particularly powerful such as during controlled respiration especially at slow breathing rates (Porta et al., 2012a) and under mechanical ventilation during general anesthesia (Bassani et al., 2013). However, it is worth stressing that, since the formation of Ω is arbitrary, results are fully dependent on the specific view underpinning its construction. Defining $\Omega = \{HP, SAP, RESP\}$ and HP as the assigned effect, the underlying view mainly accounts for baroreflex control of HP and respiratory-related influences on HP mainly mediated by the variations of the vagal outflow, while modifications of HP due to changes of peripheral resistances or sympathetic outflow independent of cardiac baroreflex are disregarded. Nevertheless, the adopted fully multivariate approach might allow future enlargement of Ω, thus virtually accounting for any correlation between the assigned effect and the presumed cause and due to the common action of sources on both.

5.5.1.3 Comparison between LP and CE Approaches for the Assessment of Complexity of HP Dynamics and Causal Relations from SAP and RESP to HP Variability

The model-free data-driven multivariate approach adopted in this study allowed the comparison between two different approaches for the assessment of complexity HP dynamics and causal relations from SAP and RESP to HP variability. The two approaches, largely exploited in the literature for the assessment of both complexity (Sugihara et al., 1996; Porta et al., 2000a,c; Pincus et al., 1993; Richman and Moorman, 2000) and causality (Granger, 1980; Schreiber, 2000; Porta et al., 2014) are based on LP and CE. The comparison of the two approaches in the context of HP variability analysis pointed out that the both the LP and CE methods found an amount of past HP samples helpful to reduce unpredictability and uncertainty of HP dynamics, $q_{HP \rightarrow HP^\circ}$, significantly different from 0. This finding suggests that exogenous sources taken into account in this study (i.e., SAP and RESP) were unable to account for all the *prima facie* causes of HP changes, thus prompting for the search for additional, significant determinants of the HP dynamics. Alternatively, resonance properties of mechanisms capable of regulating HP independently of SAP and RESP should be hypothesized.

Regardless of age and experimental conditions, the LP approach identified a total number of components helpful to reduce HP unpredictability and uncertainty to a minimum, q_{HP°, greater than the CE technique. It might be hypothesized that comparison between original and predicted HP dynamics might unveil dependencies over past samples that the direct assessment of degree of HP uncertainty cannot discover. This difference between the LP and CE approaches leads to the different ability of the two approaches in detecting the effects of STAND. Indeed, while both the LP and CE approaches detected the decrease of complexity of HP dynamics and of the strength of the causal relation from RESP to HP during REST, the increase of the strength of the causal link from SAP to HP was detected only by the LP method during STAND. Since a major involvement of cardiac baroreflex control is expected during STAND, the disappointing performance of CE might indicate an excessive parsimoniousness of CE preventing the inclusion of a sufficient number of SAP samples in the optimal embedding space. This parsimoniousness is certainly helpful to limit the rate of false detection of causality when causality is not present (i.e., false positives), but it might increase the rate of false negatives (i.e., the probability of missing causality when a causal link exists). The greater parsimoniousness of CE might also explain the reduced statistical power of the CE approach in detecting the progressive increase of complexity of HP dynamics with age during STAND (the probability of type-I error was close to the significance value) compared to the LP approach.

5.5.2 Discussion of the Experimental Findings

The second part of the discussion is mainly devoted to experimental considerations relevant to the application of a model-free data-driven multivariate technique to HP, SAP, and RESP series for the evaluation of the complexity of the cardiac control, as assessed through HP variability, and of the degree of involvement of cardiac baroreflex and cardiopulmonary pathway, as evaluated via the quantification of the strength of the casual relation from SAP and RESP to HP variability, respectively. This part discusses findings linked to orthostatic challenge and to senescence.

5.5.2.1 *Effect of Orthostatic Challenge on HP and SAP Traditional Parameters*

After pooling together all the subjects independently of age, orthostatic challenge induces a decrease of HP mean and variance and an increase of SAP mean and variance. This result is in agreement with (Cooke et al., 1999; Laitinen et al., 2004; Porta et al., 2011; Turianikova et al., 2011) considering cohorts of subjects with narrower ranges of age. This finding was interpreted as a consequence of the vagal withdrawal and/or sympathetic enhancement induced by the caudal shift of blood induced by the postural change. While the increase of tonic sympathetic activity and/or its modulation (i.e., the amplitude of the changes of sympathetic activity about its mean value) was proved (Cooke et al., 1999; Furlan et al., 2000), changes of vagal activity and its modulation were usually inferred from HP variability (Montano et al., 1994; Cooke et al., 1999; Porta et al., 2007d).

5.5.2.2 *Effect of Orthostatic Challenge on Complexity of HP Dynamics and Causal Relations from SAP and RESP to HP Variability*

This study confirms that STAND induces a significant decrease of complexity of HP dynamics (Turianikova et al., 2011). The most likely mechanism responsible for this finding is the decrease of vagal modulation directed to the heart limiting respiratory sinus arrhythmia (Montano et al., 1994; Cooke et al., 1999; Porta et al., 2007d; Turianikova et al., 2011). The reduction of vagal influences directed to the heart prevents fast HP changes, thus limiting the number of temporal scales that can be exploited by the cardiovascular control to regulate HP and, consequently, the dynamical complexity of HP variability (Porta et al., 2007b, 2012c). This finding corroborates previous results indicating that the complexity of HP dynamics is under vagal control. Indeed, it decreased gradually with the magnitude of the orthostatic challenge during graded head-up tilt (Porta et al., 2007b, 2012c), it was markedly reduced during cholinergic blockade induced by high dose of atropine (Porta et al., 2007c, 2012c), and it was unaffected by beta-adrenergic blockade induced by propranolol or after central blockade of the sympathetic outflow to the heart and vasculature carried out by clonidine (Porta et al., 2012c). Our study supports further the hypothesis of the inability of respiratory influences to impinge on the heart. Indeed, the strength of the causal relation from RESP to HP was significantly reduced during STAND (Porta et al., 2012b). This finding suggests that the reduction of the respiratory sinus arrhythmia observed during STAND (Montano et al., 1994; Cooke et al., 1999; Porta et al., 2007d; Turianikova et al., 2011) is more likely to be the result of the uncoupling of the HP dynamics from the respiratory-related fluctuations of the vagal outflow than the effect of a decrease of the gain of the transfer function between the vagal outflow and HP variability. In addition, this study suggests a further possible explanation for the decrease of complexity of HP variability during STAND. Indeed, we found that the magnitude of the causal link from SAP to HP increased during STAND (Porta et al., 2012b), thus indicating an increased impact of SAP variability on HP dynamics and, consequently, an augmented role of baroreflex in the HP regulation during STAND. The increased impact of SAP on HP during STAND played a direct role in decreasing HP complexity because it produces a larger decrement of unpredictability and of information carried by HP. The major involvement of baroreflex in regulating HP during orthostatic stress is not surprising: indeed, baroreflex is the main reflex involved in the maintenance of blood pressure levels in the presence of the reduction of venous return induced by the change of posture. This observation corroborates previous findings suggesting the increased role played by baroreflex in governing HP–SAP variability interactions during passive orthostatic stress (Nollo et al., 2002, 2005; Porta et al., 2011, 2013c). This result is particularly robust because it is independent of the type of approach actually exploited to estimate causality; indeed, it was found by both the LP and CE techniques in the present study, a model-free approach in the information domain in Porta et al. (2011) and Nollo et al. (2002), a model-based approach in the time domain in Porta et al. (2013c), and a model-based approach in the frequency domain in Nollo et al. (2005).

5.5.2.3 *Effect of Age on HP and SAP Traditional Parameters*

We confirm that at REST, the mean HP is unrelated to age (Laitinen et al., 2004), mean SAP progressively increases with age (Laitinen et al., 2004), and HP variance gradually decreases (Beckers et al., 2006; Kaplan et al., 1991; O'Brien et al., 1986). The tendency of SAP variance to increase with age at REST observed in Laitinen et al. (1999) was found to be to significant in this study. Several mechanisms have been advocated to explain these relations with age: (1) the depressed pacemaker activity of sinoatrial node myocytes (Larson et al., 2013); (2) the gradual augmentation of tonic sympathetic activity as measured from postganglionic sympathetic nerves directed to skeletal muscles (Seals and Esler, 2000; Parker Jones et al., 2003); (3) the progressive increase of norepinephrine concentrations (Ziegler et al., 1976; Parker Jones et al., 2003; Barnett et al., 1999); (4) the continuing decline of vagal modulation as assessed from the amplitude of respiratory sinus arrhythmia in the time or frequency domain (Hrushesky et al., 1984; Beckers et al., 2006); (5) the gradual alteration of the adrenoceptor function (Kelly and O'Malley, 1984); (6) the progressive diminution of the responsiveness of the sinus node to sympathetic outflow (Lakatta, 1993; Barnett et al., 1999; Laitinen et al., 2004); and (7) the regular decrease of baroreflex sensitivity (Laitinen et al., 2004; Barnett et al., 1999; Veermann et al., 1994; Parker Jones et al., 2003).

During STAND, we confirm the positive dependence of HP mean and the negative relation of HP variance on age (O'Brien et al., 1986; Barnett et al., 1999), the positive correlation of SAP mean with age (Veermann et al., 1994), and the lack of a linear relation between SAP variance and age (Veermann et al., 1994; Barnett et al., 1999). These results were explained by the reduced effect of the postural maneuver on the cardiovascular variables due to the diminished responsiveness of the sinus node to neural inputs in response to stressors (Lakatta, 1993; Esler et al., 1995; Barnett et al., 1999; Laitinen et al., 2004), by the reduced responsiveness of the vasculature to vasodilatator agents (Elliott et al., 1982) and in reaction to stimuli (Veermann et al., 1994; Barnett et al., 1999; Laitinen et al., 2004), by the increase of peripheral resistances (Laitinen et al., 2004), and by the decreased baroreflex efficiency in response to the postural challenge (Laitinen et al., 2004).

5.5.2.4 Effect of Age on Complexity of HP Dynamics and Causal Relations from SAP and RESP to HP Variability

This study confirms the gradual decrease of complexity of HP dynamics with age (Kaplan et al., 1991; Pikkujamsa et al., 1999; Takahashi et al., 2012; Viola et al., 2011; Beckers et al., 2006). The result was obtained by exploiting a multivariate set of information about the behavior of the cardiovascular control system (i.e., HP, SAP, and RESP series), thus possibly avoiding inaccuracies of the reconstruction of the system dynamics that might happen using only one signal due to the presence of subsystems unobservable from HP series. As a consequence of its multivariate nature, the exploited approach is completely different from traditional approaches using only HP series to quantify the complexity of the cardiac control (Kaplan et al., 1991; Pikkujamsa et al., 1999; Takahashi et al., 2012; Viola et al., 2011). The gradual decrease of the complexity of HP variability appears to be robust because it was detected by both the LP and CE approaches. As a new finding, STAND was associated with a progressive increase of HP complexity with age measured according to the LP approach. Since HP complexity during STAND decreased as a result of the sympathetic activation and vagal withdrawal, this finding indicates a reduced ability of the cardiovascular system to cope with the postural challenge leading to more and more limited reduction of HP complexity in response to postural challenge with age. This finding is less evident with CE (the type-I error probability is larger than the selected level of significance but close to it), although the tendency is the same (i.e., correlation coefficient is positive). Therefore, we suggest the use of complexity indexes and the response to orthostatic challenge to quantify the reduced ability of cardiovascular control of elderly subjects to cope with stressors.

Regardless of the technique exploited to assess causality at REST, we did not find any linear relation of the strength of the causal link from SAP to HP on age. This finding suggests that the importance of the causal link from SAP to HP was not modified by aging. This result might appear surprising at the first sight because it was observed that baroreflex sensitivity gradually fell with age (Barnett et al., 1999; Parker Jones et al., 2003; Laitinen et al., 1998). However, it is worth recalling that the decrease of the gain of the relation from SAP to HP does not necessarily imply diminished strength of the causal link from SAP to HP because the two indexes bring complementary information (Porta et al., 2013b,c). In addition, since at REST, the dominant direction of interactions is from HP to SAP (Porta et al., 2011, 2013b), the unmodified importance of the causal relation from SAP to HP with age stresses again the negligible involvement of the cardiac baroreflex in governing the HP–SAP variability interactions during REST. During STAND, we observed a gradual reduction of the strength of the causal link from SAP to HP with age, thus suggesting a progressively less efficient baroreflex control with age. This result was pointed out only by the LP approach likely because it is easier for this approach to explore higher dimensional phase spaces compared to the CE technique. We suggest that causality indexes from SAP to HP might be fruitfully exploited to monitor the degree of efficiency of cardiac baroreflex control and its deterioration with senescence, especially during a baroreflex challenge such as STAND.

Another relevant finding of this study is the progressive decrease with age of the strength of the causal link from RESP to HP at REST. This finding was independent of the paradigm utilized to assess causality; indeed, the same result was obtained using both the LP and CE approaches. This finding corroborates recent observations (Nemati et al., 2013; Iatsenko et al., 2013). This result might be the consequence of the progressive increase of tonic sympathetic activity and vagal withdrawal leading to a gradual uncoupling between respiratory centers and the heart. During STAND, the strength of the causal link from RESP to HP was unrelated to age. This result was independent of the technique utilized to assess causality. Since STAND induces a sympathetic activation and vagal withdrawal (Cooke et al., 1999; Furlan et al., 2000) and, consequently, a reduction of the respiratory sinus arrhythmia (Veermann et al., 1994; Javorka et al., 2008), it can be concluded that the residual respiratory sinus arrhythmia might be insufficient for tracking modification of the strength of the HP–RESP causal coupling with age or, alternatively, HP changes at the respiratory rate might be driven by SAP changes through the stimulated cardiac baroreflex instead of being the result of central respiratory influences.

5.6 Conclusions

This study applied a model-free data-driven multivariate framework for the assessment of the complexity of HP variability and its causal interactions with SAP and RESP series. The study demonstrated the practical usefulness of the approach in describing HP variability and its ability to quantify the contribution of specific physiological mechanisms to cardiovascular regulation. Indeed, the method was found helpful to monitor changes associated to the senescence process and to assess the response of the cardiovascular control to an orthostatic challenge. The approach does not require prior assumptions about the physiological mechanisms underpinning HP dynamics and its relation with SAP and RESP and produces practical indexes necessitating the setting of very few parameters, essentially limited to the number of nearest neighbors necessary for coarse graining the multivariate embedding space. Given these features, the adopted model-free data-driven multivariate approach is highly recommended in any exploratory analysis in which classical multivariate model-based approach might be inappropriate due to the presence of nonlinearities and/or the absence of any reasonable physiological hypothesis about the mathematical relations linking the cardiovascular variables. Given the promising results, the proposed indexes should be tested on larger databases of healthy and pathological individuals along with more traditional HP variability indexes with the aim at assessing their extra value.

Acknowledgments

This study was supported by the São Paulo Foundation for Research Support/Brazil, (FAPESP, process 2010/52070-4) and by a CAPES grant to A.P. (project number A012_2013) supporting his position of Special Visiting Professor at the Department of Physiotherapy, Federal University of São Carlos, São Carlos, Brazil.

References

Abarbanel, H.D.I., T.L. Carroll, L.M. Pecora et al. 1994. Predicting physical variables in time-delay embedding. *Phys. Rev. E. 49*:1840–1853.

Akselrod, S., D. Gordon, F.A. Ubel et al. 1981. Power spectrum analysis of heart rate fluctuations: A quantitative probe of beat-to-beat cardiovascular control. *Science. 213*:220–223.

Barnett, S.R., R.J. Morin, D.K. Kiely et al. 1999. Effects of age and gender on autonomic control of blood pressure dynamics. *Hypertension. 33*:1195–1200.

Baselli, G., S. Cerutti, F. Badilini et al. 1994. Model for the assessment of heart period and arterial pressure variability interactions and respiratory influences. *Med. Biol. Eng. Comput. 32*:143–152.

Bassani, T., V. Bari, A. Marchi et al. 2013. Coherence analysis overestimates the role of baroreflex in governing the interactions between heart period and systolic arterial pressure variabilities during general anesthesia. *Auton. Neurosci. Basic Clin. 178*:83–88.

Beckers, F., B. Verheyden and A.E. Aubert. 2006. Aging and nonlinear heart rate control in a healthy population. *Am. J. Physiol. 290*:H2560–H2570.

Cooke, W.H., J.B. Hoag, A.A. Crossman et al. 1999. Human responses to upright tilt: A window on central autonomic integration. *J. Physiol. 517*:617–628.

Eckberg, D.L. 1976. Temporal response patterns of the human sinus node to brief carotid baroreceptor stimuli. *J. Physiol. 258*:769–782.

Eckberg, D.L. 2003. The human respiratory gate. *J. Physiol. 548*:339–352.

Elliott, H.L., D.J. Summer, K. McLean et al. 1982. Effect of age on the responsiveness of vascular alpha-adrenoceptors in man. *J. Cardiovasc. Pharmacol. 4*:388–392.

Esler, M.D., J.M. Thompson, D.M. Kaye et al. 1995. Effects of aging on the responsiveness of the human cardiac sympathetic nerves to stressors. *Circulation. 91*:351–358.

Faes, L., S. Erla, A. Porta et al. 2013. A framework for assessing frequency domain causality in physiological time series with instantaneous effects. *Phil. Trans. R. Soc. A. 371*:20110618.

Faes, L., G. Nollo and A. Porta. 2011. Information-based detection of nonlinear Granger causality in multivariate processes via a nonuniform embedding technique. *Phys. Rev. E. 83*:051112.

Farmer, J.D. and J.J. Sidorowich. 1987. Predicting chaotic time series. *Phys. Rev. Lett. 59*:845–848.

Furlan, R., A. Porta, F. Costa et al. 2000. Oscillatory patterns in sympathetic neural discharge and cardiovascular variables during orthostatic stimulus. *Circulation. 101*:886–892.

Goldberger, A.L. 1996. Non-linear dynamics for clinicians: Chaos theory, fractals and complexity at the bedside. *Lancet. 347*:1312–1314.

Granger, C.W.J. 1980. Testing for causality. A personal viewpoint. *J. Econ. Dyn. Control. 2*:329–352.

Halamek, J., T. Kara, P. Jurak et al. 2003. Variability of phase shift between blood pressure and heart rate fluctuations. A marker of short-term circulation control. *Circulation. 108*:292–297.

Hrushesky, W.J.M., D. Fader, O. Schmitt et al. 1984. The respiratory sinus arrhythmia: A measure of cardiac age. *Science. 224*:1001–1004.

Iatsenko, D., A. Bernjak, T. Stankovski et al. 2013. Evolution of cardiorespiratory interactions with age. *Phil. Trans. R. Soc. A. 371*:20110622.

Javorka, M., Z. Trunkvalterova, I. Tonhajzerova et al. 2008. Short-term heart rate complexity is reduced in patients with type 1 diabetes mellitus. *Clin. Neurophysiol. 119*:1071–1081.

Kaplan, D.T., M.I. Furman, S.M. Pincus et al. 1991. Aging and the complexity of cardiovascular dynamics. *Biophys. J. 59*:945–949.

Kelly, J. and K. O'Malley. 1984. Adrenoceptor function and ageing. *Clin. Sci. 66*:509–515.

Laitinen, T., J. Hartikainen, L. Niskanen et al. 1999. Sympathovagal balance is major determinant of short-term blood pressure variability in healthy subjects. *Am. J. Physiol. 276*:H1245–H1252.

Laitinen, T., J. Hartikainen, E. Vanninen et al. 1998. Age and gender dependency of baroreflex sensitivity in healthy subjects. *J. Appl. Physiol. 84*:576–583.

Laitinen, T., L. Niskanen, G. Geelen et al. 2004. Age dependency of cardiovascular autonomic responses to head-up tilt in healthy subjects. *J. Appl. Physiol. 96*:2333–2340.

Lakatta, E.G. 1993. Cardiovascular regulatory mechanisms in advanced age. *Physiol. Rev. 73*:413–465.

Larson, E.D., J.R. St Clair, W.A. Summer et al. 2013. Depressed pacemaker activity of sinoatrial node myocytes contributes to the age-dependent decline in maximum heart rate. *Proc. Natl. Acad. Sci U S A.* 110:18011–18016.

Laude, D., J.L. Elghozi, A. Girard et al. 2004. Comparison of various techniques used to estimate spontaneous baroreflex sensitivity (the EuroBaVar study). *Am. J. Physiol.* 286:R226–R231.

Montano, N., T. Gnecchi-Ruscone, A. Porta et al. 1994. Power spectrum analysis of heart rate variability to assess changes in sympatho-vagal balance during graded orthostatic tilt. *Circulation.* 90:1826–1831.

Mullen, T.J., M.L. Appel, R. Mukkamala et al. 1997. System identification of closed loop cardiovascular control: Effects of posture and autonomic blockade. *Am. J. Physiol.* 272:H448–H461.

Nemati, S., B.A. Edwards, J. Lee et al. 2013. Respiration and heart rate complexity: Effects of age and gender assessed by band-limited transfer entropy. *Respir. Physiol. Neurobiol.* 189:27–33.

Nollo, G., L. Faes, A. Porta et al. 2002. Evidence of unbalanced regulatory mechanism of heart rate and systolic pressure after acute myocardial infarction. *Am. J. Physiol.* 283:H1200–H1207.

Nollo, G., L. Faes, A. Porta et al. 2005. Exploring directionality in spontaneous heart period and systolic arterial pressure variability interactions in humans: Implications in the evaluation of baroreflex gain. *Am. J. Physiol.* 288:H1777–H1785.

O'Brien, I.A.D., P. O'Hare and R.J.M. Corrall. 1986. Heart rate variability in healthy subjects: Effect of age and the derivation of normal ranges for tests of autonomic function. *Br Heart J.* 55: 348–354.

Pagani, M., F. Lombardi, S. Guzzetti et al. 1986. Power spectral analysis of heart rate and arterial pressure variabilities as a marker of sympatho-vagal interaction in man and conscious dog. *Circ. Res.* 59:178–193.

Parker Jones, P., D.D. Christou, J. Jordan et al. 2003. Baroreflex buffering is reduced with age in healthy men. *Circulation.* 107:1770–1774.

Patton, D.J., J.K. Triedman, M.H. Perrott et al. 1996. Baroreflex gain: Characterization using autoregressive moving average analysis. *Am. J. Physiol.* 270:H1240–H1249.

Pikkujamsa, S.M., T.H. Makikallio, L.B. Sourander et al. 1999. Cardiac interbeat interval dynamics from childhood to senescence. Comparison of conventional and new measures based on fractals and chaos theory. *Circulation.* 100:393–399.

Pincus, S.M., T.R. Cummins and G.G. Haddad. 1993. Heart rate control in normal and aborted-SIDS infants. *Am. J. Physiol.* 33:R638–R646.

Porta, A., F. Aletti, F. Vallais et al. 2009. Multimodal signal processing for the analysis of cardiovascular variability. *Phil. Trans. R. Soc. A.* 367:391–408.

Porta, A., G. Baselli and C. Cerutti. 2006. Implicit and explicit model-based signal processing for the analysis of short-term cardiovascular interactions. *Proc. IEEE.* 94:805–818.

Porta, A., G. Baselli, S. Guzzetti et al. 2000a. Prediction of short cardiovascular variability signals based on conditional distribution. *IEEE Trans. Biomed. Eng.* 47:1555–1564.

Porta, A., G. Baselli, O. Rimoldi et al. 2000b. Assessing baroreflex gain from spontaneous variability in conscious dogs: Role of causality and respiration. *Am. J. Physiol.* 279:H2558–H2567.

Porta, A., T. Bassani, V. Bari et al. 2012a. Accounting for respiration is necessary to reliably infer Granger causality from cardiovascular variability series. *IEEE Trans. Biomed. Eng.* 59:832–841.

Porta, A., T. Bassani, V. Bari et al. 2012b. Model-based assessment of baroreflex and cardiopulmonary couplings during graded head-up tilt. *Comput. Biol. Med.* 42:298–305.

Porta, A., P. Castiglioni, V. Bari et al. 2013a. K-nearest-neighbor conditional entropy approach for the assessment of short-term complexity of cardiovascular control. *Physiol. Meas.* 34:17–33.

Porta, A., P. Castiglioni, M. di Rienzo et al. 2012c. Short-term complexity indexes of heart period and systolic arterial pressure variabilities provide complementary information. *J. Appl. Physiol.* 113:1810–1820.

Porta, A., P. Castiglioni, M. di Rienzo et al. 2013b. Cardiovascular control and time domain Granger causality: Insights from selective autonomic blockade. *Phil. Trans. R. Soc. A.* 371:20120161.

Porta, A., A.M. Catai, A.C.M. Takahashi et al. 2011. Causal relationships between heart period and systolic arterial pressure during graded head-up tilt. *Am. J. Physiol.* 300:R378–R386.

Porta, A., L. Faes, V. Bari et al. 2014. Effect of age on complexity and causality of the cardiovascular control: Comparison between model-based and model-free approaches. *PLOS ONE. 9*:e89463.

Porta, A., L. Faes, M. Masé et al. 2007a. An integrated approach based on uniform quantization for the evaluation of complexity of short-term heart period variability: Application to 24h Holter recordings in healthy and heart failure humans. *Chaos. 17*:015117.

Porta, A., R. Furlan, O. Rimoldi et al. 2002. Quantifying the strength of the linear causal coupling in closed loop interacting cardiovascular variability signals. *Biol. Cybern. 86*:241–251.

Porta, A., T. Gnecchi-Ruscone, E. Tobaldini et al. 2007b. Progressive decrease of heart period variability entropy-based complexity during graded head-up tilt. *J. Appl. Physiol. 103*:1143–1149.

Porta, A., S. Guzzetti, R. Furlan et al. 2007c. Complexity and nonlinearity in short-term heart period variability: Comparison of methods based on local nonlinear prediction. *IEEE Trans. Biomed. Eng. 54*:94–106.

Porta, A., S. Guzzetti, N. Montano et al. 2000c. Information domain analysis of cardiovascular variability signals: Evaluation of regularity, synchronisation and co-ordination. *Med. Biol. Eng. Comput. 38*:180–188.

Porta, A., A.C.M. Takahashi, A.M. Catai et al. 2013c. Assessing causal interactions among cardiovascular variability series through a time domain Granger causality approach. In: Baccalà L. and Sameshima K. (Eds). *Methods in Brain Connectivity Inference through Multivariate Time Series Analysis*. Boca Raton, Ann Arbor, London, Tokyo: CRC Press, 223–242.

Porta, A., E. Tobaldini, S. Guzzetti et al. 2007d. Assessment of cardiac autonomic modulation during graded head-up tilt by symbolic analysis of heart rate variability. *Am. J. Physiol. 293*:H702–H708.

Richman, J.S. and J.R. Moorman. 2000. Physiological time-series analysis using approximate entropy and sample entropy. *Am. J. Physiol. 278*:H2039–H2049.

Saul, J.P., R.D. Berger, P. Albrecht et al. 1991. Transfer function analysis of the circulation: Unique insights into cardiovascular regulation. *Am. J. Physiol. 261*:H1231–H1245.

Schreiber, T. 2000. Measuring information transfer. *Phys. Rev. Lett. 85*:461–464.

Seals, D.R. and M.D. Esler. 2000. Human ageing and sympathoadrenal system. *J. Physiol. 528*:407–417.

Soderstrom, T. and P. Stoica. 1988. *System Identification*. Englewood Cliffs, NJ: Prentice Hall.

Sugihara, G., W. Allan, D. Sobel and K.D. Allan. 1996. Nonlinear control of heart rate variability in humans infants. *Proc. Nat. Acad. Sci. 93*:2608–2613.

Takahashi, A.C.M., A. Porta, R.C. Melo et al. 2012. Aging reduces complexity of heart rate variability assessed by conditional entropy and symbolic analysis. *Intern. Emerg. Med. 7*:229–235.

Task Force of the European Society of Cardiology and the North American Society of Pacing and Electrophysiology. 1996. Standard of measurement, physiological interpretation and clinical use. *Circulation. 93*:1043–1065.

Triedman, J.K., M.H. Perrott, R.J. Cohen et al. 1995. Respiratory sinus arrhythmia: Time domain characterization using autoregressive moving average analysis. *Am. J. Physiol. 268*:H2232–H2238.

Turianikova, Z., K. Javorka, M. Baumert et al. 2011. The effect of orthostatic stress on multiscale entropy of heart rate and blood pressure. *Physiol. Meas. 32*:1425–1437.

Veermann, D.P., B.P.M. Imholz, W. Wieling et al. 1994. Effects of aging on blood pressure variability in resting conditions. *Hypertension. 24*:120–130.

Viola, A.U., E. Tobaldini, S.L. Chellappa et al. 2011. Short-term complexity of cardiac autonomic control during sleep: REM as a potential risk factor for cardiovascular system in aging. *PLOS ONE. 6*:e19002.

Vlachos, I. and D. Kugiumtzis. 2010. Nonuniform state-space reconstruction and coupling direction. *Phys. Rev. E. 82*:016207.

Xiao, X., T.J. Mullen and R. Mukkamala. 2005. System identification: A multi-signal approach for probing neural cardiovascular regulation. *Physiol. Meas. 26*:R41–R71.

Ziegler, M.G., C.R. Lake and I.J. Kopin. 1976. Plasma noradrenaline increases with age. *Nature. 261*:333–334.

6

Visualization of Short-Term Heart Period Variability with Network Tools as a Method for Quantifying Autonomic Drive

Danuta Makowiec, Beata Graff, Agnieszka Kaczkowska, Grzegorz Graff, Dorota Wejer, Joanna Wdowczyk, Marta Żarczyńska-Buchowiecka, Marcin Gruchała, and Zbigniew R. Struzik

CONTENTS

6.1 Introduction

Network methods have been successfully used to capture and represent properties of multilevel complex man-made systems (Havlin et al. 2012) and living organisms (Bashan et al. 2012). The use of network representations in the characterization of time series complexity is a relatively new but quickly developing branch of time series analysis (Donner et al. 2010; Fortunato 2010). The most direct method is to map a time series into a graph in which the vertices represent signal values, while edges link values that are consecutive in a signal. The correspondence between the time series formed by consecutive cardiac interbeat intervals, so-called *RR*-intervals, and such networks was studied by Campanharo et al. (Campanharo et al. 2011). The topology in these networks appeared as a clique, that is, each state is reachable from any other in a single step. Understanding

RR-interval dynamics arising from a network with such a structure is not straightforward. It appears, in general, that information provided by a network graph strongly depends on the nature of sequences and our knowledge about the underlying dynamics (Fortunato 2010; Havlin et al. 2012). Therefore, the use of network methods, for example, visualization or/and structure decomposition, is effective only if they are used in conjunction with other sources of learning. We show how the tools developed within the scope of complex networks can be fruitfully applied to the qualification and quantification of short-term heart period dynamics. Fluctuations in *RR*-intervals are known to have a scale-invariant structure which demonstrates fractal (Kobayashi and Musha 1982; Yamamoto and Hughson 1991; Peng et al. 1995) and multifractal (Ivanov et al. 1999) properties. These fluctuations appear as a result of many component interactions acting over a wide range of time and space scale. Competing stimuli from the autonomic nervous system are assumed to be the reason for the fractal organization observed in *RR*-intervals (Struzik et al. 2004). By observing subsequent changes in *RR*-intervals—ΔRR—beat-to-beat information about the resulting force of these interactions is obtained, and important dynamical aspects about the autonomic competitive regulation can be described by changes in *RR*-intervals, namely by *RR*-increments (Makowiec et al. 2013a, 2014). Signal increments of ΔRR can be decomposed into their magnitude (absolute value) and their direction (sign). Magnitude of $|\Delta RR|$ and sign of ΔRR analysis have been used to investigate the scaling properties of *RR*-intervals (Ashkenazy et al. 2001). It has been found by detrended fluctuation analysis that magnitude series are long-range correlated, while sign series are anticorrelated (i.e., correlation follows the power-law with exponents 0.74 for $|\Delta RR|$ and 0.40 for sign(ΔRR)). Furthermore, it has also been shown that during sleep, the strength of these correlations varies depending on the stage of the sleep: rapid-eye-movement (REM) or other (non-REM) sleep stages (Kantelhardt et al. 2002). It appears that both the strongest anticorrelations in the sign signals, and largest exponents for long-range correlations for the magnitude signals are in REM sleep. Furthermore, the nonlinear properties of the heartbeat dynamics are more pronounced during REM sleep (Schmitt et al. 2009). During sleep, the heart rate is mostly regulated by the autonomic nervous system and is less influenced by physical or mental activity. Moreover, during the night, vagal (parasympathetic) predominance is present, which makes this period a useful state to observe autonomic activity (Bonnemeier et al. 2003). The nonlinear tools (Shannon entropy, corrected conditional entropy) applied to measuring heart rate variability during physiological sleep have shown that the REM stage is characterized by a likely sympathetic predominance associated with a vagal withdrawal, while the opposite trend is observed during non-REM sleep (Tobaldini et al. 2013). Previous studies have also shown that alternations in nocturnal heart rate variability have clinical importance, for example, may explain why sudden cardiac death in many cases occurs during sleep (Huikuri et al. 1994; Vanoli et al. 1995).

Heart transplantation surgery destroys the nerve connections between the organism and the graft—the donor heart is completely denervated, the vagal ganglia at the sinus node are cut off from medulla oblongata and brain-stem system signals. The regulation is driven by the intrinsic heart mechanisms and the concentration of many circulating humoral substances (e.g., adrenal catecholamines, angiotensin II, aldosterone), which follow the activity of sympathetic nerves (Klabunde 2012). The lack of vagal activity has the effect, for example, that heart transplant recipients have a resting heart rate higher than the average in healthy people, and their heart rate variability is significantly reduced (Bigger et al. 1996). The exception is a small respiratory sinus arrhythmia (Radaelli et al. 1996; Eckberg 2003), which is assumed to be an effect of the intracardiac reflex (Armour 2008; Zarzoso et al. 2013) or mechanical stretch of the sinus node. Cardiac reinnervation has been demonstrated in long-term heart transplant recipients (van de Borne et al. 2001; Porta et al. 2011; Cornelissen et al. 2012), but it seems that it is limited to the sympathetic nerves. Therefore, a comparison of the nocturnal heart rate variability in healthy young individuals and heart transplant patients gives a unique opportunity to show the impact of autonomic (especially vagal) activity on heart rate regulation. Following Ashkenazy et al. (2001), to discover in which way properties of networks constructed from *RR*-increments demonstrate nonlinear or/and linear dependences among consecutive *RR*-intervals, we investigated properties of artificially modified *RR*-interval data (Schreiber and Schmitz 2000). In the following, we argue that network methods are successful in detecting nonlinear properties in the dynamics of autonomic nocturnal regulation in short-term variability. Two modes of visualization of networks constructed from *RR*-increments are proposed. The first is based on the handling of a state space. The state space of *RR*-increments can be modified by a bin size used to code a signal and by the role of a given vertex as the representation of events occurring in a signal. The second mode relies on the matrix representation of the network on the two-dimensional plane. This approach is similar to the accepted method, known as the Poincaré plot representation of time series for evaluation of heart rate variability. The methods introduced will be applied to nocturnal Holter signals recorded from healthy young people and from cardiac transplant recipients. Thus, we obtain a way to filter out the intrinsic heart rate variability from the autonomic drive and then to quantify complexity in the short-term *RR*-interval variability related to nocturnal rest. Changes in *RR*-increments in a heart deprived of autonomic control provide insight into beat-to-beat dependences in forces governing the intrinsic heart dynamics.

6.2 Method

6.2.1 Groups and Signals Studied

Twenty-four-hour Holter electrocardiogram (ECG) recordings during a normal sleep–wake rhythm were analyzed in two study groups. The first group, the *Young*, consisted of healthy young volunteers (18 females, 18 males, ages 19–32). The second group, the *HTX*, comprised heart transplant patients (surgery at ages 28–65). Data from the *HTX* group was constructed of 20 recordings obtained from 10 patients without any signs of heart graft rejection, who had undergone surgery more than 12 months previously. The Holter recordings were first analyzed using Del Mar Reynolds Impresario software and screened for premature, supraventricular and ventricular beats, missed beats and pauses. Finally, the signals were thoroughly manually corrected and annotated.

As the method of signal preprocessing may impact the results, only long, good-quality fragments of ECG were analyzed. Since the analysis concentrates on hours of sleep, the *RR*-intervals were analyzed from 24:00 to 04:00 in the case of the *Young* group and from 22:00 to 05:00 in the case of signals from the *HTX* group. Such time intervals were long enough to build a sequence containing 10,000 *RR*-intervals obtained by joining the parts which had more than 500 normal-to-normal *RR*-intervals, that is, *RR*-intervals between two subsequent heart contractions initiated by the sinus node. What is worth noting is that all the signals constructed were built from less than seven consistent parts. Selection of the parts was independent of the sleep stage—REM or non-REM. The number of 10,000 points was chosen to ensure proper statistical relevance.

6.2.2 Signal Preprocessing

Our Holter equipment provides data with a 128 Hz sampling frequency. Therefore, the RR-intervals have a limited resolution: $1s/128 = 7.8125$ ms, which can be approximated as 8 ms. This value, denoted as Δ_0, is accepted as the signal resolution. To decrease the number of different values appearing in a sequence of RR-intervals, we use a binning procedure based on multiples of Δ_0. Namely, we always set the bin size to Δ_{bin} as $\Delta_{bin} = k\Delta_0$ for $k = 1, 2, \ldots$. The bin quantization described has the effect that RR-intervals take values which are multiples of the bin size Δ_{bin}. As a consequence, RR-increments are also multiples of Δ_{bin}, namely, $\Delta RR_t \in \{0, \pm\Delta_{bin}, \pm 2\Delta_{bin}, \pm 3\Delta_{bin}, \ldots \}$. The two types of artificially modified cardiac signals were constructed for their further use in statistical tests:

- *Shuffled* signals, which were obtained by random shuffling of RR-intervals
- *Surrogate* signals, which were calculated by randomization of phases in the Fourier transform of RR-intervals

The analysis of *shuffled* signals tests the presence of dependencies in the signals studied, while the analysis of *surrogate* signals provides information about whether these dependences are linear or not (Schreiber and Schmitz 2000). Signals of both types were prepared with the help of the TISEAN software (Hegger et al. 1999). For each cardiac signal, we prepared 10 shuffled signals (`surrogates -i0 -I`) and 10 surrogate signals (`surrogates -S -I`) with different random seeds. A network was constructed separately for each signal analyzed. Then the mean network for each of the groups of signals studied was established by collecting networks corresponding to the same class of subjects. The confidence interval (CI) for each element of the mean network was also estimated. Calculations were performed with the special software prepared by us.

6.2.3 Transition Network for *RR*-Increments

Let $RR_{\Delta_{bin}} = \{RR_0, RR_1, \ldots, RR_t, \ldots, RR_N\}$ be a time sequence of RR-intervals binned with a Δ_{bin}. Let $\Delta RR = \{\Delta RR_1, \Delta RR_2, \ldots, \Delta RR_N\}$ be a time sequence of RR-increments, that is, $\Delta RR_t = RR_t - RR_{t-1}$. Discrete values of the set ΔRR serve as states in the state space of the transition network indexed by the bin value Δ_{bin}.

Let K denote the number of different states in the network state space, and let us arrange them as follows. If the smallest state is $\Delta^{min} = \min_t \Delta RR$ and the greatest state is $\Delta^{max} = \max_t \Delta RR$, then the vertices of a network are labeled consecutively as

$$\Delta^{(1)} = \Delta^{min}, \quad \Delta^{(2)} = \Delta^{(1)} + \Delta_{bin}, \quad \ldots, \quad \Delta^{(K)} = \Delta^{max} = \Delta^{(1)} + (K-1)\Delta_{bin}. \qquad (6.1)$$

A directed edge $(\Delta^{(I)}, \Delta^{(J)})$ from a vertex $\Delta^{(I)}$ to a vertex $\Delta^{(J)}$ is established if $\Delta^{(I)}$ and $\Delta^{(J)}$ represent a pair of consecutive events in a time sequence ΔRR. Namely, there is a moment in time $t = 1, \ldots, N-1$, for which $(\Delta RR_t, \Delta RR_{t+1}) = (\Delta^{(I)}, \Delta^{(J)})$. If a given pair of increments occurs many times in ΔRR, the weight of this edge $w(\Delta^{(I)}, \Delta^{(J)})$ increases accordingly to represent counts of occurrences.

Note that the weight of the edge $w(\Delta^{(I)}, \Delta^{(J)})$ measures the size of a set consisting of the following events:

$$
\begin{aligned}
w(\Delta^{(I)}, \Delta^{(J)}) &= |\{(RR_{t-1}, RR_t, RR_{t+1}): \text{ where} \quad (6.2)\\
\Delta^{(I)} = RR_t - RR_{t-1}, \qquad \Delta^{(J)} &= RR_{t+1} - RR_t \quad \text{for } t = 1, \dots N-1\}|
\end{aligned}
$$

This means that

if $\Delta^{(I)} \cdot \Delta^{(J)} > 0$, both increments are negative or both are positive, we observe a run of accelerations or decelerations, accordingly

if $\Delta^{(I)} \cdot \Delta^{(J)} < 0$, we observe an alternation between an acceleration and a deceleration or vice versa

This completes the construction of the transition network from a given time series. The resulting network is directed and weighted. The sums of weights of edges adjacent to a given vertex (total number of *incoming* and total number of *outgoing* edges) provide the basic network characteristics (called the *in* degree and *out* degree, respectively), which quantify the role of the vertex in a network. But a network constructed from time series is specific in that each *outgoing* edge from a given vertex is accompanied by an edge *incoming* to this vertex (with the exception of vertices representing the first and last events in consistent parts of a signal), which implies that the *in* and *out* degrees of each vertex can be considered to be equal to each other. This degree, if normalized by the length of time series, is directly related to the probability p that an event represented by $\Delta^{(I)}$ occurs in a signal.

The modular structures, also called the community structure in networks, have been shown to be relevant to the understanding of the structure and dynamics of the system studied (Havlin et al. 2012). However, this problem has been found to be difficult and has not yet been satisfactorily solved (Kumpula et al. 2008; Fortunato 2010). Here, we propose to investigate modularity in the transition network by the so-called *p-core graph* (Seidman 1983; Kumpula et al. 2008). The *p*-core graph is constructed from a given network by the removal of all the vertices with a probability less than p. Then, all the edges which connected these deleted vertices with the other parts of a network are removed. The sum of normalized weights in the resulting subgraph is called the *volume of the p-core graph*. A decay in this volume with an increasing p value is known as the network disintegration (Makowiec et al. 2013b).

6.2.4 Transition Network Graph

Visualization of a transition network is challenging because usually a transition network consists of many vertices which are densely, often completely, interconnected. The plot of such a network may be barely readable. Therefore, the graph organization requires a special effort.

There are parameters in the method which have to be thoroughly tuned:

Δ_{bin}—the bin size which is used in preprocessing RR-intervals and which determines the number of states in the state space

p—the probability of neglected events, which also allows a reduction in the number of states

Since states in the state space are ordered according to the values of their labels, see Equation 6.1, we plot them in a circle arranged clockwise according to increasing value of the vertex label from $\Delta^{\min}$ to $\Delta^{\max}$. Moreover, if we call two vertices Δ-neighboring when the magnitude of difference between their labels is equal to Δ, then we can code transitions between Δ-neighboring vertices by colors.

Here, we use the following color code:

- Violet to mark 0-neighboring vertices, that is, loops describing events of two adjacent accelerations or decelerations of the same value; the case of the $0 \rightarrow 0$ loop denotes the situation when three consecutive *RR*-intervals have the same value.
- Green to mark Δ_{bin}-neighboring vertices, that is, transitions to the nearest neighbors in the state space; they denote the smallest possible observable changes in subsequent accelerations and/or decelerations within a given binning.
- Blue to mark transitions for $2\Delta_{\mathrm{bin}}$-neighboring vertices.
- Red to mark transitions between $3\Delta_{\mathrm{bin}}$-neighboring vertices.
- Yellow to mark the transitions linking $4\Delta_{\mathrm{bin}}$-neighboring vertices.
- Black to mark transitions of a size larger than $4\Delta_{\mathrm{bin}}$ which, for example, in the case of $\Delta_{\mathrm{bin}} = 8$ ms means changes of at least of 40 ms.

Moreover, we use also the width of an edge to visualize the weight of a given transition.

In the following, we use the popular software PAJEK (Batagelj and Mrvar 1998) to plot graphs of transition networks.

6.2.5 Matrix Representation of a Transition Network

Adjacency matrixes and transition matrixes are standard representations of any network (Fortunato 2010). For a transition network with K vertices, the adjacency matrix $\mathbf{A}$ is a $K \times K$ matrix. The number of the outgoing edges from vertex $\Delta^{(I)}$ to vertex $\Delta^{(J)}$ is counted and designated as $A_{(I)(J)}$. If there is no edge between these vertices, then $A_{(I)(J)} = 0$. Hence

$$A_{(I)(J)} = \begin{cases} w(\Delta^{(I)}, \Delta^{(J)}) & \text{total number of edges from } \Delta^{(I)} \text{ to } \Delta^{(J)}; \\ 0 & \text{in other cases.} \end{cases}$$

In the following, we normalize counts $w(\Delta^{(I)}, \Delta^{(J)})$ by the total number of events. As a result, $A_{(I)(J)}$ stands for the probability of a given transition. When referring to a signal with *RR*-increments, $A_{(I)(J)}$ stands for the probability that the value $\Delta^{(J)}$ occurs after $\Delta^{(I)}$ in a signal. The transition matrix $\mathbf{T}$ is obtained by dividing elements of each row $(I) : (1), \ldots, (K)$ of the matrix $\mathbf{A}$ by the total weight of vertex $\Delta^{(I)}$. Thus,

$$T_{(I)(J)} = \frac{w(\Delta^{(I)}, \Delta^{(J)})}{\sum_{\Delta^{(J)}} w(\Delta^{(I)}, \Delta^{(J)})}.$$

Therefore, $\mathbf{T}$ describes a Markov walk on a network where a walker being in vertex $\Delta^{(I)}$ moves to $\Delta^{(J)}$ with a probability $T_{(I)(J)}$.

It appears that the contour plots of adjacency and transition matrices provide a readable visualization of transition networks obtained from *RR*-increments even in the case when the bin size is equal to the resolution of signals. Manipulations in the range of the axes allow one to pass through the whole range of values obtained. However, when departing from $(0,0)$, less probable events with larger standard errors are estimated. The large variations between neighboring points lead to an unclear picture if the plots are constructed from signals binned with a small bin size. Therefore, in the following, we limit our interest to the ranges of *RR*-increments which contain the most probable events, ignoring the remaining ones. In the case of the *Young* group, the range is $(-100, 100)$ and for the *HTX* group the range is $(-30, 30)$.

Each point $(\Delta^{(I)}, \Delta^{(J)})$ of the contour plots can be resolved into the three *RR*-interval patterns as described by Equation (6.2). Moreover, these events can be translated into codes of short-term variability proposed by Porta et al. (2007): 0V—0 variation, 1V—1 variation, 2LV—2 likely variations, and 2UV—2 unlikely variations. The relation between three *RR*-interval patterns and their description by 0, 1, or 2 variations is shown in Figure 6.1.

6.3 Results

6.3.1 Graphs of Transition Networks for the *Young* Group

In the presentation of our results, we first refer to some graphs which demonstrate the possibilities of the introduced visualization method. In particular, these graphs clarify the influence of the parameters Δ_{bin} and p on the graph shape. In Figure 6.2, there are six graphs which represent networks obtained from the signals of the *Young* group (Figure 6.2a through d) and their surrogates (Figure 6.2e and f). The left column networks were prepared with signals binned with $\Delta_{\text{bin}} = 8$ ms, while the right column graphs come from signals binned with $\Delta_{\text{bin}} = 64$ ms. The graphs in the first and third rows show vertices

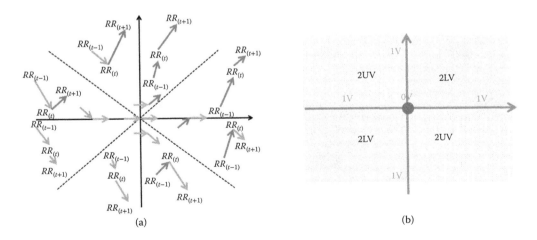

(a)   (b)

FIGURE 6.1
The patterns of changes in *RR*-intervals corresponding to particular parts of the matrix representation of a network of *RR*-increments (a) and their interpretation as variations 0V, 1V, 2LV, and 2UV—codes proposed by Porta et al. (2007) (b). Red arrows indicate decelerations, green arrows denote accelerations, and blue arrows correspond to no-change events.

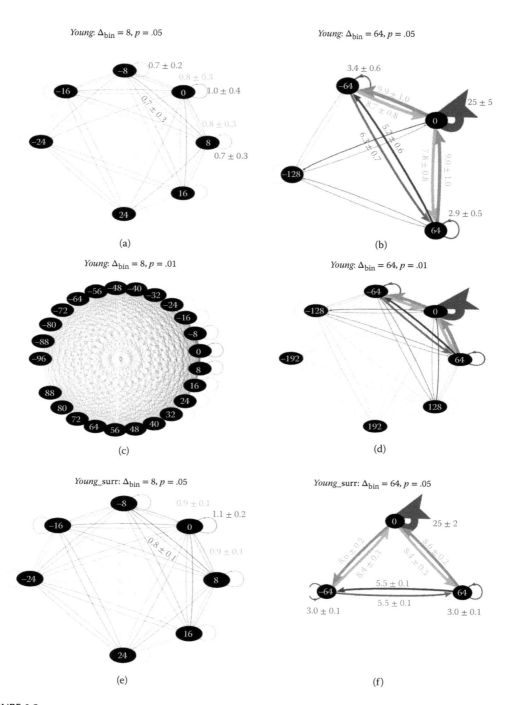

FIGURE 6.2
The *p*-core graphs with $p = 5\%$ (a, b, e, and f) and $p = 1\%$ (c and d) of the mean networks obtained from signals of young persons binned in $\Delta_{bin} = \Delta_0 = 8$ ms (a, c, and e) and $\Delta_{bin} = 8\Delta_0 = 64$ ms (b, d, and f), and surrogates obtained from signals from young persons (e and f). The crucial transitions—the thickest edges—are described by the mean of probability given in percentages ±95% CI. (c and d have the same weights as a and b, respectively). The colors of the values match the colors of the edges.

which correspond to deceleration/acceleration events appearing in a signal with probability $p > 5\%$. The graphs in the second row contain vertices representing more rare events because only vertices with $p > 1\%$ are plotted. All the graphs are complete, which means that each vertex is connected to all the others. The color of the edges corresponds to the size of the change in the way defined in Section 6.2.4. The weight of an edge is represented by its width. The global weights of the most important transitions are described additionally by giving their probability value in percentages and $\pm 95\%$ CI. We see that the $(0, 0)$ transition is the most frequent in all the graphs, namely the transition from no-change to no-change occurs the most often. However, the probability of observing such an event is different depending on the binning applied to the signals. The bin size works like a magnifying glass, making it possible to perceive the event in greater detail. For example, vertex 0 in the network constructed from signals binned at 64 ms (Figure 6.2b) represents the whole p-core graph (a) obtained at $p = 5\%$. The graphs in Figure 6.2 specify the ingredients of heart period variability. The widths of arrows, hence the numbers in the graphs, describe the roles played by the particular changes in the overall heart dynamics. Then, a clinician can decide whether the structure of such a decomposition is regular or whether it exhibits some peculiar patterns since different pathophysiologic processes alter the heart period variability. Figure 6.2 also gives graphs obtained from networks constructed from surrogates of cardiac signals of the *Young* group—see parts (Figure 6.2e and f). It follows that with 5% accuracy and at $\Delta_{bin} = 8$ ms, the basic spectrum of events constituting the cardiac dynamics is similar to the spectrum of events resulting from the linear dynamics left in the surrogate signals. This might indicate that dynamical relationships among the most important events are of a linear type. However, when the analysis is performed with $\Delta_{bin} = 64$ ms, we see that the cardiac graph is significantly different from the graph of the surrogates. The difference lies in the presence of the vertex -128, which indicates that nonlinear mechanisms are present and they are involved in sharp accelerations. Surprisingly, the lack of a symmetrical vertex representing decelerations $+128$ may additionally point to the complex mechanisms engaged only in sharp accelerations. Graphs obtained for the shuffled signals of the *Young* group are not presented because they are barely readable. Moreover, when signals are binned with Δ_0, the p-core graph of $p = 5\%$ consists of only a few vertices (Figure 6.2a), while the number of vertices grows sharply, if we decrease the probability p to 1% (Figure 6.2c). Hence, the graph in Figure 6.2a, rather superficially describes the dynamics of the system, since a slight change in any parameter strongly influences the graph shape. This is a typical observation with complex dynamics. This is different in the case of signals binned with $\Delta_{bin} = 64$ ms; compare Figure 6.2b and d. Therefore, the volume of a given p-core graph gives an important message about how dynamical forces presented by a graph are meaningful for the overall dynamics of the system studied. Here, the volumes of the p-cores presented in Figure 6.2 are (a): $27 \pm 14\%$, (b): $89.1 \pm 1.0\%$, (c): $84.7 \pm 1.4\%$, (d): $97.1 \pm 0.2\%$, (e): $26.3 \pm 3.2\%$, (f): $76.2 \pm 1.0\%$ (mean $\pm 95\%$CI).

6.3.2 Graphs of Transition Networks for *HTX* Group

The signals with *RR*-intervals obtained from patients after *HTX* are plain in the sense that consecutive *RR*-increments do not differ much. Therefore, it becomes possible to present readable p-core graphs even when p is low, for example, $p = 1\%$, and the bin size is equal to the signal resolution $\Delta_{bin} = 8$ ms. Moreover, graphs obtained from modified *HTX* signals, their surrogates and shuffled signals, are also clear. All these graphs are shown in Figure 6.3.

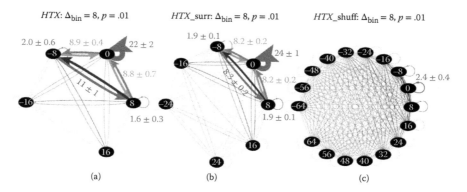

FIGURE 6.3
The p-core subgraphs of the mean transition networks obtained from signals from *HTX* (a) and their surrogates (b), and shuffled signals (c) at $p = 0.01$ in bin $\Delta_0 = 8$ ms. The most important transitions—the thickest edges—are described by their probabilities given in percentages ±95% CI.

Figure 6.3 demonstrates the following:

- How different the graph obtained from *HTX_shuffled* is from all the other graphs. This indicates that adjacent *RR*-intervals resulting from intrinsic mechanisms of variability are strongly correlated.

- There is similarity between graphs representing signals *HTX* and *HTX_surrogates*. However, note that there is a noticeable difference in the probability of transitions between no-change vertex 0 and vertices $0, \pm 8$. This observation may indicate that dependences between *RR*-intervals cannot be approximated by linear relationships.

- There is a similarity between graphs of *HTX* and those of the *Young* which are binned at an interval eight times longer than the *HTX* series; see Figure 6.2d. This approximate similarity may give rise to the conjecture that the variability driven by autonomic regulation enhances eight times the magnitude of fluctuations of the intrinsic heart period variability.

6.3.3 Network Disintegration

The decay of the volume of the p-core when p is increasing can provide information about the collective structures in the system dynamics. Figure 6.4 shows these decays for all signals studied binned at $\Delta_{\text{bin}} = 8$ ms. It appears that the network formed from signals of the *HTX* group is significantly more resistant to the vertex removal than all the other networks. This network decays the slowest. Moreover, its p-core volume stays unchanged at $83.2 \pm 1.3\%$ for $8\% < p < 18\%$. This firmed core is built from transitions between the three vertices 0 and ± 8. A similar network core also emerges from the network constructed from surrogate signals of the *HTX* group. Its volume of $76.8 \pm 1.5\%$ is significantly lower than the volume of the network constructed from original cardiac signals (by Mann–Whitney U test, $p = .011$) for all p in the interval described. This fact may indicate that the network organization resulting from the cardiac signals relies on important nonlinear dependences.

On the contrary, a similar property does not hold in the case of the disintegration of the network constructed from the *Young* group signals. The volume of the p-core decays in the

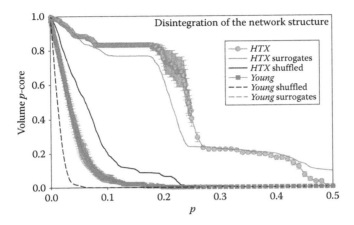

FIGURE 6.4
Network disintegration by the volume of p-core resulting from subsequent removal of vertices with probability less than p.

same way in both networks: the network made from cardiac signals and the network made from surrogate signals. The disintegration of both networks goes fast, for example at $p = 10\%$, the network volume is about $5 \pm 2\%$ in both cases. Obviously, the networks obtained from shuffled signals decay more quickly when compared to the networks produced from cardiac series (Figure 6.4).

6.3.4 Adjacency and Transition Matrices for the *Young* Group

Figure 6.5 shows contour plots of both matrices: adjacency **A** and transition **T** obtained from signals recorded from the *Young* group. Together, the plots obtained from surrogates of these signals and shuffled RR-intervals are presented. All the plots represent signals binned at Δ_0 and for changes smaller than 100 ms for **A** and smaller than 70 ms in case of **T**.

From the plots in Figure 6.5, it is evident that shuffled RR-intervals provide different matrix representations. The meaningful smaller probability of events corresponding to small accelerations or decelerations (i.e., probability of events around $(0,0)$) is a noticeable effect of the independence of RR-intervals. Moreover, the symmetry in these matrices is different from symmetries which are present in other plots. These symmetric features can be explained by elementary counting of the sets built from the three RR-interval events of the specific type. Since the state space of RR-intervals is discrete and limited, the values of RR_t for any $t = 1, 2, \ldots, N$ take one of the values from the set of K' different values:

$$RR^{(1)} = \min RR_{\Delta_{bin}} < RR^{(2)} = RR^{(1)} + \Delta_{bin} < \quad \cdots < \quad RR^{(K')} = \max RR_{\Delta_{bin}}. \tag{6.3}$$

For simplicity, let us assume that all events of Equation 6.3 are equally probable, $p(RR^{(I)}) = K'/N$. Then, the number of possible monotonically growing three-element sequences $(RR^{(I)}, RR^{(J)}, RR^{(M)})$ with $I < J < M$ constructed from these values, namely patterns of the 2LV type, is $K'(K' - 1)(K' - 2)/3$. On the other hand, from each sequence of the 2LV type, one can construct two different three-element sequences of the 2UV type. Hence, the total probability of events of the 2UV type is twice as large as of the 2LV type. In the case when

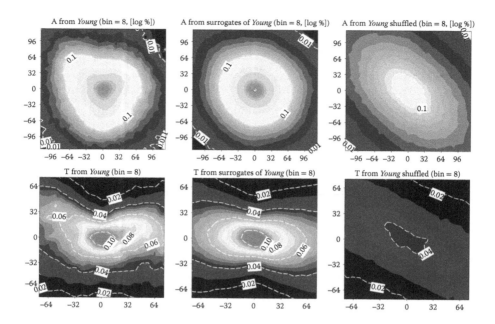

FIGURE 6.5
Adjacency matrices **A** (first row) and transition matrices **T** (second row) for cardiac signals of the *Young* group (left column), for their *surrogates* (middle column) and *shuffled* signals (right column). Contour representations of **A** show logarithms of **A** values given in percentages from 0.001% to 1%. Contours representing **T** are plotted in linear scale from 0.0 to 0.1 with step 0.02.

events from the list described in Equation 6.3 are not distributed uniformly, the calculations are more demanding, but finally they lead to the conclusion that if $\Delta^{(I)}\Delta^{(J)} < 0$, then events $(\Delta^{(I)}, \Delta^{(J)})$ are more probable than $(-\Delta^{(I)}, \Delta^{(J)})$ or $(\Delta^{(I)}, -\Delta^{(J)})$.

In addition, comparing **A** matrices obtained from cardiac signals and their surrogates, Figure 6.5 first row, we see:

1. There is a small deficiency of events close to $(0,0)$ in cardiac signals when compared to signals with surrogates.

2. There are three regions in **A** in which cardiac signals dominate their surrogates. They can be described as three *RR*-interval events of the type:

   (a) 2LV, but related only to large decelerations

   (b) 1V, when after a small change, a large acceleration occurs

   (c) 2UV, but only for a large deceleration after a large acceleration

   By large changes above, we mean *RR*-increments greater than 30 ms.

6.3.5 Adjacency and Transition Matrices for *HTX* Group

In the absence of any influence of the autonomic nervous system, the network representation of *RR*-increments consists of considerably fewer vertices than for a typical healthy person, as has been already shown in Figure 6.3. Figure 6.6 presents results aimed at

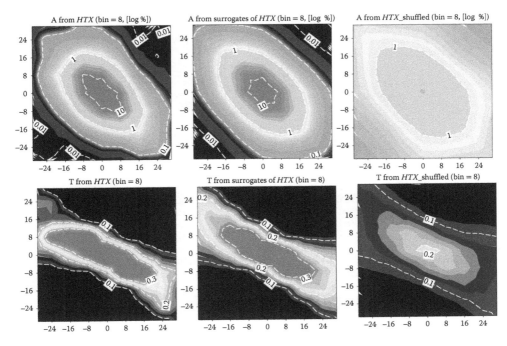

FIGURE 6.6
Adjacency matrices **A** (first row) and transition matrices **T** (second row) for cardiac signals of *HTX* group (left column), for their *surrogates* (middle column) and *shuffled* signals (right column). Values of **A** are shown as logarithms of percentages from 0.01% to 10%. **T**s are plotted in a linear scale from 0.0 to 0.3 with step 0.1.

widening our understanding of the nonlinear effects of the intrinsic mechanisms controlling the heart contractions. Note that the contour plots in Figure 6.6 are in different scales from the plots representing signals of the *Young* group in Figure 6.5. We see in Figure 6.6 similar symmetric features in all three plots with **A** matrices, namely that alternating changes with $\Delta^{(I)} \cdot \Delta^{(J)} < 0$ are more dominant than monotonic changes. Following our discussion in the previous subsection about the imprints of randomness, this observation may imply stochastic independence of the underlying dynamics. However, the cardiac dynamics is more concentrated around transitions from a no-change event to the smallest increments possible, namely to $\pm 8, \pm 16$ ms, than if it resulted from random sources. Furthermore, a closer analysis of **A** (compare Figure 6.3a and b) reveals that the system represented by the cardiac signals is less likely to stay in the no-change vertex, and changes of size 16 ms between vertices representing transitions of +8 and −8 ms in size occur more often in the cardiac signals [$p(8, -8) = p(-8, 8) = 11 \pm 1\%$] than in their surrogate series [$p(8, -8) \approx p(-8, 8) \approx 8.4 \pm 0.2\%$]. Additionally, a comparison between the corresponding **T** matrices provides important distinctions between cardiac signals and their surrogates in the system reaction after the larger accelerations, namely, if $\Delta < -16$ ms. It appears that when accelerating, the system is more resistant to a pendulum-like reaction. This has the effect that the *RR*-interval is able to retain the shorter rhythm for the next contraction. In Figure 6.7, we show plots of differences between matrix graphs arising from cardiac signals of the *Young* group when the signals are binned with $\Delta_{\text{bin}} = 64$ ms, and the *HTX* group. We see that a similarity is apparent between the dynamics underlying these two systems. The basic distinction relies on events of the 2LV type, where two subsequent accelerations

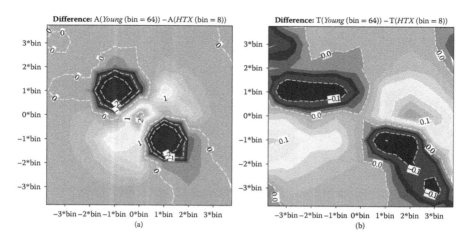

FIGURE 6.7

Difference between adjacency matrices (a) and transition matrices (b) obtained from cardiac signals of the *Young* group when the signals were binned with $\Delta_{bin} = 64$ ms and from recordings of the *HTX* group. Values of differences in **A** are in percentages. The more reddish areas are the regions of greater cardiac superiority. The more blue areas are the regions of greater superiority of surrogates.

or two subsequent decelerations are involved. Since such persistence could be involved in some overall purpose like actual bodily needs, the next supposition can be formulated as follows. While the intrinsic heart control mechanisms are devoted to keeping the homeostasis, the control of the autonomic nervous system aims at satisfying physical demands.

6.4 Conclusions

Network structure methods are able to visualize, describe, and differentiate heart rate dynamics in healthy young subjects and *HTX* patients. The resulting plots can be considered as an alternative way of assessing heart rate variability. Our method, based on beat-to-beat dependencies, provides the spectrum of short-term correlations. This spectrum resolves the heart rate variability at the required accuracy (if tuned by p the probability of neglected events) and/or zoomed (by changes in the bin size Δ_{bin}). Using these methods, the general dynamical properties of heart rate can be defined as correlated or not correlated (employing the comparison of raw and shuffled signals), and linearly or nonlinearly correlated (comparing raw signals and signals with shuffled phases of the Fourier transform). The essential feature of complex dependencies in nocturnal heart rhythm in our group of healthy young persons is related to large *RR*-increments, both decelerations and accelerations. This feature manifests itself in that large accelerations are more likely antipersistent, while large decelerations are more likely persistent. This observation also seems to be an important indicator of healthy heart rate.

Moreover, since the vagal part of autonomic regulation is considered responsible for large *RR*-increments, we may hypothesize that vagal activity is a crucial source of complexity in short-term heart rate variability. In healthy young individuals, the change in vagal tone during sleep (e.g., change from high vagal activity to its withdrawal between non-REM and REM sleep stages) allows us to observe the specific patterns of heart rate dynamics. We interpret the nonlinear relationship observed between consecutive accelerations and decelerations in the case of bigger changes (accelerations and decelerations of more than 35 ms) as an effect of vagal activity. Although in *HTX* patients, heart rate regulation is mostly intrinsic with no autonomic control, the relationship between consecutive accelerations and decelerations is also observed, but in this case, the scale of changes is much lower. *RR*-increments vary as fluctuations around a homeostatic state. However, the organization of this homeostatic state in the case of raw signals shows that it involves dynamical forces more strongly than if the dynamics were driven by linear forces only. In posttransplant patients, the nonlinear dependencies are also characterized by the appearance of sequences made of bigger (>20 ms) accelerations followed by smaller decelerations (<10 ms). This means that an increase in heart rate is not so effective as in healthy individuals but is still possible. We hypothesize that this pattern of heart rate in *HTX* patients may be a result of gradual sympathetic reinnervation.

Acknowledgments

The authors Danuta Makowiec, Zbigniew R. Struzik, Beata Graff, Dorota Wejer, and Agnieszka Kaczkowska acknowledge the financial support of the National Science Centre, Poland, UMO: 2012/06/M/ST2/00480.

This work was partially realized under the SKILLS project of the Foundation for Polish Science (172/UD/SKILLS/2012) and was cofinanced by the European Union through the European Social Fund.

References

Armour, J.A. 2008. Potential clinical relevance of the "little brain" on the mammalian heart. *Exp Physiol.* 95:165–76.

Ashkenazy, Y., Ivanov, P.Ch., Havlin, S., and Peng, C.-K. 2001. Magnitude and sign correlations in heartbeat functions. *Phys Rev Lett.* 86:1900–3.

Bashan, A., Bartsch, R.P., Kantelhardt, J.W., Havlin, S., and Ivanov, P.C. 2012. Network physiology reveals relations between network topology and physiological function. *Nat Commun.* 3:702.

Batagelj, V., and Mrvar. A. 1998. Pajek: A program for large network analysis. *Connections.* 21:47–57.

Bigger Jr, J.T., Steinman, R.S., Rolnitzky, L.M., Fleiss, J.L., Albrecht, P., and Cohen, R.J. 1996. Power law behavior of *RR*-interval variability in healthy middle-aged persons, patients with recent acute myocardial infarction, and patients with heart transplants. *Circulation.* 93:2142–51.

Bonnemeier, H., Richardt, G., Potratz, J., Wiegand, U.K., Brandes, A., Kluge, N., and Katus, H.A. 2003. Circadian profile of cardiac autonomic nervous modulation in healthy subjects: Differing effects of aging and gender on heart rate variability. *J Cardiovasc Electrophysiol.* 14(8):791–9.

van de Borne, P., Neubauer, J., Rahnama, M., Jansens, J.L., Montano, N., Porta, A., Somers, V.K., and Degaute, J.P. 2001. Differential characteristics of neural circulatory control: Early versus late after cardiac transplantation. *Circulation.* 104:1809–13.

Campanharo, A.S.L.O., Sirer, M.I., Malmgren, R.D., Ramos, F.M., and Amaral, L.A.N. 2011. Duality between time series and networks. *PLOS ONE.* 6(8):e233378.

Cornelissen, V.A., Vanhaecke, J., Aubert, A.E., and Fagard, R.H. 2012. Heart rate variability after heart transplantation: A 10-year longitudinal follow-up study. *J Cardiol.* 59:220–24.

Donner, R.V., Zou, Y., Donges, F.F., Marwan, N., and J. Kurths. 2010. Recurrence networks—A novel paradigm for nonlinear time series analysis. *New J Phys.* 12:1–40. http://iopscience.iop.org/1367-2630/12/3/033025.

Eckberg, D.L. 2003. The human respiratory gate. *J Physiol.* 548:339–52.

Fortunato, S. 2010. Community detection in graphs. *Phys Rep.* 486:75–174.

Havlin, S., Kenett, D.Y., Ben-Jacob, E., Bunde, A., Cohen, R., Hermann, H., Kantelhardt, J.W., Kertész, J., Kirkpatrick, S., Kurths, J., Portugali, J., and Solomon, S. 2012. Challenges in network science: Applications to infrastructures, climate, social systems and economics. *Eur Phys J Spec Top.* 214:273–93.

Hegger, R., Kantz, H., and T. Schreiber. 1999. Practical implementation of nonlinear time series methods: The TISEAN package. *Chaos.* 9:413–34. Software accessible from www.mpipks-dresden.mpg.de/~tisean/Tisean_3.0.1.

Huikuri, H.V., Niemelä, M.J., Ojala, S., Rantala, A. Ikäheimo, M.J., and Airaksinen, K.E. 1994. Circadian rhythms of frequency domain measures of heart rate variability in healthy subjects and patients with coronary artery disease. *Circulation.* 90:121126.

Ivanov, P.C., Amaral, L.A., Goldberger, A.L., Havlin, S., Rosenblum, M.G., Struzik, Z.R., and Stanley, H.E. 1999. Multifractality in human heartbeat dynamics. *Nature.* 399:461–5.

Kantelhardt, J.W., Ashkenazy, Y., Ivanov, P.Ch., Bunde, A., Havlin, S., Penzel, T., Peter, J.H., and Stanley, H.E. 2002. Characterization of sleep stages by correlations in the magnitude and sign of heartbeat increments. *Phys Rev E.* 65:051908.

Klabunde, R.E. 2012. *Cardiovascular Physiology Concepts.* Baltimore, MD: Lippincott Williams & Wilkins.

Kobayashi, M., and Musha T. 1982. 1/f fluctuation of heartbeat period. *IEEE Trans Biomed Eng.* 29: 456–7.

Kumpula, J.M., Kivelä, M., Kaski, K., and Saramäki, J. 2008. A sequential algorithm for fast clique percolation. *Phys Rev E.* 78:026109.

Makowiec, D., Struzik, Z.R., Graff, B., Wdowczyk-Szulc, J., Zarczynska-Buchnowiecka, M., Gruchala, M., and Rynkiewicz, A. 2013a. Complexity of the heart rhythm after heart transplantation by entropy of transition network for *RR*-increments of time intervals between heartbeats. *Conf Proc IEEE Eng Med Biol Sci.* 2013:6127–30.

Makowiec, D., Struzik, Z.R., Graff, B., Wdowczyk-Szulc, J., Zarczynska-Buchowiecka, M., and Kryszewski, S. 2013b. Community structure in networks representation of increments in beat-to-beat time intervals of the heart in patients after heart transplantation. *Acta Phys Pol B.* 44:1219–33.

Makowiec, D., Struzik, Z.R., Graff, B., Zarczynska-Buchowiecka, M., and Wdowczyk, J. 2014. Transition network entropy in characterization of complexity of the heart rhythm after heart transplantation. *Acta Phys Pol B.* 45:1771–82.

Peng, C.-K., Havlin, S., Stanley, H.E., and Goldberger, A.L. 1995. Quantification of scaling exponents and crossover phenomena in nonstationary heartbeat time series. *Chaos.* 5:82–7.

Porta, A., Catai, A.M., Takahashi, A.C.M., Magagnin, V., Bassani, T., Tobaldini, E., van de Borne, P., and Montano, N. 2011. Causal relationship between heart period and systolic arterial pressure during graded head-up tilt. *Am J Physiol Regul Integr Comp Physiol.* 300:R378–86.

Porta, A., Tobaldini, E., Guzzetti, S., Furlan, R., Montano, N., and Gnecchi-Ruscone, T. 2007. Assessment of cardiac autonomic modulation during graded head-up tilt by symbolic analysis of heart rate variability. *Am J Physiol Heart Circ Physiol.* 293:H702–8.

Radaelli, A., Valle, F., Falcone, C., Calciati, A., Leuzzi, S., Martinelli, L., Goggi, C., Viganò, M., Finardi, G., and Bernardi, L. 1996. Determinants of heart rate variability in heart transplanted subjects during physical exercise. *Eur Heart J.* 17:462–71.

Schmitt, D.T., Stein, P.K, and Ivanov, P.Ch. 2009. Stratification pattern of static and scale-invariant dynamic measures of heartbeat fluctuations across sleep stages in young and elderly. *IEEE Trans Biomed Eng.* 56(5):1564.

Schreiber, T., and Schmitz, A. 2000. Surrogate time series. *Physica D.* 142:346–82.

Seidman, S.B. 1983. Network structure and minimum degree. *Soc Netw.* 5:269–87.

Struzik, Z.R., Hayano, J., Sakata, S., Kwak, S., and Yamamoto, Y. 2004. 1/f scaling in heart rate requires antagonistic autonomic control. *Phys Rev E Stat Nonlin Soft Matter Phys.* 70:050901.

Tobaldini, E., Nobili, L., Strada. S., Casali, K.R., Braghiroli, A., and Montano, N. 2013. Heart rate variability in normal and pathological sleep. *Front Physiol.* 4:294.

Vanoli, E., Adamson, P.B., Ba-Lin, M.P.H., Pinna, G.D., Lazarra, R., and Orr, W.C. 1995. Heart rate variability during specific sleep stages. A comparison of healthy subjects with patients after myocardial infarction. *Circulation.* 91(7):1918–22.

Yamamoto, Y., and Hughson, R.L. 1991. Coarse-graining spectral analysis: New method for studying heart rate variability. *J Appl Physiol.* 71:1143–50.

Zarzoso, M., Ryseavaite, K., Milstein, M.L., Calvo, C.J., Kean, A.C., Atienza, F., Pauza, D.H., Jalife, J., and Noujaim, S.F. 2013. Nerves projecting from the intrinsic cardiac ganglia of the pulmonary veins modulate sinoatrial node pacemaker function. *Cardiovasc Res.* 99:566–75.

7

Analysis and Preprocessing of HRV—Kubios HRV Software

Mika P. Tarvainen, Jukka A. Lipponen, and Pekka Kuoppa

CONTENTS

7.1 Introduction

Heart rate variability (HRV) is a commonly used tool when trying to assess the functioning of cardiac autonomic regulation. It has been used in a multitude of studies related to cardiovascular research and different human well-being applications, as an indirect tool to evaluate the functioning and balance of the autonomic nervous system (ANS) [1]. One of the main clinical scenarios where HRV has been found valuable is the risk stratification of sudden cardiac death after acute myocardial infarction [1–4]. In addition, decreased HRV is generally accepted to provide an early warning sign of diabetic cardiovascular autonomic neuropathy [1,2], the most significant decrease in HRV being found within the first

5–10 years of diabetes [5,6]. Besides these two main clinical scenarios, HRV has been studied with relation to several cardiovascular diseases, renal failure, physical exercise, occupational and psychosocial stress, gender, age, drugs, alcohol, smoking, and sleep [1,2,7–10].

Both sympathetic and parasympathetic branches of the ANS are involved in the regulation of heart rate (HR). Sympathetic nervous system (SNS) activity increases the HR and decreases the HRV, whereas parasympathetic nervous system (PNS) activity decreases the HR and increases the HRV [11]. The control of the autonomic output involves several interconnected areas of the central nervous system, which form the so-called central autonomic network. In addition to this central control, arterial baroreceptor reflex as well as respiration are known to induce quick changes in the HR. Typically, the most conspicuous oscillatory component of HRV is the respiratory sinus arrhythmia (RSA), where the vagus nerve stimulation is being cut off during inhalation, and thus, the HR increases during inhalation and decreases during exhalation. This high frequency (HF) component of HRV is thus centered at respiratory frequency and is considered to range from 0.15 to 0.4 Hz. Another conspicuous component of HRV is the low frequency (LF) component ranging from 0.04 to 0.15 Hz. The HF component is mediated almost solely by the PNS activity, whereas the LF component is mediated by both SNS and PNS activities and is also affected by baroreflex activity [1,3,11]. The origin of the LF oscillations is however considered to be dominated by the SNS and the normalized power of the LF component could be used to assess sympathetic efferent activity [12,13].

This chapter introduces the commonly used time-domain, frequency-domain, and nonlinear HRV analysis methods, also giving some ideas as to how to extend these methods for analysis of nonstationary HRV time series. The computations of these analysis methods are described with enough detail to be able to make correct interpretations of the results and to understand the interdependencies between the different parameters. In the presentation of the HRV analysis methods, we focus on the ones available on the Kubios HRV software [14,15] (available at http://www.kubios.com), which is an easy to use software package making the various HRV analysis methods usable by physiologists and clinicians all over the world.

In addition to the presentation of the analysis methods, some important issues in the assessment of HRV time series are presented. These include two preprocessing steps and estimation of the RSA component. The two preprocessing steps, which both can have a major impact on the assessment of HRV, are (1) correction of ectopic and other aberrant beats and (2) removal of the very low frequency (VLF) trend from the HRV time series. The effects of these preprocessing steps are illustrated with real data in order to fully understand their impact on HRV analysis results and possible misinterpretations. The effect of respiratory rate on the HRV is then demonstrated and ways to incorporate this in the HRV analysis are described.

7.2 HRV Time Series

The HRV time series is a series of consecutive heartbeat time intervals, that is, time intervals between consecutive R-waves in an electrocardiogram (ECG) or simply RR intervals. The R-wave occurrence times can be detected using a QRS detection algorithm such as the well-known Pan–Tompkins algorithm [16]. The term normal-to-normal (NN) is sometimes used when referring to these beat-to-beat intervals, merely to indicate that the consecutive

QRS complexes result from normal SA-node depolarization, excluding for example premature ventricular beats and other arrhythmic events. Throughout this chapter, the term RR is used to denote beat-to-beat intervals resulting from the normal sinoatrial (SA)-node depolarization.

Derivation of RR interval time series from ECG is illustrated in Figure 7.1. If we assume that the ECG recording includes $N+1$ heartbeats, then the RR interval series has N data points

$$RR = (RR_1, RR_2, \ldots, RR_N) \tag{7.1}$$

This time series is not equidistantly sampled, but needs to be presented as a function of time, that is, the nth RR interval is observed at time t_n. Equidistant sampling is assumed by standard spectral estimation techniques such as those based on discrete Fourier transform or autoregressive (AR) modeling. This aspect has not been considered in all the early HRV studies where the spectrum is calculated directly from the RR interval tachogram (see Figure 7.1). When using the tachogram for spectrum estimation, an assumption of equidistant sampling is erroneously made, which can cause distortion to the spectrum and the spectrum can not be considered to be a function of frequency but rather is a function of cycles per beat [17,18].

One commonly used approach to take care of the nonequidistant sampling of the RR time series is to use interpolation methods in converting the nonequidistantly sampled time series to equidistantly sampled time series [1]. Several different interpolation methods

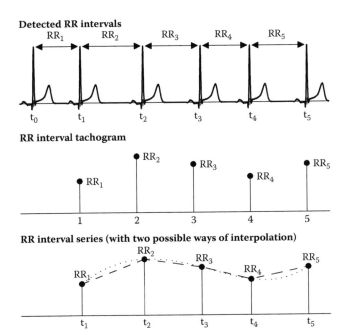

FIGURE 7.1
Derivation of RR interval time series: detection of RR intervals from ECG (top panel), RR interval tachogram (middle panel), and interpolated RR interval time series (bottom panel). In the bottom panel, linear (dashed line) and cubic spline interpolation (dotted line) trajectories of the nonequidistantly sampled RR time series are illustrated.

have been applied for this task among which cubic spline interpolation, providing smooth interpolation over the beat-to-beat intervals, has been used in several studies and is also adopted in the Kubios HRV software package. After interpolation, standard spectrum estimation methods can be applied to assess the HRV spectra. The interpolation rate should be selected high enough to avoid aliasing, basically at least as high as the baseline HR. Typical choices for the interpolation rate are 2–4 Hz. Regardless of the interpolation rate, the baseline HR needs to be high enough when compared to the respiratory rate in order to avoid aliasing in the RSA component [19]. For example, a respiratory rate of 0.3 Hz can be observed successfully (without aliasing) from RR time series only if the HR is higher than 36 beats/min (0.6 Hz). Normally, this is not an issue because respiratory rate is decreased in rest and increases during exercise, that is, the changes are parallel to those in the HR.

Other approaches for HRV spectral estimation, which do not assume equidistant sampling, include the Lomb–Scargle periodogram [20–22], the integral pulse frequency modulation (IPFM) model [17,23], and the point-process model [24]. The Lomb–Scargle periodogram is a generalization of discrete Fourier transform, which does not assume equidistant sampling. The IPFM models the neural modulation of the SA node from the beat occurrence times (sequence of delta functions). According to this model, the modulating signal is integrated until a reference level is achieved after which an impulse is emitted and the integrator is set to zero. The spectrum for the sequence of delta functions, also called spectrum of counts, is finally computed using the estimated modulation signal. The point-process model relies on the assumption that the stochastic properties of the RR intervals are governed by an inverse Gaussian renewal model.

7.3 Time-Domain Analysis Methods

The time-domain analysis methods described below are computationally simple linear methods that are applied directly in the time domain to the series of consecutive RR interval values. All of these time-domain methods are included in the Kubios HRV software and are summarized in Section 7.1.

Given the N point beat-to-beat RR interval time series $RR = (RR_1, RR_2, \ldots, RR_N)$, the mean RR interval $(\overline{RR})$, and the mean HR $(\overline{HR})$ are computed as

$$\overline{RR} = \frac{1}{N} \sum_{j=1}^{N} RR_j \quad \text{and} \quad \overline{HR} = \frac{1}{N} \sum_{j=1}^{N} \frac{60}{RR_j} \tag{7.2}$$

It should be noted that the mean HR $(\overline{HR})$ is not equal to $60/\overline{RR}$ due to the nonlinear relationship between beat-to-beat RR interval and HR values. This means that the distributions of these two time series are also different as illustrated in Figure 7.2.

In addition to mean values, several parameters that measure the variability within the beat-to-beat RR interval values have been defined. The standard deviation of RR intervals (SDNN) is defined as

$$SDNN = \sqrt{\frac{1}{N-1} \sum_{j=1}^{N} (RR_j - \overline{RR})^2} \tag{7.3}$$

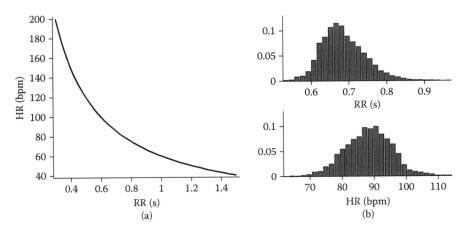

FIGURE 7.2
Interrelationship between RR interval and heart rate. (a) Mathematical relationship between RR interval and HR. (b) Illustrations of RR interval and HR time series histograms extracted from 1-hour HRV recording of healthy female subject.

Both short-term and long-term HRV influence SDNN, and thus, it is a measure of overall HRV. Short-term, beat-to-beat HRV is better captured by the standard deviation of successive RR interval differences (SDSD) defined by

$$SDSD = \sqrt{E\left\{\Delta RR_j^2\right\} - E\left\{\Delta RR_j\right\}^2} \tag{7.4}$$

If the RR series is stationary $E\{\Delta RR_j\} = E\{RR_{j+1}\} - E\{RR_j\} = 0$ and SDSD is approximated by the root mean square of successive differences (RMSSD) parameter, which is defined as

$$RMSSD = \sqrt{\frac{1}{N-1} \sum_{j=1}^{N-1} (RR_{j+1} - RR_j)^2} \tag{7.5}$$

Another HRV parameter calculated from successive RR interval differences is the NN50, which is defined as the number of successive intervals differing more than 50 ms and is often reported as a percentage value (pNN50), that is,

$$NN50 = \text{nbr of } \left\{ RR_{j+1}, RR_j; j = 1 \cdots N-1 \,|\, (RR_{j+1} - RR_j) > 50\,\text{ms} \right\} \tag{7.6}$$

$$pNN50 = \frac{NN50}{N-1} \times 100\% \tag{7.7}$$

In addition to the above time-domain measures of HRV, there are two geometric measures that are commonly used to assess HRV data. These are the HRV triangular index (HRVi) and the triangular interpolation of the RR interval histogram (TINN). Both of these geometric measures are calculated from the RR interval histogram. HRVi is obtained by dividing the integral of the histogram (i.e., the total number of RR intervals) by the height of the histogram (i.e., the number of RR intervals at the modal bin). The value of this parameter is affected by the selected bin width, and thus, a bin width of $1/128$ seconds was recommended in [1] to obtain comparable results between different studies. TINN is defined as the baseline width of a triangle fitted on the RR interval histogram. HRVi measures the peakedness of the RR interval distribution, smaller values of HRVi indicating a more peaked distribution. TINN, on the other hand, estimates the baseline width of the RR interval distribution, thus providing an estimate of overall HRV.

7.4 Frequency-Domain Analysis Methods

The frequency-domain measures of HRV assess the HRV time series in the frequency domain, that is, through power spectral density (PSD) analysis. In the Kubios HRV software, the spectrum of the RR interval time series is estimated using two standard approaches: Welch's periodogram based on discrete Fourier transform and AR spectrum estimation. Both of these spectrum estimation methods assume equidistant sampling, and thus, the RR interval time series is interpolated using cubic spline interpolation (the default interpolation rate in Kubios HRV being 4 Hz) prior to spectrum estimation. Let us denote the interpolated RR interval time series with $x = (x_1, x_2, \ldots, x_L)$, where L is the length of the interpolated series.

7.4.1 Welch's Periodogram

A periodogram power spectrum estimate is defined as the squared absolute value of signals discrete Fourier transform [35], that is,

$$P_x(f_k) = \frac{1}{Lf_s} \left| \sum_{j=0}^{L-1} x_j e^{-i2\pi jk/L} \right|^2 \tag{7.8}$$

where L is the length of the signal, f_s is the sampling frequency, and $f_k = \frac{k}{L}f_s$, $k = 0 \ldots L - 1$. It can be shown that the periodogram is an asymptotically unbiased estimate of the spectrum, meaning that the expected value of the periodogram approaches the true spectrum when data length approaches infinity. However, the periodogram is not a consistent estimate of the spectrum because the variance of the periodogram is approximately equal to true spectral power and does not approach zero when data length approaches infinity.

The variance of the periodogram can be reduced by using certain periodogram modifications such as Welch's periodogram. In this periodogram modification, the signal is divided into overlapping segments, each segment is windowed to decrease the leakage effect, and the periodograms of these windowed segments are finally averaged to reduce the variance. Welch's periodogram is defined as

$$P_{\text{Welch}}(f_k) = \frac{1}{M} \sum_{m=1}^{M} \left(\frac{1}{Df_s U} \left| \sum_{j=0}^{D-1} w_j x_j^{(m)} e^{-i2\pi jk/D} \right|^2 \right) \tag{7.9}$$

where $x_j^{(m)} = x_{(m-1)(D-s)+j}$ is the mth overlapping segment (segment length D points and overlap s points), M is the number of overlapping segments and w_j is the window function (in Kubios HRV, a smooth Hanning window is used). The periodogram of each segment needs to be scaled with the segment length (D) and, sampling frequency (f_s) as well as the energy of the window function ($U = 1/D \sum_{j=0}^{D-1} w_j^2$) in order for the Parsevals theorem (preservation of energy) to hold. If the individual segment periodograms are independent (observations of spectrum), the variance of Welch's periodogram is reduced in relation to the number of segments M due to averaging, that is, to minimize variance M should be as high as possible. The number of segments can be increased by decreasing segment length (D) or by increasing overlap (s) between successive segments. By increasing segment overlap the correlation between the segments increases, and thus, the variance is not expected to decrease in relation to increase in M. Furthermore, decreasing of the segment length leads to decrease in frequency resolution. In the Kubios HRV software, the default value for segment overlap is 50% and the segment length needs to be defined based on the length of the available data.

7.4.2 AR Spectral Estimate

In the AR spectrum estimation approach, the interpolated RR time series is modeled with an AR model of specific order and the spectrum estimate can be produced from the estimated model parameters. An AR model of order p is given by

$$x_t = \sum_{j=1}^{p} a_j x_{t-j} + e_t \tag{7.10}$$

where a_j ($j = 1 \ldots p$) is the AR(p) parameters and e_t is the model residual. The AR model can be considered as one-step prediction equations where the current value of the time series is predicted as a weighted sum of p previous values, the weights being the AR parameters to be solved. Equation 7.10 also has a system interpretation where e_t (a noise process) is the input and x_t is the output of an infinite impulse response (IIR) system defined by the AR parameters. Parameters of the AR model can be estimated, for example, by solving the set of linear equations, $t = 1 \ldots L$ in 7.10, using least squares (LS) estimation, that is, minimizing the squared norm of the model residual terms. In the Kubios HRV software, the AR parameters are estimated using a combined forward and backward prediction LS solution [35].

The AR spectrum estimate can be obtained from the estimated AR parameters and is defined as

$$P_{AR}(f) = \frac{\sigma_e^2 / f_s}{\left| 1 + \sum_{j=1}^{p} a_j e^{-i2\pi j f / f_s} \right|^2} \tag{7.11}$$

where σ_e^2 is the variance of model residual, f_s is the sampling rate, and a_j are the AR parameters. Equation 7.11 rises from the system interpretation of the AR model, where σ_e^2 / f_s is the spectrum of a white noise process and the remaining part (on the right-hand side of Equation 7.11) is the spectrum of the IIR system defined by the AR parameters. The model residual e_t is white noise only when the AR model is fitted into a pure AR process. Real-world signals are, however, rarely AR processes that cause bias to the AR spectrum estimate, but this bias can be minimized by choosing the AR model order optimally.

The basic idea in optimal AR model order selection is to observe the improvement in model fit (decrease of σ_e^2) as a function of model order p. The optimal model order is obtained from the point where the curve σ_e^2 as a function of p levels off. Detection of this point is not always easy and several model order selection criteria, such as Akaikes information criteria (AIC), final prediction error (FPE), and minimum description length (MDL), have been developed to simplify this selection. For HRV analysis, it has been recommended that an AR model order not less than $p = 16$ should be used [36].

Figure 7.3 illustrates the effect of the model order on the AR spectrum quality. Three different model order selection criteria (AIC, FPE, and MDL) are computed for a 5-minute RR interval data recording from a healthy male subject during supine rest. It is observed that all three criteria level off at around order $p = 16$ which could thus be taken to the optimal model order. The AR spectrum with model order 16 does show similar structure to the Fourier fast transform (FFT)-based spectrum (Welch's periodogram computed with 150-second window and 50% overlap), but a higher model order ($p = 24$) produces even better correspondence between the two spectrum estimation techniques. However, if an order substantially lower than what is indicated by the model order selection criteria (e.g., $p = 8$) is selected, the AR model can not fully model the oscillations within the RR time series (i.e., the model residual is not white noise) and the spectrum estimate is thus missing details.

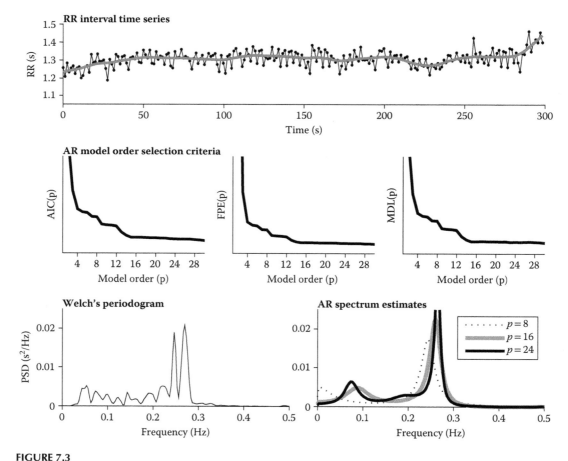

FIGURE 7.3
An illustration of autoregressive (AR) model order selection showing how the AR spectrum estimate compares to Welch's periodogram at different model orders.

One property, which is especially advantageous in assessing HRV spectrum, is that the AR spectrum estimate can be decomposed into distinct spectral components [37]. The decomposition is based on the factored form of Equation 7.11 given by

$$P_{AR}(f) = \frac{\sigma_e^2/f_s}{\prod_{j=1}^{p}(z - \alpha_j)(z^{-1} - \alpha_j^*)}, \quad z = e^{i2\pi f/f_s} \quad (7.12)$$

where α_j is the roots of the AR polynomial given in the denominator of Equation 7.11 and α_j^* is the complex conjugates of the roots. Each root produces a peak in the spectrum and the power of the spectral peak depends on how close to the unit circle the root is in the complex domain. The spectral component produced by a single root α_j can be estimated by assuming the effect of other roots is constant in the vicinity of frequency f_j, where the specific root α_j is positioned. The sum of the spectral components of all roots should be equal to the overall AR spectrum.

7.4.3 Parameterization of the Spectrum

The HRV spectrum is typically divided into VLF (0–0.04 Hz), LF (0.04–0.15 Hz), and HF (0.15–0.4 Hz) bands. This division is based on the current physiological understanding regarding cardiovascular regulatory systems. For example, the HF component is known to reflect parasympathetic nervous activity, whereas the LF component is affected by both SNS and PNS activations. Changes in cardiac autonomic regulation can thus be evaluated from these spectral features. Standard frequency-domain parameters computed from HRV spectra are summarized in Table 7.1 and their computations are described below.

Let us next denote the power spectrum estimate, computed using any relevant method (e.g., Welch's periodogram or AR spectrum), as $P(f_k)$, where f_k is the discrete frequencies between zero and the Nyquist frequency (half of the sampling frequency). The power within some specific frequency band is computed by integrating the spectrum, that is, by evaluating the area under the curve as illustrated in Figure 7.4. The powers of VLF, LF, and HF bands are thus computed from

$$P_{VLF} = \sum_{f_k \in [0-0.04]\,Hz} P(f_k)\Delta f \quad (7.13)$$

$$P_{LF} = \sum_{f_k \in [0.04-0.15]\,Hz} P(f_k)\Delta f \quad (7.14)$$

$$P_{HF} = \sum_{f_k \in [0.15-0.4]\,Hz} P(f_k)\Delta f \quad (7.15)$$

where $\Delta f = f_k - f_{k-1}$ is the bin width of a bar chart representing the spectrum and $P(f_k)$ is the heights of the columns in the bar chart (see Figure 7.4). As mentioned in Section 7.4.2, the AR spectrum can be divided into distinct spectral components as illustrated in Figure 7.4. In such case, the band powers are not computed by summing over frequencies within a prespecified frequency band as in Equations 7.13 through 7.15, but summing over the frequency components lying within a prespecified frequency band. The absolute band powers described above are usually given in units ms^2 or s^2 and a logarithm is often taken from the absolute power values in order to make these values normally distributed (e.g., over the patient population) for statistical analyses.

TABLE 7.1

Summary of Standard HRV Parameters Divided into Time-Domain, Frequency-Domain, and Nonlinear Categories

Parameter	(Units)	Description of the Parameter
Time-Domain Parameters		
Mean RR	(ms)	The mean of the beat-to-beat RR intervals
Mean HR	(bpm)	The mean of beat-to-beat heart-rate values in beats per minute
SDNN	(ms)	Standard deviation of RR intervals
RMSSD	(ms)	Square root of the mean-squared differences between successive RR intervals
NN50	(beats)	Number of successive RR intervals that differ more than 50 ms
pNN50	(%)	Percentage of successive RR intervals differing more than 50 ms (NN50 divided by the total number of RR intervals)
HRVi		HRV triangular index, obtained by dividing the area of the RR interval histogram by the number of RR intervals at the modal bin of the histogram [1]
TINN	(ms)	Triangular interpolation of RR interval histogram, which provides the baseline width of a triangle fitted to the histogram [1]
Frequency-Domain Parameters		
VLF power	$(ms^2, \%)$	Spectral power of the VLF component (typically ranging from 0 to 0.04 Hz) presented in absolute units (ms^2) or in percentage of total power (%): $$\text{VLF power } (\%) = \text{VLF power } (ms^2)/\text{Total power } (ms^2) \times 100\%$$
LF power	$(ms^2, \%, \text{n.u.})$	Spectral power of the LF component (typically ranging from 0.04 to 0.15 Hz) presented in absolute units (ms^2), percentage of total power (%) or normalized units (n.u.): $$\text{LF power } (\%) = \text{LF power } (ms^2)/\text{Total power } (ms^2) \times 100\%$$ $$\text{LF power } (\text{n.u.}) = \text{LF power } (ms^2)/[\text{Total power } (ms^2) - \text{VLF power } (ms^2)] \times 100\%$$
HF power	$(ms^2, \%, \text{n.u.})$	Spectral power of the HF component (typically ranging from 0.15 to 0.4 Hz) presented in absolute units (ms^2), percentage of total power (%) or normalized units (n.u.): $$\text{HF power } (\%) = \text{HF power } (ms^2)/\text{Total power } (ms^2) \times 100\%$$ $$\text{HF power } (\text{n.u.}) = \text{HF power } (ms^2)/[\text{Total power } (ms^2) - \text{VLF power } (ms^2)] \times 100\%$$
LF/HF		Ratio between LF and HF component powers
Peak frequency	(Hz)	LF and HF component peak frequencies (frequency corresponding to the maximum power within the frequency band)
Nonlinear Parameters		
SD1, SD2	(ms)	Standard deviation of the Poincaré plot perpendicular to the line-of-identity (SD1) and along the line-of-identity (SD2) [25,26]
α_1, α_2		Slopes of short term (α_1) and long-term (α_2) fluctuations in DFA [27,28]
ApEn		Approximate entropy [29,30]
SampEn		Sample entropy [30]
D2		Correlation dimension [31,32]
Lmean, Lmax	(beats)	Mean and maximum line lengths of diagonal lines in RP [33,34]
REC, DET	(%)	Recurrence rate (percentage of recurrence points in RP) and determinism (percentage of recurrence points which form diagonal lines in RP)
ShanEn		Shannon entropy of diagonal line lengths probability distribution

DET, determinism; HF, high frequency; HR, heart rate; HRV, heart rate variability; LF, low frequency; RP, recurrence plot; REC, recurrence rate; RMSSD, root mean square of successive differences; TINN, triangular interpolation of RR interval histogram; VLF, very low frequency.

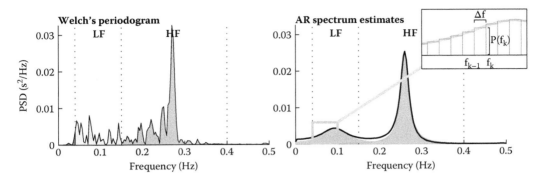

FIGURE 7.4
Computation of LF and HF powers from power spectral density estimates.

The relative powers of the VLF, LF, and HF bands can be presented in percentage values as

$$P_{\text{VLF}}(\%) = \frac{P_{\text{VLF}}(\text{ms}^2)}{P_{\text{Total}}(\text{ms}^2)} \times 100\% \tag{7.16}$$

$$P_{\text{LF}}(\%) = \frac{P_{\text{LF}}(\text{ms}^2)}{P_{\text{Total}}(\text{ms}^2)} \times 100\% \tag{7.17}$$

$$P_{\text{HF}}(\%) = \frac{P_{\text{HF}}(\text{ms}^2)}{P_{\text{Total}}(\text{ms}^2)} \times 100\% \tag{7.18}$$

In addition, the relative powers of the LF and HF bands can be presented in normalized units (n.u.) as

$$P_{\text{LF}}(\text{n.u.}) = \frac{P_{\text{LF}}(\text{ms}^2)}{P_{\text{Total}}(\text{ms}^2) - P_{\text{VLF}}(\text{ms}^2)} \times 100\% \tag{7.19}$$

$$P_{\text{HF}}(\text{n.u.}) = \frac{P_{\text{HF}}(\text{ms}^2)}{P_{\text{Total}}(\text{ms}^2) - P_{\text{VLF}}(\text{ms}^2)} \times 100\% \tag{7.20}$$

and the power ratio between them can be simply computed as

$$\text{LF/HF} = \frac{P_{\text{LF}}(\text{ms}^2)}{P_{\text{HF}}(\text{ms}^2)} \tag{7.21}$$

The relative powers of different frequency components and the LF/HF ratio are useful when examining the proportion of LF to HF, which is known to reflect sympatho-vagal balance. One advantage in using relative powers is that the high interindividual variability known to exist in the absolute HRV power values is not an issue, because the values are normalized with the total power.

7.5 Nonlinear Analysis Methods

Considering the complex regulation of the cardiovascular system, it is quite obvious that the HRV time series features cannot be fully captured using linear methods. Therefore, various nonlinear methods have been applied to HRV to fully capture the characteristics of the beat-to-beat variability. However, nonlinearity of a method per se is not a guarantee of capturing useful information from the HRV time series. Furthermore, the physiological interpretation of the results obtained using nonlinear methods is sometimes difficult. Therefore, it is important to compare the results from nonlinear methods against those obtained from the standard linear methods.

In Kubios HRV software, nonlinear properties of HRV can be assessed using measures such as Poincaré plot, approximate (ApEn) and sample entropy (SampEn), correlation dimension, detrended fluctuation analysis (DFA), and recurrence plot (RP) analysis. The nonlinear methods implemented in Kubios are summarized in Table 7.1 and described shortly in the following.

7.5.1 Poincaré Plot Analysis

The Poincaré plot is a graphical presentation of the correlation between consecutive RR intervals, that is, a plot of RR_{j+1} as a function of RR_j [25,26]. The shape of the plot is quantified by fitting an ellipse into the data points (RR_j, RR_{j+1}) oriented along the line of identity (LOI) where $RR_j = RR_{j+1}$. The width and length of the ellipse are determined by the standard deviations of the points perpendicular to and along the LOI as illustrated in Figure 7.5. The standard deviation perpendicular to the LOI is denoted by SD1 and standard deviation along the LOI by SD2. SD1 is considered to reflect short-term (beat-to-beat) variability, which is mainly caused by RSA. It can be shown that the SD1 is related to the time-domain measures SDSD (or RMSSD) by [25]

$$SD1 = \sqrt{\frac{SDSD^2}{2}} \simeq \sqrt{\frac{RMSSD^2}{2}} \tag{7.22}$$

The standard deviation along the LOI denoted by SD2, on the other hand, measures overall variability, that is, aggregate of short-term and long-term variabilities and has been shown to be related to the time-domain measures SDNN and SDSD (or RMSSD) by [25]

$$SD2 = \sqrt{2\,SDNN^2 - \frac{SDSD^2}{2}} \simeq \sqrt{2\,SDNN^2 - \frac{RMSSD^2}{2}} \tag{7.23}$$

The ratio of these two standard deviations, that is, SD1/SD2 can thus be considered to yield a nonlinear index for the balance between short-term beat-to-beat variability and longer term variability.

7.5.2 Entropy Measures

ApEn and SampEn are two commonly used entropy measures, both measuring the complexity or irregularity of the signal [29,30]. A generalization of SampEn is provided by multiscale entropy (MSE) described after ApEn and SampEn. These three entropy measures are included in the Kubios HRV software. Another entropy measure that has drawn

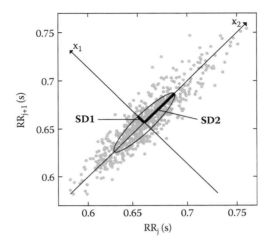

FIGURE 7.5
Parametrization of the Poincaré plot with the ellipse fitting procedure. SD1 and SD2 are standard deviations at directions x_1 and x_2, where x_2 is the line of identity (LOI) having $RR_j = RR_{j+1}$.

attention lately is Renyi entropy, which is also an MSE measure including Shannon entropy as a special case [38].

Considering the values of ApEn or SampEn, large values indicate high irregularity whereas smaller values indicate a more regular signal. The computations of these entropy values starts by forming length m embedding vectors u_j:

$$u_j = \left(RR_j, RR_{j+1}, \dots, RR_{j+m-1} \right), \quad j = 1, 2, \dots, N-m+1 \qquad (7.24)$$

where m is the embedding dimension and N is the number of beats. Then, for every u_j, the relative number of vectors u_k, for which the distance to u_j is small enough, is calculated. At this point, the computations of ApEn and SampEn diverge, but in both measures the distance between any two vectors u_j and u_k is defined as the maximum absolute element-wise difference:

$$d(u_j, u_k) = \max \left\{ |RR_{j+n} - RR_{k+n}| \, \middle| \, n = 0, \dots, m-1 \right\} \qquad (7.25)$$

In ApEn, the relative number of vectors u_k for which $d(u_j, u_k) \leq r$ is defined as

$$C_j^m(r) = \frac{\text{nbr of } \left\{ u_k \, \middle| \, d(u_j, u_k) \leq r \right\}}{N-m+1} \quad \forall k \qquad (7.26)$$

The value of $C_j^m(r)$ is always between $1/(N-m+1) \leq C_j^m(r) \leq 1$. ApEn is obtained by first averaging the natural logarithms of every $C_j^m(r)$ as

$$\Phi^m(r) = \frac{1}{N-m+1} \sum_{j=1}^{N-m+1} \ln C_j^m(r) \qquad (7.27)$$

Equations 7.24 through 7.27 are then reevaluated for embedding dimension $m+1$ and ApEn is obtained as

$$\text{AppEn}(m, r, N) = \Phi^m(r) - \Phi^{m+1}(r). \tag{7.28}$$

In SampEn, the self-comparison of u_j is excluded when computing $C_j^m(r)$, that is, Equation (7.26) is replaced with

$$C_j^m(r) = \frac{\text{nbr of } \left\{ u_k \,\middle|\, d(u_j, u_k) \le r \right\}}{N - m} \quad \forall k \neq j \tag{7.29}$$

where now $0 \le C_j^m(r) \le 1$. SampEn is obtained by first averaging the terms $C_j^m(r)$ with

$$\Phi^m(r) = \frac{1}{N - m + 1} \sum_{j=1}^{N-m+1} C_j^m(r) \tag{7.30}$$

and then (after reevaluating the same for embedding dimension $m+1$) evaluating

$$\text{SampEn}(m, r, N) = \ln\left(\frac{\Phi^m(r)}{\Phi^{m+1}(r)} \right) \tag{7.31}$$

The values of ApEn and SampEn depend on three factors, the embedding dimension m, the tolerance value r, and number of beats N. Both entropy measures are estimates for the negative natural logarithm of the conditional probability that a time series of length N, having repeated itself within a tolerance r for m points, will also repeat itself for $m+1$ points. In the Kubios HRV software, the default values for the embedding dimension and tolerance are $m=2$ and $r=0.2\,\text{SDNN}$. Fixing the tolerance value on standard deviation of the time series enables comparison of different time series acquisitions. Finally, it should be mentioned that the length N of the time series also has an effect on the entropy measures, but when N increases both ApEn and SampEn approach their asymptotic values.

7.5.2.1 Multiscale Entropy

MSE is an extension of SampEn in the sense that it provides sample entropy values as a function of a scale factor [39]. A course-graining process is applied to extract different scales from the original RR interval time series. Computation of MSE involves the following two steps:

1. Several course-grained time series are extracted from the measured RR data by averaging the beat-to-beat data within nonoverlapping windows of increasing length τ. In the Kubios HRV software, the scale factor τ is selected to range between $\tau = 1, 2, \ldots, 20$ and the length of the course-grained time series is N/τ (N being the number of beats).

2. SampEn is calculated for each course-grained time series and the MSE is obtained by presenting the SampEn values as a function of the scale factor τ. MSE for scale factor $\tau = 1$ involves no course graining and returns standard SampEn.

7.5.3 Correlation Dimension

The correlation dimension is also a measure of the complexity or strangeness of the data, and is expected to give information on the minimum number of dynamic variables needed to model the complex system [31,32]. The computation of the correlation dimension starts similarly as for the entropy measures described above, that is, length m embedding vectors are first formed according to Equation 7.24 and then the relative number of vectors u_k for which the distance to u_j is below a prespecified tolerance is computed according to Equation 7.26. The distance between two embedding vectors u_j and u_k is now, however, defined as

$$d(u_j, u_k) = \sqrt{\sum_{l=1}^{m} \left(u_j(l) - u_k(l) \right)^2}$$

(7.32)

The average of the terms $C_j^m(r)$ (computed according to Equation 7.26) is then computed according to Equation 7.30. The correlation dimension, denoted with D_2, is defined as the limit value

$$D_2(m) = \lim_{r \to 0} \lim_{N \to \infty} \frac{\log \Phi^m(r)}{\log r}$$

(7.33)

In practice, this limit value is approximated by the slope of the regression curve $(\log r, \log \Phi^m(r))$ [32]. Specifically, the slope is calculated from the linear part of the log–log plot as shown in Figure 7.6. The slope of the regression curves tend to saturate on the finite value of D_2 when m is increased, but for higher values of m longer data sequences would be required. In the Kubios HRV software, the default value for the embedding dimension is $m = 10$.

7.5.4 Detrended Fluctuation Analysis

DFA evaluates correlations within the RR interval time series. The correlations can be extracted for different time scales as described below [27,28]. First, the RR time series is

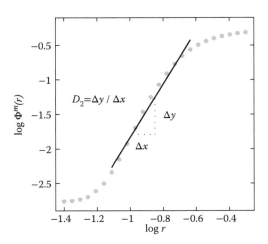

FIGURE 7.6
Approximation of the correlation dimension D_2 from a $(\log r, \log \Phi^m(r))$ plot.

integrated according to

$$y(k) = \sum_{j=1}^{k} \left(RR_j - \overline{RR} \right), \quad k = 1, \ldots, N \tag{7.34}$$

which is simply the cumulative sum of zero mean RR interval values. This integrated series is then divided into length n nonoverlapping segments and within each segment a local trend is estimated by fitting a LS line into the segment data points. The integrated series $y(k)$ is then detrended by subtracting the local trends $\overline{y_n}(k)$ segment-by-segment. The root mean square value of the integrated and detrended RR series is then calculated as

$$F(n) = \sqrt{\frac{1}{N} \sum_{k=1}^{N} \left(y(k) - \overline{y_n}(k) \right)^2} \tag{7.35}$$

The computation of $F(n)$ is repeated over different segment lengths (scales) and typically $F(n)$ increases as a function of n. The presence of fractal scaling is assessed by looking at a linear relationship of $\log F(n)$ and $\log n$. In HRV research, the scales are usually divided to reflect short-term and long-term fluctuations. The default values in the Kubios HRV software for the scales are $4 \le n \le 12$ for short-term and $13 \le n \le 64$ for long-term fluctuations. The short- and long-term fluctuations are then characterized by the slopes α_1 and α_2 of linear regression lines fitted separately in the log–log graph ($\log F(n)$, $\log n$) on scales $4 \le n \le 12$ and $13 \le n \le 64$ as illustrated in Figure 7.7.

The different values of α are interpreted as follows [27]:

> $0 < \alpha < 0.5$: Indicates correlation where large RR interval values are likely to be followed by small values and vice versa
>
> $\alpha = 0.5$: White noise

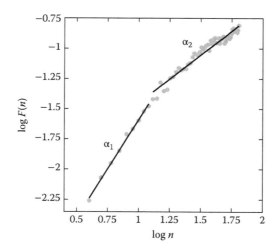

FIGURE 7.7
Computation of the detrended fluctuation analysis (DFA) short-term and long-term fluctuation slopes (α_1 and α_2, respectively) from a ($\log n$, $\log F(n)$) plot.

0.5 < α < 1: Indicates persistent long-term correlation where the large RR interval values are likely to be followed by large values and vice versa

α = 1: 1/f noise

1 < α < 1.5: Indicates different kinds of correlated noise

α = 1.5: Brownian noise (integration of white noise)

Furthermore, the value of α can also be considered as an indicator of RR interval time series smoothness, that is, the larger the value of α the smoother the time series.

7.5.5 RP Analysis

RP analysis is yet another nonlinear method for assessing the complexity of RR time series [33,34,40]. Similar to the entropy measures computation, embedding vectors

$$u_j = \left(RR_j, RR_{j+\tau}, \ldots, RR_{j+(m-1)\tau} \right), \quad j = 1, 2, \ldots, N - (m-1)\tau \tag{7.36}$$

where m is the embedding dimension and τ is the embedding lag, are extracted from the RR time series. Vectors u_j can be considered to represent the RR time series trajectory in m-dimensional space. The RP is a symmetric binary matrix such that the value in the jth row and kth column RP(j, k) is

$$RP(j,k) = \begin{cases} 1, & d(u_j - u_k) \leq r \\ 0, & \text{otherwise} \end{cases} \tag{7.37}$$

where $d(u_j - u_k)$ is the Euclidean distance between u_j and u_k given in Equation 7.32 and r is a fixed threshold. An example of RP for HRV data if presented in Figure 7.8. Short line segments of ones parallel to the main diagonal, which are typical for RP matrices of correlated data, are clearly observed. The lengths of the diagonal line segments are related

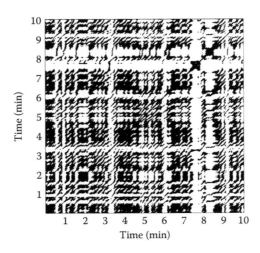

FIGURE 7.8
Recurrence plot matrix for 10-minute RR time series (black = 1 and white = 0).

to the duration for which two embedding vectors are close to each other. In Kubios HRV, the default values are for the embedding dimension $m = 10$ and threshold $r = \sqrt{m}\text{SDNN}$ (embedding delay is fixed to $\tau = 1$).

Several parameters for quantifying the RP have been proposed in [33], some of which are summarized here. Recurrence rate (REC) gives the ratio of ones and zeros in the RP matrix, that is,

$$\text{REC} = \frac{1}{(N-m+1)^2} \sum_{j=1}^{N-m+1} \sum_{k=1}^{N-m+1} \text{RP}(j,k) \tag{7.38}$$

where $N - m + 1$ is the number of rows and columns in the RP matrix when $\tau = 1$. In addition, several parameters assessing the lengths of the diagonal lines have been proposed. To exclude recurrences caused by nondiagonal trajectory movements, a threshold of minimum diagonal line length $l_{min} = 2$ is applied. Furthermore, the longest observed diagonal line (excluding the main diagonal) is denoted with l_{max}. Divergence (DIV) is defined as the inverse of $l_{min} = 2$, that is,

$$\text{DIV} = \frac{1}{l_{max}} \tag{7.39}$$

and it has been shown to correlate with the largest positive Lyapunov exponent [40]. The average diagonal line length (l_{mean}), on the other hand, can be computed from

$$l_{mean} = \frac{\sum_{l=l_{min}}^{l_{max}} lN_l}{\sum_{l=l_{min}}^{l_{max}} N_l} \tag{7.40}$$

where N_l is the number of length l lines. The determinism (DET) of the time series is defined as

$$\text{DET} = \frac{\sum_{l=l_{min}}^{l_{max}} lN_l}{\sum_{j,k=1}^{N-m+1} \text{RP}(j,k)} \tag{7.41}$$

Finally, the Shannon information entropy of the line length distribution is defined as

$$\text{ShanEn} = -\sum_{l=l_{min}}^{l_{max}} n_l \ln n_l \tag{7.42}$$

where n_l is the number of length l lines scaled with the total number of lines, that is,

$$n_l = \frac{N_l}{\sum_{j=l_{min}}^{l_{max}} N_j} \tag{7.43}$$

7.6 Considerations in the Assessment of HRV

This section tackles the three following important issues related to HRV analysis:

1. What is the effect of trend on HRV analysis? Often HR shows gradual increase or decrease during the recording period, which give rise to trend or baseline changes

in the RR interval time series. It is not always easy to understand how the trend a effects different HRV parameters and how to handle it.

2. How do we handle incorrect beat detections, ectopic, and other aberrant beats? Almost always (at least in longer recordings) RR interval recordings include one or more such artifacts. It is commonly understood that only normal-to-normal RR intervals (originating from sinus rhythm) should be included in the analysis, but the effect that even one single abnormal beat can have on different HRV parameters is not easy to perceive.

3. What is the effect of respiration on HRV and how do we take this into account in HRV analysis? RSA is one of the two main components of HRV and quite often the RSA component is evaluated using standard assumptions of respiratory frequency.

In each of these three cases, illustrative examples are given to help the reader understand the effects that these issues have on HRV analysis and avoid the possible pitfalls of misinterpretation of HRV analysis results.

7.6.1 The Effect of Trend and Artifacts on HRV Analysis

Accurate estimation of different HRV parameters necessitates a sufficiently long ECG recording. In principle, the recording should last at least 10 times the wavelength of the investigated frequency component. This would indicate that the HF component of HRV (RSA component) can be reliably estimated from as short as 1-minute data segments (if the LF bound of the RSA component is at 0.15 Hz). The LF component would then need approximately twice as long of a data segment to be assessed, whereas many of the nonlinear parameters require at least 5 minutes of data to have reasonable accuracy. In order to standardize different studies investigating short-term HRV, 5-minute recordings have been recommended unless the nature of the study dictates otherwise [1]. However, recordings should be free from artifacts or other disruptive components to optimally assess the normal beat-to-beat HRV.

7.6.1.1 Very Low Frequency Trend Components of HRV

An HRV time series often includes nonstationarities like slow linear or more complex trends, that is, changes in the average HR. These baseline changes of HR can be noticeable even within short-term recordings and they can have quite significant effects on different HRV parameter values as illustrated below. The origins for such nonstationarities in HRV are discussed, for example, in [11]. One approach to get around the nonstationarity problem is to systematically test for nonstationarities and select only stationary segments for analysis as suggested in [41]. The representativeness of these stationary segments in comparison with the whole HRV signal was, however, questioned in [42]. The representativeness of the selected segment is actually one common dilemma among HRV researchers, that is, dealing with nonstationarities like slow trends or occasional HRV anomalies caused, for example, by atypical breathing patterns or unexpected postural changes. In general, it is advisable to visually verify that the selected segment does not include atypical HRV patterns or clear outliers and that the segment is representative in comparison with the whole HRV signal.

To deal with VLF trends of arbitrary form, we have proposed a smoothness priors regularization-based method for trend removal [43]. In this method, we do not need to set any model for the trend. The only assumption is smoothness of the trend, which is implemented by adding a smoothness prior regularization term (smoothness induced by a second-order difference operator) into a standard LS minimization problem. If we denote a length L RR interval time series as $x = (x_1, x_2, \ldots, x_L)$ and consider that it consists of two components

$$x = x_{\text{Stat}} + x_{\text{Trend}} \tag{7.44}$$

where x_{Stat} is the stationary part of the RR series and x_{Trend} is the trend. Using the smoothness priors regularization (for details see [43]), the estimate for the trend and detrended RR series are obtained in the form

$$x_{\text{Trend}} = \left(I + \lambda^2 D_2^T D_2\right)^{-1} x \tag{7.45}$$

$$x_{\text{Stat}} = x - x_{\text{Trend}} \tag{7.46}$$

where I is an identity matrix and D_2 is a second-order difference matrix. In MATLAB® (http://www.mathworks.com), the trend estimation can be performed in a few simple lines:

```
L = length(x);
lambda = 500;
I = speye(L);
D2 = spdiags(ones(L-2,1)*[1 -2 1],[0:2],L-2,L);
xTrend = (I+lambda^2*D2'*D2)\x;
xStat = x-xTrend;
```

When applied to equidistantly sampled time series, the smoothness priors detreding method was shown to be equal to a time-varying highpass filter [43]. The amplitude response of this filter is presented in Figure 7.9, which illustrates the time-varying amplitude response (Figure 7.9a) and the amplitude response for different values of the smoothing parameter λ (Figure 7.9b). It is observed that the form of the amplitude response is mostly constant, but the beginning and end of the RR data is processed differently. Thus, the method is not comparable to the simple learning tools interoperability (LTI) highpass

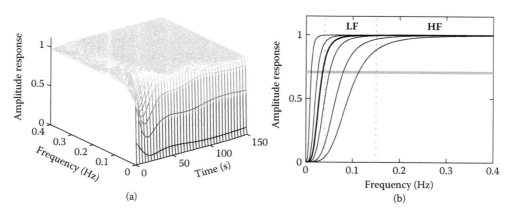

(a)   (b)

FIGURE 7.9
(a) Time-varying amplitude response for the smoothness priors detrending method when sampling frequency of the data is 4 Hz and smoothing parameter $\lambda = 500$. (b) Amplitude responses (constant part) for different values of λ (from left to right $\lambda = 5000, 1000, 500$ [bold line], 250, 100, 50 and cutoff frequencies are 0.016, 0.029, 0.035, 0.051, 0.080, and 0.113 Hz, respectively).

filter and the beginning and end of the data are estimated nicely without any tricks. Smoothness of the trend (or the cutoff frequency for trend removal) is adjusted by the smoothing parameter; bigger values of λ produce smoother trend estimates (lower cutoff frequency for detrending).

7.6.1.2 Artifacts in HRV Recordings

The artifacts in HRV recording can be divided into technical and physiological artifacts. The technical artifacts include missing beat detections or misplaced beat detections. The performance of the QRS detection algorithm has a direct effect on the number of these artifacts. Low signal-to-noise ratio due to poorly fastened electrodes or movement artifacts increases the number of misdetections. Physiological artifacts include premature ventricular beats (ectopic beats) and other arrhythmic events. Several different correction methods for handling such artifacts have been proposed within the past few decades. The proposed methods involve deletion, interpolation, or filtering techniques to edit the artifact beats. A recent review of HRV artifact correction methods can be found in [44].

In Kubios HRV, there are two possibilities for correcting artifacts. If an ECG has been recorded, then one should always fix artifacts caused by R-wave misdetections by editing the R-wave peak detections from the ECG data using the tools available for that. Any changes made to the R-wave detections are saved on the MATLAB MAT file while saving the results of the analysis. The MAT file can be reopened in Kubios, which enables the user to return to the file without losing the changes made to the R-wave detections. If ECG is not measured or the artifacts cannot be corrected by editing R-wave detections, Kubios HRV offers simple artifact correction options. The user can select between very low, low, medium, strong, and very strong correction levels. The different correction levels define thresholds (very low = 0.45 sec, low = 0.35 sec, medium = 0.25 sec, strong = 0.15 sec, very strong = 0.05 sec) for detecting the RR intervals differing abnormally from the local mean of the RR interval. These correction thresholds are for HR of 60 beats/min; for higher HRs the thresholds are decreased (because the variability is expected to decrease when HR increases). Detected artifacts are corrected by applying a piecewise cubic spline interpolation method.

7.6.1.3 The Effects on HRV Analysis

Next, we examine briefly the impact that trend or small number of artifacts within the RR interval time series can have on different HRV analysis parameters. To do this, we selected a 5-minute ECG recording of a healthy young male subject measured during supine rest. The ECG data did not originally include any abnormal beats. The beat-to-beat RR intervals were extracted from the ECG using the built-in QRS detector of Kubios HRV software and authenticity of beat detections were visually verified. The original RR interval time series and its Fourier spectrum (estimated using Welch's periodogram method) are presented in Figure 7.10a. The trend was then removed using the smoothness priors method ($\lambda =$ 1000). The detrended RR time series and its Fourier spectrum as shown in Figure 7.10b. The reduction of the VLFs (frequencies below 0.04 Hz) is evident.

Two artifacts were then produced in the RR time series by removing one beat detection (simulating a missed beat detection) and by bringing forward one beat detection (simulating a premature ventricular contraction). These simulated artifacts and corresponding Fourier spectra are shown in Figures 7.10c and d. It is observed that the two simulated artifacts cause an observable increase in spectral power in both the LF and HF bands. It is worth noting also that for the artifact-free data, the HRV spectrum shows a quite nice peak around 0.28 Hz, which was the respiratory frequency of the subject as assessed from

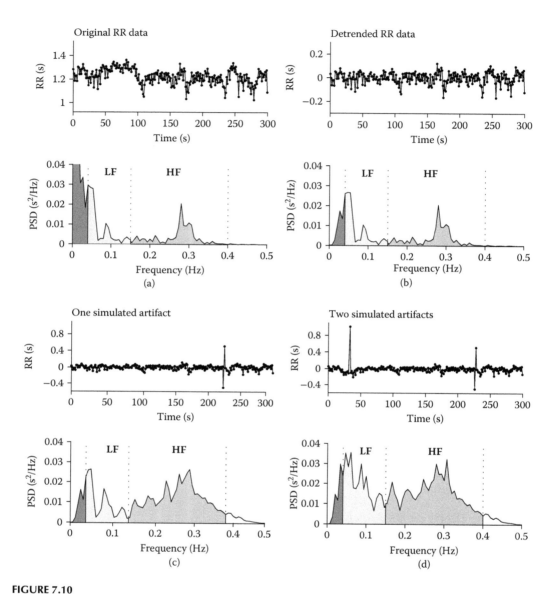

FIGURE 7.10
RR interval time series and Fourier spectra for (a) original 5-minute artifact-free RR interval time series, (b) detrended RR time series, (c) RR time series including one simulated artifact (premature ventricular beat), and (d) RR time series with two artifacts (one missed peak detection and one premature ventricular beat).

the ECG using the ECG derived respiration (EDR) methodology [45]. For the data with the simulated artifacts, the RSA component is not as easily distinguished due to spectral leakage.

The effect of the trend and the simulated artifacts shown in Figure 7.10 on commonly used short-term HRV analysis parameters is illustrated in Table 7.2. Naturally, the trend removal mainly affects parameters such as SDNN, TINN, and Poincaré SD2, which all reflect long-term variability. The peaked artifacts, which appear as clear outliers within the

TABLE 7.2

The Effect of Trend and Artifacts (Illustrated in Figure 7.10) on HRV Analysis Parameters

Parameter	(Units)	Original RR Data[a]	Detrended RR Data[b]	One Simulated Artifact[c]	Two Simulated Artifacts[d]
Time-Domain Parameters					
Mean RR	(ms)	1222	1222	1222	1227
SDNN	(ms)	63.9	50.1	67.8	96.7
RMSSD	(ms)	60.1	59.9	99.6	141.7
pNN50	(%)	43.5	43.5	43.9	44.9
HRVi		15.44	11.76	10.74	11.71
TINN	(ms)	298	238	690	1024
Frequency-Domain Parameters					
VLF power	(ms^2)	2046	374	336	480
LF power	(ms^2)	862	826	1101	2122
HF power	(ms^2)	822	822	3144	3859
LF power	(n.u.)	51.2	50.1	25.9	35.4
HF power	(n.u.)	48.8	49.9	73.9	64.4
LF/HF		1.05	1.00	0.35	0.55
Nonlinear Parameters					
Poincaré plot, SD1	(ms)	42.6	42.4	70.6	100.4
Poincaré plot, SD2	(ms)	79.3	56.3	64.7	92.8
ApEn		0.99	1.06	1.18	1.17
SampEn		1.73	2.12	1.75	1.36
Correlation dimension, D2		3.70	4.24	4.12	3.67
DFA, α_1		1.04	0.96	0.76	0.66
DFA, α_2		0.93	0.41	0.37	0.29

DFA, detrended fluctuation analysis; HF, high frequency; HRV, heart rate variability; LF, low frequency; VLF, very low frequency.

[a] Original normal-to-normal RR interval data as shown in Figure 7.10a.
[b] Original RR data after removing the trend using the smoothness priors method as shown in Figure 7.10b.
[c] Detrended RR data with one simulated artifact as shown in Figure 7.10c.
[d] Detrended RR data with two simulated artifacts as shown in Figure 7.10d.

RR time series, cause a major increase in HRV parameters reflecting strength of variability in one way or another, that is, SDNN, RMSSD, TINN, LF and HF absolute powers, and Poincaré indices SD1 and SD2 all increase. Nonlinear measures of HRV complexity or predictability such as ApEn and SampEn, correlation dimension, and detrended fluctuation analysis parameters do not show such clear changes. Based on the data of only one subject, we cannot of course say much about the sensitivity of different HRV parameters to artifacts. However, it is easy to understand (and was shown here as well) that parameters measuring the HRV amplitude or power in one way or another are significantly affected by outliers such as missed peak detections or ectopic beats. Therefore, such outliers should always be either corrected or excluded from analysis.

7.6.2 Analysis of RSA

The most conspicuous component of HRV is usually the HF component ranging from 0.15 to 0.4 Hz. The HF component is commonly known as the RSA due to how this higher frequency oscillatory component is originated. During inhalation, the vagus nerve is unstimulated resulting in lowered vagal (parasympathetic) input to the heart. Therefore, the HR increases during inhalation and then again decreases during exhalation. In addition to respiratory rate, the depth of respiration also affects HR regulation.

The effect of respiration on the HRV time series and spectral components (LF and HF components) is illustrated in Figure 7.11, which shows an RR interval recording of a healthy young male subject during a controlled breathing test. During the test, the subject breathed at constant rates for 3-minute periods by following a visual control given on a computer screen. The respiratory rates carried out in the test were 0.3, 0.2, 0.17, 0.12, and 0.1 Hz (proceeding from highest to lowest). At the beginning and the end of the test, the subject breathed spontaneously.

Lowered respiratory rate has been associated with increased HRV [46,47], which is also illustrated in Figure 7.11. The increase in the RSA component power (HF component

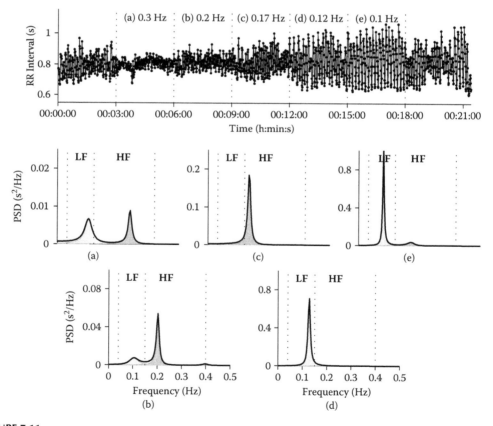

FIGURE 7.11
RR interval time series and autoregressive spectrum estimates for altered respiratory rates. The controlled respiratory frequencies were (a) 0.3 Hz, (b) 0.2 Hz, (c) 0.17 Hz, (d) 0.12 Hz, and (e) 0.1 Hz. Each controlled respiratory rate was maintained for 3 minutes; the beginning and the end of the recording consisted of spontaneous breathing.

observed a clear spectral peak at respiratory frequency) for lower respiratory rates is substantial (note the increasing y-axis scale on the spectral plots). This figure illustrates plainly how important it is to know a subject's respiratory rate for HRV analysis. For example, if one would interpret the HRV spectrum presented in Figure 7.11e without knowing the respiratory rate, they could report a strong LF component and weak HF (RSA) component indicating high sympatho-vagal balance, even though the weak HF component observed would truly be just a harmonic component induced by overlapping LF and HF components at 0.1 Hz. When there is a risk that the LF and HF components might overlap, spectral decomposition approaches, such as those presented in [37,48], are useful for estimating these component powers more reliably.

7.7 Conclusions

In this chapter, we have introduced the commonly used time-domain, frequency-domain, and nonlinear HRV analysis methods. All the presented analysis methods are available in Kubios HRV software, which is available at http://www.kubios.com [15]. Kubios HRV supports several input data formats for ECG data and beat-to-beat RR interval data. The software has a built-in QRS detection algorithm and easy-to-use tools for artifact correction, trend removal, and analysis sample selection (i.e., selecting one or more time periods from the data for analysis). The software includes several adjustable settings, which are necessary to optimize the methods for different kinds of HRV data. The main purpose of Kubios HRV software is to provide a reliable and easy-to-use analysis tool for researchers who use HRV recording in their studies and have the necessary knowledge to interpret and report the results. Thus, Kubios HRV provides the user only the values of the various HRV analysis parameters, whereas finding the appropriate interpretation or meaning of the results is left to the user.

HRV is known to provide quantitative information of ANS, that is, of the balance between sympathetic and parasympathetic tones. Decrease in HRV is related to increased sympatho-vagal balance, that is, sympathetic tone is emphasized compared to parasympathetic tone, and vice versa. Some of the HRV analysis parameters have quite clear interpretation regarding the division between sympathetic and parasympathetic activities. This division is done easiest using frequency-domain parameters, that is, LF and HF component powers. The HF component is known to originate solely from parasympathetic neural activity, whereas the LF component is affected by both sympathetic and parasympathetic but predominated by sympathetic neural activity. Therefore, the HF power both in absolute units as well as in percentage or normalized units indicates parasympathetic neural activity, and LF/HF ratio or LF power in percentage or normalized units can all be used as indices of sympatho-vagal balance.

Some division between sympathetic and parasympathetic neural activities can also be done from the HRV time-domain parameters. For example, the time-domain parameters that evaluate RR interval differences between successive beats, such as RMSSD, NN50, and pNN50, can all be considered to be more affected by parasympathetic neural activity, simply because the HF (HF component) oscillations of parasympathetic origin are affected more on successive beat interval differences than the slower (LF component) oscillations. The SDNN, on the other hand, which is the standard deviation of beat intervals, reflects overall variability without any clear division between sympathetic and parasympathetic neural activities, except of course the fact that HRV is overall higher when parasympthetic tone is emphasized (rest and digest) compared to when sympathetic tone is emphasized (fight or flight). Nonlinear measures of HRV are often hardest to interpret, that is, hardest to relate to known physiology. However, some of the nonlinear parameters have been observed to capture HRV features undetectable by standard linear parameters, and thus, nonlinear parameters may provide additional information of clinical significance.

One challenge in interpreting HRV findings is the comparability between the multitude of studies reporting HRV analysis results. The guidelines for HRV analysis published in 1996 [1] have been somewhat followed in the majority of HRV studies, which makes comparing of studies easier. However, over 20 years have passed since these guidelines were published and several new methodologies (especially nonlinear analysis methods) for HRV analysis have been proposed ever since. The preprocessing steps like artifact correction and trend removal described in this chapter should always be carefully considered and reported because they both have significant effects on the HRV analysis results. Finally, respiratory frequency has a direct influence on HRV, and thus, respiration should ideally always be measured along with the HRV.

References

1. Task Force of the European Society of Cardiology and the North American Society of Pacing and Electrophysiology. Heart rate variability—Standards of measurement, physiological interpretation, and clinical use. *Circulation*, 93(5):1043–1065, March 1996.
2. U.R. Acharya, K.P. Joseph, N. Kannathal, C.M. Lim, and J.S. Suri. Heart rate variability: A review. *Medical & Biological Engineering & Computing*, 44:1031–1051, 2006.
3. T. Laitio, J. Jalonen, T. Kuusela, and H. Scheinin. The role of heart rate variability in risk stratification for adverse postoperative cardiac events. *Anesthesia and Analgesia*, 105(6):1548–1560, 2007.
4. O. Pradhapan, M.P. Tarvainen, T. Nieminen, R. Lehtinen, K. Nikus, T. Lehtimäki, M. Kähönen, and J. Viik. Effect of heart rate correction on pre- and post-exercise heart rate variability to predict risk of mortality—An experimental study on the FINCAVAS cohort. *Frontiers in Physiology*, 5(Article 208):1–9, 2014.
5. A.I. Vinik, T. Erbas, and C.M. Casellini. Diabetic cardiac autonomic neuropathy, inammation and cardiovascular disease. *Journal of Diabetes Investigation*, 4(1):4–8, 2013.
6. M.P. Tarvainen, T.P. Laitinen, J.A. Lipponen, D.J. Cornforth, and H.F. Jelinek. Cardiac autonomic dysfunction in type 2 diabetes—Effect of hyperglycemia and disease duration. *Frontiers in Endocrinology*, 5(Article 130):1–9, 2014.
7. C.M.A. van Ravenswaaij-Arts, L.A.A. Kollée, J.C.W. Hopman, G.B.A. Stoelinga, and H.P. van Geijn. Heart rate variability. *Annals of Internal Medicine*, 118(6):436–447, 1993.
8. M. Malik and A.J. Camm. Components of heart rate variability—What they really mean and what we really measure. *American Journal of Cardiology*, 72(11):821–822, 1993.
9. J. Pumprla, K. Howorka, D. Groves, M. Chester, and J. Nolan. Functional assessment of heart arte variability: Physiological basis and practical applications. *International Journal of Cardiology*, 84:1–14, 2002.
10. J. Achten and A.E. Jeukendrup. Heart rate monitoring—Applications and limitations. *Sports Medicine*, 33(7):517–538, 2003.
11. G.G. Berntson, J.T. Bigger Jr., D.L. Eckberg, P. Grossman, P.G. Kaufmann, M. Malik, H.N. Nagaraja, S.W. Porges, J.P. Saul, P.H. Stone, and M.W. Van Der Molen. Heart rate variability: Origins, methods, and interpretive caveats. *Psychophysiology*, 34:623–648, 1997.

12. M. Pagani, N. Montano, A. Porta, A. Malliani, F.M. Abboud, C. Birkett, and V.K. Somers. Relationship between spectral components of cardiovascular variabilities and direct measures of muscle sympathetic nerve activity in humans. *Circulation*, 95:1441–1448, 1997.

13. R. Furlan, A. Porta, F. Costa, J. Tank, L. Baker, R. Schiavi, D. Robertson, A. Malliani, and R. Mosqueda-Garcia. Oscillatory patterns in sympathetic neural discharge and cardiovascular variables during orthostatic stimulus. *Circulation*, 101:886–892, 2000.

14. J-P. Niskanen, M. P. Tarvainen, P. O. Ranta-aho, and P. A. Karjalainen. Software for advanced HRV analysis. *Computer Methods and Programmes in Biomedicine*, 76(1):73–81, 2004.

15. M.P. Tarvainen, J.-P. Niskanen, J.A. Lipponen, P.O. Ranta-aho, and P.A. Karjalainen. Kubios HRV—Heart rate variability analysis software. *Computer Methods and Programs in Biomedicine*, 113(1):210–220, 2014.

16. J. Pan and W.J. Tompkins. A real-time QRS detection algorithm. *IEEE Transactions on Biomedical Engineering*, 32(3):230–236, March 1985.

17. R.W. DeBoer, J.M. Karemaker, and J. Strackee. Comparing spectra of a series of point events particularly for heart rate variability data. *IEEE Transactions on Biomedical Engineering*, 31(4):384–387, April 1984.

18. J. Mateo and P. Laguna. Improved heart rate variability signal analysis from the beat occurrence times according to the IPFM model. *IEEE Transactions on Biomedical Engineering*, 47(8):985–996, August 2000.

19. H. Witte, U. Zwiener, M. Rother, and S. Glaser. Evidence of a previously undescribed form of respiratory sinus arrhythmia (RSA)—The physiological manifestation of "cardiac aliasing". *Pflügers Archiv: European Journal of Physiology*, 412:442–444, 1988.

20. N.R. Lomb. Least-squares frequency analysis of unequally spaced data. *Astrophysical Space Science*, 39:447–462, 1976.

21. J.D. Scargle. Studies in astronomical time series analysis. II. Statistical aspects of spectral analysis of unevenly spaced data. *Astrophysical Journal*, 263:835–853, 1982.

22. G.D. Clifford and L. Tarassenko. Quantifying errors in spectral estimates of HRV due to beat replacement and resampling. *IEEE Transactions on Biomedical Engineering*, 52(4):630–638, 2005.

23. R. Bailón, G. Laouini, C. Grao, M. Orini, P. Laguna, and O. Meste. The integral pulse frequency modulation model with time-varying threshold: Application to heart rate variability analysis during exercise stress testing. *IEEE Transactions on Biomedical Engineering*, 58(3):642–652, 2011.

24. R. Barbieri and E.N. Brown. Application of dynamic point process models to cardiovascular control. *BioSystems*, 93:120–125, 2008.

25. M. Brennan, M. Palaniswami, and P. Kamen. Do existing measures of Poincaré plot geometry reflect nonlinear features of heart rate variability? *IEEE Transactions on Biomedical Engineering*, 48(11):1342–1347, 2001.

26. S. Carrasco, M.J. Caitán, R. González, and O. Yánez. Correlation among Poincaré plot indexes and time and frequency domain measures of heart rate variability. *Journal of Medical Engineering & Technology*, 25(6):240–248, November/December 2001.

27. C.-K. Peng, S. Havlin, H.E. Stanley, and A.L. Goldberger. Quantification of scaling exponents and crossover phenomena in nonstationary heartbeat time series. *Chaos*, 5:82–87, 1995.

28. T. Penzel, J.W. Kantelhardt, L. Grote, J.-H. Peter, and A. Bunde. Comparison of detrended uctuation analysis and spectral analysis for heart rate variability in sleep and sleep apnea. *IEEE Transactions on Biomedical Engineering*, 50(10):1143–1151, October 2003.

29. Y. Fusheng, H. Bo, and T. Qingyu. Approximate entropy and its application in biosignal analysis. In M. Akay (ed.), *Nonlinear Biomedical Signal Processing: Dynamic Analysis and Modeling*, volume II, chapter 3, pp. 72–91. New York, NY: IEEE Press, 2001.

30. J.A. Richman and J.R. Moorman. Physiological time-series analysis using approximate entropy and sample entropy. *American Journal of Physiology: Heart and Circulatory Physiology*, 278:H2039–H2049, 2000.

31. S. Guzzetti, M.G. Signorini, C. Cogliati, S. Mezzetti, A. Porta, S. Cerutti, and A. Malliani. Nonlinear dynamics and chaotic indices in heart rate variability of normal subjects and heart-transplanted patients. *Cardiovascular Research*, 31:441–446, 1996.

32. B. Henry, N. Lovell, and F. Camacho. Nonlinear dynamics time series analysis. In M. Akay, (ed.) *Nonlinear Biomedical Signal Processing: Dynamic Analysis and Modeling*, volume II, chapter 1, pp. 1–39. New York, NY: IEEE Press, 2001.

33. C.L. Webber Jr. and J.P. Zbilut. Dynamical assessment of physiological systems and states using recurrence plot strategies. *Journal of Applied Physiology*, 76:965–973, 1994.

34. J.P. Zbilut, N. Thomasson, and C.L. Webber. Recurrence quantification analysis as a tool for the nonlinear exploration of nonstationary cardiac signals. *Medical Engineering & Physics*, 24:53–60, 2002.

35. S.L. Marple. *Digital Spectral Analysis*. London: Prentice-Hall International, 1987.

36. A. Boardman, F.S. Schlindwein, A.P. Rocha, and A. Leite. A study on the optimum order of autoregressive models for heart rate variability. *Physiological Measurement*, 23:325–336, 2002.

37. M.P. Tarvainen, S.D. Georgiadis, P.O. Ranta-aho, and P.A. Karjalainen. Time-varying analysis of heart rate variability signals with Kalman smoother algorithm. *Physiological Measurement*, 27(3):225–239, 2006.

38. D. Cornforth, M.P. Tarvainen, and H.F. Jelinek. How to calculate Renyi entropy from heart rate variability, and why it matters for detecting cardiac autonomic neuropathy. *Frontiers in Bioengineering and Biotechnology*, 2(Article 34):1–8, 2014.

39. M. Costa, A.L. Goldberger, and C.-K. Peng. Multiscale entropy analysis of biological signals. *Physical Reviews E*, 71:021906, 2005.

40. L.L. Trulla, A. Giuliani, J.P. Zbilut, and C.L. Webber Jr. Recurrence quantification analysis of the logistic equation with transients. *Physics Letters A*, 223(4):255–260, 1996.

41. E.J.M. Weber, C.M. Molenaar, and M.W. van der Molen. A nonstationarity test for the spectral analysis of physiological time series with an application to respiratory sinus arrhythmia. *Psychophysiology*, 29(1):55–65, January 1992.

42. P. Grossman. Breathing rhythms of the heart in a world of no steady state: A comment on Weber, Molenaar, and van der Molen. *Psychophysiology*, 29(1):66–72, January 1992.

43. M.P. Tarvainen, P.O. Ranta-aho, and P.A. Karjalainen. An advanced detrending method with application to HRV analysis. *IEEE Transactions on Biomedical Engineering*, 49(2):172–175, February 2002.

44. M.A. Peltola. Role of editing of RR intervals in the analysis of heart rate variability. *Frontiers in Physiology*, 3(Article 148):1–10, 2012.

45. R. Bailón, L. Sörnmo, and P. Laguna. A robust method for ECG-based estimation of the respiratory frequency during stress testing. *IEEE Transactions on Biomedical Engineering*, 53(7):1273–1285, 2006.

46. H. Song and P. Lehrer. The effects of specific respiratory rates on heart rate and heart rate variability. *Applied Psychophysiology and Biofeedback*, 28(1):13–23, 2003.

47. B. Aysin and E. Aysin. Effect of respiration in heart rate variability (HRV) analysis. In *Proceedings of the 28th Annual International Conference of the IEEE Engineering in Medicine and Biology Society*, pp. 1776–1779, 2006.

48. P. Kuoppa, J.A. Lipponenand, and M.P. Tarvainen. Dynamic modeling of respiratory sinus arrhythmia component from HRV with multivariate Kalman smoother. In *Proceedings of the 35th Annual International Conference of the IEEE Engineering in Medicine & Biology Society*, pp. 1684–1687, 2013.

8

Multiscale Complexity Measures of Heart Rate Variability—A Window on the Autonomic Nervous System Function

David J. Cornforth and Herbert F. Jelinek

CONTENTS

8.1 Introduction

Cardiac rhythm is controlled by membrane properties of the sinoatrial node and the activity of the neurohormonal and autonomic nervous system (ANS) modulation (Valensi et al., 2002; Vinik et al., 2003). There are two extrinsic ANS influences that determine the natural rhythm of the human heart, known as the sympathetic and parasympathetic signals. Generally, sympathetic activity decreases the interbeat (RR) intervals and decreases heart rate variability (HRV), whereas parasympathetic activity increases the RR intervals and increases HRV (Berntson et al., 1997).

In order to investigate the ANS modulation of HR, we examined cardiac autonomic neuropathy (CAN), a disease often presenting as a complication of diabetes, which affects the ANS. CAN is characterized by peripheral nerve damage leading to abnormal regulation of the heartbeat by the ANS (Tarvainen et al., 2013; Pop-Busui, 2010) and may manifest in up to 60% of individuals with type-2 diabetes at different stages during disease progression (Ziegler et al., 1992). One would expect CAN to be characterized by changes in the HRV, so an important question is whether CAN is detected from an analysis of HRV using only the beat-to-beat interval.

8.2 Measures of HRV

HRV is concerned only with changes in the time between successive heartbeats. It is non-invasive and easy to obtain from a surface lead III electrocardiogram (ECG) recording for short recording periods or from Holter data if longer recording periods are required as may be the case for analyzing circadian changes. The RR intervals are extracted from the ECG as a time series. A variety of measures can then be derived from this and fall into three categories: time series measures, frequency domain measures, and complex or non-linear measures (TFESC, 1996; Sacre et al., 2012; Khandoker et al., 2009). All of these can be derived from the RR interval time series through suitable mathematical functions. It remains to ask what further processing is appropriate in order to reveal details of the operation of the ANS, and in the context of this chapter, to determine which measures are able to discriminate between healthy participants and stages of CAN progression in patients.

Research efforts have been ongoing to develop advanced algorithms for the characterization of HRV. This is important since standard measures can lead to incorrect interpretation of pathology (Rodriguez et al., 2007; Goldberger and West, 1987). The aim of nonlinear methods is to address the nonlinearity and nonstationarity as well as complexity of HR time signals. Several methods, multiscale entropy (MSE), multifractal detrended fluctuation analysis (MFDFA), and multiscale Rényi (MSRényi) entropy, have been extensively applied (Stanley et al., 1999; Ivanov et al., 1999; Costa et al., 2003; Ihlen, 2012). However, whether these algorithms have similar or different sensitivities in classifying pathology has only recently been investigated. To date, some studies have shown that there is a reduction in HRV with progression of CAN, which may be related to continued increases in blood sugar levels (Tarvainen et al., 2014; Jelinek et al., 2007; Karmakar et al., 2013).

8.2.1 Nonlinear Measures

Nonlinear methods include fractal analysis and entropy measures. Nonlinear analysis methods have recently enjoyed increased interest from researchers and are acknowledged as providing information complimentary to that resulting from linear measures, for identifying risk of future morbidity and mortality in diverse patient groups (Francesco et al., 2012; Kunz et al., 2012; Pivatelli et al., 2012; Schiecke et al., 2014). Fractal analysis examines scale invariance within the time series formed by the intervals between heartbeats. There is a variety of fractal measures, depending on the methods used to obtain the estimate, as well as multiscale versions of these measures. For example, sample entropy considers sequences of RR intervals of a given length. This length can be altered to provide additional measures. Rényi entropy is a generalization of Shannon entropy, where an exponent determines the order of the entropy measures obtained, and a width parameter determines the pattern length over which comparison occurs. Thus, both sample entropy and Rényi entropy can be implemented as multiscale measures.

Multiscale measures provide a series of measures, rather than a single measure, as a function of some scaling factor. The way in which multiple scales are implemented differs between the methods examined here. MSE examines RR intervals at a number of different scales in order to provide multiple measures based on the same time series. MFDFA and the MSRényi entropy are multiscale in the sense that a parameter is used to control the order or power that a quantity is raised to. This can take multiple values and so provides multiple measures.

8.2.1.1 Multiscale Sample Entropy

The entropy $H(X)$ of an RR interval time series $\{x_1, ..., x_n\}$ expresses the uncertainty of the n intervals as a random variable X, where

$$H(X) = -\sum_{i=1}^{n} p(x_i) \log p(x_i) \tag{8.1}$$

The probability p_i may be estimated from the RR interval data by discretizing the range of values for X and dividing the number of times that X falls within its discretizing band by n. This is the histogram method. However, there is no need to be limited to considering a single RR interval as the variate x. Instead, a sequence of m contiguous RR intervals $X_m(i) = \{x_i, ..., x_{i+m-1}\}$ can be examined, which allows the estimation of a probability for $X_m(i)$. The probability of each unique $X_m(i)$ is then calculated. In this application of multiscale analysis, the histogram method rapidly becomes impractical, as the sequence length m is increased and consequently the number of unique sequences increases. Instead, the probability may be estimated by counting the number of sequences, which are similar when their elements x_i are compared and the difference is less than a threshold r. This is the method commonly used in estimation of the *sample entropy*. The number of sequences $c_m(i)$ are counted having length m and starting at $j(j \neq i)X_m(j)$ where each scalar comparison $|xi - xj| \leq r$. The total number of sequences of length m across the entire series is given by

$$c_m = \sum_{i=1}^{n-m+1} c_m(i) \tag{8.2}$$

The sample entropy can then be seen as the probability that a sequence of RR intervals of length m that repeats itself within a threshold r will also repeat itself if the sequence length is extended to $m+1$. Sample entropy calculates the negative logarithm of the ratio of two measures A and B:

$$\text{SampEn} = -\log \frac{A}{B} \tag{8.3}$$

where $B = c_m$ is the number of matches from sequences of RR intervals of length m and $A = c_{m+1}$ is a similar measure calculated using sequences of length $m+1$ (Richman and Moorman, 2000).

MSE extends this concept by using coarse-grained copies of the original data series:

$$y_j^\tau = \frac{1}{\tau} \sum_{i=(j-1)\tau+1}^{j\tau} x_i \tag{8.4}$$

where τ is the scale factor and $1 \leq j \leq n/\tau$, and the x_i of Equation 8.2 is replaced by y_j, so that MSE is a function of the scale (Richman and Moorman, 2000; Costa et al., 2002, 2005). The implementation of the algorithm used in this work was from PhysioNet (2017).

8.2.1.2 Multifractal Detrended Fluctuation Analysis

Detrended fluctuation analysis (DFA) is a fractal-like measure that examines the self-similarity properties of a time series, in this case a sequence of RR intervals. In the following discussion, we follow the implementation of Ihlen (2012) for determining the multifractal

DFA. For the convenience of the reader, we have provided a summary of Ihlen's work translated from MATLAB® code into a series of equations. The MATLAB code is available online (MATLAB Central, 2014).

A given sequence of RR intervals $\{x_1, ..., x_n\}$ is transformed into a random walk by subtracting the mean from each value and calculating the cumulative sum as

$$X_k = \sum_{i=1}^{k} (x_i - \bar{x}) \tag{8.5}$$

The transformed series, X_k, is divided into sequences of length s and a straight line is fitted to each sequence by minimizing the sum of the squared errors to provide a slope and offset. It is possible to use higher order polynomials to fit the segments, but in our work, we always use a linear fit. The root mean square (rms) error of the fit ε_v is calculated for each segment v of length m as

$$\varepsilon_v = \sqrt{\sum_{i=mv}^{m(v+1)} (X_i - \acute{X}_i)^2} \tag{8.6}$$

where $\acute{X}_i$ is the estimated value of X_i. The mean rms error is found for all segments of length m as

$$\varepsilon_m = \sqrt{\frac{1}{n/m} \sum_{v=1}^{n/m} \varepsilon_v^2} \tag{8.7}$$

Using the graphical technique for estimation of the fractal dimension, the values of ε_m are plotted against the scale m, using a logarithmic scale for both axes, and the slope of the resulting curve is calculated. This slope is the result of the process of DFA.

In order to derive a multifractal measure for DFA, Equation 8.3 is modified by substituting an exponent q that can be varied as a parameter of the method:

$$\varepsilon_{q,m} = \left(\frac{1}{n/m} \sum_{v=1}^{n/m} \varepsilon_v^q \right)^{1/q} \tag{8.8}$$

where n/m is the number of segments in the complete series of length m.

8.2.1.3 Rényi Entropy

The Rényi entropy is naturally a multiscale measure, as it generalizes the Shannon entropy and includes the Shannon entropy as a special case (Rényi, 1960). The ability of Rényi entropy to discriminate levels of cardiac risk using different scales has been demonstrated (Kurths et al., 1995). Rényi entropy H is defined as

$$H(\alpha) = \frac{1}{1-\alpha} \log_2 \left(\sum_{i=1}^{n} p_i^\alpha \right) \tag{8.9}$$

where p_i is the probability that a random variable takes a given value out of n values and α is the exponent or order of the entropy measure. When α is varied this provides the multiscale measure. $H(\alpha)$ is simply the logarithm of n. As α increases, the measures become more sensitive to the values occurring at higher probability and less to those occurring at lower probability, which provides a picture of the RR length distribution within a signal. However, the entropy requires an estimate of probabilities, and there are a number of ways in which this can be determined. Previous work described two main methods of estimating probabilities: the histogram method and the density method (Cornforth et al., 2014). That work showed that the density method is superior in terms of providing a measure that can discriminate different classes of CAN, while providing a measure that is complimentary to, rather than duplicating, the standard deviation of the RR intervals.

The histogram method estimates the probability that an RR interval assumes a value within a given range. For each range, there will be a number of RR intervals assuming this value, and this can be used to estimate the probability p_i of Equation 8.9. An example is shown in Figure 8.1. Here, the RR intervals have been detrended and normalized to have a mean of zero. The histogram method has advantages in terms of its low computational effort and its ability to allow a simple visualization of the distribution of RR values. However, its reliance on bins introduces an artificial discretization, leading to a boundary problem where an individual value may be included in one bin or the other depending on a very small perturbation. This can be ameliorated by using a smoothing method that spreads data points into adjacent bins, but does not take into account how close a particular data point was to the bin boundary. In addition, this method is problematic when the assumption of a single RR interval is relaxed. If it is desired to estimate the probability of a sequence of RR intervals, rather than a single RR interval, other methods may be required.

The density method also estimates a probability, but does this in a continuous, rather than a discrete space. The density method allows one to estimate the probability of a sequence of RR intervals of length m by considering the sequence as a point in an m-dimensional space. This method uses a notional density of space around a point, which is compared to all other sequences, also represented as points in the same space. Points are compared using a distance measure, and the two sequences are considered to be similar if the distance in each dimension is less than a given threshold. This is the method used in the calculation of sample entropy described above, which counts all sequences that are closer

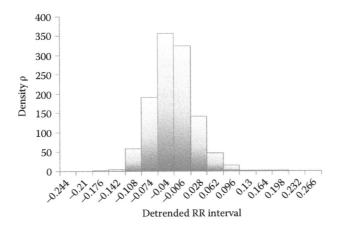

FIGURE 8.1
An example of a histogram of detrended RR intervals.

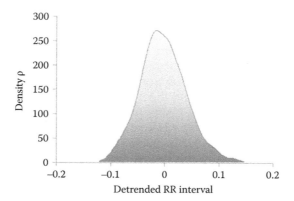

FIGURE 8.2
A probability density function calculated from the same data as Figure 8.1. Notice that a continuous, rather than a discretizing, estimate of the density has been obtained.

to a chosen sequence given a specific threshold r. However, this depends on choosing a suitable value for the threshold, so still retains the problem of a discretization.

In order to provide a truly continuous measure of probability, an adjustment to the above method may be used to remove the need for a hard threshold. Here, a Gaussian kernel is centered on each point (representing a sequence of m RR intervals in m-dimensional space), and a contribution is added for each of the other points, based on the distance between the points. This results in a "score" for each point, which can be converted into a probability. This is small if all other points are far away, leading to a low probability, and large if the point has many close neighbors, leading to a high probability. This score or density measure is calculated for the sequence of RR intervals with index i, as the sum of all contributions from other sequences with index j:

$$\rho_i = \frac{1}{\sigma\sqrt{2\pi}} \sum_{i=1}^{n} e^{-\frac{\text{dist}_{ij}^2}{2\sigma^2}} \tag{8.10}$$

using a distance measure

$$\text{dist}_{ij}^2 = \sum_{k=1}^{m} (x_{i+k} - x_{j+k})^2 \tag{8.11}$$

where σ is the dispersion of the function and replaces the threshold r. This provides a continuous rather than a discretized estimate of probability, and an example is shown in Figure 8.2, which was calculated from the same data used in Figure 8.1.

8.3 Empirical Comparison

The work reported here used data from the Charles Sturt Diabetes Complications Screening Group (DiScRi), Australia (Jelinek et al., 2006). The study was approved by the Charles Sturt University Human Ethics Committee and written informed consent was obtained from all participants. All recordings were obtained in a temperature-stable environment following a 5- to 10-minute rest period in a supine position by all participants. The sampling rate was set to 400 samples/sec and recordings preprocessed according to the method described by Tarvainen et al. (2002). A 20-minute lead II ECG recording was taken from participants attending the clinic, using a Maclab Pro with Chart 7 software (ADInstruments, Sydney). Participants were comparable for age, gender, and HR, and after initial screening, those with heart disease, presence of a pacemaker, kidney disease, or polypharmacy (including multiple antiarrhythmic medication) were excluded from the study. The same conditions were used for each participant. The status of CAN was defined using the Ewing battery criteria (Khandoker et al., 2009; Javorka et al., 2008; Ewing et al., 1985), and each participant was assigned as either without CAN (71 participants), early CAN (67 participants), or definite CAN (11 participants). From the 20-minute recording, a 15-minute segment was selected from the middle in order to remove start-up artifacts and movement at the end of the recording. From this shorter recording, the RR intervals were extracted. No other information was used in this study. The RR interval series for each participant was detrended, and the measures used were determined from these data (Tarvainen et al., 2013).

The MSE was calculated using the default parameters of sequence length $m = 2$, threshold $r = 0.15$, and coarse-graining factors 1–10. As the recordings are only 15 minutes in length, this restricts the length of sequence m and the scale of coarse graining τ. Note that when $\tau = 1$, the measure is equivalent to the sample entropy without multiscaling. The MFDFA was calculated using integer values of order from −5 to +5. A range of scaling exponents similar to MFDFA, α from −5 to +5 was used to determine the MSRényi entropy. The MSRényi entropy was then calculated using sequence length $m = 16$ and $\sigma = 0.16$ (see Section 8.2.1.3). For each measure, a Mann–Whitney test was performed to compare the normal to the early CAN group, the early to the definite CAN group, and the definite CAN to the normal group.

8.4 Results

Figure 8.3 shows the results of a comparison of disease classes using MSE calculated from RR intervals. The x-axis shows the scale factor τ of Equation 8.4 from 1 to 10, that is, the level of coarse graining applied to RR intervals. The y-axis shows the Area Under the receiver operating characteristic curve (AUC). The minimum value of AUC is 0.5, indicating a result no better than random chance, and the maximum value is 1, indicating perfect separation of the classes (Mason and Graham, 2002). Each line shows a comparison between two of the participant groups. The three comparisons are normal versus early, early versus definite, and definite versus normal. Only three results are greater than 0.6, and these are all for normal versus early comparisons, using a scale factor τ of 1 (equivalent to the sample entropy), 6, and 8 RR intervals. All other points show little difference from 0.5, the level corresponding to random choice between classes. These results offer little evidence that MSE is able to discriminate classes of participants and may not be useful in a clinical setting.

Results for MFDFA are shown in Figure 8.4 with a scaling factor range q between −5 and +5 (Ihlen, 2012). High values of AUC were obtained for comparisons between normal and definite, especially for negative values of q, suggesting that this approach is able to yield results that are useful in discrimination of CAN from normal suggesting this may be a useful clinical measure.

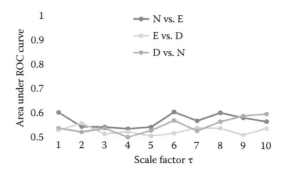

FIGURE 8.3

Results of comparison between different classes of participants using multiscale entropy (MSE), expressed as Area Under the receiver operating characteristic Curve (AUC).

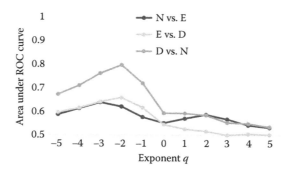

FIGURE 8.4

Results of comparison between different classes of participants using multifractal detrended fluctuation analysis (MFDFA) variables calculated from RR interval series, expressed as Area Under the receiver operating characteristic Curve (AUC).

The best measures for discriminating classes of CAN were for $q = -2$. As an intuitive explanation for this negative exponent, we observe that this is related to the standard deviation of the reciprocal of rms errors. The relative success of the measures for negative q suggests that the transformation involved in the inverse maps these values of rms error into a space where disease classes are more distinct.

AUC values greater than 0.8 can be considered to have clinical significance, and thus, this method shows some promise for the detection of CAN in a clinical setting. Several of the tests comparing early CAN with other classes provided results above 0.6, suggesting detection of early CAN may be possible.

The result of calculating AUC for Rényi entropy based on probabilities calculated using the density method is shown in Figure 8.5. The range of exponents α for the MSRényi calculation varied from −5 to +5 (Equation 8.9). All of the comparisons between normal and CAN showed that high values of AUC results greater than, or close to, 0.8 indicate clinical usefulness. MSRényi results were more consistent across classes than the other methods studied, with results associated with negative α decreasing with disease progression and vice versa. The difference between negative and positive values for the exponent α has

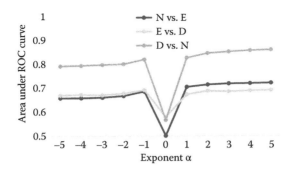

FIGURE 8.5
Results of comparison between different classes of participants using MFDFA variables calculated from RR interval series. Results are shown as Area Under the receiver operating characteristic Curve (AUC).

been explored in previous work (Cornforth et al., 2014). That work showed that although positive values of α provide higher discrimination of classes, with corresponding lower *p* values, the entropy values resulting from positive exponents were highly correlated with the standard deviation. While the standard deviation is a useful measure of HRV, it falls into the category of linear measures of HRV discussed above and is correspondingly simpler to calculate than Rényi entropy. In terms of clinical practice, the standard deviation has also been shown to be less discriminatory for disease condition (Goldberger and West, 1987), and therefore, the Rényi entropy results based on positive exponents of α are of less interest. The measures based on negative exponents of α are more interesting since they clearly discriminate between classes but may provide information complimentary to that derived from time-domain measures such as the standard deviation. More work is required to understand the meaning of negative exponents in multiscale or multifractal analysis.

Results comparing early CAN with the other classes show promise in discriminating the early stages of CAN and thus a combination of HRV measures to discriminate between CAN subtypes and CAN progression may provide useful clinical information when it includes results from both linear and nonlinear measures (Tarvainen et al., 2014; Cornforth et al., 2014).

8.5 Conclusion

CAN is a disease that involves nerve damage leading to abnormal control of HR. CAN affects the heart rhythm and in turn, leads to associated arrhythmias and heart attack. An open question is to what extent this condition is detectable by the measurement of HRV. An even more desirable avenue of research is to detect CAN in its early, preclinical stage, with the hope that this can lead to improved treatment and treatment outcomes.

Nonlinear analysis methods have been shown to offer increased sensitivity for identifying risk of future morbidity and mortality in cardiac patients. In particular, Rényi entropy has shown significant differentiation of cardiovascular disease.

References

Berntson, G.G., J.T. Bigger Jr., D.L. Eckberg, P. Grossman, P.G. Kaufmann, M. Malik, H.N. Nagaraja, S.W. Porges, J.P. Saul, P.H. Stone, and M.W. van der Molen. 1997. Heart rate variability: Origins, methods, and interpretive caveats. *Psychophysiology* 34:623–648.

Cornforth, D.J., M.P. Tarvainen, and H.F. Jelinek. 2014. How to calculate Rényi entropy from heart rate variability, and why it matters for detecting cardiac autonomic neuropathy. *Frontiers in Bioengineering and Biotechnology* 2:34. doi:10.3389/fbioe.2014.00034.

Costa, M., A.L. Goldberger, and C.K. Peng. 2002. Multiscale entropy analysis of complex physiologic time series. *Physical Review Letters* 89:068102.

Costa, M., A.L. Goldberger, and C.K. Peng. 2003. Multiscale entropy analysis: A new measure of complexity loss in heart failure. *Journal of Electrocardiology* 36(Supplement 1):39–40.

Costa, M., A.L. Goldberger, and C.K. Peng. 2005. Multiscale entropy analysis of biological signals. *Physical Review E* 71:021906.

Ewing, D.J., C.N. Martyn, R.J. Young, and B.F. Clarke. 1985. The value of cardiovascular autonomic functions tests: 10 years' experience in diabetes. *Diabetes Care* 8:491–498.

Francesco, B., B. Maria Grazia, G. Emanuele et al. (2012). Linear and nonlinear heart rate variability indexes in clinical practice. *Computational and Mathematical Methods in Medicine* 2012:219080. doi:10.1155/2012/219080.

Goldberger, A.L. and B.J. West. 1987. Fractals in physiology and medicine. *Yale Journal of Biological Medicine* 60:421–435.

Ihlen, E.A.F. 2012. Introduction to multifractal wavelet and detrended fluctuation analyses. *Frontiers in Physiology* 3:141. doi:10.3389/fphys.2012.00141.

Ivanov, P., L.A.N. Amaral, A.L. Goldberger, S. Havlin, M. Rosenblum, Z.R. Struzik, and H.E. Stanley. 1999. Multifractality in human heartbeat dynamics. *Nature* 399:461–465.

Javorka, M., Z. Trunkvalterova, I. Tonhajzerova, J. Javorkova, K. Javorka, and M. Baumert. 2008. Short-term heart rate complexity is reduced in patients with type 1 diabetes mellitus. *Clinical Neurophysiology* 119:1071–1081.

Jelinek, H.F., P. Pham, Z.R. Struzik, and I. Spence. 2007. Short term ECG recording for the identification of cardiac autonomic neuropathy in people with diabetes mellitus. In *Proceedings of the 19th International Conference on Noise and Fluctuations*, Tokyo, Japan: IEEE Press.

Jelinek, H.F., C. Wilding, and P. Tinley. 2006. An innovative multi-disciplinary diabetes complications screening programme in a rural community: A description and preliminary results of the screening. *American Journal of Public Health* 12:14–20.

Karmakar, C.K., A.H. Khandoker, H.F. Jelinek, and M. Palaniswami. 2013. Risk stratification of cardiac autonomic neuropathy based on multi-lag Tone-Entropy. *Medical and Biological Engineering and Computing* 51(5):537–546.

Khandoker, A.H., H.F. Jelinek, and M. Palaniswami. 2009. Identifying diabetic patients with cardiac autonomic neuropathy by heart rate complexity analysis. *Biomedical Engineering Online* 8:3. doi:10.1186/1475-925X-8-3.

Kunz, V.C., E.N. Borges, R.C. Coelho, L.A. Gubolino, L.E.B. Martins, and E. Silva. 2012. Linear and nonlinear analysis of heart rate variability in healthy subjects and after acute myocardial infarction in patients. *Brazilian Journal of Medical and Biological Research* 45(5):450–458.

Kurths, J., A. Voss, P. Saparin, A. Witt, H.J. Kleiner, and N. Wessel. 1995. Quantitative analysis of heart rate variability. *Chaos* 5(1):88–94.

Mason, S.J. and N.E. Graham. 2002. Areas beneath the relative operating characteristics (ROC) and relative operating levels (ROL) curves: Statistical significance and interpretation. *Quarterly Journal of the Royal Meteorological Society* 128:2145–2166.

MATLAB Central. 2014. Multifractal Detrended Fluctuation Analyses. http://www.mathworks.com.au/matlabcentral/fileexchange/38262-multifractal-detrended-fluctuation-analyses (Accessed on 21 Oct 2014).

PhysioNet. 2017. *The research resource for complex physiologic signals.* http://www.physionet.org/ (Accessed on 13 May 2017).

Pivatelli, F.C., M.A. dos Santos, G.B. Fernandes et al. 2012. Sensitivity, specificity and predictive values of linear and nonlinear indices of heart rate variability in stable angina patients. *International Archives of Medicine* 5:31. doi:10.1186/1755-7682-5-31.

Pop-Busui, R. 2010. Cardiac autonomic neuropathy in diabetes. *Diabetes Care* 33:434–441.

Rényi, A. 1960. On measures of information and entropy. In *Proceedings of the Fourth Berkeley Symposium on Mathematics, Statistics and Probability*, Berkeley, CA, USA, 20 June–30 July:547–561.

Richman, J.S. and J.R. Moorman. 2000. Physiological time-series analysis using approximate entropy and sample entropy. *American Journal of Physiology, Heart and Circulatory Physiology* 278:H2039–H2049.

Rodriguez, E., J.C. Echeverria, and J. Alvarez-Ramirez. 2007. Detrended fluctuation analysis of heart intrabeat dynamics. *Physica A: Statistical Mechanics and Its Applications* 384(2):429–438.

Sacre, J.W., C.L. Jellis, T.H. Marwick, and J.S. Coombes. 2012. Reliability of heart rate variability in patients with type 2 diabetes mellitus. *Diabetic Medicine* 29:e33–40.

Schiecke, K., M. Wacker, D. Piper, F. Benninger, M. Feucht, and H. Witte. 2014. Time-variant, frequency-selective, linear and nonlinear analysis of heart rate variability in children with temporal lobe epilepsy. *IEEE Transactions on Biomedical Engineering* 61(60):1798–1808, June 2014. doi:10.1109/TBME.2014.2307481.

Stanley, H.E., L.A.N. Amaral, A.L. Goldberger, S. Havlin, P.Ch. Ivanov, and C.K. Peng. 1999. Statistical physics and physiology: Monofractal and multifractal approaches. *Physics A Statistical Mechanics and Its Applications* 270:309–324.

Tarvainen, M.P., D.J. Cornforth, P. Kuoppa, J.A. Lipponen, and H.F. Jelinek. 2013. Complexity of heart rate variability in type 2 diabetes effect of hyperglycemia. In *Proceedings of the 35th Annual International Conference of the Engineering in Medicine and Biology Society (EMBS)*, Osaka, Japan, 3–7 July:5558–5561.

Tarvainen, M.P., T.P. Laitinen, J.A. Lipponen, D.J. Cornforth, and H.F. Jelinek. 2014. Cardiac autonomic dysfunction in type 2 diabetes—Effect of hyperglycemia and disease duration. *Frontiers in Endocrinology* 5:130.

Tarvainen, M.P, P.O. Ranta-Aho, and P.A. Karjalainen. 2002. An advanced detrending method with application to HRV analysis. *IEEE Transactions on Biomedical Engineering* 49(2):172–175.

TFESC, NASPE. 1996. Heart rate variability: Standards of measurement, physiological interpretation, and clinical use. *Circulation* 93:1043–1065.

Valensi, P.E., N.B. Johnson, P. Maison-Blanche, F. Estramania, G. Motte, and P. Coumel. 2002. Influence of cardiac autonomic neuropathy on heart rate variability dependence of ventricular repolarization in diabetic patients. *Diabetes Care* 25:918–923.

Vinik, A.I., R.E. Maser, B.D. Mitchell, and R. Freeman. 2003. Diabetic autonomic neuropathy. *Diabetes Care* 26:1553–1579.

Ziegler, D., F.A. Gries, M. Spuler, and F. Lessmann. 1992. Diabetic cardiovascular autonomic neuropathy multicenter study group. The epidemiology of diabetic neuropathy. *Journal of Diabetes Complications* 6:49–57.

9

BP and HR Interactions: Assessment of Spontaneous Baroreceptor Reflex Sensitivity

Tatjana Lončar-Turukalo, Nina Japundžić-Žigon, Olivera Šarenac, and Dragana Bajić

CONTENTS

9.1 Introduction

The arterial baroreceptor reflex (BRR) is a key neurogenic control mechanism of the arterial blood pressure (BP) that acts as a negative feedback corrector. It counteracts BP deviations from a reference set point by modulating heart rate (HR) and peripheral resistance. The BRR is crucial for maintaining BP during postural challenge, including active standing and passive upright tilt (Eckberg 2008). By contrast, the BRR is suppressed during exercise and stress to allow simultaneous increase of BP and HR required for "fight and flight" response (Raven et al. 2005; Bajic et al. 2010). Remodeling of the autonomic nervous system (ANS) control of the cardiovascular system, and of the baroreceptor function, occurs in cardiovascular diseases (La Rovere et al. 2008). Permanent resetting of the BRR characterizes primary hypertension, while reduction of BRR sensitivity (BRS) has been found to predict bad outcomes (Di Rienzo et al. 2009). Deregulation of BP in neurologic disorders associated with ANS dysfunction (dysautonomia) is due to impairment of BRR function.

The need to evaluate BRR function, both as a diagnostic tool and as an assessment of the efficacy of treatment, has driven the development of novel techniques for spontaneous BRR assessment. The main advantage of spontaneous BRR assessment is that it precludes the use of vasoactive drugs (vasoconstrictors and vasodilators) that interfere with cardio-vascular autonomic response and represent a significant risk for the patient. Therefore, methods aimed to estimate spontaneous BRR (sBRR) sensitivity from spontaneous fluc-tuations of BP have been developed. However, clinical application of new techniques is hindered for several reasons. First, the assessment of spontaneous BRR requires continu-ous BP measurement with equipment that is not available in most clinical settings. Second, the equipment for continuous noninvasive BP measurement provides implementation of sBRR assessment procedures, whose complexity precludes easy recognition by medical practitioners. Finally, the establishment of reference values for integration of more intuitive methodological approaches into commercially available devices is still a matter requiring further scrutiny. For all these reasons, the widespread validation of sBRR in clinical settings is delayed.

In the following sections, basic physiological knowledge on the BRR and its pathophys-iological relevance are briefly described. This is followed by the elaboration of methods for assessment of sBRR sensitivity/gain. An insight into the methodology of the most fre-quently used method for evaluation of sBRS, the sequence technique, from the user point of view, is given. Recommendations are provided for the valid clinical application of the sequence technique. These include the necessity of signal quality assessment prior to anal-ysis and the rules for sequence identification. New temporal sequence parameters for the assessment of the sBRR set point and sBRR operating range are suggested, and their use-fulness is demonstrated in physiological experimentation in rats. Finally, an efficient pro-cedure for the evaluation of the degree of randomness in the spontaneous cardiovascular fluctuations is proposed.

9.1.1 Physiological Background of BRR

BP and HR interact on a beat-to-beat basis to maintain adequate circulation to all organs, especially the brain. The BP and HR fast interactions have been shown to be mediated via the ANS, that is, the BRR. Receptors that sense changes in BP, the baroreceptors, are located in large arteries of the thorax and the neck, most densely in the aortic arch and the carotid sinuses. The information about the change of BP is transmitted via the vagus nerve (X) and the glossopharyngeal nerve (IX) to the nucleus of the solitary tract (NTS) in the medulla oblongata and further to the hypothalamus. The main integration of the auto-nomic response directed to peripheral blood vessels and the heart occurs in the rostral ven-trolateral medulla (RVLM) for the sympathetic outflow and in the vagal nuclear complex (nucleus ambiguus, dorsal vagal nucleus) for the parasympathetic outflow. There are two possible scenarios for BP changes (Figure 9.1). Scenario 1 assumes that BP increases. In this

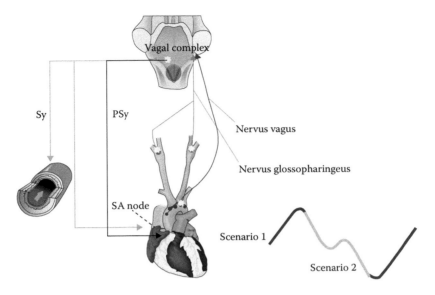

FIGURE 9.1
Baroreceptor reflex (BRR) arch. Sy: sympathetic efferent branches of the BRR; PSy: parasympathetic efferent branch of the BRR. Scenario 1: when blood pressure (BP) is perturbed toward an increase (red), the BRR will increase the parasympathetic tone to the heart and withdraw the sympathetic tone to the heart and the blood vessels. This will slow down the heart and induce peripheral vasodilation, both of which will restore basal values of BP. Scenario 2: when BP is perturbed toward a decrease (green), the BRR will reduce vagal outflow to the heart and enhance sympathetic outflow to the heart and the blood vessels. This will accelerate the heart, vasoconstrict blood vessels, and increase BP.

case, the BRR shifts the autonomic cardiovascular control to the vagus and withdraws sympathetic influence to the cardiovascular system. The vagal activation will slow down the heart and withdrawal of sympathetic influence will lead to arterial vasodilation and reduction of the peripheral resistance. Altogether, this will produce a decrease of BP and restoration of basal values. Scenario 2 supposes that BP decreases. In this case, the BRR shifts the autonomic balance to the sympathetic control of the cardiovascular system, which will increase HR and peripheral resistance, and restore the basal level of BP. As a consequence of the BRR, functioning BP and HR will oscillate around the set point. The period of BP and HR oscillations induced by the BRR ranges from seconds to hours, and contributes to both short-term and long-term BP and HR variability (HRV).

Since perturbations of BP elicit HR response, HR oscillations are delayed with respect to BP oscillations, for the time needed for transmission and the processing of information by the ANS. It has been shown that the responses directed to the heart mediated by sympathetic and parasympathetic efferent nerves have different time lags. Parasympathetic nerves respond to rapid rises in BP and produce an almost immediate slowing of the heart, with 200–600 ms delay in humans (Seidel et al. 1997). On the other hand, sympathetically mediated cardiovascular effects are more sluggish and occur with a delay of 2–3 seconds in humans. Under basal physiological conditions, the HR is controlled mainly by parasympathetic, that is, vagal activity (La Rovere et al. 2008), while exercise and stress increase sympathetic influence on the cardiovascular system.

9.1.2 Pathophysiological Relevance

Cardiovascular diseases are accompanied by BRR remodeling. In primary hypertension, the BRR works around a higher BP set-point value due to the chronic hyperadrenergic state. Depressed sensitivity of the BRR was found to parallel deterioration of the clinical status of cardiovascular patients and to predict poor survival. Reduced BRS (cardiac vagal branch) has been found to be an independent marker of the risk of mortality and major adverse cardiovascular events in hypertensive patients (La Rovere et al. 2001; Ormezzano et al. 2008; Narkiewicz and Grassi 2008), moderate-to-severe chronic heart failure (Mortara et al. 1997), obstructive sleep apnea (Ryan et al. 2007), and myocardial infarction (La Rovere et al. 2001).

The Autonomic Tone and Reflexes After Myocardial Infarction (ATRAMI) clinical trial demonstrated that besides conventional markers, such as depressed left ventricular ejection fraction (LVEF) and the presence of nonsustained ventricular tachycardia (NSVT), markers of reduced vagal activity, such as depressed BRS and HRV, are strong predictors of cardiac mortality after myocardial infarction (La Rovere et al. 2001). It was suggested that the use of BRS and HRV significantly improves the sensitivity of risk stratification in myocardial infarction survivors. The ATRAMI study demonstrated that depressed BRS indicates more accurately patients at the risk of total or arrhythmic mortality, who, according to the traditional risk stratification markers, were not included in the high-risk population (Wellens et al. 2014). On the other hand, BRS has been found to be a modest risk stratification marker for a sudden cardiac death in patients with nonischemic dilated cardiomyopathy (Goldberger et al. 2014).

An impairment of the BRR function characterizes degenerative neurologic disorders (primary dysautonomia) and secondary dysautonomia induced by autoimmune disorders, diabetes mellitus, Parkinson's disease, and multiple sclerosis. Moreover, some drugs as well as brain injuries can be a cause of autonomic deregulations and malfunction of the BRR. In these patients, the inability of the BRR to control BP during postural challenge will trigger syncope (Fu and Levine 2014). On the other hand, some disorders may be accompanied by BRR overcompensation that elicits a hypertensive crisis that can cause serious complications (Fessel and Robertson 2006).

9.2 BRS Assessment—Brief Review

The complex BRR control has a time-dependent gain and nonlinear characteristics along the negative feedback path. The assessment of the overall BRR function is challenging due to the complexity of the most effective BRR branch: the regulation of the peripheral resistance in the body (Di Rienzo et al. 2009). Thus, the assessment of BRR effectiveness is usually simplified to the evaluation of BRR gain only from the BRR branches directed to the heart.

For the assessment of BRR gain, the changes of HR and BP in time (or on beat-to-beat basis) should be available. HR can be determined from the recorded ECG by measuring the interval between the peak of the QRS waves (RR interval [RRI]), as HR is inversely proportional to the RRI. The changes in BP on beat-to-beat basis can be presented by changes in maxima of the BP waveform during one beat, that is, systolic BP (SBP). The BRR gain/sensitivity (measured in ms/mmHg) reflects the relative change in the RRI following a unitary change in BP. BRS is modulated in time by central influences to enable the cardiovascular response to the daily challenges (Smyth et al. 1969; Di Rienzo et al. 1997). Thus, techniques enabling its dynamic assessment have flourished, complementing traditionally available pharmacological techniques producing static BRS estimates.

As the BRR aims to buffer short-term BP variations, an evaluation of its influence on HR, that is, RRIs, can be achieved by inducing the changes in BP that provoke an RRI response, and then by characterizing the RR–SBP relationship. Limited means are available to uncover the RR–BP relationship, since the physiological subsystems cannot easily be isolated from their environment without altering their normal behavior. Additionally, the variation of physiological control parameters is physiologically limited. Consequently, the RR–SBP relationship can only be analyzed in a limited homeostatic range. In the analysis of the HR BRR, the control variable BP can be varied by introduction of loading doses of short-acting vasoactive drugs: vasodilators (e.g., sodium nitroprusside), which provoke a fall in BP, and vasoconstrictors (e.g., phenylephrine), which induce a rise in BP. Over these imposed arterial pressure changes, the RR–SBP relationship is a sigmoid with a threshold, an approximately linear part, and a saturation point. The baseline operating BP point, which the BRR tends to maintain, is localized in an almost linear sigmoid region (Hunt and Farquhar 2005). Different methods can be used to estimate a static reflex gain, but usually linear regression is applied and BRS is calculated as a slope of the fitted line. It has to be noted that if BP fluctuates, BRS may also change as the function of frequency of BP oscillations around a set point.

The techniques for BRS estimation can be roughly divided into traditional techniques, yielding static BRS estimates obtained in a laboratory environment, and modern techniques providing dynamic BRS estimates from spontaneous BP and HR fluctuations.

9.2.1 Traditional Techniques—Static Approach

This first technique to assess BRS used in physiology was developed by Smyth in 1969. The *Oxford method* introduced by Smyth induces the increase in BP by bolus injections of vasoactive medication phenylephrine with minimal effect on the sinoatrial node. This method is focused on the HR BRR branch and measures changes in RRIs provoked by induced changes in BP. The limitation of the Oxford method is that only vasoconstrictors are used, exploring only a limited part of the RR–SBP sigmoidal curve and mainly the vagal component of the BRR. The *modified Oxford method* introduced the use of vasodilators to produce a fall in the BP and a response of the sinoatrial node partly mediated by sympathetic branches (Rudas et al. 1999). BRS is estimated by the means of linear regression between SBP and one-beat-delayed RRI values in the time span between the beginning and the end of the induced change in BP.

There are several limitations of the pharmacological approaches. The methodology requires stable laboratory conditions and drug implementation through intravenous cannulation, which limits its applicability both in experimental and clinical settings. The major limitation is the lack of selectivity in the response to the induced BP changes. Stimulation of the BP also simultaneously stimulates some other reflex receptors, for example, cardiopulmonary receptors, which may interfere with arterial baroreceptors. The use of vasoactive drugs may affect the properties of baroreceptors, the central nervous system (CNS) part of the reflex arc, and the response of the sinus node (La Rovere et al. 2008).

To induce the changes in BP without the use of vasoactive drugs, other noninvasive alternatives are possible: Valsalva maneuver, the neck chamber technique that leads to a lower body negative pressure in humans and stimulates the ANS response. The *Valsalva maneuver* is carried out by performing a forced expiration against a closed glottis or obstruction.

This kind of straining is usually used to test the cardiac function and the autonomic control of the heart. The induced changes in BP are followed by an adequate change in RR response, which are used to calculate BRS under linear regression. The *neck chamber technique* is based on the application of measurable positive or negative pneumatic pressure in the neck region to enable selective activation or deactivation of the carotid baroreceptors. This method is easier to use than the pharmacological methods and better tolerated by the subjects, producing a satisfactory range of BP changes in both directions (Eckberg et al. 1975). However, all of these *"traditional"* techniques require standardized environmental conditions, provide a limited insight into BRR function, and evaluate RRI changes due to BP changes induced by external stimulation. These induced graded changes in BP enable an investigation of the whole sigmoidal stimulus–response curve resulting in static BRS estimates in stable controlled conditions. However, the procedure brings about considerable risk of untoward cardiovascular events and is contraindicated in people with cardiorespiratory disease. In addition, this static BRS estimation does not reflect BRS under spontaneous behavior and has no information on dynamic changes of BRS (Di Rienzo et al. 2001).

9.2.2 Modern Techniques—Dynamic Approach

In the 1980s, the first methods appeared to quantify HR BRR gain without pharmacological or mechanical perturbations. These methods aimed to estimate BRS from spontaneous BP fluctuations over several hours, or over a short stationary segments 5 to 10 minutes long. Since the spontaneous changes of BP are small, it is supposed that BP fluctuates in the vicinity of the BRR set point, thus in the approximately linear region of the RR–SBP sigmoid. Modern techniques can be classified as: time-domain techniques, frequency-domain (spectral) techniques, and model-based techniques.

9.2.2.1 Time-Domain Techniques

The most popular time-domain method is the sequence technique introduced by Di Rienzo et al. (1985) and further described in Bertinieri et al. (1988). The method is based on the computerized scanning of beat-to-beat series of SBP and RRI values in search of spontaneous SBP monotonic pressure changes (SBP ramps) over at least three or more consecutive heartbeats followed by unidirectional RR monotonic changes (RR ramp). When the SBP ramp and the related RR ramp fulfill conditions with respect to the minimal value of the sequence length, amplitude change, and/or correlation coefficient, the BRR sequence (BS) is formed. The delay of the RR ramps with respect to the SBP ramps is evaluated according to the estimated BRR time delay from a change in SBP to a reflex response in RR. BRS is estimated as the mean of the regression line slopes between the SBP and RR values included in each sequence. The BRR origin of these spontaneous fluctuations was confirmed by sinoaortic denervation in cats, resulting in a significant decrease in the number of sequences (86%) (Bertinieri et al. 1988; Di Rienzo et al. 2001). BRS obtained with the sequence technique is highly correlated with BRS obtained by the Oxford method (Parlow et al. 1995).

The dual sequence method is the brief modification of the sequence technique (Malberg et al. 2002). The delay of SBP and RR is modified and allowed to be up to three beats, instead of the former fixed one-beat delay (in humans). This modification allowed identification of delayed BRR response and more BS.

The cross-correlation baroreflex sensitivity (xBRS) method proposed in Westerhof et al. (2004) requires the resampled SBP and RR series at 1 Hz. The regression is carried out on the values included in the 10-second window, with a delay between SBP and RR series that maximizes their cross-correlation. Subsequently, the starting window point slides 1 second to the next SBP and RR sample. Finally, the geometric average of these local estimates over the available recording is taken as a BRS estimate. Since a 10-second window is applied, different effects can be included and they cannot be separated.

The events technique introduced in Gouveia et al. (2009) proposes the use of BRR events (BEs), segments with high SBP–RR correlation regardless of the value and sign of SBP and RR amplitude changes. BEs are variable in length and BRS is estimated as the global regression slope of the SBP and RR values identified in all BE. The global estimator and relaxed conditions of BE validation compared with BS improve robustness and reproducibility of the BRS estimation.

9.2.2.2 Frequency-Domain Techniques

The spectral analysis of SBP and RR series has also been used successfully to obtain BRS estimates. The spectral estimates of SBP and RRI series are obtained and their spectra and cross-spectra are analyzed. The evaluation of BRS by spectral methods is based on the assumption that spontaneous oscillations of BP would elicit oscillation around the same frequency in RR series due to the BRR feedback mechanism (La Rovere et al. 2008). The main frequency bands considered in humans are the LF band (0.04 Hz–0.15 Hz) centered on the 0.1 Hz frequency of the Mayer waves and the HF band (0.15 Hz–0.4 Hz).

The α method (Pagani et al. 1988) determines BRS as the square root of the ratio between RR and SBP spectral power estimated in a frequency region around 0.1 Hz, or at the respiratory frequency (around 0.3 Hz) in humans. Measurements are retained only if the coherence between the two signals is greater than 0.5. The transfer function method, originally proposed by Robbe et al. (1987), estimates BRS as the average value of the gain of the transfer function between SBP and RRI in the 0.07–0.14 Hz frequency range in humans. This method also considers only those points where the coherence is greater than 0.5 in order to guarantee reliable transfer function estimates. The limitations of frequency-based methods are associated with requirements for reliable spectral estimation: 5 to 10 minute long stationary recordings, filtering or manual inspection, and removal of artifacts and ectopic activity.

The major disadvantage of the time- and frequency-domain methods as originally proposed is the open-loop assumption, with SBP as an input and RR as an output. They neglect the closed-loop anatomical structure of the arterial BRR arch. The feed-forward effect of HR (i.e., RRIs) on BP acts simultaneously with the BRR. The time-domain and spectral methods cannot reveal whether observed changes in the SBP and RRIs are the result of feedback (BRR) or feed-forward interaction (Starling and Windkessel effects). Therefore, their major limitation is the inability to acknowledge causality (Porta et al. 2000a).

9.2.2.3 Model-Based Techniques

The main aim of the model-based techniques is the evaluation of BRR gain capable of imposing causality, that is, evaluating the fraction of RR variability driven by BP changes. The models should take into account the sources of RR variability acting independently of BP (Porta et al. 2000a). The autoregressive (AR) multivariate techniques, based on simplified models of the entire cardiovascular system, can provide a closed-loop evaluation of the interactions between RR and SBP (Barbieri et al. 2001). One of the first closed-loop models proposed by Baselli et al. (1988) identifies the interaction between RR and SBP and considers that respiration influences BP mechanically and consequently RRIs through a feedback loop. Patton et al. (1996) compared measures of open-loop HR BRR gain in the time domain with closed-loop autoregressive moving average (ARMA) analysis and concluded that ARMA modeling yielded lower BRS estimates, but closely correlated with time-domain estimates. Barbieri et al. (1997) suggested a trivariate model including respiration as the third signal and Porta et al. (2000a) introduces respiration as an exogenous signal modeled as an AR process acting independently on RR and SBP signals. The model proposed by Nollo et al. (2001) describes the causal relationship between RRI and SBP by dividing the RRI variability in SBP-related and -unrelated parts. Barbieri et al. (2001) applies the time-domain, spectral, and AR approach, concluding that the absolute values of obtained estimates highly correlate but differ in absolute values, with open-loop estimates overshooting the closed-loop results more than 30%.

Barbieri et al. (2005) developed a statistical model of human heartbeat intervals to study heartbeat dynamics. The model was built taking into consideration the point-process nature of the RRIs, their dependence on autonomic influences directed to the sinoatrial node, and time-variant characteristics of these influences introducing nonstationary conditions. The idea is further developed to include BP as a covariate in the heartbeat interval point-process model (Chen et al. 2011). The closed-loop bivariate parametric AR model provides dynamic assessment of the BRR gain within the feedback BP–RR transfer function and estimation of the feed-forward RR–BP frequency response. The estimation of BRS based on the linear bivariate system assumes a purely linear RR and BP relationship, which is valid around the BP set point. Although this methodology has its limitations (sensible initialization of model parameters, neglecting of respiration influences), it enables an estimation of BRS in a dynamic fashion, instantaneous HR, HRV, the coherence, and cross-bispectrum, which may be used for ambulatory monitoring in clinical practice (Chen et al. 2011).

9.2.3 Comparison of Different BRS Estimation Techniques

BRS estimates provided by modern techniques differ in absolute values when compared with static methods. The methodological diversity is deepened with variations in implementation procedures of these techniques, significantly affecting reproducibility of the results. These ambiguities inspired a comparative study carried out on the EUROBAVAR data set consisting of noninvasive recordings obtained in a nonhomogeneous population of 21 subjects, two of which had established BRR failure (Laude et al. 2004). Within this study, 21 different techniques were compared including spectral analysis (11 procedures), the sequence method (7 procedures), and one exogenous model with the AR input method (XAR). The study enables insight into BRS estimates obtained by different methods, the influence of different implementations of one method on BRS estimates, ability of the methods to detect BRR failure in patients, and reproducibility of the procedures.

Without the gold standard, this kind of comparative study can only assess the individual performance of each method and determine the equivalent procedures. The EUROBAVAR study shows that BRS estimates obtained by spectral and sequence technique are closely correlated and clustered. Moreover, the results indicate that different implementation procedures and changes in parameters relevant to these methods do not affect agreement between the procedures. The EUROBAVAR study further suggests that an effort should be made to tune the techniques in order to improve the detection of BRR impairment (Laude et al. 2004).

The availability of techniques for spontaneous BRS assessment and their clinical potential reported in clinical studies indicates the potential relevance in everyday clinical practice. Some of the techniques are already incorporated in commercially available equipment and their valid use largely depends on the availability of reference values, as well as on awareness of their methodological limitations. For further methodological details, the indicated references should suffice, and comprehensive reviews can be found in Parati et al. (2000), Laude et al. (2004), and La Rovere et al. (2008). Reference values for patients after myocardial infarction and in patients with heart failure for traditional and some time and frequency methods are summarized in La Rovere et al. (2008).

9.2.4 Nonlinear Approach to HR and BP Interactions

Complex interaction of cardiovascular variables and control mechanisms result in the nonlinear nature of BP and HR dynamics. BRR feedback control includes some nonlinear features (Di Rienzo et al. 2009) such as the baroreceptor sensing mechanism, sigmoid RR–SBP relationship, stochastic resonance phenomenon (Hidaka et al. 2000; Soma et al. 2003), and resetting phenomenon (McCubbin et al. 1956; Seagard et al. 1992).

BP and heart period interactions have been studied using nonlinear approaches to complement the BRS estimation techniques, offering new indices reflecting patterns, similarity, synchronization, and time delays. To quantify the BP and RR interactions, joint symbolic dynamics methods have been used (Baumert et al. 2005, 2015). Symbolic dynamics offers flexible transformation rules and word formation, revealing and quantifying physiologically relevant patterns in RR–BP dynamic interaction. Although some studies show additional value of symbolic analyses, a systematic comparison for establishing clinical research value has not yet been conducted (Baumert et al. 2015). Besides, the optimal threshold values for symbolization procedures require further investigation.

Fischer and Voss (2014) proposed three-dimensional segmented Poincaré plot analysis (SPPA3) suitable for coupling analysis between two and three different systems. SPPA enhances Poincaré plot analysis to retain the nonlinear features of systems' dynamics by observing the three-dimensional phase space subdivided into $12 \times 12 \times 12$ equal cubelets according to the predefined range of signals. The method is based on probability of occurrence of data points in each cubelet, for which reliable estimation longer recordings are required (30 minutes).

Quantification of RR–BP interactions can be done using other nonlinear approaches, cross-sample entropy (Richman and Moorman 2000), cross-multiscale entropy (Costa et al. 2002), information-domain synchronization index (IDSI) (Porta et al. 2000b), and information-based similarity index (Yang et al. 2003). These methods were applied to detected BRR impairment in young patients with subclinical autonomic dysfunction in type 1 diabetes mellitus in Javorka et al. (2011), revealing some discrimination potential. Nevertheless, the significance of the estimated nonlinear measures requires further study.

The BRR mechanism has been mainly analyzed using linear approaches, relying on the assumption that the RR–BP relationship is linear around the BP set point. Linear analysis is based on solid theoretical grounds and provides methodological approaches with very clear interpretation. Complex interaction with other cardiovascular control mechanisms and nonlinear features of the BRR control loop justify the use of the nonlinear approaches. While the linear methods offer limited information about the underlying complex processes, the nonlinear approach suffers from the course of dimensionality (Wessel et al. 2000). Long stationary time series are required for the reliable estimation of nonlinear descriptors, a condition rarely met in the clinical practice. Additionally, nonlinear indices usually lack the clear interpretation offered by linear descriptors.

9.3 The Sequence Method—Implementation Procedure

9.3.1 Importance of the Signal Quality Assessment

The sequence method requires two input streams: RRI data and SBP time series. These data are derived from acquired electrocardiogram (ECG) and BP data. Alternatively, in animal experimentation, if only direct BP measurements are available, the interval between two successive BP maxima (pulse interval [PI]) can be used instead of the RRI series.

However, the derivation of these two data streams is not a straightforward task. Regarding RR extraction, automatic ECG delineation has been evolving for more than 40 years. Nowadays, when computational power does not present an issue, performance of the ECG delineation methods is the only objective for further enhancements. An exception to this rule would be ECG analysis in battery-driven devices, where rational energy consumption is the basic limitation. There are numerous ECG delineation algorithms available, including novel ones based on wavelet transforms, artificial neural networks, filter banks, genetic algorithms, and so on. The basic principles of QRS detection using these and many more methods are reviewed in Kohler et al. (2002), where the full list of references is given to obtain the details on each method. On the contrary, there are only several published algorithms on BP waveform delineation. Since pressure detection algorithms are necessary for most types of pulse oximeters and devices that monitor cardiac output, most of these algorithms are proprietary, developed by medical device companies. Consequently, researchers implement their own algorithms that lack the performance, robustness, and generality of ECG parameterization techniques. Most of these algorithms are not even rigorously validated.

The feature extraction and detection parts of the BP delineation algorithm depend on the way the BP is recorded. BP can be recorded directly from the radial or brachial artery using an intra-arterial catheter resulting in continuous BP waveform. A noninvasive alternative approach is BP monitoring on beat-to-beat basis using Finapres technology, for example.

Direct BP measurement potentially introduces complications and requires technical expertise to be implemented. Nonetheless, arterial catheterization with continuous pressure transduction remains the accepted standard for BP monitoring in hospitals. In experimental animals, the techniques for measuring BP have improved considerably over the past decade. Methods for direct measurement of BP are generally preferred because of their ability to continuously monitor dynamic BP changes. BP can be directly measured in experimental animals using radiotelemetry techniques or via indwelling catheters connected to externally mounted transducers.

Seemingly easy, the derivation of the RRI data and BP features presents a challenging task for real-time analysis, especially considering fast morphological and pattern changes induced by pathology, respiration, movements, and inevitable noise components. Generally, ECG and BP delineation are already included in advanced commercial devices for cardiovascular assessment, or the software tools are publicly available on Internet. The time series of cardiovascular variability, which are extracted with these demanding delineation procedures, should be plotted and carefully examined for possible misdetections. The preprocessing procedures depend on the analysis requirement, but removal of artifacts and ectopic beats seem to be a universal demand. The automatic procedures eliminate the artifacts and arrhythmias using filtering procedures over RR to output the series of normal-to-normal intervals (NN). One adaptive filtering algorithm presented in Wessel et al. (2000) can be used for RR/PI series filtering with the MATLAB® implementation freely available at http://tocsy.pik-potsdam.de/. However, this filtering procedure cannot be applied in real time, but only after signal acquisition, and it also does not apply to SBP time series.

To illustrate the necessity of visual examination and/or preprocessing of series of cardiovascular variability prior to any further analysis, we present an example of an extracted HR series in beats per minute (bpm) from radiotelemetry recording of a laboratory rat (Figure 9.2). The BP recording sampled at 1000 Hz served as the source trace for PI and SBP extraction. The HR trace in the upper panel, extracted by commercially available

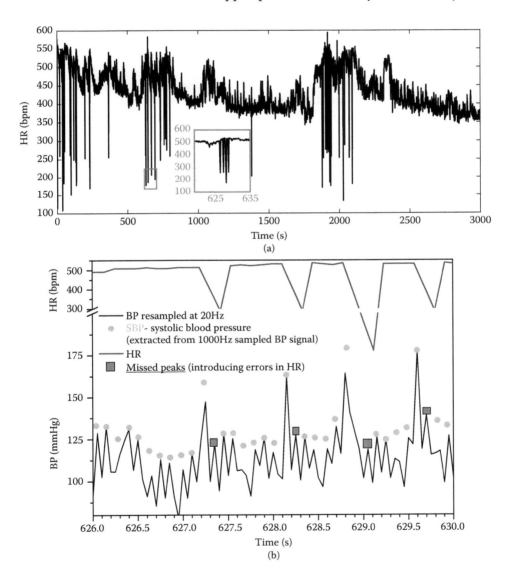

FIGURE 9.2
(a) HR series in beats per minute (bpm) with one of the erroneous parts enlarged. (b) The enlarged part with HR and resampled BP trace reveling that four errors in HR result from four beat omissions. *Source*: Bajic, D. et al., Biomedical signals in BANs: Pre-channel issues, In *Proceedings of European Wireless 2011*, Vienna, Austria, VDE Verlag, Berlin, Offenbach. Reprinted with permission.

software, reveals the omissions in the BP delineation procedure, which is confirmed in the bottom panel. The lower trace of the bottom panel in Figure 9.2 is BP originally recorded at 1000 Hz, but resampled for export at 20 Hz for the faster visual verification of the peak detection procedure. The resampled BP trace helps identify the sources of errors in the extracted HR signal, which include omission of a beat, double beat recognition, and noise corrupting part of BP signal. Each correctly detected peak is marked with a light gray dot, while the misdetections producing errors in HR signals are marked with dark gray squares. Any frequency or time-domain analysis of the compromised signal parts would yield disputable and erroneous results.

9.3.2 The Sequence Identification Procedure

The sequence method analysis is performed by an examination of beat-to-beat SBP and RR time series in search of spontaneous sequences of three or more consecutive heartbeats in which SBP and RR strictly monotonically change in the same direction. If SBP progressively increases and, usually with a species-specific BRR delay, RRI progressively lengthens, then RR+/SBP+ increasing (positive) sequences are obtained. Vice versa, if SBP progressively decreases and RRI shortens, then RR/SBP decreasing (negative) sequences are found (Di Rienzo et al. 2001).

When studying the reflex neural control of the sinus node, using RR (or PI extracted from BP in animal experimentation when ECG is not available) is more appropriate than HR, according to Iellamo (2001) and Waki et al. (2006). This is primarily because the relationship between the frequency of stimulation of vagal efferent nerves and RR (or PI) interval responses is linear, while the relationship between HR and vagal stimulation is hyperbolic (Parker et al. 1984; Daly 1997).

The progressive beat-by-beat increase in SBP is *called positive (increasing) SBP ramp*, whereas the progressive decrease in SBP is called the *negative (decreasing) SBP ramp*. These ramps present the input to the baroreceptors, while the corresponding progressive change in RR or PI (*RR [PI] ramp*) is taken as the response of the BRR to the SBP input (Di Rienzo et al. 2001).

Not all of the SBP–RR segments exhibiting concordant monotonic increase are considered BSs. The BS is formed only if the SBP ramp and the related RR ramp fulfill the conditions with respect to the minimal values of sequence length, amplitude change, and/or correlation coefficient. The parameters required for determination of whether a BS is identified are as follows:

M_{min}—the minimal sequence length in interbeat intervals (IBIs) or alternatively $M_{min}+1$ (SBP, RR) pairs (beats)

d_{SBP}—the minimal amplitude change between consecutive SBP values

d_{RR}—the minimal amplitude change between consecutive RRI (or d_{PI} if PI time series is used)

r_{min}—the minimal correlation coefficient of the linear SBP–RR regression line (additional or alternative condition)

The threshold values set in humans for these parameters are $d_{SBP} = 1$ mmHg, while d_{RR} ranges from 1 to 6 ms, with the most usual value being 5 ms (Di Rienzo et al. 2001; Laude et al. 2004; Gouveia et al. 2009). A minimal correlation coefficient of the linear SBP–RR regression line r_{min} can be set as an additional or alternative condition. If applied, its usual value is 0.7 or 0.8 (Laude et al. 2004; Gouveia et al. 2009). According to some studies, d_{SBP}, d_{RR}, and r_{min} in small animals can be set to zero (Oosting et al. 1997; Laude et al. 2008, 2009). Even in humans, some studies suggest the amplitude threshold d is not needed if a value of 0.8 is imposed on the r_{min} (Laude et al. 2004).

The latency introduced by the BRR, τ (beats), determines the delay of the RR ramps with respect to the SBP ramps. It is species dependent: in humans, it is usually set to one beat, and in rats between three and five beats (Laude et al. 2004, 2008; Bertinieri et al. 1988; Oosting et al. 1997; Di Rienzo et al. 2001; Porta et al. 2002; Baselli et al. 1994).

9.3.3 BRS Estimate and the Temporal Features

For each validated BRR sequence BS_i, $i = 1, \ldots, I$, consisting of $M_i > M_{min}(\text{IBI})$, BRS_i is estimated as the slope of the linear regression line of SBP and RR values, obtained using the ordinary least-squares method. In Figure 9.3, the sequence of length $M_i = 3(\text{IBI})$ recorded from a male Wistar rat is presented. The regression line is dotted. Its slope presents the local BRS_i estimate. The global BRS estimate is obtained by averaging the slopes of all the BS found:

$$\text{BRS} = \frac{1}{I} \sum_{i=1}^{I} \text{BRS}_i \qquad (9.1)$$

Temporal sequence parameters and additional BRR features can be extracted from the sequence method analysis. These can be used to compare experimental groups or as intraindividual comparisons, based on the analysis of available SBP and RR time series. In

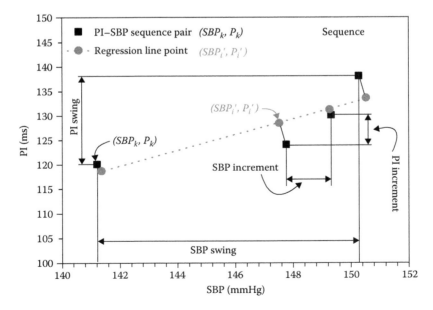

FIGURE 9.3
An example of the baroreflex sequence of length 3(IBI) (four SBP–PI pairs) from the SBP–PI series of a male Wistar rat. SBP and PI increment and swing parameters are illustrated. The slope of the dotted regression line is taken as the local BRS estimate.

cases when RRI series is not available, PI series can be used instead without any changes in the parameter definition. These features include the following:

N_S—number of sBRR sequences per minute; normalization should be done if recordings of different duration are compared.

N_R—number of SBP ramps per minute.

BEI—sBRR effectiveness index is the ratio between the number of SBP ramps followed by a concomitant reflex RRI modulation and the overall number of SBP ramps observed in a given time window (proposed in Di Rienzo et al. 2001).

N_{SBP-RR}—mean number of SBP–RR pairs in one sequence (beats).

S_{SBP}—SBP swing is the mean difference (in mmHg) between the highest and lowest SBP value in one sequence (Figure 9.3).

S_{RR}—RR swing is the mean difference (in ms) between the highest and lowest RR value in one sequence (Figure 9.3).

Δ_{SBP} and Δ_{RR}—SBP and RR increment—absolute SBP and RR increments (in mmHg and ms, respectively) are the mean absolute difference between the successive SBP and RR values in one sequence (Figure 9.3).

sBRR Operating Range (*sequence coverage area* [SCA])—a rectangle region in the SBP–RR plane between the lowest and the highest sequence points in both dimensions without 5% outlier points (proposed in Bajic et al. 2010).

sBRR Upper and Lower Limit—the average value of the first and the last vigintile in both dimensions (SBP$_{LL}$, SBP$_{UL}$, RR$_{LL}$, and RR$_{UL}$), as proposed in Bajic et al. (2010). A vigintile is a quantile of order 0.05, or 5% of outlier points.

sBRR Set Point—calculated as a median value of all SBP–RR sequence points.

The last three temporal parameters are introduced in Bajic et al. (2010) and shown in Figure 9.4. The two areas in Figure 9.4 correspond to the two phases in the experiment where a Wistar rat was exposed to mild emotional stress mimicked by a short-lasting exposure to an air-jet from a pressurized bottle directed to the back of its head. The air-jet induced a typical startle reaction followed by an escape. An example of concomitant changes of SBP and PI is shown in Figure 9.5. The details on this investigation can be found in Bajic et al. (2010).

9.4 The Caveats of the Sequence Technique

The sequence method is the most frequently used technique for BRS assessment for its noninvasive nature, ease of implementation, and understandable formulation. However, several questionable issues might appear in a practical application of this technique.

9.4.1 Reference Threshold Values

The main limitation of the sequence technique in the case of autonomic dysfunction is the absence of BS, whose validation requires conforming to several criteria concerning length,

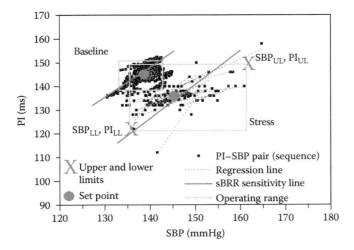

FIGURE 9.4
Features of the spontaneous BRR (sBRR) under baseline conditions and during exposure to stress. Note a decrease of sBRR sensitivity (expressed as a mean regression of all sequences), increase of sBRR operating range (rectangle surface in SBP–PI plane between the lower and upper limits), and resetting of the sBRR (set point calculated as median value of all SBP–PI sequence points). *Source*: Bajic, D. et al., *Stress.*, 13, 142–154, 2010. Copyright © 2010, Informa Helathcare. Reproduced with permission of Informa Healthcare.

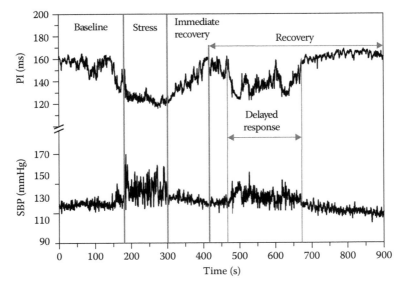

FIGURE 9.5
Time course of SBP and PI changes in a rat exposed to air-jet stress. Exposure to air-jet induces simultaneous increases in SBP and shortening of PI followed by three distinct dynamic regions of SBP and PI changes during recovery: fast (immediate recovery), slow (recovery), and delayed response. *Source*: Bajic, D. et al., *Stress.*, 13, 142–154, 2010. Copyright © 2010, Informa Healthcare. Reproduced with permission of Informa Healthcare.

threshold (minimal amplitude change), and/or minimum correlation between SBP and RR/PI samples included in potential BS. The sequence method applies only to one-fourth of available beats, leaving the rest of the recording out of the analysis (Bertinieri et al. 1988). Moreover, these criteria should be relaxed or changed when different species are analyzed, such as dogs, cats, rats, and mice. If the strict criteria for BS validation hold, the sequence method is likely to fail in patients with impaired BRR (Davies et al. 2001). Several thresholds required for sequence identification are set in the study in anesthetized cats (Bertinieri et al. 1988 and transferred to humans without evidence on their optimality (Davies et al. 2001). The alternations in threshold values changes the number of the sequences found and thus the BRS estimate.

To overcome this limitation, a set of reference threshold values optimal for the use in humans is required. Davies et al. (2001) found that by decreasing BP and RRI amplitude thresholds in patients with congestive heart failure (CHF), the agreement of the sequence method estimates with traditional techniques is optimized. Another possible methodological improvement, recently proposed in Gouveia et al. (2009), is a replacement of BS with BE validated based only on correlation coefficient criteria. This comparative study has shown that the events technique provides a BRS estimate that correlates with the basic sequence method estimates. Longer BEs incorporate an average of 50% of all beats into analysis and provide BRS estimates in cases without identified BS.

9.4.2 BRR Sequences or Random Occurrences?

Another important issue regarding the sequence technique is the nonselective inclusion of all the sequences meeting the imposed criteria in BRS estimation. One side of this problem is, as discussed earlier, that the sequence method is not able to evaluate the fraction of RR variability driven by SBP changes (Porta et al. 2000a). Consequently, the produced BRS estimate lumps the properties of both the feedback and feed-forward path. This drawback can be surpassed by using model-based approaches that assume a closed-loop RR–SBP relation (Barbieri et al. 2001).

The other side of the problem is whether these sequences reflect true physiological RR and SBP (BRR or non-BRR) interactions or accidental, random occurrences. By *random occurrence*, we consider a chance alignment of increasing or decreasing SBP samples, followed by a chance alignment of unidirectional RR/PI ramp. The differences among successive samples are usually small and due to random fluctuations (noise), but occasionally they would be aligned, fulfilling the criteria of the BS with a minimal length. This problem may not be so evident in humans, since the strict criteria for sequence validation would largely disable the inclusion of these random occurrences. Yet, even in humans, this may happen if the minimum length of the BS is set to three beats. The major problem arises when the sequence technique is applied on animal experimentation data: the smaller the animal, the more relaxed are the criteria for sequence validation. When it comes to rats or mice, the only criteria is the sequence length (three or four beats) (Oosting et al. 1997; Laude et al. 2008). Unfortunately, these criteria include a significant number of random occurrences. If no amplitude threshold is required for BS validation, it is highly probably that some of such chance alignments are counted as BSs. Since animal experimentation is often used in pharmacological experimentation for drug testing and elucidating its effects, reliable estimates on the functioning of the main short-term BP regulator are clearly valuable.

To test the hypothesis of whether a sequence obtained from the time series presents a physiological response, the method of surrogate data is used (Theiler et al. 1992). The method of surrogate data successfully explores the underlying patterns within data (Blaber et al. 1995). Two different types of surrogate data can be used, depending on the type of investigated SBP–RR interactions. The hypothesis that sequences are real physiological responses of the RRI to changes in SBP, and not a random alignment, can be tested by replacing the RRI time series with isospectral surrogate data. Briefly, isospectral surrogate data can be obtained by inverse Fourier transform of the original series spectra, keeping the amplitudes but randomizing the phases, thus removing the phase relationship between SBP and RRI data. If temporal signal features are observed, isodistributional (ID) surrogate data present *"the control experiment"* to estimate the degree to which observed interactions may be due to completely random fluctuations (noise) in the data. ID surrogates are generated by randomly permuting the temporal order of the original signal samples, presenting a set of independent and identically distributed (i.i.d.) random variables with the same mean, variance, and distribution as the original time series.

The authors of the classic review paper (Schreiber and Schmitz 2000) recommend that the actual testing using surrogate data should be carried out as a rank test. This means that for achieving the level of significance $(1 − \alpha)$ 100% in a two-sided test, a total of $S = (2K/\alpha) − 1$ surrogate sequences have to be generated, where S is a positive integer. For example, for a significance level of 95%, at least 39 surrogate sequences have to be generated. Larger K values give a more sensitive test, yet the authors suggest using $K = 1$ in order to minimize the computational effort of generating surrogates. This recommendation means that, for each original SBP–RRI series pair, 39 surrogate pairs have to be generated. For each surrogate pair, the sequence technique parameters have to be calculated in order to estimate the time averages for surrogate data. These computations present an excessive and unavoidable effort.

Considering the frequent usage of the sequence technique and the following exhausting surrogate testing, we have developed the Markov model outlined below to derive formulae for the temporal sequence parameters (distribution, length, and number of sequences) in ID surrogate data. The obtained expressions present ensemble averages of these sequence method parameters, that is, their expected numbers, as a function of the minimal sequence length, the amplitude thresholds, and the observed SBP–RR time series length N (Loncar-Turukalo et al. 2011).

9.4.2.1 The Markov Model

To describe the temporal statistics of sBRR sequences, the model must "count" successive occurrences of the increasing or the decreasing signal amplitudes. The signal samples will be denoted x_i, $i = 1, \ldots, N$, and the amplitude changes of consecutive signal samples $\Delta_i = x_{i+1} − x_i$, $i = 1, \ldots, N − 1$ form a signal of successive differences, which we refer to as Δ-signal. A difference can be positive, negative, or "idle."

$$\Delta_i = \begin{cases} \text{positive,} & x_{i+1} − x_i > d \\ \text{idle,} & |x_{i+1} − x_i| \leq d \quad, \quad d \geq 0, \ i = 1, \ldots, N − 1 \\ \text{negative,} & x_{i+1} − x_i < −d \end{cases} \tag{9.2}$$

The amplitude range of the biological signals is physiologically limited, thus the same is valid for their ID surrogates. For this reason, it can be shown that for a certain number i of the successive differences with the same sign, the probability that the $L + 1$th difference in the row will have the same sign will be almost zero. When the samples are shuffled, such as in ID surrogate data, the probability of occurrence of the longer ramps is further decreased.

The proposed model is a discrete, homogenous, and ergodic Markov chain describing successive increases and decreases of amplitudes in pairs of ID surrogate data, with a bounded number of states, L (Figure 9.6).

The states of the model in Figure 9.6 are labeled from $n = 1$ to $n = L$, counting either the consecutive Δ-signal samples or $(\Delta_{\text{SBP}}, \Delta_{\text{PI}})$ sequence pairs of the same sign (states $n > 1$). The state 1 corresponds to the Δ-signal sample (or $(\Delta_{\text{SBP}}, \Delta_{\text{PI}})$ pair) that is either idle or different from the previous one.

Transition probabilities $p_{n+1,n} = \Pr\{\Delta_k \in (n+1) | \Delta_{k-1} \in n\}$ reflect the likelihood that the sample Δ_k will retain the same sign (and thus transit to the state $n + 1$) as the previous sample Δ_{k-1} (belonging to state n, as nth successive difference in the row). The model state equations are

$$P(n) = P(1) \cdot \prod_{i=1}^{n-1} p_{i+1,i}, \quad n = 2, \dots, L; \quad \sum_{n=1}^{L} P(n) = 1 \tag{9.3}$$

The occurrences of ramps in different ID surrogate series are independent. The sequence state probability is the joint probability that a particular SBP surrogate Δ-signal sample and its PI counterpart are both the nth one in a row and of the same sign; therefore, the following holds:

$$P_{\text{SEQ}}(n) = \frac{P(n)^2}{2}, \quad n = 2, \dots, L, \quad P_{\text{SEQ}}(1) = 1 - \sum_{i=2}^{L} P_{\text{SEQ}}(i) \tag{9.4}$$

The ramp passes through the state n if its length exceeds or is equal to n (Figure 9.6). The probability that a sample Δ_i is an element of the ramp of length l is called the "ramp probability," $h(l)$. The state probability $P(n)$ comprises all the probabilities $h(l), l \geq n$ of ramps longer than or equal to n.

$$P(n) = \sum_{l=n}^{L} h(l), \quad n = 1, \dots, L \tag{9.5}$$

The same analogy is valid for sequences and we introduce "sequence probability" $h_{\text{SEQ}}(l)$.

The string of length k is a subset of k model states starting at an arbitrary model position (unlike the ramp that starts at the first model position), see Figure 9.6. The relationship

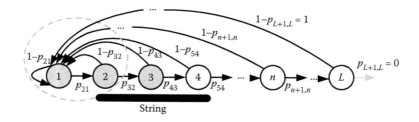

FIGURE 9.6
Model that counts successive Δ-signals of the same sign in ID surrogate data; gray states: a ramp of length $l = 3$; underlined states: a string of length $k = 3$. *Source*: Loncar-Turukalo, T. et al., *IEEE Transactions on Biomedical Engineering*, 58, 16–24, 2011. Reprinted with permission. © 2011 IEEE.

between the probability of string of length k, $S(k)$ and state probabilities $P(n)$ is given by

$$S(k) = \sum_{n=k}^{L} P(n), \quad k = 1, \ldots, L \tag{9.6}$$

The expression for string probabilities as a function of length n and the amplitude threshold d are given in Table 9.1 (Loncar-Turukalo et al. 2011).

It is easy to show that the string probability, if the amplitude threshold d is set to zero, is equal to

$$S(n, d = 0) = \frac{2}{(n+1)!}, \quad n \geq 1 \tag{9.7}$$

Knowing the string probabilities $S(n, d)$ and the relations (Equations 9.3 through 9.6), state, ramp, and transition probabilities can be derived. Setting the amplitude threshold to zero ($d = 0$), these probabilities can be expressed as

$$P(n, d = 0) = \frac{2 \cdot (n+1)}{(n+2)!}, n \geq 1, \quad P_{SEQ}(n, d = 0) = \frac{4 \cdot (n+1)^2}{[(n+2)!]^2}, n > 1 \tag{9.8}$$

$$h(n, d = 0) = \frac{2[(n+1)^2 + n]}{(n+3)!}, \quad h_{SEQ}(n, d = 0) = \frac{4[(n+1)^2(n+3)^2 - (n+2)^2]}{[(n+3)!]^2} \tag{9.9}$$

$$p_{n+1,n} = \frac{(n+2)}{(n+1)(n+3)}; \quad p_{SEQn+1,n} = \frac{(n+2)^2}{(n+1)^2(n+3)^2} \tag{9.10}$$

When the sequence technique is applied with amplitude thresholds, two different threshold values d_{SBP} and d_{Pi} have to be applied to the surrogates of the PI and SBP series (Table 9.1). Also, the state probabilities $P_{PI}(n)$ and $P_{SBP}(n)$ of the corresponding surrogates are not the same. Then the probabilities $P_{SEQ}(n)$ are evaluated as follows:

$$P_{SEQ}(n, d_{SBP}, d_{PI}) = \frac{P_{SBP}(n, d_{SBP}) \cdot P_{PI}(n, d_{PI})}{2} \tag{9.11}$$

TABLE 9.1

String Probabilities $S(n, d)$

n	$S(n, d)$
2	$\frac{2}{3!} - \frac{d}{a} + \frac{3 \cdot d^2}{4 \cdot a^2}$
3	$\frac{2}{4!} - \frac{d}{2 \cdot a} + \frac{d^2}{a^2} - \frac{2 \cdot d^3}{3 \cdot a^3}$
4	$\frac{2}{5!} - \frac{d}{6 \cdot a} + \frac{5 \cdot d^2}{8 \cdot a^2} - \frac{25 \cdot d^3}{24 \cdot a^3} + \frac{125 \cdot d^4}{192 \cdot a^4}$
5	$\frac{2}{6!} - \frac{d}{24 \cdot a} + \frac{d^2}{4 \cdot a^2} - \frac{3 \cdot d^3}{4 \cdot a^3} + \frac{9 \cdot d^4}{8 \cdot a^4} - \frac{27 \cdot d^5}{20 \cdot a^5}$

Source: From Loncar-Turukalo, T. et al., *IEEE Transactions on Biomedical Engineering*, 58, 16–24, 2011. Reprinted with permission. © 2011 IEEE.

Note: The parameter a is equal to $\hat{\sigma} \cdot \sqrt{3}$, where $\hat{\sigma}$ is the standard deviation estimated from the original data.

The increasing and decreasing sequences in ID surrogate data are expected to occur with the same probability. To describe them separately, the string, state, and sequence probabilities must be reduced to half whereas the transition probabilities remain the same.

9.4.2.2 The Temporal Sequence Parameters in ID Surrogate Data

The model provides formulae for the temporal parameters of sBRR sequences in ID surrogates, as functions of the recording length N (i.e., number of SBP–PI pairs), a minimal sequence length M (IBI) (i.e., $M+1$ SBP–PI pairs), and amplitude thresholds d_{SBP} and d_{PI} (here expressed as d) (Loncar-Turukalo et al. 2011). The formulae can be applied either to refer to a single ID surrogate series, resulting in the expected values for ramps, or they can be applied to the pairs of SBP–PI ID surrogate data to provide these averages for sequences.

- $T(M)$: expected ramp (or sequence) length in ID surrogate data, expressed in number of IBI, if M is the minimal sequence length:

$$T(M,d) = M - 1 + \frac{\displaystyle\sum_{n=M}^{L} P(n,d)}{\displaystyle\sum_{n=M}^{L} (1 - p_{n+1,n}) \cdot P(n,d)} \tag{9.12}$$

- $H_N(n)$: the length histogram is the expected number of ramps (or sequences) of length n(IBI) in a record of duration N SBP–PI ID surrogate pairs:

$$H_N(n) = (N-1) \cdot h(n,d), \quad n = 1, \ldots, L \tag{9.13}$$

- $N_S(M,N)$: total number of ramps (sequences) in a record of ID surrogates data of length N, when the minimal sequence length is set to M(IBI):

$$N_S(M,N,d) = (N-1) \cdot P(M,d) \tag{9.14}$$

- $BEI(M)$: BRR effectiveness index, defined as the ratio of the number of sequences in pairs of SBP–RR ID surrogate data and the number of ramps in the SBP ID surrogate:

$$BEI(M) = N_{S\_SEQ}(M,N,d)/N_{S\_SBP\_RAMP}(M,N,d) \tag{9.15}$$

The thorough validation of these formulae is done in recording of laboratory rats (Loncar-Turukalo et al. 2011). Having HR five times as fast as humans, the recordings in rats provide longer stationary segments necessary for reliable estimation of probabilities for longer sequences. The results obtained from this validation are presented in Tables 9.2 through 9.4. The sequence method is applied without amplitude thresholds, according to Oosting et al. (1997). The details on the experimental protocol and the data used for the model validation can be found in Loncar-Turukalo et al. (2011). However, the temporal sequence parameters in ID surrogate data of human SBP and RR series are accurately predicted by the model as well (Loncar-Turukalo et al. 2010).

If the model is used to calculate the expected value of BRR-like sequences in ID surrogate data pairs, an excellent level of agreement between formulae value (the first row), and the

TABLE 9.2

State Probabilities $P_{SEQ}(n, d = 0), n = 1, \ldots, 4$ for Sequences

	$P_{SEQ}(1) \pm \sigma$	$P_{SEQ}(2) \pm \sigma$	$P_{SEQ}(3) \pm \sigma$	$P_{SEQ}(4) \pm \sigma$
Equation 9.8	0.967	0.03125	0.00222	9.65×10^{-5}
Surrogate	0.968 ± 0.00062	0.02985 ± 0.00051	0.00198 ± 0.00011	$0.000074 \pm 0.00001**$
Original	0.972 ± 0.00722	0.024 ± 0.00561	0.00323 ± 0.0016	0.00049 ± 0.00043

Source: From Loncar-Turukalo, T. et al., *IEEE Transactions on Biomedical Engineering*, 58, 16–24, 2011. Reprinted with permission. © 2011 IEEE.

Note: Expected value (Equation 9.8) and time averages estimated from ID surrogates. Values estimated from real data (original) is presented as an illustration.
The statistical significance of the values as evaluated by Equation 9.8 vs. SURROGATE, was assessed using repeated measures ANOVA test at levels $p < 0.05$ (∗), $p < 0.01$ (∗∗), $p < 0.005$ (∗∗∗).

TABLE 9.3

Number of Sequences $H_{1000}(n)$ of length $n = 1, \ldots, 5$, Normalized per 1000 SBP–PI Pairs

	$H_N(2) \pm \sigma$	$H_N(3) \pm \sigma$	$H_N(4) \pm \sigma$	$H_N(5) \pm \sigma$
Equation 9.13	29.03	2.126	0.0936	0.00277
Surrogate	28.66 ± 0.42	2.009 ± 0.097	0.0827 ± 0.0146	0.00331 ± 0.00081
Original	$20.739 \pm 4.53**$	$2.742 \pm 1.237*$	$0.4458 \pm 0.4389**$	$0.19395 \pm 0.07592**$

Source: From Loncar-Turukalo, T. et al., *IEEE Transactions on Biomedical Engineering*, 58, 16–24, 2011. Reprinted with permission. © 2011 IEEE.

Note: The statistical significance of ORIGINAL versus SURROGATES was assessed using a repeated-measures ANOVA test at levels $*p < .05$, $**p < .01$, $***p < .005$.
Expected value (Equation 9.13), the time averages estimated from ID surrogates and the number found in original SBP–PI data.

TABLE 9.4

Correlation Coefficient $r(n)$ of Sequences of Length $n = 2, \ldots, 5$

	$r(2) \pm \sigma$	$r(3) \pm \sigma$	$r(4) \pm \sigma$	$r(5) \pm \sigma$
Surrogate	0.91 ± 0.005	0.90 ± 0.001	0.376 ± 0.07	0.03 ± 0.015
Original	0.92 ± 0.01	0.93 ± 0.02	$0.92 \pm 0.05**$	$0.92 \pm 0.09**$

Source: From Loncar-Turukalo, T. et al., *IEEE Transactions on Biomedical Engineering*, 58, 16–24, 2011. Reprinted with permission. © 2011 IEEE.

Note: The statistical significance of original versus surrogates was assessed using repeated measures ANOVA test at levels $*p < .05$, $**p < .01$, $***p < .005$.

averages calculated from generated surrogates (the second row) is observed (Table 9.2). The time averages calculated from the original SBP–PI pairs are added in the third row for comparison.

The number of sequences of the specific length per 1000 SBP–PI pairs (histogram $H_{1000}(n)$) is presented in Table 9.3, again in accordance with the expected values calculated by the formula and the time averages of the generated ID surrogate data set. The sequences of length $n(IBI) \geq 3$ (i.e., sequences of length four or more SBP–PI pairs) in the original data significantly outnumber the corresponding sequences in ID surrogate data.

The statistical differences in the number of sequences motivated the analysis of the correlation coefficient in sequences of different length, as a measure of the linear association between the corresponding samples that form a sequence (Table 9.4). In ID surrogate pairs, the correlation coefficient significantly drops with the increase of the sequence length. In the original data, the correlation coefficient preserves the high values. The correlation coefficient of the sequences in the SBP–RR series exceed the threshold set to $r_{min} = 0.8$. In surrogate data, only 37% of $n = 4$ sequences, 3% of $n = 5$ sequences, and no $n = 6$ sequences exceed $r_{min} = 0.8$. This high linear coupling of long SBP–PI sequences, nonexistent in random data, suggests their strong relationship with physiological events, regardless of their origin (Rothlisberger et al. 2003).

While calculating the sequence histogram $H(n)$, it was noticed that the sequences of length $n(\text{IBI}) = 3$ (four SBP–PI pairs) in original data have high correlation coefficient $r(n)$ and significantly outnumber the sequences in ID surrogate data (Tables 9.3 and 9.4). This high linear coupling of long SBP–PI sequences does not exist in random and surrogate data. It suggests that the longer sequences are more likely to be an outcome of physiological events. Conversely, all the sequences of length $n = 2$ (IBI) (i.e., three SBP–PI pairs) have a high correlation coefficient, both in original and in random or surrogate data. This implies that it is difficult to estimate whether sequences of length $n = 2(\text{IBI})$ are due to random or to physiological fluctuations. This finding reinforces a proposal from Oosting et al. (1997) that the threshold that specifies minimal sequence length in rats should be set to at least $M = 3$ (IBI), that is, to four SBP–PI pairs. Thus, the number of sequences would be reduced, but the likelihood that a sequence is an outcome of an sBRR event is increased.

The validation study on humans showed that the number of long sequences is significantly larger in original data, with very high correlation coefficient, which rules out the possibility of accidental occurrences (Loncar-Turukalo et al. 2010). This may serve as an indication of the minimal sequence length $M = 3$ (IBI) (four SBP–PI pairs), for which correlation between streams of random data is lost. This analysis suggests that the threshold for correlation coefficient $r_{min} = 0.8$ can be used in combination with the increased minimal sequence length $M = 3$ (IBI) to validate the sequence, since the chance of random occurrences with such properties is negligible. These results further reinforce the idea suggested in Gouveia et al. (2009) that instead of BSs, BE can be used with a threshold imposed only on the correlation coefficient among SBP–RR data points belonging to the event segment. Our study confirms that long segments with high correlation coefficients are rare in random data.

9.5 Conclusions

The need to evaluate BRR function both as a diagnostic tool and as an assessment of the efficacy of the existing treatment has driven the development of new techniques for sBRR assessment, and its gain/sensitivity (sBRS). This chapter provides an insight into analysis of spontaneous BP and HR fluctuations and possibilities of computer-aided assessment of BRR function. The overview of available methods and the corresponding references should lead the reader to their more detailed methodological description. Within the chapter, details are provided on the sequence method, the most frequently used technique for BRS assessment for its noninvasive nature, ease of implementation, and understandable formulation. The use of the sequence method requires careful preprocessing and clear rules for sequence identification, depending both on the species and adopted methodological procedure. However, questions remain on the reference values and interpretation of the obtained results, and we have tried to refer the reader to some comprehensive overviews of reference values available in the literature.

The importance of spontaneous BRR investigation and popularity of the sequence technique has yielded numerous methodological variants of the originally proposed procedure in order to obtain more reliable estimates, especially in BRR failure patients. We have addressed this issue, introducing the reader to the available methods and methodological studies based on the sequence technique, which aim to overcome the problem of spontaneous BRS assessment. Two major limitations have been studied: the absence of BSs and the random sequence occurrences. In the cases where BSs are absent, the possible options are to relax the strict criteria for sequence validation, or to preserve only the correlation coefficient threshold leading to an assessment based on BE (Gouveia et al. 2009)

Regarding the question of automatic inclusion of random sequences in BRS estimation, their presence can be estimated by running the surrogate data test. To avoid the exhausting surrogate testing, we contributed a Markov-based model and resulting set of formulae for the straightforward calculation of the expected number of random sequence occurrences, distribution of their lengths, and their average duration in ID surrogate data of arbitrary length N. The formulae are functions of particular sequence parameters: the minimal sequence length M (expressed in IBI), the amplitude thresholds d_{SBP} and d_{PI}, and the time series length N. The derived expressions can be easily implemented to check the expected number of random sequence occurrences among the overall number of the sequences found in the original SBP–RR time series. The presented analysis has also confirmed that applying the minimal sequence length $M = 3$ (IBI) and the threshold for correlation coefficient $r_{min} = 0.8$ rules out the random sequence occurrences.

The more comprehensive approach to BRS estimation requires the use of model-based techniques for sBRS estimation capable of imposing causality, that is, evaluating the fraction of RR variability driven by BP changes. These models also take into account sources of RR variability acting independently of BP. Nonlinear approaches have been addressed as a potential tool to complement linear approaches, which offer limited information about the underlying complex processes. However, the systematic comparison for establishing clinical research value of nonlinear indices is still missing (Baumert et al. 2015). Dynamic BRS estimations have revealed time-variant BRR control, dependent on physiological conditions, and the importance of continuous BRR monitoring. Analysis and monitoring of nonstationary dynamics of BRR regulatory mechanisms continues to be an active research topic.

References

Bajic, D., Loncar-Turukalo, T., and Milovanovic, B. 2011. Biomedical signals in BANs: Pre-channel issues. In *Proceedings of European Wireless 2011*, Vienna, Austria, VDE Verlag, Berlin, Offenbach.

Bajic, D., Loncar-Turukalo, T., Stojicic, S. et al. 2010. Temporal analysis of the spontaneous baroreceptor reflex during mild emotional stress in the rat. *Stress* 13(2):142–154.

Barbieri, R., Bianchi, A. M., Triedman, J. K. et al. 1997. Model dependency of multivariate autoregressive spectral analysis: Quantifying cardiovascular control using bivariate and trivariate models. *IEEE Engineering in Medicine and Biology Magazine* 16(5):74–85.

Barbieri, R., Matten, E. C., Alabi, A. A., and E. N. Brown. 2005. A point-process model of human heartbeat intervals: New definitions of heart rate and heart rate variability. *American Journal of Physiology Heart and Circulatory Physiology* 288:H424–H435.

Barbieri, R., Parati, G., and J. P. Saul. 2001. Closed- versus open-loop assessment of heart rate barore-flex. *IEEE Engineering in Medicine and Biology Magazine* 20:33–42.

Baselli, G., Cerutti, S., Badilini, F. et al. 1994. Model for the assessment of heart period and arterial pressure variability interactions and respiration influences. *Medical and Biological Engineering and Computing* 32:143–152.

Baselli, G., Cerutti, S., Civardi, S., Malliani, A., and M. Pagani. 1988. Cardiovascular variability signals: Towards the identification of a closed-loop model of the neural control mechanisms. *IEEE Transactions on Biomedical Engineering* 35(12):1033–1046.

Baumert, M., Baier, V., Truebner, S., Schirdewan, A., and Voss, A. 2005. Short- and long-term joint symbolic dynamics of heart rate and blood pressure in dilated cardiomyopathy. *IEEE Transactions on Biomedical Engineering* 52:2112–2115.

Baumert, M., Javorka, M., and M. Kabir. 2015. Joint symbolic dynamics for the assessment of cardiovascular and cardiorespiratory interactions. *Philosophical Transactions of the Royal Society A* 373:20140097.

Bertinieri, G., di Rienzo, M., Cavallazzi, A. et al. 1988. Evaluation of baroreceptor reflex by blood pressure monitoring in unanesthetized cats. *American Journal of Physiology* 254:H377–H383.

Blaber, A. P., Yamamoto, Y., and R. L. Hughson. 1995. Methodology of spontaneous baroreflex relationship assessed by surrogate data analysis. *American Journal of Physiology* 268:H1682–H1687.

Chen, Z., Purdon, P. L., Grace Harrell, G. et al. 2011. Dynamic assessment of baroreflex control of heart rate during induction of propofol anesthesia using a point process method. *Annals of Biomedical Engineering* 39(1):260–276.

Costa, M., Goldberger, A. L., and C. K. Peng. 2002. Multiscale entropy analysis of complex physiologic time series. *Physical Review Letters* 89(6):068102.

Daly, M. 1997. Peripheral arterial chemoreceptors and respiratory cardiovascular integration. *Monographs of the Physiological Society* 46. Oxford: Oxford Medical Publications.

Davies, L. C., Francisa, D. P., Scotta, A. C. et al. 2001. Effect of altering conditions of the sequence method on baroreflex sensitivity. *Journal of Hypertension* 19(7):1279–1289.

Di Rienzo, M., Bertinieri, G., Mancia, G., and A. Pedotti. 1985. A new method for evaluating the baroreflex role by a joint pattern analysis of pulse interval and systolic blood pressure series. *Medical and Biological Engineering and Computing* 23(suppl. I):313–314.

Di Rienzo, M., Castiglioni, P., Mancia, G., Pedotti, A., and G. Parati. 2001. Advancements in estimating baroreflex function. *IEEE Engineering in Medicine and Biology Magazine* 20(2):25–32.

Di Rienzo, M., Parati, G., Castiglioni, P. et al. 2001. Baroreflex effectiveness index: An additional measure of baroreflex control of heart rate in daily life. *American Journal of Physiology—Regulatory, Integrative and Comparative Physiology* 280:744–751.

Di Rienzo, M., Parati, G., Mancia, G., Pedotti, A., and P. Castiglioni. 1997. Investigating baroreflex control of circulation using signal processing techniques. *IEEE Engineering in Medicine and Biology Magazine* 16(5):86–95.

Di Rienzo, M., Parati, G., Radaelli, A., and P. Castiglioni. 2009. Baroreflex contribution to blood pressure and heart rate oscillation: Time scales, time variant characteristics and nonlinearities. *Philosophical Transactions of the Royal Society A* 367:1301–1318.

Eckberg, D. L. 2008. Arterial baroreflex and cardiovascular modeling. *Cardiovascular Engineering* 8:513.

Eckberg, D. L., Cavanaugh, M. S., Mark, A. L. et al. 1975. A simplified neck suction device for activation of carotid baroreceptors. *Journal of Laboratory and Clinical Medicine* 85:167–173.

Fessel, J. and D. Robertson. 2006. Orthostatic hypertension: When pressor reflexes overcompensate. *Nature Clinical Practice Nephrology* 2(8):424–431.

Fischer, C. and A. Voss. 2014. Three-dimensional segmented poincaré plot analyses SPPA3 investigates cardiovascular and cardiorespiratory couplings in hypertensive pregnancy disorders. *Frontiers in Bioengineering and Biotechnology* 2(51).

Fu, Q. and B. D. Levine. 2014. Pathophysiology of neurally mediated syncope: Role of cardiac output and total peripheral resistance. *Autonomic Neuroscience* 184:24–26.

Goldberger, J. J., Subačius, H., Patel, T., Cunnane, R., and A. H. Kadish. 2014. Sudden cardiac death risk stratification in patients with nonischemic dilated cardiomyopathy. *Journal of the American College of Cardiology* 63(18):1879–1889.

Gouveia, S., Rocha, A., Laguna, P., and P. Lago. 2009. Time domain baroreflex sensitivity assessment by joint analysis of spontaneous SBP and RR series. *Biomedical Signal Processing and Control* 4:254–261.

Hidaka, I., Nozaki, D., and Y. Yamamoto. 2000. Functional stochastic resonance in the human brain: Noise induced sensitization of baroreflex system. *Physical Review Letters* 85:3740–3743.

Hunt, B. and W. Farquhar. 2005. Nonlinearities and asymmetries of the human cardiovagal baroreflex. *American Journal of Physiology—Regulatory, Integrative and Comparative Physiology* 288:R1339–1346.

Iellamo, F. 2001. Neural mechanisms of cardiovascular regulation during exercise. *Autonomic Neuroscience: Basic and Clinical* 90:66–75.

Javorka, M., Lazarova, Z., Tonhajzerova, I. et al. 2011. Baroreflex analysis in diabetes mellitus: Linear and nonlinear approaches. *Medical and Biological Engineering and Computing* 49(3): 279–288.

Kohler, B., Hennig, C., and R. Orglmeister. 2002. The principles of software QRS detection. *IEEE Engineering in Medicine and Biology Magazine* 21(1):42–57.

La Rovere, M.T., Pinna, G.D., Hohnloser, S. H. et al. 2001. Baroreflex sensitivity and heart rate variability in the identification of patients at risk for life-threatening arrhythmias: Implications for clinical trials. *Circulation* 103: 2072–2077.

La Rovere, M. T., Pinna, G. D., and G. Raczak. 2008. Baroreflex sensitivity: Measurements and clinical implications. *Annals of Noninvasive Electrocardiology* 13(2):191–207.

Laude, D., Elghozi, J. L., Girard, A. et al. 2004. Comparison of various techniques used to estimate spontaneous baroreflex sensitivity (the EUROBAVAR study). *American Journal of Physiology—Regulatory, Integrative and Comparative Physiology* 286:R226–R231.

Laude, D., Baudrie, V., and J. L. Elghozi. 2008. Applicability of recent methods used to estimate spontaneous baroreflex sensitivity to resting mice. *American Journal of Physiology—Regulatory, Integrative and Comparative Physiology* 294:R142–R150.

Laude, D., Baudrie, V., and J. L. Elghozi. 2009. Tuning the sequence technique. *IEEE Engineering in Medicine and Biology Magazine* 28(6):30–34.

Loncar-Turukalo, T., Japundzic Zigon, N., and D. Bajic. 2011. Temporal sequence parameters in isodistributional surrogate data: Model and exact expressions. *IEEE Transactions on Biomedical Engineering* 58(1):16–24.

Loncar-Turukalo, T., Milovanovic, B., and D. Bajic. 2010. Markov model and entropy of sequences in isodistributional surrogate data. In *Proceedings of 8th International Symposium on Intelligent Systems and Informatics*, 53–56.

Malberg, H., Wessel, N., Hasart, A., Osterziel, H., and A. Voss. 2002. Advanced analysis of spontaneous baroreflex sensitivity, blood pressure and heart rate variability in patients with dilated cardiomyopathy. *Clinical Science* 102:465–473.

McCubbin, J. W., Green, J. H., and I. H. Page. 1956. Baroreceptor function in chronic renal hypertension. *Circulation Research* 4:205–210.

Mortara, A., La Rovere, M. T., Pinna, G. D. et al. 1997. Arterial baroreflex modulation of heart rate in chronic heart failure: Clinical and hemodynamic correlates and prognostic implications. *Circulation* 96:3450–3458.

Narkiewicz, K. and G. Grassi. 2008. Impaired baroreflex sensitivity as a potential marker of cardiovascular risk in hypertension. *Journal of Hypertension* 26:1303–1304.

Nollo, G., Porta, A., Faes, L. et al. 2001. Causal linear parametric model for baroreflex gain assessment in patients with recent myocardial infarction. *American Journal of Physiology Heart and Circulatory Physiology* 280:H1830–H1839.

Oosting, J., Struijker-Boudier, H. A. J., and B. J. A. Janssen. 1997. Validation of a continuous baroreceptor reflex sensitivity index calculated from spontaneous fluctuations of blood pressure and pulse interval in rats. *Journal of Hypertension* 15:391–399.

Ormezzano, O., Cracowski, J. L., Quesada, H. et al. 2008. Evaluation of the prognostic value of barore-flex sensitivity in hypertensive patients: The EVABAR study. *Journal of Hypertension* 26:1373–1378.

Pagani, M., Somers, V., Furlan, R. et al. 1988. Changes in autonomic regulation induced by physical training in mild hypertension. *Hypertension* 12:600–610.

Parati, G., Di Rienzo, M., and G. Mancia. 2000. How to measure baroreflex sensitivity: From the cardiovascular laboratory to daily life. *Journal of Hypertension* 18:7–19.

Parker, P., Celler, B. G., Potter E. K., and D. I. McCloskey. 1984. Vagal stimulation and cardiac slowing. *Journal of the Autonomic Nervous System* 11:226–231.

Parlow, J, Viale, J. P., Annat, G., Hughson, R., and L. Quintin. 1995. Spontaneous cardiac baroreflex in humans: Comparison with drug-induced responses. *Hypertension* 25:1058–1068.

Patton, D. J., Triedman, J. K., Perrott, M. H., Vidian, A. A., and J. P. Saul. 1996. Baroreflex gain: Characterization using autoregressive moving average analysis. *American Journal of Physiology* 39:H1240–H1249.

Porta, A., Baselli, G., Rimoldi, O., Malliani, A., and M. Pagani. 2000a. Assessing baroreflex gain from spontaneous variability in conscious dogs: Role of causality and respiration. *American Journal of Physiology Heart and Circulatory Physiology* 279:H2558–H2567.

Porta, A., Furlan, R., Rimoldi, O., Pagani, M., Malliani, A., and P. van de Borne. 2002. Quantifying the strength of the linear causal coupling in closed loop interacting cardiovascular variability signals. *Medical and Biological Engineering and Computing* 86: 241–251.

Porta, A., Guzzetti, S., Montano, N. et al. 2000b. Information domain analysis of cardiovascular vari-ability signals: Evaluation of regularity, synchronization and co-ordination. *Medical and Biolog-ical Engineering and Computing* 38:180–188.

Raven, P. B., Fadel, P. J., and S. Ogoh. 2005. Arterial baroreflex resetting during exercise: A current perspective. *Experimental Physiology* 91(1):37–49.

Richman, J. S. and J. R. Moorman. 2000. Physiological time-series analysis using approximate entropy and sample entropy. *American Journal of Physiology* 278:H2039–H2049.

Robbe, H. W. J., Mulder, L. J. M, Ruddel, H. et al. 1987. Assessment of baroreceptor reflex sensitivity by means of spectral analysis. *Hypertension* 10:538–543.

Rothlisberger, B. W., Badra, L. J., Hoag, J. B. et al. 2003. Spontaneous 'baroreflex sequences' occur as deterministic functions of breathing phase. *Clinical Physiology and Functional Imaging* 23:307–313.

Rudas, L., Crossman, A. A., Morillo, C. A. et al. 1999. Human sympathetic and vagal barore-flex responses to sequential nitroprusside and phenylephrine. *American Journal of Physiology* 276:H1691–1698.

Ryan, S., Ward, S., Heneghan, C., and W. T. McNicholas. 2007. Predictors of decreased spontaneous baroreflex sensitivity in obstructive sleep apnea syndrome. *Chest* 131:1100–1107.

Schreiber, T., and A. Schmitz. 2000. Surrogate time series. *Physica D* 142: 346–382.

Seagard, J. L., Gallemberg, L. A., Hopp, F. A., and C. Dean. 1992. Acute resetting in two functionally different types of carotid baroreceptors. *Circulation Research* 70:559–565.

Seidel, H., Herzel, H., and D. L. Eckberg. 1997. Phase dependancies of the human barore-receptor reflex. *American Journal of Physiology Heart and Circulatory Physiology* 272:H2040–2053.

Smyth, H. S., Sleight, P., and G. W. Pickering. 1969. Reflex regulation of arterial pressure during sleep in man: A quantitative method of assessing baroreflex sensitivity. *Circulation Research* 24:109–121.

Soma, R., Nozaki, D., Kwak, S., and Y. Yamamoto. 2003. 1/f noise outperforms white noise in sensi-tizing baroreflex function in the human brain. *Physical Review Letters* 91:078101.

Theiler, J., Eubank, S., Longtin, A., Galdrikian, B., and J. D. Farmer. 1992. Testing for nonlinearity in time series: The method of surrogate data. *Physica D* 58:77–94.

Waki, H., Katahira, K., Polson, J. W. et al. 2006. Automation of analysis of cardiovascular autonomic function from chronic measurements of arterial pressure in conscious rats. *Experimental Physi-ology* 91:201–213.

Wellens, H. J. J, Schwartz, P. J., Lindemans, F.W. et al. 2014. Risk stratification for sudden cardiac death: Current status and challenges for the future. *European Heart Journal* 35(25):1642–1651.

Wessel, N., Voss, A., Malberg, H. et al. 2000. Nonlinear analysis of complex phenomena in cardiological data. *Herzschrittmachertherapie & Elektrophysiologie* 11:159–173

Westerhof, B. E., Gisolf, J., Stok, W. J., Wesseling, K. H., and J. M. Karemaker. 2004. Time-domain cross-correlation baroreflex sensitivity: Performance on the eurobavar data set. *Journal of Hypertension* 33(7):1371–1380.

Yang, A. C. C., Shu-Shya, H., Huey-Wen, Y., Goldberger, A. L., and C. K. Peng. 2003. Linguistic analysis of the human heartbeat using frequency and rank order statistics. *Physical Review Letters* 90:108103.

10

Tone–Entropy Analysis of Heart Rate Variability in Cardiac Autonomic Neuropathy

Chandan Karmakar, Ahsan H. Khandoker, Herbert F. Jelinek, and Marimuthu Palaniswami

CONTENTS

10.1 Introduction

Diabetes mellitus (DM) affects more than 366 million people around the world (Alam et al. 2009). One of the serious clinical complications of DM is cardiovascular autonomic neuropathy (CAN), which gradually results in abnormalities of heart rate (HR) control and vascular dynamics (Kuehl and Stevens 2012; Vinik and Ziegler 2007). The occurrence of confirmed CAN in diabetes patients is approximately 20%, and increases up to 65% with age and diabetes duration (Spallone et al. 2011). Ewing et al. reported a mortality rate of 53% after 5 years in a cohort of diabetic patients with CAN versus 15% in the control group (i.e., diabetic patients without CAN) (Ewing et al. 1980). CAN progression may lead to severe postural hypotension, exercise intolerance, enhanced intraoperative instability, increased incidence of silent myocardial infarction, and ischemia (Vinik and Ziegler 2007). Around 75% of people with diabetes die from cardiovascular disease such as heart attack and stroke, which includes autonomic neuropathy as a cause (Krolewski et al. 1977; Nathan et al. 2005). Early detection of CAN in diabetic patients and intervention is therefore of prime importance to reduce the increased mortality of diabetes patients. The presence and severity of CAN are difficult to diagnose at the subclinical stage due to the absence of overt symptoms. As a result, it creates a potential negative impact on the quality of life of patients and those with the preclinical asymptomatic disease (Spallone et al. 2011; Vinik and Ziegler 2007). To enable early treatment intervention and improved outcomes requires accurate and sensitive measures for detecting subclinical CAN.

10.1.1 Cardiovascular Symptoms of CAN

A decrease in heart rate variability (HRV) during deep breathing or exercise may be a sign of autonomic neuropathy and is associated with a high risk of coronary heart disease in patients with or without diabetes (May et al. 2000). Resting tachycardia is an early sign, as is loss of HR variation during deep breathing (Ewing et al. 1980). Limited exercise tolerance is due to impaired sympathetic and parasympathetic responses that normally augment cardiac output and redirect peripheral blood flow to skeletal muscles. A prolonged corrected QT interval (QTc) indicates an imbalance between the right and left sympathetic innervation (Veglio et al. 1999). The abnormal circadian pattern of blood pressure (BP) is another symptom of CAN, which rises during the night and falls in the early morning. This abnormal pattern has been shown to correlate with postural hypotension due to CAN (Nakano et al. 1991). Blunted symptoms of coronary artery disease and lack of pain because of damaged afferent nerves appear in diabetic patients with CAN (Airaksinen and Koistinen 1992).

10.2 Clinical Practice for CAN Detection and Staging

The gold standard for the detection and staging of CAN is the noninvasive autonomic nervous system test battery proposed by Ewing et al. There are five different tests in the Ewing battery assessment. A brief description of the five tests (Vinik and Erbas 2001) is given in Sections 10.2.1 through 10.2.5.

10.2.1 Valsalva Maneuver

The Valsalva maneuver is performed by having the participant exhale for 15 seconds, while maintaining an expiratory pressure of 40 mmHg. Expiratory pressure can be measured by having the patient blow into a mouthpiece connected to a pressure transducer. The maneuver is performed at least three times in order to maximize participant compliance and ensure reproducibility. The Valsalva ratio is an index of HR or interbeat length

(RR interval [RRI]) changes associated with parasympathetic response to forced exhalation. The Valsalva ratio is taken as the maximum RRI in the 30 seconds following expiration divided by the minimum RRI during the maneuver. A ratio of longest to shortest RRI of less than 1.2 is abnormal.

10.2.2 Deep Breathing

Respiratory sinus arrhythmia is assessed by performance of six deep breaths per minute at a frequency of 0.1 Hz. The timed breathing is performed with the aid of a metronome or verbal cues. The response is taken as the mean of the differences between the maximum and minimum instantaneous HR for each cycle. A minimum of three breaths is required for inclusion. A difference in HR of less than 10 beats/minute is abnormal. An expiration:inspiration RR can also be determined and is abnormal if the ratio > 1.17.

10.2.3 The 30:15 Lying to Standing Ratio

This is performed by rising from the supine to a standing position. The 30:15 ratio is then the RRI at the 30th beat divided by the RRI at the 15th beat immediately after standing. A 30:15 ratio of less than 1.03 is considered abnormal.

10.2.4 Orthostasis

Change in systolic BP is calculated as the difference between the systolic BP 2 minutes after standing and the mean systolic BP for the 20 beats immediately prior to standing. A fall of more than 30 mmHg is abnormal.

10.2.5 Sustained Handgrip

Participants hold a pressure gauge and exert maximal compression force to determine the maximal grip force. For the test, the required force exerted by the participant is adjusted to 30% of the maximal grip for 5 minutes. Change in diastolic BP is calculated as the difference between the maximal diastolic BP before releasing the handgrip and the mean diastolic BP for the 20 beats immediately prior to commencing the handgrip. A rise of less than 16 mmHg in the contralateral arm is abnormal.

The major drawbacks of the Ewing battery are: (1) it requires patient cooperation (Ewing et al. 1985), (2) it is unable to be performed when comorbidities are present in the patient such as heart or lung disease (Pagani 2000), and (3) it is less sensitive to changes associated with cardiac autonomic neuropathy compared to spectral methods (Ewing and Clarke 1982). A widely accepted alternative to address the abovementioned limitations are the HRV-based techniques, since the change in HRV is regarded as one of the early signs of CAN (Spallone et al. 2011). HR and cardiac function are regulated through a complex autonomic neuronal network. Figure 10.1 shows the progression of CAN in diabetic subjects and indicates that decreased HRV and cardiac autonomic imbalance can be considered as suitable HRV phenomena for detection of CAN at the subclinical stage. Therefore, a progression of autonomic denervation that leads to the development of decreased HRV and cardiac autonomic imbalance, despite being subclinical, can be detected using validated methods (Camm et al. 1996).

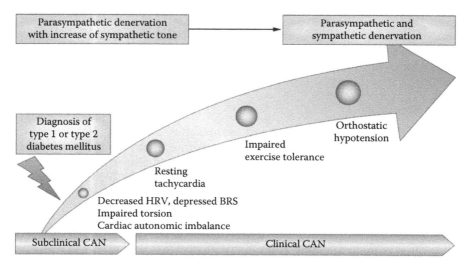

FIGURE 10.1
Progression of cardiac autonomic neuropathy. The earliest detectable subclinical signs of CAN are impaired spectral analysis of HRV and abnormal BRS, which can be present at the time of diagnosis of diabetes mellitus. Initial parasympathetic denervation enables augmentation of sympathetic tone in the early stages of CAN. Over time, sympathetic denervation follows and correlates clinically with the development of resting tachycardia and impaired exercise tolerance. The presence of orthostatic hypotension often indicates the presence of advanced or severe CAN. BRS, baroreflex sensitivity; CAN, cardiovascular autonomic neuropathy; HRV, heart rate variability. (Adapted from Kuehl, M. and M. J. Stevens, *Nature Reviews Endocrinology*, 8, 405–416, 2012.)

10.3 Limitations of Traditional HRV Methods for Diagnosis of CAN

Conventionally used time- and frequency-domain parameters of HRV are not always suitable for measurement of reduced HRV activity because of the nonstationarity characteristic of the electrocardiogram (ECG) recordings and the presence of nonlinear phenomena in the HR signal. Spectral analysis methods also lack sensitivity for detecting asymptomatic/preclinical CAN (Karmakar et al. 2013). Positron emission tomography (PET) and single-photon emission computed tomography (SPECT) are two nuclear medicine imaging techniques used for the real-time assessment of cardiac autonomic innervation and might become a more utilized method to diagnose as well as monitor the progression of CAN (Kuehl and Stevens 2012). But the availability of this diagnostic tool is limited due to high cost, lack of availability outside of large metropolitan centers, and trained operator requirements.

Therefore, methods that are noninvasive and independent of patient cooperation are preferable in the detection and staging of CAN. Only a few studies have applied new parameters based on nonlinear dynamics theory to HRV analysis in DM patients (Ziegler 1994; Costa et al. 2005; Flynn et al. 2005; Khandoker et al. 2009; Cornforth et al. 2015). A previous study has shown that sympathovagal balance can be detected even in the time domain through the tone–entropy (T–E) (Oida et al. 1997). Tone was verified to reflect the sympathovagal balance by a pharmacological experiment where tone changed in value consistently and in an HR recovery experiment after exercise where the parasympathetic division became predominant (Oida et al. 1997). The T–E evaluation process is neither influenced by the time period of data acquisition nor by the baseline HR. In addition, the T–E data processing has no signal deformation process such as a filtering, window, or limiting process. A very important advantage is that there is no need to control respiration rate in the T–E method, allowing data to be obtained in a natural process (Oida et al. 1999). Since CAN is reported to be associated with alteration of sympathovagal balance, T–E may be a better marker for detection and staging of CAN. The conventional T–E method of quantifying HRV uses successive RRIs with the implicit assumption that the current beat is influenced by the immediately preceding beat. However, the delay of such influence is affected by the variation of baroreflex sensitivity and therefore can be greater than one beat (Cavalcanti and Belardinelli 1996; Ottesen 1997). For example, the baroreflex sensitivity is reduced in chronic renal failure (CRF) patients (Tomiyama et al. 1980), which augments the delay in the HR response. Therefore, a heartbeat influences not only the beat immediately following it but also up to 6–10 beats downstream (Lerma et al. 2003). Lerma was the first to show this with several researchers confirming higher lag being associated with disease processes (Lerma et al. 2003; Martinez-Garcia et al. 2012). Thus, successive RRI duplets will likely underestimate the role of the autocovariance function of RRIs, that is, the ability of heartbeats to influence a train of succeeding beats. Moreover, the autocovariance function of RRIs captures additional aspects of HRV (e.g., nonlinearity) that are otherwise masked by the strong correlation between successive beats if lag 1 (n vs. $n+1$ beats) T–E is used. Therefore, multilag T–E analysis can overcome the limitations of the present practice of single lag T–E analysis in HRV studies.

10.4 T–E Method

A RRI or period is defined as the time difference between two consecutive R peaks of the ECG signal. Let the RRIs time series **RR** be defined as

$$RR \equiv (RR_1, RR_2, \ldots, RR_N) \tag{10.1}$$

where N is the number RRIs. HR acceleration and inhibition can be determined from the difference of consecutive RRIs. If RR_{i+1} is shorter than RR_i then there is an acceleration of the HR. Therefore, acceleration of the heart is expressed as a plus difference and inhibition as a minus difference of RRIs. However, to reduce the impact of HR variation over a wide range of time and patients, using a normalized variation in RRI is preferred to monitor the variability. In conventional T–E analysis, percentile change of the successive RRIs with respect to the first RRI is expressed as the percentage index (PI) and defined as

$$PI(i) = \frac{RR_i - RR_{i+1}}{RR_i} \times 100 \tag{10.2}$$

The *tone* is defined as a first-order moment (arithmetic average) of this **PI** time series as

$$\text{Tone} = \frac{1}{N-1} \sum_{i=1}^{N-1} PI(i) \tag{10.3}$$

Tone is the balance between accelerations ($PI > 0$) and inhibitions ($PI < 0$) of the HR and represents the sympathovagal balance faithfully as shown in previous studies (Amano et al. 2005; Oida et al. 1997). *Entropy* is defined from the probability distribution of **PI** by using Shannon's formula (Shannon 1948):

$$\text{Entropy} = -\sum_{i=1}^{n} p(i) \log_2 p(i) \tag{10.4}$$

where $p(i)$ is a probability of **PI** having values in the range $i < \textbf{PI} < i+1$, where i is an integer. The entropy evaluates total acceleration–inhibition activities, or total heart period variations, in a familiar unit of bit.

10.4.1 Multilag T–E Analysis of HRV Signal

For multilag T–E analysis, we have introduced the lag (m) in Equation 10.2 (Section 10.4), used to derive the **PI** time series from the **RR** time series signal. Hence, in the multilag T–E analysis, *PI* is expressed as the percentile change of the ith and $i+m$th RRIs with respect to the ith RRI and is defined as

$$PI(i) = \frac{RR_i - RR_{i+m}}{RR_i} \times 100 \tag{10.5}$$

where m is an integer and $m = 1$ represents the conventional T–E analysis.

10.4.2 Effect of Data Length on Multilag T–E Measurement

An important benefit of conventional (lag 1) T–E evaluation is that it is not influenced by the time period of data acquisition. However, increasing lag time reintroduces the sensitivity to recording length. Therefore, we analyzed the variation of *T–E* values with varied length of RRI data (from 50 to 900 beats) and a range of lags ($1 \leq m \leq 8$).

10.4.3 Patients and ECG Signals

After standard exclusion criteria were applied to ensure that any changes in HRV detected were due to the severity of cardiac autonomic neuropathy, 41 patients with type 2 DM were included in the study. Fifteen patients had definite CAN (CAN+), while the remaining 26 were negative for CAN (CAN−), that is, they did not have clinical signs and symptoms of CAN. The detailed demography of patients is shown in Table 10.1.

Exclusion criteria included those with a history of cardiac pathology, hypertension, or use of antihypertensive or antiarrhythmic medication, and those with less than 85%

TABLE 10.1

Subject Demography of CAN+ and CAN− Groups

Group	Total Subject	Age (Years) (Mean ± SD)	Gender (F, M)
CAN−	26	64 ± 11	20, 6
CAN+	15	55 ± 15	7, 8

qualified sinus beats. ECGs were recorded over 20 minutes using a lead-II configuration (Maclab ADInstruments, Australia) and recorded on Macintosh Chart Version 5 with a sampling rate set at 400 Hz and a notch filter at 50 Hz. ECG signals were edited using the MLS310 HRV module (version 1.0, ADInstruments, Australia) included with the Chart software package. A 45 Hz low-pass filter and a 3 Hz high-pass filter were applied prior to determining the RRIs. Ectopic beats were identified visually and deleted from the ECG recording. QRS peaks were determined using the algorithm developed by Pan and Tomkin (Pan and Tompkins 1985) and RRIs calculated. The presence of CAN+ was assessed using the complete Ewing battery (Ewing et al. 1985).

10.4.4 ROC Area Analysis

In order to retain the relative importance of the selected HRV features, a receiver-operating curve (ROC) analysis was used (Hanley and McNeil 1982), with the area under the curve for each feature represented by the ROC area. A ROC area value of 0.5 indicates that the distributions of the features are similar in the two groups with no discriminatory power. Conversely, a ROC area value of 1.0 would mean that the distribution of the features of the two groups does not overlap at all. The ROC is obtained by automatic selection of different thresholds or cutoff points and calculating the sensitivity/specificity pair for each one of the cutoff points. The area under the ROC curve was approximated numerically using the trapezoidal rules (Hanley and McNeil 1982) where the larger the ROC area is, the better the discriminatory performance.

10.4.5 Classification of CAN Patients

A quadratic discriminant (QD) classifier was applied to test the ability of T–E values together in detecting CAN+ subjects. The beat sequence length $len = 250$ and lag $m = \{1, 2, 3\}$ was taken for the T–E calculation based on the ROC results for all lengths and lags. A leave-one-out cross-validation scheme was adopted to evaluate the generalization ability of the classifiers. Cross-validation procedures have been used in a number of classification evaluations, particularly for limited data sets (Ripley 1996). In this scheme, the classifier was trained using 40 records and tested on the remaining record. This was repeated 41 times, so that each record was left out for one round of training and testing.

The following three measures of accuracy, sensitivity, and specificity were used to assess the performance of the classifiers (Chan et al. 2002; Pang et al. 2003):

$$\text{Accuracy} = \frac{TP + TN}{TP + FP + TN + FN} \times 100$$
$$\text{Sensitivity} = \frac{TP}{TP + FN} \times 100 \tag{10.6}$$
$$\text{Specificity} = \frac{TN}{TN + FP} \times 100$$

where TP is the number of true positives, that is, the classifier identifies a patient that was labeled as CAN+; TN is the number of true negatives, that is, the classifier identifies a patient that was labeled as CAN−; FP is false CAN+ identifications; and FN is false CAN− identifications. Accuracy indicates overall detection accuracy. Sensitivity is defined as the ability of the classifier to accurately recognize a CAN+, whereas specificity indicates the classifier's ability not to generate a false negative (CAN−). All results were statistically analyzed using analysis of variance (ANOVA) and assuming unknown and different variance for testing the hypothesis regarding the mean. The mean of tone values for data length $len = 900$ and other lengths ($len = 50 - 850$) are assumed equal. The same test was applied to the hypothesis for entropy values.

A nonparametric Kruskal–Wallis test was applied to investigate the significance between age distributions of subjects of the CAN– and CAN+ groups. The effect size—in essence how much overlap is there between two groups—was investigated using Cohen's d value (Cohen 1988). Following this, the power analysis was carried out to justify the repeatability of the difference in T–E values found between two groups for a small sample size. This provides the probability that the null hypothesis (there is no difference in T–E values between CAN– and CAN+ groups) is wrong. A large size for Cohen's d value represents less degree of overlap between two groups and vice versa. On the other hand, a small p value indicates that the null hypothesis can be rejected.

10.5 Results

Mean T–E values for both the CAN– and CAN+ group for all lags ($1 \leq m \leq 8$) and beat sequence lengths ($50 \leq len \leq 900$) are shown in Figure 10.1. Mean tone values were lower for all lags and beat sequence lengths in the CAN– compared to the CAN+ group. In addition, mean tone values in the CAN– group consistently decreased with increasing lag for all beat sequence lengths. In contrast, the mean tone values associated with a specific lag tended to increase with increasing length of the ECG analyzed (not consistent at every lag). Similarly, the mean tone values in the CAN+ group decreased with increasing lag for any sequence length greater than 150 beats. However, there was no consistent relationship between the mean tone values at a specific lag and sequence length.

Mean entropy values were higher in the CAN– than CAN+ group for all lags and beat sequence lengths (Figure 10.2). The mean entropy values in the CAN– group were mostly increased (except $m = \{6, 7\}$ and $len = 50$; $m = 6$ and $len = 500$) with increasing lags. Similarly, the mean entropy values for a specific lag increased for most lags investigated with an increasing recording length of the ECG (beat sequence length). The mean entropy values of the CAN+ group increased (except lag $= \{8\}$ and $len = 50$) with increasing lags, while the mean entropy value for a specific lag showed an increasing trend only up to $len = 200$ where this trend disappeared.

The association between T–E-related estimates of HRV and beat sequence lengths for varying lags was analyzed and shown in Figure 10.3 for the associations of two extreme examples of beat sequence lengths ($len = 50$, Figures 10.3a and b; $len = 900$, Figures 10.3c and d). Similarly, we analyzed the association between T–E-related estimates of HRV and lag for varying beat sequence lengths. Figure 10.4 shows these associations for two lags.

ROC areas are calculated to measure the performance of *tone* and *entropy* features in differentiating between CAN– and CAN+ for all lags and beat sequence lengths. ROC areas of *tone* for all lags and beat sequence lengths $len \geq 250$ are summarized in Table 10.3. The maximum ROC area ($= 0.95$) between CAN– and CAN+ using *tone* is found for $m = 2$ and $len = \{450 \text{ and } 800\}$. For any beat sequence lengths, the maximum ROC area for classifying the CAN– and CAN+ groups is found for lag $m = 2$. Beat sequence length of $len = 400$ for lag $m = 3$ also resulted in a maximum ROC.

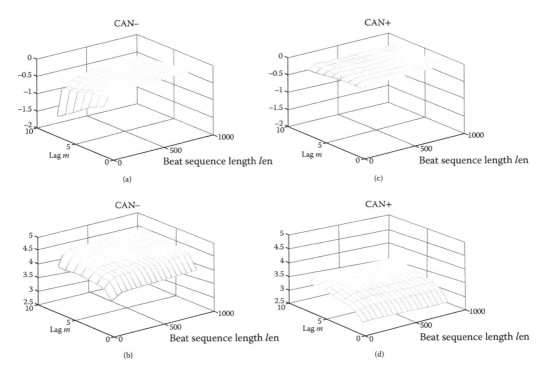

FIGURE 10.2
Mean *tone* and entropy *values* for the CAN− and CAN+ group for all lags ($1 \leq m \leq 8$) and beat sequence lengths ($50 \leq len \leq 900$). (Adapted from Karmakar, C. K. et al., *Medical and Biological Engineering and Computing*, 51, 537–546, 2013.)

ROC areas of *entropy* for all lags and beat sequence lengths $len \geq 250$ are summarized in Table 10.3. The hypothesis and method for selecting length $len \geq 250$ are discussed in detail in the next section. The maximum ROC area ($=0.97$) between CAN− and CAN+ using *entropy* is found for $m = 3, len = 750$ and $m = \{2, 3\}$ and $len = \{800, 850$ and $900\}$. Maximal ROC results were also found for other combinations of length and lag as shown in Table 10.2.

In this study, we have used the QD with leave-one-out (LOO) testing methodology to quantify the accuracy of T–E values in discriminating CAN+ from CAN−. LOO allows determination of how accurately an unknown recording is classified into the correct class (CAN− or CAN+). The beat sequence length $len = 250$ was used for classification, as T–E values become consistent (i.e., variation of mean becomes minimal) over multiple lags at length $len \geq 250$. In addition, lag $m = 1–3$ was selected as the maximum ROC area between CAN− and CAN+ was found at lag 2 and 3 (see Table 10.2) and the result needs to be compared to lag 1 or conventional T–E analysis. Results of the LOO cross-validation tests (accuracy, sensitivity, and specificity) of the QD classifier are summarized in Figure 10.5 and Table 10.3. For beat sequence length $len = 250$, the accuracy reached 100% at a lag $m = \{2, 3\}$. The effect size and power (one-tailed and two-tailed) for T–E parameters at lag $m = \{1–3\}$ and for length $len = 250$ is shown in Table 10.4.

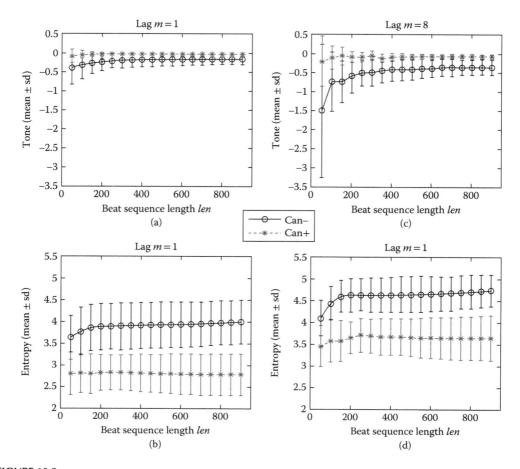

FIGURE 10.3
Tone–entropy values in the CAN– and CAN+ group associated with beat sequence length. (a) and (b) show T–E *with respect to* increasing length at lag 1 and (c) and (d) show T–E for lag 8. (Adapted from Karmakar, C. K. et al., *Medical and Biological Engineering and Computing*, 51, 537–546, 2013.)

10.6 Discussion

Linear and nonlinear analyses of RRIs have been applied for some time for the classification of cardiovascular disease and cardiac autonomic neuropathy in particular. These methods differ in terms of their appropriateness for analysis of the RRI time series, which is non-stationary and nonlinear, and also with respect to the information they provide including their sensitivity and specificity (Alam et al. 2009; Costa et al. 2005; Ewing and Clarke 1982; Huikuri et al. 2009; Lombardi et al. 2001). For many of the current methods, the assumption is that for all consecutive beats, each beat only has influence on the subsequent beat, whereas it has been shown that each beat in a time series can have an influence on up to 10 beats downstream (Lerma et al. 2003). This opened up the question of finding a method that allows measuring of this multilag characteristic of RRI time series and its usefulness in clinical application.

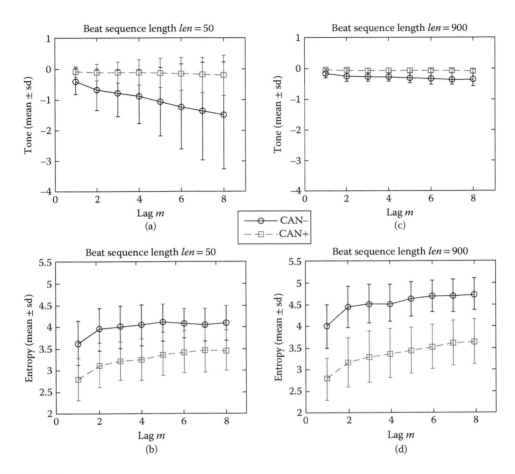

FIGURE 10.4
Tone–entropy response to changing lag in patients with definite CAN and negative CAN–. (a) and (b) show the T–E response for sequences 50 beats long, whereas (c) and (d) show the T–E response for sequences 900 beats long. (Adapted from Karmakar, C. K. et al., *Medical and Biological Engineering and Computing*, 51, 537–546, 2013.)

The results discussed in this chapter and previously published confirm the finding of Lerma et al. (2003) and Cornforth et al. (2015) that a current beat can influence a beat further downstream and extend this work by applying multilag analysis to cardiac autonomic neuropathy. Our approach using multilag T–E values of HRV can be used to correctly identify a patient as CAN+ or CAN−, which takes into consideration the influence an individual beat has on subsequent beats in the time series. The physiological interpretations of T–E in various experimental settings were previously reported (Khandoker et al. 2010; Oida et al. 1997). Lower tone values (negative) indicate that vagal activity predominates in the sympathovagal balance in a healthy population at rest (Bootsma et al. 1994; Oida et al. 1997; Tulppo et al. 2001). This is also reflected in higher entropy values in the healthy (CAN−) population. Higher tone (nearing zero) and lower entropy values indicate that parasympathetic efferent pathways progressively withdraw their activity (Khandoker et al. 2010). The major findings of the study are discussed in the following subsections.

TABLE 10.2

ROC Areas of *Tone* and *Entropy* for Different Lags and Beat Sequence Lengths

No of Beats	Parameter	Lags							
		1	2	3	4	5	6	7	8
250	Tone	0.88	**0.93**	0.90	0.82	0.85	0.82	0.85	0.82
	Entropy	0.90	**0.95**	**0.95**	0.85	0.90	0.90	0.90	0.85
300	Tone	0.85	**0.90**	0.88	0.78	0.75	0.82	0.75	0.70
	Entropy	0.88	**0.93**	0.90	0.82	0.90	0.90	0.88	0.82
350	Tone	0.85	**0.90**	0.85	0.63	0.70	0.75	0.65	0.53
	Entropy	0.88	0.90	0.90	0.78	0.88	**0.93**	0.88	0.78
400	Tone	0.85	0.93	**0.93**	0.85	0.88	0.85	0.85	0.85
	Entropy	0.88	0.90	0.90	0.78	0.82	**0.93**	0.85	0.80
450	Tone	0.85	**0.95**[a]	0.88	0.82	0.88	0.85	0.82	0.82
	Entropy	**0.90**	0.90	0.90	0.78	0.82	**0.90**	0.85	0.78
500	Tone	0.85	**0.93**	0.88	0.82	0.82	0.85	0.82	0.80
	Entropy	**0.90**	0.90	0.88	0.78	0.82	0.88	0.85	0.78
550	Tone	0.85	**0.88**	0.85	0.72	0.75	0.85	0.78	0.72
	Entropy	0.90	**0.93**	**0.93**	0.78	0.82	0.88	0.85	0.80
600	Tone	0.88	**0.93**	0.88	0.78	0.78	0.85	0.80	0.70
	Entropy	0.90	**0.93**	0.90	0.75	0.82	0.88	0.85	0.75
650	Tone	0.88	**0.93**	0.88	0.70	0.78	0.82	0.78	0.72
	Entropy	0.90	**0.93**	**0.93**	0.75	0.82	0.88	0.85	0.72
700	Tone	0.88	**0.93**	0.88	0.82	0.80	0.85	0.82	0.78
	Entropy	0.90	**0.95**	**0.95**	0.78	0.85	0.90	0.85	0.78
750	Tone	0.90	**0.93**	0.93	0.88	0.82	0.85	0.85	0.78
	Entropy	0.90	0.95	**0.97**[b]	0.80	0.82	0.93	0.85	0.78
800	Tone	0.90	**0.95**[a]	0.93	0.88	0.90	0.93	0.90	0.88
	Entropy	0.93	**0.97**[b]	**0.97**[b]	0.80	0.93	0.95	0.88	0.78
850	Tone	0.88	**0.93**	0.90	0.80	0.82	0.85	0.80	0.60
	Entropy	0.90	**0.97**[b]	**0.97**[b]	0.80	0.93	0.97	0.88	0.78
900	Tone	0.88	**0.93**	0.90	0.82	0.82	0.88	0.85	0.82
	Entropy	0.90	**0.97**[b]	**0.97**[b]	0.78	0.88	0.95	0.85	0.78

Note: Boldfaced numbers represent maximum ROC area for *tone* or *entropy* for corresponding beat sequence length.

[a] Maximum ROC area of *tone* for all lags and beat sequence lengths.

[b] Maximum ROC area of *entropy* for all lags and beat sequence lengths.

10.6.1 Physiological Understanding of T–E Measurement

Physiologically, tone was reported to reflect the sympathovagal balance by a pharmacological experiment where tone changed in value consistently in an HR recovery experiment after exercise where parasympathetic rebound is observed (Javorka et al. 2008). On the other hand, entropy was considered as the total amount of sympathovagal activity. The nature of T–E was examined in eight healthy volunteers by autonomic perturbation experiments. For these studies, we employed the data set of previous studies (Kamen et al. 1996; Brennan et al. 2002) because it contained data from the participants over a wide range of

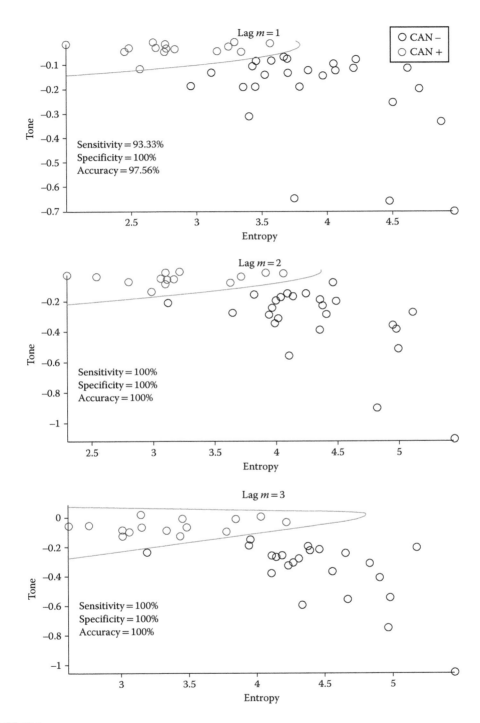

FIGURE 10.5
Classification performance of the quadratic classifier between CAN– and CAN+ subjects using tone and entropy features with beat sequence lengths *len* = 250 and lags *m* = {1, 2, 3}. (Adapted from Karmakar, C. K. et al., *Medical and Biological Engineering and Computing*, 51, 537–546, 2013.)

TABLE 10.3

Sensitivity, Specificity, and Accuracy Obtained Using QD Classifier with *Tone* and *Entropy* Feature to Classify CAN+ from CAN− Using the Minimum Beat Sequence Length $len = 250$ and Lags $m = \{1, 2, 3\}$

Classifier	Lag m	Sensitivity (%)	Specificity (%)	Accuracy (%)
	1	93.33	100.00	97.56
QD	2	100.00	100.00	100.00[a]
	3	100.00	100.00	100.00[a]

[a] Shows the maximum classification accuracy found between CAN+ and CAN−.

TABLE 10.4

Effect Size (Cohen's d) and Power (One-Tailed and Two-Tailed) Values of *Tone* and *Entropy* Features of CAN− and CAN+ Subjects for Beat Sequence Length $Len = 250$ and Lags $m = \{1, 2, 3\}$

Parameter	Lag	Effect Size (Cohen's d)	Power (One-Tailed)	Power (Two-Tailed)
Tone	1	1.2113	0.9828	0.9611
	2	1.4662	0.9982	0.9946
	3	1.6036	0.9996	0.9985
Entropy	1	2.1350	1.0000	1.0000
	2	2.2820	1.0000	1.0000
	3	2.1764	1.0000	1.0000

autonomic conditions. This first data set described by Kamen et al. (1996) and Brennan et al. (2002) consisted of eight healthy participants (four females, four males) aged between 20 and 40 years (means $\pm$ SD:31.2 ± 6.2). Each participant underwent three autonomic perturbations: (1) baseline study with subjects in the supine position in a quiet environment; (2) 70° head–up tilt, which increases sympathetic activity and decreases parasympathetic activity; (3) atropine infusion (atropine sulphate, 1.2 mg), which markedly decreases parasympathetic nervous system activity. In all, 24 records were collected, each containing 1000 RRIs.

Figure 10.6 illustrates a typical example of RRIs, PI time series, and their histograms selected from each group. Alteration of the distributions is clearly discernible. Individual and averaged data of T–E in T–E space, where the tone is plotted on the ordinate and entropy on the abscissa is shown in Figure 10.7. Rectangles show mean $\pm$ SE. The tone was found to be negative in the resting control baseline (B). The negative tone increased for 70° tilt (T) and further increased to nearly zero (-0.0017 ± 0.0011) for blockade by atropine (A). Entropy decreased for tilt and blockade by atropine. Parasympathetic blockade made the tone almost zero. When both autonomic divisions were blocked, the tone became zero (Oida et al. 1997). Entropy decreased below 2 bits (1.939 ± 0.268) for the functionally denervated heart. In contrast, entropy was high at rest. It was shown in a previous study (Javorka et al. 2008) that the increase in entropy corresponds to autonomic recovery in the heart reflecting total cardiac autonomic efferent activity.

In Figure 10.8, the results of the autonomic perturbation experiments (dotted rectangles) are superimposed on the T–E scatter plot of the clinical data. Dotted rectangle represents

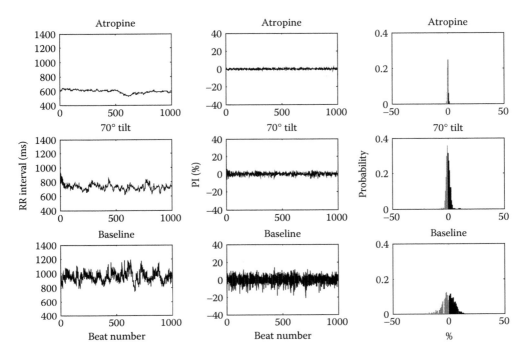

FIGURE 10.6
Typical heart period (RR intervals) time series (left), PI time series deduced from left (center), and its probability distributions in histogram (right) selected in each group (atropine, 70° tilt, and baseline). In histograms, filled bars represent accelerations (*PI* > 0), and open bars inhibitions of the heart (*PI* < 0), respectively. Abbreviations are defined in the text. (Adapted from Khandoker, A. H. et al., *Medical Engineering and Physics*, 32, 161–167, 2010.)

mean ± SE of each group. The control baseline (*B*) and tilt group (*T*) of the autonomic perturbation experiments were found to overlap with the *N* and eCAN+ groups. The definite CAN group approached the region of parasympathetic blockade (*A*). These results are aligned with the effect of CAN progression on the autonomic nervous system, which is shown in Figure 10.1.

10.6.2 Changes of T–E Values at Different Lags

For any beat sequence length ($50 \leq len \leq 900$), the mean tone value for the CAN− group decreased with increasing lag. This indicates that the parasympathetic influence of the current beat decreases with increasing lag (distant heartbeats) in the CAN− group. A similar response was found for the CAN+ group with a minimum beat sequence length of 200 beats. Therefore, tone can be considered as a measurement of sympathovagal balance at multiple lags with the early lag (approximately one to five beats) predominantly indicating parasympathetic influence.

For any beat sequence length ($50 \leq len \leq 900$), the mean entropy values in the CAN− group increased (except $m = \{6, 7\}$ and $len = 50$; $m = 6$ and $len = 500$) with increasing lag (Figure 10.2). Higher entropy values indicate that the degree of both sympathetic and parasympathetic activity increases with increasing lag in CAN− patients. Similarly, the mean entropy values in the CAN+ group tend to increase (except lag $m = \{8\}$ and $len = 50$)

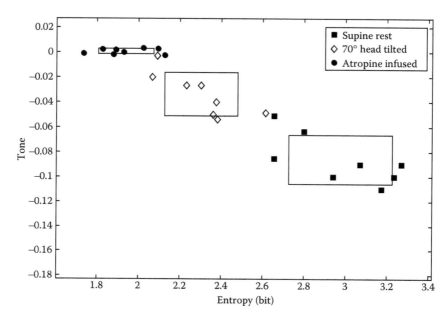

FIGURE 10.7
Evaluated tone and entropy in T–E space, ensemble averages by open rectangles (averages ± SE), and individuals by symbols. A, T, and B are significantly ($p < .01$) different among each other. (Adapted from Khandoker, A. H. et al., *Medical Engineering and Physics*, 32, 161–167, 2010.)

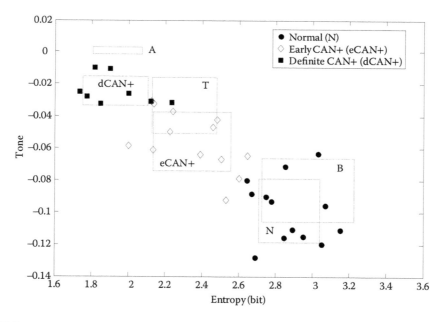

FIGURE 10.8
Evaluated tone and entropy in T–E space, ensemble averages by open rectangles (averages ± SE), and individuals by symbols. N, $eCAN+$, and $dCAN+$ are significantly ($p < .01$) different among each other. (Adapted from Khandoker, A. H. et al., *Medical Engineering and Physics*, 32, 161–167, 2010.)

with increasing lag. The increase in entropy with increasing lag for both the CAN– and CAN+ group suggests that the correlation between parasympathetic and sympathetic function decreases with increasing lag. Our results show that the parasympathetic influence has a range up to lag 5 and then decreases as the sympathetic influence increases. Therefore, at higher lag, the variance of entropy decreases and becomes more stable as it mainly reflects the sympathetic and endocrine components.

The influence of a heartbeat on other beats downstream from it may be a function of sinus arrhythmia as proposed by Lerma et al. (2003) and Shi et al. (2009) with Poincaré plot analysis. Using Poincaré plot analysis, HRV measures, which are influenced by respiratory sinus arrhythmia, change their pattern at a lag value of 6 or 7 (Shi et al. 2009). However, since in our study, the pattern of T–E values did not change (from increasing to decreasing or vice versa), physiological factors other than respiratory sinus arrhythmia may influence T–E values at higher lags. Alternatively, this finding may be a function of the different HRV analysis used here compared to the Poincaré method described in Lerma et al. (2003). This requires further investigation by evaluating the baroreflex activity in conjunction with multilag T–E analysis and comparing the results to different HRV algorithms.

10.6.3 Changes of T–E Values with Incremental Beat Sequence Lengths

We have observed the association between the T–E estimation and varying the length of beat sequences. Conventional T–E analysis (lag 1) is reported as an evaluation process, which is not influenced by the time period of data acquisition. We have demonstrated here the effect of varying beat sequence length on T–E values at higher lags when using the multilag T–E algorithm.

The distribution of both T–E values changes with length for both CAN– and CAN+ groups. This change can be either due to the length/number of beats used for analysis or due to changes in function of the autonomic nervous system. To reduce the influence of beat sequence length on the T–E parameters, we have defined the minimum length for reliable T–E analysis. The hypothesis behind the minimum beat sequence length is that the minimum length should be the length for which the mean of the distribution of the parameters (T–E) is insignificantly different to the mean of the distribution for maximum data length. We have tested the hypothesis using an ANOVA analysis between T–E values at beat length 900 (maximum for this study) and beat lengths down to 50 beats. The ANOVA analysis was performed for all lags. For the CAN– group the tone value is insignificantly different for beat lengths ≥ 250 compared to shorter lengths. In contrast, the entropy values in the CAN+ group at length 50 showed the same mean distribution as with length 900. Therefore, we selected a minimum length of 250 beats to make the T–E measurement consistent.

10.6.4 Detection of CAN in Diabetic Subjects Using T–E Analysis

It should be noted that the mean tone values are lower in the CAN– group than in the CAN+ group for all lags and beat sequence lengths. From a pathophysiological perspective, this indicates that the parasympathetic predominance found in normal beat regulation is reduced in CAN+ patients to some extent. Our finding supports our previous results that heart function with respect to CAN+ resembled that of the parasympathetically denervated heart (Khandoker et al. 2010). The change in the predominance of the parasympathetic activity, measured using tone, is best captured at lag $m = 2$ or $m = 3$ rather than $m = 1$.

Another important finding is that the mean entropy values are higher in the CAN− group than in the CAN+ group for all lags and beat sequence length. Entropy is a measurement of total autonomic activity (Khandoker et al. 2010; Oida et al. 1997) and in CAN+ subjects this total activity consisting of the sympathetic and parasympathetic influence is less than in CAN− subjects. However, the reduction in entropy values in the CAN+ group may be attributed to either a withdrawal of vagal activity, which is reflected by the increased tone, or increased sympathetic activity. This is again consistent with our previous findings (Khandoker et al. 2010; Oida et al. 1997; Shi et al. 2009; Tulppo et al. 2001). From a pathophysiologial perspective, the higher activity of the parasympathetic system in maintaining a steady HR and the associated higher firing rate of the parasympathetic nerves increase the likelihood of free radical damage of the nerve terminals and a reduction in the magnitude of the parasympathetic influence on HR. The change in neural activity measured by entropy is best captured at lag $m = \{2, 3\}$ leading to higher accuracy when classifying CAN using entropy.

Use of multilag T–E analysis introduces a novel analysis of cardiovascular function with respect to autonomic modulation and can be used to obtain better results in classifying CAN− and CAN+ patients. From the results of this study, we can conclude that CAN− and CAN+ can be better differentiated at lag $m = \{2, 3\}$ than at lag $m = 1$. Moreover, the data length used for multilag T–E analysis is 250 beats (ECG signal of less than 5 minutes), which is shorter than the minimum data length required of many time- and frequency-domain analyses as well as nonlinear algorithms (Teich et al. 2000). Cardiac autonomic neuropathy manifests as a deterioration of autonomic modulation at two or three beats, which is in line with findings that the parasympathetic response of HR occurs within two to five beats. The results of this study suggest that multilag T–E is a sensitive indicator of sympathovagal balance and activity that may be helpful in detecting CAN.

Although the number of subjects are small in each group of this study, Cohen's d value was large for length $len = 250$ and lags $m = \{1 - 3\}$, which indicates that the two groups are substantially different and is reflected in the power (Table 10.4). Therefore, we conclude that the difference in T–E values among CAN− and CAN+ groups as well as the classification results found in this study can be repeated or extended for a broader population.

10.7 Conclusion

The results of the conventional T–E analysis indicate the significant alteration of the autonomic system with the severity of CAN in a clear way. The T–E analysis classification could be useful in recognizing early and definite CAN in diabetic as well as in other patient groups and individuals at risk of cardiac autonomic neuropathy such as those with a family history of diabetes or cardiac disease or the elderly.

In addition, alteration of autonomic nervous system function measured by multilag T–E can be used to identify CAN subjects with higher accuracy than the conventional T–E method with shorter ECG recording length.

Further research on a larger sample size is required to further elucidate the findings of this study and effectiveness of multilag T–E analysis for differentiation between mild and definite CAN+ in diabetic patients. In the future, it may be worth looking at how the T–E analysis method performs on subjects with borderline Ewing scores. Nevertheless, the importance of our findings lies in that the T–E results associated with normal (*N*), *eCAN,* and *dCAN* overlap with the results obtained when autonomic function was changed experimentally. Therefore, we propose that our research is the first that reports a robust validation of an alternative test to the Ewing battery that both indicates the pathophysiological changes in heart function regulation and correlates with the clinical findings of the Ewing battery.

References

Airaksinen, K. E. J. and M. J. Koistinen. 1992. Association between silent coronary-artery disease, diabetes, and autonomic neuropathy—Fact or fallacy. *Diabetes Care* 15(2):288–292.

Alam, I., M. J. Lewis, J. Morgan, and J. Baxter. 2009. Linear and nonlinear characteristics of heart rate time series in obesity and during weight-reduction surgery. *Physiological Measurement* 30(7): 541–557.

Amano, M., E. Oida, and T. Moritani. 2005. Age-associated alteration of sympatho-vagal balance in a female population assessed through the tone-entropy analysis. *European Journal of Applied Physiology* 94(5–6):602–610. doi: 10.1007/s00421-005-1364-x.

Bootsma, M., C. A. Swenne, H. H. Vanbolhuis, P. C. Chang, V. M. Cats, and A. V. G. Bruschke. 1994. Heart-rate and heart-rate-variability as indexes of sympathovagal balance. *American Journal of Physiology* 266(4):H1565–H1571.

Brennan, M., M. Palaniswami, and P. Kamen. 2002. Poincare plot interpretation using a physiological model of HRV based on a network of oscillators. *American Journal of Physiology-Heart and Circulatory Physiology* 283(5):H1873–H1886.

Camm, A. J., M. Malik, J. T. Bigger, G. Breithardt, S. Cerutti, R. J. Cohen, P. Coumel, E. L. Fallen, H. L. Kennedy, R. E. Kleiger, F. Lombardi, A. Malliani, A. J. Moss, J. N. Rottman, G. Schmidt, P. J. Schwartz, and D. Singer. 1996. Heart rate variability—standards of measurement, physiological interpretation, and clinical use. *Circulation* 93(5):1043–1065.

Cavalcanti, S. and E. Belardinelli. 1996. Modeling of cardiovascular variability using a differential delay equation. *IEEE Transactions on Biomedical Engineering* 43(10):982–989. doi: 10.1109/10.536899.

Chan, K. L., T. W. Lee, P. Sample, M. H. Goldbaum, R. N. Weinreb, and A. T. J. Sejnowski. 2002. Comparison of machine learning and traditional classifiers in glaucoma diagnosis. *IEEE Transactions on Biomedical Engineering* 49(9):963–974.

Cohen, J. 1988. *Statistical Power Analysis for the Behavioral Sciences.* 2nd ed. Hillsdale, NJ: Lawrence Erlbaum Associates.

Cornforth, D., H. F. Jelinek, and M. Tarvainen. 2015. A comparison of nonlinear measures for the detection of cardiac autonomic neuropathy from heart rate variability. *Entropy* 17(3):1425–1440.

Costa, M., A. L. Goldberger, and C. K. Peng. 2005. Multiscale entropy analysis of biological signals. *Physical Review E* 71(2).

Ewing, D. J., I. W. Campbell, and B. F. Clarke. 1980. The natural history of diabetic autonomic neuropathy. *Quarterly Journal of Medicine* 49(193):95–108.

Ewing, D. J. and B. F. Clarke. 1982. Diagnosis and management of diabetic autonomic neuropathy. *British Medical Journal* 285(6346):916–918.

Ewing, D. J., C. N. Martyn, R. J. Young, and B. F. Clarke. 1985. The value of cardiovascular autonomic function tests—10 years experience in diabetes. *Diabetes Care* 8(5):491–498.

Flynn, A. C., H. F. Jelinek, and M. Smith. 2005. Heart rate variability analysis: A useful assessment tool for diabetes associated cardiac dysfunction in rural and remote areas. *Australian Journal of Rural Health* 13(2):77–82. doi: 10.1111/j.1440-1854.2005.00658.x.

Hanley, J. A. and B. J. McNeil. 1982. The meaning and use of the area under a receiver operating characteristic (ROC) curve. *Radiology* 143(1):29–36.

Huikuri, H. V., J. S. Perkiomaki, R. Maestri, and G. D. Pinna. 2009. Clinical impact of evaluation of cardiovascular control by novel methods of heart rate dynamics. *Philosophical Transactions of the Royal Society A—Mathematical Physical and Engineering Sciences* 367(1892):1223–1238.

Javorka, M., Z. Trunkvalterova, I. Tonhaizerova, J. Javorkova, K. Javorka, and M. Baumert. 2008. Short-term heart rate complexity is reduced in patients 14 with type 1 diabetes mellitus. *Clinical Neurophysiology* 119(5):1071–1081.

Kamen, P. W., H. Krum, and A. M. Tonkin. 1996. Poincare plot of heart rate variability allows quantitative display of parasympathetic nervous activity in humans. *Clinical Science* 91(2): 201–208.

Karmakar, C. K., A. H. Khandoker, H. F. Jelinek, and M. Palaniswami. 2013. Risk stratification of cardiac autonomic neuropathy based on multi-lag Tone-Entropy. *Medical and Biological Engineering and Computing* 51(5):537–546. doi: 10.1007/s11517-012-1022-5.

Khandoker, A. H., H. F. Jelinek, T. Moritani, and M. Palaniswami. 2010. Association of cardiac autonomic neuropathy with alteration of sympatho-vagal balance through heart rate variability analysis. *Medical Engineering and Physics* 32(2):161–167. doi: 10.1016/j.medengphy.2009. 11.005.

Khandoker, A. H., H. F. Jelinek, and M. Palaniswami. 2009. Identifying diabetic patients with cardiac autonomic neuropathy by heart rate complexity analysis. *Biomedical Engineering Online* 8:3.

Krolewski, A. S., A. Czyzyk, D. Janeczko, and J. Kopczynski. 1977. Mortality from cardiovascular-diseases among diabetics. *Diabetologia* 13(4):345–350.

Kuehl, M. and M. J. Stevens. 2012. Cardiovascular autonomic neuropathies as complications of diabetes mellitus. *Nature Reviews Endocrinology* 8(7):405–416.

Lerma, C., O. Infante, H. Perez-Grovas, and M. V. Jose. 2003. Poincare plot indexes of heart rate variability capture dynamic adaptations after haemodialysis in chronic renal failure patients. *Clinical Physiology and Functional Imaging* 23(2):72–80.

Lombardi, F., T. H. Makikallio, R. J. Myerburg, and H. V. Huikuri. 2001. Sudden cardiac death: Role of heart rate variability to identify patients at risk. *Cardiovascular Research* 50(2):210–217.

Martinez-Garcia, P., C. Lerma, and O. Infante. 2012. Baroreflex sensitivity estimation by the sequence method with delayed signals. *Clinical Autonomic Research* 22(6):289–297.

May, O., H. Arildsen, E. M. Damsgaard, and H. Mickley. 2000. Cardiovascular autonomic neuropathy in insulin-dependent diabetes mellitus: Prevalence and estimated risk of coronary heart disease in the general population. *Journal of Internal Medicine* 248(6):483–491.

Nakano, S., K. Uchida, T. Kigoshi, S. Azukizawa, R. Iwasaki, M. Kaneko, and S. Morimoto. 1991. Circadian-rhythm of blood-pressure in normotensive NIDDM subjects—Its relationship to microvascular complications. *Diabetes Care* 14(8):707–711.

Nathan, D. M., P. A. Cleary, J. Y. C. Backlund, S. M. Genuth, J. M. Lachin, T. J. Orchard, P. Raskin, B. Zinman, and DCCT EDIC Study Research Group. 2005. Intensive diabetes treatment and cardiovascular disease in patients with type 1 diabetes. *New England Journal of Medicine* 353(25):2643–2653.

Oida, E., T. Kannagi, T. Moritani, and Y. Yamori. 1999. Aging alteration of cardiac vagosympathetic balance assessed through the tone-entropy analysis. *Journals of Gerontology Series a-Biological Sciences and Medical Sciences* 54(5):M219–M224. doi: 10.1093/gerona/54.5.M219.

Oida, E., T. Moritani, and Y. Yamori. 1997. Tone-entropy analysis on cardiac recovery after dynamic exercise. *Journal of Applied Physiology* 82(6):1794–1801.

Ottesen, J. T. 1997. Modelling of the baroreflex-feedback mechanism with time-delay. *Journal of Mathematical Biology* 36(1):41–63. doi: 10.1007/s002850050089.

Pagani, M. 2000. Heart rate variability and autonomic diabetic neuropathy. *Diabetes Nutrition and Metabolism* 13(6):341–346.

Pan, J. and W. J. Tompkins. 1985. A real-time QRS detection algorithm. *IEEE Transactions on Biomedical Engineering* 32(3):230–236.

Pang, C. C. C., A. R. M. Upton, G. Shine, and M. V. Kamath. 2003. A comparison of algorithms for detection of spikes in the electroencephalogram. *IEEE Transactions on Biomedical Engineering* 50(4):521–526.

Ripley, B. D. 1996. *Pattern Recognition and Neural Networks.* Cambridge, New York: Cambridge University Press.

Shannon, C. E. 1948. A mathematical theory of communication. *Bell System Technical Journal* 27(3): 379–423.

Shi, P., Y. S. Zhu, J. Allen, and S. J. Hu. 2009. Analysis of pulse rate variability derived from photoplethysmography with the combination of lagged Poincare plots and spectral characteristics. *Medical Engineering and Physics* 31(7):866–871.

Spallone, V., D. Ziegler, R. Freeman, L. Bernardi, S. Frontoni, R. Pop-Busui, M. Stevens, P. Kempler, J. Hilsted, S. Tesfaye, P. Low, P. Valensi, and Toronto Consensus Panel Diabet. 2011. Cardiovascular autonomic neuropathy in diabetes: Clinical impact, assessment, diagnosis, and management. *Diabetes-Metabolism Research and Reviews* 27(7):639–653.

Teich, M. C., B. L. Steven, M. J. Bradley, V.-R. Karin, and H. Conor. 2000. Heart rate variability: Measures and models. In *Nonlinear Biomedical Signal Processing*, 159–213. John Wiley & Sons, Inc.

Tomiyama, O., T. Shiigai, T. Ideura, K. Tomita, Y. Mito, S. Shinohara, and J. Takeuchi. 1980. Baroreflex sensitivity in renal failure. *Clinical Science* 58(1):21–27.

Tulppo, M. P., R. L. Hughson, T. H. Makikallio, K. E. J. Airaksinen, T. Seppanen, and H. V. Huikuri. 2001. Effects of exercise and passive head-up tilt on fractal and complexity properties of heart rate dynamics. *American Journal of Physiology-Heart and Circulatory Physiology* 280(3):H1081–H1087.

Veglio, M., M. Borra, L. K. Stevens, J. H. Fuller, and P. C. Perin. 1999. The relation between QTc interval prolongation and diabetic complications. The EURODIAB IDDM Complication Study Group. *Diabetologia* 42(1):68–75.

Vinik, A. I. and T. Erbas. 2001. Recognizing and treating diabetic autonomic neuropathy. *Cleveland Clinic Journal of Medicine* 68(11):928–930, 932, 934–944.

Vinik, A. I. and D. Ziegler. 2007. Diabetic cardiovascular autonomic neuropathy. *Circulation* 115(3):387–397.

Ziegler, D. 1994. Diabetic cardiovascular autonomic neuropathy—Prognosis, diagnosis and treatment. *Diabetes-Metabolism Reviews* 10(4):339–383.

11

Heart Rate Variability Analysis in Exercise Physiology

Kuno Hottenrott and Olaf Hoos

CONTENTS

11.1 Introduction

The autonomous regulation of heart rate (HR) and its acute and chronic adaptation to exercise constitutes a classical and important field of cardiovascular research (Rosenblueth and Simeone 1934; Robinson et al. 1966). Since the end of the twentieth century the application of heart rate variability (HRV) analysis in sports has grown in importance because of the introduction of accurate electrocardiogram (ECG) measurements of beat-to-beat variability with portable devices (Laukkanen and Virtanen 1998). HRV-related research in exercise science and sports medicine has mainly focused on the general autonomic response to exercise training in people of different ages and fitness levels. Additionally, extensive research has been conducted considering general aspects and mechanisms of autonomic cardiovascular regulation during exercise and recovery. Over the past years especially, the monitoring of training load and recovery as well as the early detection of overreaching and overtraining via HRV analysis has gained significant attention. These aspects are essential for an effective optimization of short-, mid-, and long-term training processes.

11.2 HRV and Endurance Training

11.2.1 Cross-Sectional Studies

Several epidemiological and population-based trials show that physical activity influences the autonomic nervous system (e.g., Fagard et al. 1999; Horsten et al. 1999; Rennie et al. 2003). In physically active Swedish woman aged 31–68 years, Horsten et al. (1999) found a significantly higher overall variability (standard deviation of all NN intervals [SDNN]) and low-frequency (LF) power (+30%) in comparison to their inactive peers of the same sex. Additionally, the British Whitehall II Trial confirmed a 20% increase of the high-frequency (HF) power over the lowest quartile of the cohort in subjects of the highest activity quartile (Rennie et al. 2003). Most cross-sectional studies also confirmed that athletes compared to untrained subjects are characterized by a higher overall variability (SDNN, TP: total power of all NN intervals) and increased values in time- and frequency-based parameters (RMSSD: root mean square of successive differences, SD1: standard deviation of the Poincaré plot data around the horizontal axis, HF: high-frequency power) at rest, which usually go along with nonpathological bradycardia (De Meersman 1993; Goldsmith et al. 1992; Sztajzel et al. 2008). In 24-hour ECG recordings HF power in athletes was increased fourfold over untrained peers (Goldsmith et al. 1992). Additionally, the amplitude of respiratory sinus arrhythmia (RSA), which was assessed via short-term recordings (3 minutes) at a rate of six breaths per minute, increased by 60% and indicated a higher vagal nerve activity when comparing 72 male runners, aged 15–83 years to 72 age- and weight-matched sedentary control subjects (De Meersman 1993). Especially endurance athletes seem to show this favorable shift toward increased overall variability and vagal activity (Sztajzel et al. 2008).

In contrast, other findings question this simple and straightforward relation between physical activity, aerobic capacity, and increased HRV (e.g., Sacknoff et al. 1994; Martinelli et al. 2005; Melanson 2000). For example, Sacknoff et al. (1994) found reduced HF power in athletes ($n = 12$), although they had a higher overall variability (SDNN) than controls ($n = 18$) in supine position. A more recent study expressed a similar disparity between time and frequency analysis as trained cyclists' SDNN was increased by 50%, while spectral power was similar to untrained controls (Martinelli et al. 2005). Although time- and frequency-domain measures of HRV may be greater in active than sedentary individuals, it seems that HRV does not necessarily increase in a dose-dependent manner with increasing levels of physical activity (Melanson 2000).

First, these somewhat conflicting results may at least be partially caused by different approaches of physical activity, training status, and aerobic fitness on the one hand and modulation of HR on the other hand. For example, vagal-related HRV measures analyzed at rest under controlled breathing were shown to be positively correlated with aerobic power in terms of VO_2max ($r = 0.53, p < .001, n = 55$), but not with weekly training load (Buchheit and Gindre 2006), which was rather related to heart rate recovery (HRR) ($r = 0.55, p < .001, n = 55$). Moreover, when power at the ventilatory threshold is used as a criterion for aerobic endurance capacity, a relation to cardiovascular autonomic control may not be detectable (Bosquet et al. 2007). Additionally, interindividual differences of breathing frequency can lead to misinterpretations of the HRV spectrum estimates (Camann and Michel 2002), especially when breathing is not controlled during HRV measurement at rest.

Second, physiological long-term adaptations to exercise play an important role. A saturation effect of vagal-related HRV measures and a dissociation with resting HR was shown in trained individuals (Kiviniemi et al. 2004). This can be attributed to the saturation of acetylcholine receptors at the myocyte level (Malik and Camm 1993). Additionally, as intrinsic changes in sinus automaticity and AV node conduction changes may be present in endurance athletes, bradycardia is not necessarily caused by autonomic influences (Stein et al. 2002).

11.2.2 Longitudinal Studies

The majority of studies with a longitudinal design have investigated effects of endurance training in the short to medium term (3 weeks up to 1 year). Most of these interventions confirmed that moderate aerobic exercise (Carter et al. 2003; Melanson and Freedson 2001; Tulppo et al. 2003) in contrast to resistance training (Forte et al. 2003; Madden et al. 2006) leads to (higher) increases of overall and vagal nerve-mediated HRV parameters at rest. This usually goes along with a reduction of resting HR. For example, Carter et al. (2003) reported increases in overall variability in the frequency domain and a reduction of HR at rest and during submaximal exercise in male and female recreational endurance runners in the third ($n = 12$) and fifth decade of their life ($n = 12$). These adaptations to 3 months of aerobic exercise were independent of sex and age. Similar effects were observed in untrained subjects after 8 weeks of moderate aerobic training (at 70%–80% of HRmax), including 6×30–60-minute sessions per week (Tulppo et al. 2003). Apart from increased bradycardia and a shift of spectral power toward the HF band, this study reported a reduction of the short-term fractal scaling component alpha1, determined by detrended fluctuation analysis (DFA), after the training period. The exercise-induced alterations of autonomic regulation of HR toward vagal dominance are supported by a meta-analysis of trials including training periods of at least 4 weeks (Sandercock et al. 2005). Twelve studies (298 cases) reported a change in RR intervals with an overall effect size of $d = 0.75$, although a subanalysis revealed a trend toward smaller responses of RR intervals in older subjects. A potentially limited HRV adaptation among the elderly was shown by Perini et al. (2002). The authors found no change of HRV in 70-year-old subjects after 8 weeks of aerobic training, although increases in physical fitness (maximal power output [Pmax]: +25%) and aerobic power (VO_2max: +18%) were observed. In this respect, either a longer intervention period up to 6 months (Levy et al. 1998) or modifications in exercise intensity (Okazaki et al. 2005) and/or modality might be necessary to improve the HRV response in the elderly. In particular, a combined strength and endurance training seems to elicit higher benefits on HR dynamics during rest and at moderate exercise in older men than endurance training alone (Karavirta et al. 2009). This is in line with the observation of increased HRV during submaximal (absolute) exercise intensities after aerobic training (Leicht et al. 2003; Martinmäki et al. 2008). However, HRV parameters usually remain unchanged when the comparisons are based on relative exercise intensity (% Pmax or HRmax). Not all studies provide evidence for beneficial effects of aerobic training on HRV at rest (Bonaduce et al. 1998; Boutcher and Stein 1995) and during exercise (Carter et al. 2003). For example, Bonaduce et al. (1998) were unable to detect changes in time- and frequency-domain measures of HRV in both waking and sleeping hours (24-hour ECG) after intensive training (20 hours) in elite cyclists, although aerobic power increased and resting HR decreased.

Consequently, regular endurance training does not increase HRV per se. On the other hand, there seems to be a relation between the individual training response of the cardiovascular system and HRV. A high vagal activity at rest may provide a favorable condition for continuous improvements of maximal oxygen uptake throughout the training process (Hautala et al. 2009) and may therefore be used as an important variable in training monitoring (see Section 11.6).

Apart from the influence of different indices used to detect training-induced changes of HRV, beneficial effects strongly depend on the continuous interaction of variables of training load (volume, duration, intensity, and frequency) and individual psychophysiological capacities to cope with exercise stress throughout the training process (Borresen and Lambert 2008; Buchheit 2014; Hottenrott et al. 2006). Adjusting only one variable, for example, training duration, does not guarantee improvements in vagal modulation of HR (Uusitalo et al. 2004).

Hence, this specific dose–response relationship between training load and the HRV response (Iwasaki et al. 2003) implies that training must be tailored toward subjects' individual age, sex, training status, and training goal in order to be efficient (Hottenrott et al. 2006, 2014).

11.3 HRV During Exercise

11.3.1 General Aspects

The underlying mechanisms for the autonomic regulation of HR during exercise are the reduced parasympathetic and increased sympathetic modulation of the sinus node, which regulate nonpathological tachycardia during exercise. The sympathovagal modulation during exercise changes as a function of intensity with the central command, circulating catecholamines, and the exercise pressor reflex being the most relevant physiological mechanisms that mediate these changes (Iellamo 2001; Williamson 2010). A significant withdrawal of vagal activity occurs immediately at the beginning of physical exercise and continuously decreases from light to moderate intensities. The continuous rise of the HR at heavy and severe exercise intensity is mainly due to increased sympathetic modulation. Whether a total withdrawal of vagal activity occurs at exhaustion is not clear, as there is some evidence for small parasympathetic effects on HR that may persist even during high-intensity exercise (Kannankeril et al. 2004).

Although some authors investigated HRV during static/isometric contractions (Iellamo et al. 1999; Taylor et al. 1995; Weippert et al. 2013), the majority of previous laboratory studies have focused on acute effects of dynamic exercise on HRV parameters. Among these trials, the test designs were very different, including both single and multiple steady-state exercises at different intensities and duration as well as incremental and ramp protocols on different ergometer devices. Additionally, the problem of nonstationarity of RR intervals during exercise conditions as well as a wide range of HRV processing and analysis further complicate this issue (Lewis and Short 2010; Sandercock and Brodie 2006).

11.3.2 Effects of Exercise Intensity and Aerobic Fitness on HRV

Although the findings on HRV during dynamic exercise are not consistent due to the above mentioned differences in exercise protocols and HRV methodologies, changes in absolute values of amplitude-related HRV parameters of time and frequency analysis seem to provide a functional dependency with exercise intensity and aerobic fitness (Figure 11.1).

As visualized in Figure 11.1, most studies show an almost exponential decrease of absolute values of overall variability (SDNN or TP as the sum of LF and HF power), HF and LF power and standard time-dependent measures of HRV (RMSSD), standard deviation of the averages of NN intervals in 5-minute segments (SDANN), standard deviation of differences between adjacent NN intervals (SDSD), mean squared differences (MSD) from rest to moderate to heavy exercise intensity (Casties et al. 2006; Hautala et al. 2003; Karapetian et al. 2008; Lewis and Short 2010; Tulppo et al. 1996, 1998). This particular trend has also been incorporated in HRV decay constants for LF and HF bandwidths (Lewis and

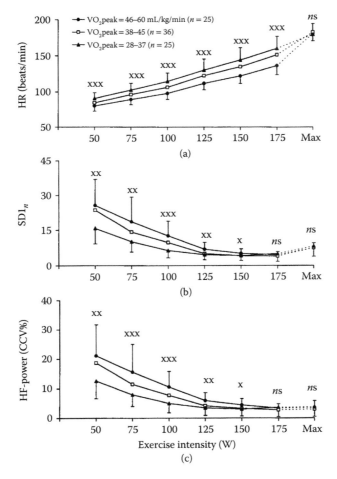

FIGURE 11.1
HR (a), 2-D vector analysis of Poincaré plots (SD1n) (b), and HF power (c) in three fitness groups (age matched) during exercise. Values are means and SD. Kruskal–Wallis H-tests were used at each exercise intensity level (among all three groups) followed by post hoc analysis (Mann–Whitney U-test) between good fitness group and poor fitness group. Annotations are as follows: x indicates $p \leq .05$, xx indicates $p \leq .01$, xxx indicates $p \leq .001$, and ns indicates not significant, for high fitness group compared with poor fitness group. (Reprinted from Tulppo, M. P. et al., *Am J Physiol.*, 274, H427, 1998. With permission.)

Short 2007). Although this general trend applies to subjects of different age and fitness levels, athletes with higher aerobic fitness additionally show higher HRV values in time and frequency domain at light (absolute) exercise intensities (Figure 11.1). Our own data support the almost exponentially decreasing trend of time- and frequency-dependent HRV measures of vagal activity with increasing exercise intensity (expressed in % VO_2peak, Figure 11.2). With progressing exercise severity HR increases linearly, while RMSSD and natural logarithm of high-frequency power (lnHF) decrease in an exponential manner reaching asymptotic values slightly above 60% VO_2peak (Figure 11.2). However, it should be noted that in contrast to absolute exercise, intensities groups of low and high aerobic fitness levels cannot be differentiated from each other, when relative intensity (e.g., % VO_2peak) is used as a reference.

From a methodological point of view, the reductions of absolute amplitude-based time and frequency parameters during exercise imply that an unfavorable signal-to-noise ratio may be reached even at moderate intensities. Although it seems favorable to use relative spectral power, whereby data can be normalized to total spectral power (LF and HF in % or normalized units [n.u.], excluding very LF [VLF] bandwidth) or to pre-exercise baseline values, previous findings on the development of spectral power density distributions (in % and n.u.) during exercise are inconsistent (Sandercock and Brodie 2006). Older studies applying classical spectral analysis methods on hardly comparable exercise loads have shown a variety of changes in relative HF and LF power (in % or n.u.) with increasing intensity: the authors found a decrease in both values, changes in opposite direction (decrease in HF, increase in LF or vice versa) or no significant change in relative power distributions (LF/HF ratio) at all (Arai et al. 1989; Bernardi et al. 1990; Casadei et al. 1995; Hagerman et al. 1996; Perini et al. 1990, 2000). More recent findings confirm a biphasic trend of the LF/HF ratio, which includes an increase at low intensity and a gradual decrease at moderate-to-high intensity exercise (Hautala et al. 2003). Additionally, time-variant spectral analysis methods rather consistently indicate that relative HF power tends to be higher than relative LF power at high exercise intensities (Blain et al. 2005; Cottin et al. 2004). The underlying mechanisms of these changes in spectral power distribution have already been mentioned earlier. Bernardi et al. (1989) attributed the HF oscillations during intense exercise primarily to nonneural, respiratory mechanisms, because the central frequency of HF power is strongly correlated with respiratory frequency. Consequently, for HRV spectral analysis during exercise it seems favorable to use time-variant spectral methods and an extended HF bandwidth up to 1 Hz. Alternatively, a time-variant cut-off frequency corresponding to the actual breathing frequency, which is clearly exceeding the Task Force recommendations (HF: 0.15–0.4 Hz) for resting HRV measurements (Cottin et al. 2006; Lewis and Short 2010), should be selected for accurate HRV spectral analysis during exercise.

Besides time- and frequency-domain measures, the evolution of nonlinear HRV methods seems promising for gaining new insights into HR dynamics during exercise. While the above mentioned nearly exponential decrease of standard amplitude-based HRV measures during graded exercise hardly allows the differentiation between heavy to severe exercise intensities, the short-term scaling exponent alpha1 of DFA is not affected by such limitations. During incremental exercise, alpha1 consistently develops in a biphasic manner: Depending on the resting value (usually between 1.0 and 1.5), stable or slightly rising values of alpha1 up to 1.5 have been reported at very low to mild intensities indicating a strongly correlated structure of HR dynamics due to a vagal withdrawal. Conversely, from moderate-to-high intensity exercise, alpha1 decreases almost linearly (Casties et al. 2006; Hautala et al. 2003; Platisa et al. 2008).

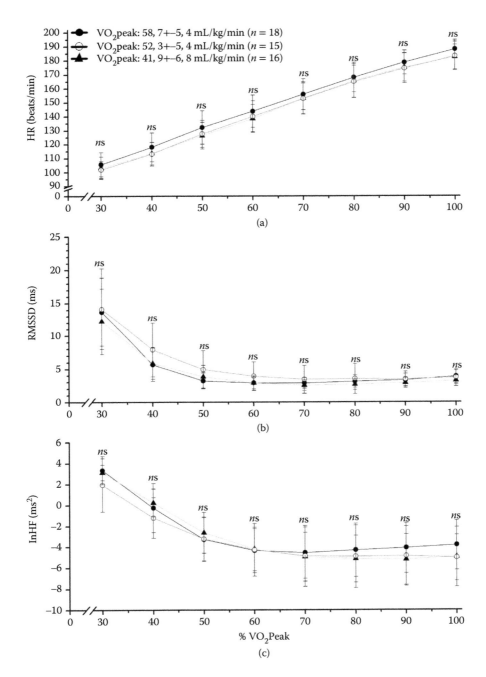

FIGURE 11.2

Heart rate (in beats/minute, upper panel), root mean square of successive differences (RMSSD in milliseconds, middle panel), and natural logarithm of high-frequency power of spectral analysis (lnHF in ms^2, lower panel) during incremental exercise in athletes of three different aerobic fitness levels (high, medium, and low). ns indicates not significant between different fitness levels (two-way mixed ANOVA [aerobic power × relative intensity] with Tukey's honest significant difference (HSD)/Bonferroni used as post hoc test). (Modified from Hoos, O., *Dynamics and Complexity of Heart Rate Regulation During Endurance Exercise*, Philipps-Universität Marburg, Habilitationsschrift, Marburg, 2010.)

These consistent findings suggest that the correlative structure of RR intervals is, in principle, first maintained or slightly increased and then decreases gradually from moderate to severe intensities, indicating that the signal character becomes more and more random (<0.5) until finally an uncorrelated state is reached. These changes in correlation properties of heart beat dynamics during exercise have been explained by a random walk model with stochastic feedback (Ivanov et al. 1998; Karasik et al. 2002; Platisa and Gal 2008).

Our own data support and extend these findings as there is a gradual decrease of alpha1 during graded exercise denoted by significant changes compared to the pevious intensity level (**), whereby degree and progression of uncorrelated HR dynamics significantly differ between trained and untrained subjects (Figure 11.3). Additionally, a crossover phenomenon may be present, as with intensities above 70% VO$_2$peak both trained groups (medium and high level) show a more pronounced reduction in alpha1 compared to the untrained state. This is similar to findings from a recent study with a longitudinal design (Karavirta et al. 2009), as the authors reported a more pronounced reduction of alpha1 at moderate intensities (equal to 60%–70% of maximum power [Pmax]) after a concurrent strength and endurance training. Although the underlying mechanism is still not known, the differences in decay rate of alpha1 may be related to lower intrinsic HRs (IHR) in

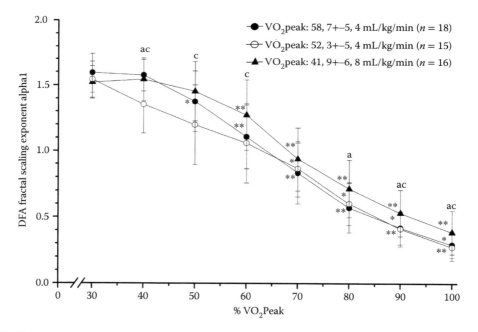

FIGURE 11.3
Short-term scaling exponent alpha1 of the detrended fluctuation analysis (DFA) during incremental exercise (% VO$_2$max) in athletes of three different aerobic fitness levels (high, medium, and low). *$p \leq .05$, **$p \leq .01$ in comparison to previous intensity level; (a) $p \leq .05$ between high and low; (b) $p \leq .05$ between high and medium; (c) $p \leq .05$ between low und medium fitness levels (two-way ANOVA [aerobic power × relative intensity] for repeated measures and Tukey's honest significant difference (HSD)/Bonferroni used as post hoc test). (Modified from Hoos, O., *Dynamics and Complexity of Heart Rate Regulation During Endurance Exercise*, Philipps-Universität Marburg, Habilitationsschrift, Marburg, 2010.)

trained subjects corresponding to a later occurrence of peak values in alpha1–intensity curves during incremental tests as these peak values may be used as a surrogate measure for IHR (Platisa et al. 2008). More work in this area is needed to further corroborate these findings and to elucidate physiological mechanisms underlying changes in nonlinear HR dynamics during exercise.

11.3.3 Detection of HRV Thresholds

Performance diagnostics and training prescription by means of ventilatory and metabolic thresholds constitute an important field of exercise physiology. In order to detect HRV-related thresholds during exercise and to prove their relation to the transition from aerobic to anaerobic energy resources two different approaches were established. The first one is straightforward and seeks to determine the exercise intensity at which a plateau of standard time-dependent measures of HRV (SDNN, RMSSD, or modifications) or parameters of the Poincaré plot (SD1) occur (Karapetian et al. 2008; Tulppo et al. 1996). The verification of this approach for both genders as well as groups of different age and fitness levels led to a commercially available HR device, which derives the lower limit of an exercise intensity zone for effective aerobic training from the above mentioned HRV plateau (Laukkanen et al. 1998). More recently, Karapetian et al. (2008) found that the deflection point of standard time-dependent measures of HRV (SDNN and MSD) with subsequent plateau formation correlates with the first lactate or ventilatory threshold ($0.82 \leq r \leq 0.89$) during graded exercise. Based on Bland–Altman criteria for comparison of methods, the HRV threshold provides sufficient agreement with the aerobic threshold from a practical perspective. However, as mentioned earlier, this approach may be critical in some cases as the HRV plateau develops within a range of low signal-to-noise ratio.

The second approach is based on advanced time variant spectral methods (Hilbert transform, short-term Fourier transform [STFT]) and analyses the changes in instantaneous HF oscillations during graded exercise and their correlation with ventilatory parameters (Anosov et al. 2000; Cottin et al. 2006). This approach takes advantage of the already mentioned strong association of breathing frequency and depth with the instantaneous central frequency and power of spectral HF bandwidth of HRV. In healthy subjects and trained athletes, the estimation of both ventilatory thresholds (first ventilatory or aerobic threshold: VT1, second ventilatory or anaerobic threshold: VT2) by STFT provides sufficient accuracy ($r > 0.9$), when the two thresholds of the product of HF peak (fHF) and spectral power in the extended HF band (0.15 Hz to maximal breathing frequency [bfmax]), which occur with increasing exercise intensity, are determined (Cottin et al. 2006, 2007). This applies to both treadmill testing as well as cycling when VT1 and VT2 are detected by the Wasserman method investigating breakpoints in minute ventilation over oxygen uptake (VE/VO$_2$) and minute ventilation over carbon dioxide output (VE/VCO$_2$)–intensity curves (Wasserman et al. 1973). The second increase of spectral power in HF band is associated with mechanical stimulation of the sinus node and mechanoelectric feedback mechanisms, respectively (Cottin et al. 2006, 2007). The latest findings in this field suggest that both methodological approaches cannot be applied to all subject groups without limitations. However, the time-variant spectral method seems to be more accurate in patients with cardiac disease and diabetes (Mourot et al. 2012; Quinart et al. 2014).

11.4 Postexercise HRV

11.4.1 General Aspects

HRR immediately after exercise characterizes the reduction of HR within a defined period of time. HRR is functionally related to vagal reactivation as well as sympathetic withdrawal (Coote 2010) and constitutes an important predictor of mortality (Cole et al. 1999). The reduction in HR and especially cardiac parasympathetic reactivation following a training session seem to be associated with the recovery process of different organ systems. Therefore, it might be used to assess changes in autonomic input to different organs and the blood flow required to restore homeostasis (Stanley et al. 2013).

Previous studies using pharmacological blockade have confirmed that vagal reactivation dominates within the first few minutes after exercise (Kannankeril and Goldberger 2002; Kannankeril et al. 2004), whereas a coordinated cardiac sympathovagal interaction in conjunction with the clearance of circulating catecholamines dominates in the following minutes and hours of recovery (Coote 2010). HRV analysis of immediate, mid-, and long-term recovery from exercise may therefore help to gain insight into the sympathovagal background of exercise recovery and the autonomic responses to different training loads. Although there is a large body of studies, the heterogeneity of subjects' fitness levels, exercise intensities, durations, and modalities of the preceding exercise as well as the variety of methods used for HRV analysis and the corresponding measuring intervals complicate a systematic comparison of previous findings.

11.4.2 HRV Response to a Single Exercise Bout—Linear and Nonlinear Dynamics

The body of evidence suggests that most time- and frequency-domain HRV measures (especially SDNN, RMSSD, SD1, SD2, TP, and HF) made during the acute recovery phase are reduced after low-intensity exercise (Gladwell et al. 2010; Martinmäki and Rusko 2008; Ng et al. 2009; Parekh and Lee 2005; Seiler et al. 2007; Terziotti et al. 2001). This is even more pronounced after heavy to severe exercise bouts (Casties et al. 2006; Buchheit et al. 2009; Kaikkonen et al. 2008, 2010) and endurance competitions (Cornolo et al. 2005; Hautala et al. 2001; Murrell et al. 2007).

HRV indices rise back to or even above baseline values during short-, mid- or long-term recovery (1 minute to 72 hours). Thereby, the temporal structure of the recovery process is highly individual. Within 1–4 minutes after all-out exercise, there already is a very prominent impact of vagal reactivation (Kannankeril et al. 2004). While absolute variability is strongly reduced at the beginning of recovery, RMSSD and spectral power in HF and LF bandwidth and LF/HF ratio increase (Arai et al. 1989; Goldberger et al. 2006; Martinmäki and Rusko 2008; Perini et al. 1990). From 15 minutes to 1–3 hours, vagal-related HRV indices further increase and LF/HF ratio decreases (Casties et al. 2006; Cornelissen et al. 2010; Martinmäki and Rusko 2008; Mourot et al. 2004; Parekh and Lee 2005; Seiler et al. 2007; Terziotti et al. 2001). Even after intense exercise bouts and endurance competitions, these indices are usually restored within 48–72 hours (Al Haddad et al. 2009; Cornolo et al. 2005; Murrell et al. 2007; Niewiadomski et al. 2007). Some authors reported an overcompensation of vagal-related HRV indices after very intense or prolonged exercise when sufficient recovery time was provided (Hautala et al. 2001; James et al. 2002; Mourot et al. 2004; Terziotti et al. 2001). This rebound effect is directly related to plasma volume adaptations (Buchheit et al. 2009).

In summary, these findings strongly suggest that HRV recovery is highly influenced by the interaction of training intensity and duration. Studies investigating both factors clearly imply that exercise intensity has the highest impact on HRV recovery (Parekh and Lee 2005; Kaikkonen et al. 2007, 2010; Seiler et al. 2007).

Regarding exercise intensity, the aerobic threshold may denote a threshold for autonomic nervous system (ANS)/HRV recovery in highly trained athletes (Seiler et al. 2007). Almost independent from the exercise duration, loads below the aerobic threshold elicit a faster recovery of the autonomic nervous system than higher exercise intensities (Gladwell et al. 2010; Martinmäki and Rusko 2008). As displayed in Figure 11.4, this notion is further supported by our own data. In comparison to 20 minutes of light aerobic exercise (E1), 20 minutes of exercise at threshold-intensity (E2) significantly extend the suppression of vagal modulation during acute recovery, while prolonged aerobic exercise (E3) does not. Additionally, the training method (interval vs. prolonged exercise) may also play an important role, because in comparison to interval sessions, continuous exercise protocols of similar intensity and duration ($\sim 85\%$ VO_2max over 21 minutes) seem to extend the required recovery time (Kaikkonen et al. 2008).

In a recent meta-analysis, Stanley et al. (2013) show generalized vagal recovery kinetics (15 minutes postexercise) after three different exercise intensities (low: below aerobic threshold, $<70\%$ VO_2max; threshold-like: $70\%–82\%$ VO_2max, high: above anaerobic threshold $>82\%$ VO_2max) in relation to pre-exercise baseline levels. Their findings support the dominant effect of exercise intensity on acute HRV recovery as the authors found an increase of (A) 116%/hour after low-intensity exercise, (B) 80%/hour after threshold-intensity exercise, and (C) 40%/hour after high-intensity exercise. In contrast, there was no clear relationship between exercise duration and cardiac parasympathetic recovery (Stanley et al. 2013).

Apart from exercise intensity, HRV recovery depends on the individual fitness level. In this respect, cross-sectional studies found that trained subjects usually show a faster vagal reactivation after exercise than untrained subjects (Mourot et al. 2004; Seiler et al. 2007). By using a longitudinal design, Yamamoto et al. (2001) confirmed a faster vagal reactivation in cyclists after only 1 week of moderate endurance training (at 80% VO_2max, 4×40 minutes/week) and a further enhancement of vagal indices of HR after continuing training for 6 weeks.

Figure 11.5 illustrates the generalized influence of different fitness levels (adjusted for exercise intensity) as recovery time courses of vagal-related HRV measures are different between inactive subjects and moderately as well as highly trained athletes. While postexercise suppression of cardiac parasympathetic activity is nearly diminished after 15 minutes in highly trained subjects, moderately trained athletes and inactive subjects require at least 40 minutes and 90 minutes, respectively, for a comparable vagal reactivation (Stanley et al. 2013).

Furthermore, HRV recovery and vagal reactivation are influenced by postexercise recovery conditions. Especially by using an active cool-down (Takahashi et al. 2002), supine position (Takahashi et al. 2000) and/or cold water immersion (Al Haddad et al. 2010), the increase of vagal-related HRV indices after exercise is enhanced.

Until now, a general consensus on the nonlinear dynamics of RR intervals during recovery has not been reached as only a few studies have focused on nonlinear HRV indices (Casties et al. 2006; Javorka et al. 2002; Platisa and Gal 2008; Platisa et al. 2008). However, available findings suggest that the short-term scaling exponent alpha1 increases independently from training status during recovery (Casties et al. 2006; Platisa and Gal

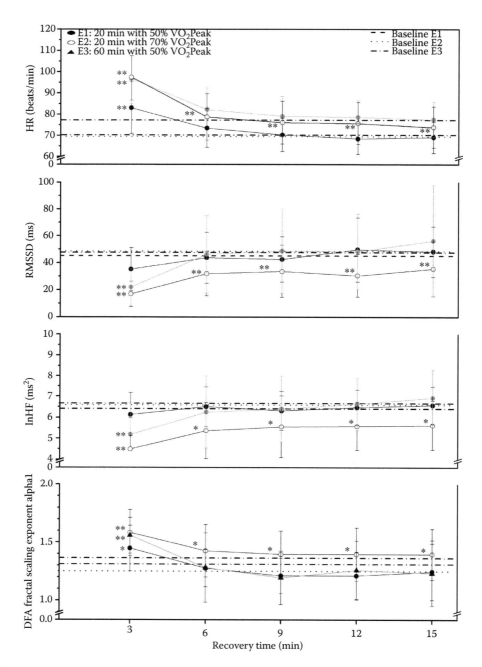

FIGURE 11.4

Time course of heart rate, linear (RMSSD, lnHF) and nonlinear (DFA alpha1) parameters of HRV during immediate recovery after different exercise protocols in moderately trained athletes ($n = 17$; VO_2peak = 49.9 ± 7.3 mL/min/kg). E1: 20 minutes below aerobic threshold; E2: 20-minute anaerobic-threshold intensity; E3: 60 minutes below aerobic threshold; $*p \leq .05$, $**p \leq .01$ in comparison to baseline (two-way ANOVA [exercise mode × recovery time] for repeated measures and Bonferroni post hoc test). (Modified from Hoos, O., *Dynamics and Complexity of Heart Rate Regulation During Endurance Exercise*, Philipps-Universität Marburg, Habilitationsschrift, Marburg, 2010.)

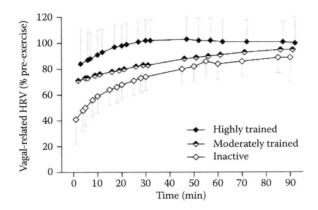

FIGURE 11.5
Influences of athletes fitness/training status, adjusted for exercise intensity, on mean parasympathetic activity (± standard deviation) during the acute recovery period (up to 90 minutes). (Reprinted from Stanley, J. et al., *Sports Med.*, 43, 1259–1277, 2013. With permission.)

2008; Platisa et al. 2008), whereas this does not apply to alpha2 (Platisa and Gal 2008). Alpha1 has been reported to return to baseline values after an immediate overcompensation phase of about 30 minutes (Casties et al. 2006). Similarly, in untrained subjects sample entropy (SampEn) is first reduced and regularity of RR intervals is increased, but rises back to baseline after 30 minutes of recovery (Javorka et al. 2002; Platisa et al. 2008). Furthermore, values of the largest Lyapunov exponent and minimum embedding dimension (MED) remain increased even after 50 minutes of recovery (Casties et al. 2006). These preliminary results suggest that more regulating systems are involved in the reorganization of heart beat dynamics during recovery than during resting conditions. Further research is needed to verify this assumption.

11.5 HRV Analysis as a Tool for Prevention of Overtraining

11.5.1 General Aspects

Performance improvements in athletes require frequent expositions to intensive and extensive training stimuli. As a consequence, training-induced fatigue may persist until the next exercise session. This accumulation of stress is not uncommon in elite athletes and leads to insufficient recovery/functional overreaching (FOR). Whereas performance may still remain at high level in this state, it is lower than the athletes' personal best. In the event that training is continued without recovery, there is a high possibility of developing nonfunctional overreaching (NFOR), which goes along with significant performance deficits (Ackel-D'Elia et al. 2010; Lehmann et al. 1997; Meeusen et al. 2013). In this state, several weeks or even months of highly dynamic and individual recovery are necessary to successfully return to a performance- enhancing training period. Regeneration processes are characterized by heterochronous reactions of different, interacting organ systems and biological signals of high complexity and dynamics. Often the overtraining syndrome (OTS) can only be diagnosed retrospectively. Its symptoms comprise performance deficits, persistent fatigue, lack of motivation, mood changes (with depressive periods), muscle pain, loss of appetite, concentration difficulties as well as increased susceptibility to infections (Budgett 1998; Roose et al. 2009; Shephard 2001). Due to the wide variety of symptoms, exercise scientists seek to identify early indicators and predictors of risk for the OTS. NFOR, a transient state of overload with decreased performance for weeks to months, is also known to decrease adrenal sensitivity to adrenocorticotropic hormone (ACTH) (cortisol release), which is closely related to the activity of the autonomous nervous system (Lehmann et al. 1997). Consequently, frequent assessments of vagal activity provide high potential for the early detection of FOR and NFOR. Figure 11.6 shows the relation between training and overtraining in the sense of a training–overtraining continuum including states of functional and NFOR.

11.5.2 Detection of Overreaching and Overtraining via Resting HRV

The OTS has a multifactorial etiology characterized by physiological, psychological, biochemical, neuroendocrine and neurovegetative disturbances. A subtle balance between exercise stress and recovery is necessary to elicit optimal adaptations and performance improvements in high-performance athletes. The dose–response relationship between training load and HRV adaptations was confirmed by a laboratory study with six untrained subjects (Pichot et al. 2002). The authors showed that overload led to a stagnation of parasympathetic indices associated to a progressive increase in sympathetic activity, whereas a recovery week induced a significant rebound of parasympathetic activity. Sufficient recovery periods are of high importance in competitive sport, because one exercise session with overload does not necessarily affect HRV (Bernardi et al. 1997; Cornolo et al. 2005; Hautala et al. 2001; Sztajzel et al. 2006). In contrast, frequent or chronic overload

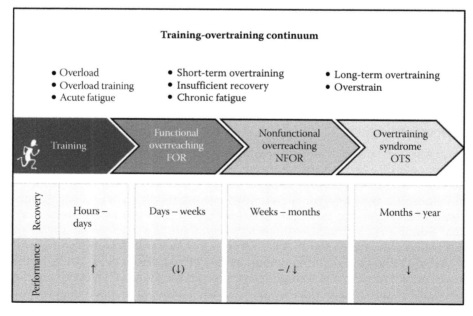

FIGURE 11.6
Training–overtraining continuum. (Modified from Hottenrott, K. and T. Gronwald, *Leistungssport.*, 5, 9–13, 2014.)

in training and competition decreases HRV (Earnest et al. 2004; Iellamo et al. 2002). This offers great potential for the prevention of overtraining, as the use of HRV measurements allow the early detection of functional limitations of the autonomous nervous system (Uusitalo 2001). Previous work suggests that changes in vagal activity are related to altered individual activity levels and training status. In this respect, physical activity correlates inversely with vagal modulation (Hottenrott et al. 2006) and positively with sympathetic activity (Fraga et al. 2007; Mueller 2007). After several weeks of endurance training, vagal modulation of the HR increases significantly in both untrained subjects and elite athletes. Similarly, an overload period up to 3 weeks (W1, W2, and W3) can also result in elevated vagal activity in supine and standing position (Figure 11.7), while the athlete's performance is compromised. Recently, Le Meur et al. (2013) showed that vagal activity in standing position decreased after a recovery week and running performance increased above initial values in the FOR group, whereas no change was observed in controls.

This state would count as FOR, when performance can be restored to or above baseline after a short recovery period (1 week). In case of temporarily decreased vagal activity during the overload period with subsequent rises in HRV during recovery, the athletes state has to be determined as FOR, too. This was often observed in highly trained athletes, who are already characterized by a high vagal activity (Figure 11.8). However, a critical state is reached, when vagal modulation does not increase despite reductions of training load

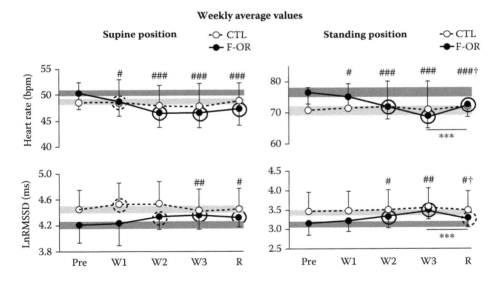

FIGURE 11.7
Heart rate (HR) and heart rate variability (HRV) variables (mean T 90% CI) at baseline (PRE) and during the 3 weeks of the experimental training program (W1, W2, and W3) and the 1-week taper (recovery [R]) for the control group (Ctrl, classic training) and for the functionally overreached group (F-OR, overload training). Results are presented for supine position and standing position (weekly average values). Gray areas represent the smallest worthwhile change for each group (light gray: Ctrl; dark gray: F-OR). Dotted and straight circles around symbols denote likely (i.e., 75%–95% chance that the true value of the statistic is practically meaningful) to very likely or almost certain (i.e., 95% chance that the true value of the statistic is practically meaningful) within-condition difference from baseline (PRE), respectively. Between-group difference in change versus Pre: #likely, ##very likely, and ###almost certain. Within-group changes versus W3: *likely, **very likely, and ***almost certain. Between-group difference in the change during the taper: †likely, ††very likely, and †††almost certain. (Reprinted from Le Meur, Y. et al., *Med Sci Sports Exerc.*, 45, 2061–2071, 2013. With permission.)

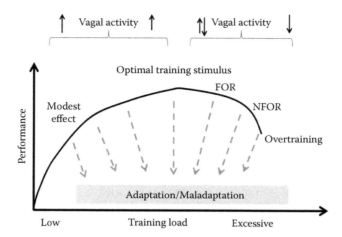

FIGURE 11.8
Vagal activity in relation to performance and training load. (Modified from Hottenrott, K. and T. Gronwald, *Leistungssport.*, 5, 9–13, 2014.)

over several days. By retrospective analysis, Plews et al. (2012) showed that this specific development of HRV indicates NFOR, and competitive performance may be significantly reduced.

In case the training process is continued without recovery periods, there is a high risk of developing the OTS. The transition from FOR to NFOR and overtraining is transient and therefore, the states are difficult to distinguish, especially in elite athletes with high vagal activity (Buchheit 2014). In order to correctly assess levels of fatigue and regeneration, the measurement of additional variables/parameters is required.

Example: Cyclist (Master athlete)

The following case (see figure 11.9) illustrates changes of vagal modulation associated within one week of high training volume. The cyclist (aged 57 years) passes a total of 1100 km in 6 days, which equals 183 km per day. A recovery day was not scheduled during this training period.

Spectral analysis of baseline values (collected before training) indicated sympathovagal balance as LF/HF ratio was about 1. After 195 km cycling on the first day of training, a reduction of HF power was observed during measurement of HRV in supine position on the next morning. Following the third day of training, vagal HRV indices dropped below baseline values and the LF/HF ratio rose to 2.2. This ratio further increased to 2.7 after the fifth day of training (Figure 11.9). At the same time, RMSSD was decreased below baseline values (21.2 ms vs. 49.0 ms). Until the fifth day of training, the cyclist reported a fatigue level of 1 (no fatigue) to 2 (low fatigue). Only on the last day, his rating of fatigue increased to 3 (medium fatigue). This indicates a discrepancy between objectively measured variables (HRV) and subjective ratings of perceived fatigue. The intensified training period was followed by 1 week of recovery. After 2 days, an increase of vagal activity was confirmed and on the fifth day of recovery baseline values were reached. However, the LF/HF ratio should only be interpreted when HRV was assessed during standardized breathing patterns, because varying respiration rates affect spectral power distributions between HF- and LF-bandwidths, e.g., a low respiration rate may increase LF power and decrease HF power. In elite athletes, who maintain a high vagal activity (very low resting HR), NFOR

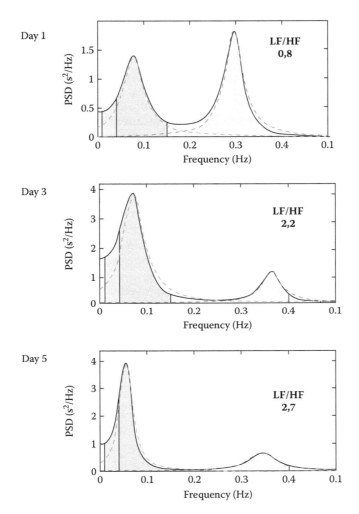

FIGURE 11.9
Spectral power density of 6-minute RR measurements in supine position. Displayed are baseline, third and fifth training day of a cyclist aged 57 years (own data extracted from Hottenrott and Haubold (2006). Colors: light purple indicates low frequency (LF), light yellow indicates high frequency (HF) spectral power, and dotted lines indicate the estimated spectral components from the autoregressive modeling (model order: 20) of spectral analysis.

can hardly be detected by using HRV. This may be at least in part be due to the saturation effect of vagal-related HRV indices (Kiviniemi et al. 2004) and long-term monitoring with at least 3 measurements per week are warranted to describe the athletes' HRV fingerprint for individual recovery prescriptions (Buchheit 2014).

11.5.3 HRV and Orthostatic Stress—A Diagnostic Tool

First, the orthostatic test requires the athlete to rest for 5–10 minutes in supine position in a quiet, slightly darkened room. Second, he or she is requested to quickly change into standing position and to maintain a relaxed posture for 3–5 minutes. Switching from supine to upright position imposes stress by gravitational pooling of the blood in the splanchnic venous reservoir and leg veins (Stewart et al. 2006). Consequently, the autonomic nervous system is required to maintain the hemodynamics to avoid cerebral hypoperfusion. This goes along with specific changes of vagal activity, so that the orthostatic stress test provides a practical method for the detection of overload and overtraining. Figure 11.10 displays the temporal course of the HR during the orthostatic stress test. Healthy subjects show a reaction of the sympathetic branch of the ANS, meaning that passive head-up tilt testing increases HR, while blood pressure decreases. In exercise science, an orthostatic test usually requires active standing-up, which leads to a higher magnitude of changes in HR and blood pressure.

In a longitudinal study, Schmitt et al. (2013) recorded RR intervals in standing and supine position. By using a validated questionnaire, the athlete's state was either classified as "fatigue" or "no fatigue." The authors found that in supine position fatigue was associated with increased HR, LF/HF and LF in normalized units, while LF, HF, TP and HF in normalized units decreased. In standing position, HR also increased and LF, HF, and TP decreased in athletes reporting fatigue. Hence, the orthostatic test can be used to assess the autonomous nervous system's response to training.

Based on previous findings (Buchheit 2014; Plews et al. 2012, 2013; Le Meur et al. 2013) and our own experiences in coaching elite athletes (Hottenrott, 2007), we show a schematic framework for typical training-induced changes that can be seen in a tachogram during orthostatic testing. Figure 11.11a displays the HR during orthostatic testing in healthy athletes with uncompromised performance. The HR is low in supine position and rises

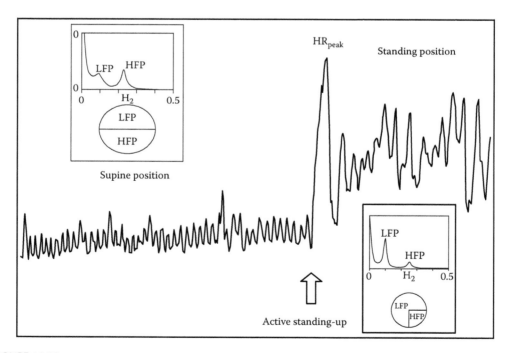

FIGURE 11.10

Typical tachogram of the heart rate in supine position, active standing-up and standing position. In healthy subjects, spectral power density depicts a ratio of low frequency (LF) to high frequency (HF) of 50%–50% in supine position and 75%–25% in standing position, respectively. (Modified from Task Force, *Circulation.*, 93, 1043–1065, 1996.)

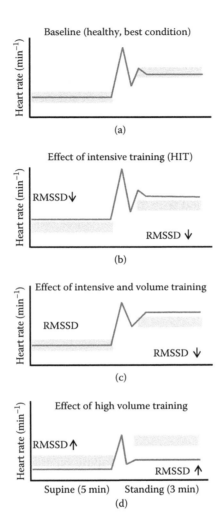

FIGURE 11.11
Training-induced changes of vagally-mediated HRV measures (RMSSD) displayed in a tachogram of orthostatic testing (schematic diagram). Shaded areas always refer to the reference HR fluctuations from Panel (a). Panel (a) HR/RMSSD baseline measurement. Panel (b) HR/RMSSD in response to HIT. Panel (c) HR/RMSSD in response to high intensity and high volume training. Panel (d) HR/RMSSD in response to high volume training.

rapidly during active standing-up. Subsequently, a counter-regulation occurs. When there is high circulation stability, HR in standing position remains higher than the HR in supine position. Standing position also induces a threefold to fourfold decrease of vagal HRV indices from high baseline values (supine position). High-intensity training over several days can lead to sympathetic overreaching, which can be identified by increased HR and decreased vagal activity in both supine and standing position (Figure 11.11b). Furthermore, high-volume training combined with some intensive sessions induces similar changes of baseline values, whereas there is a lower counter-regulatory response. Consequently, the HR difference between supine and standing position is reduced (Figure 11.11c). Changes of the tachogram can also be seen after a week of high-volume training (> 100% of baseline training duration) at low exercise intensity (Figure 11.11d).

This kind of training may lead to parasympathetic overtraining, which manifests itself by a low HR and high HRV in both supine and standing position. Due to a high vagal activity, there is (almost) no HR difference between both positions. The following example (see Figure 11.12) illustrates training-induced alterations of the HR and vagal activity in an orthostatic test (3 minutes in supine position, 2 minutes in standing position).

Example: female middle- and long-distance runner (TOP 10, Germany)

The V800 HR monitor (Polar Electro) was used to record HRV daily over 5 minutes in supine position and over 3 minutes in standing position immediately after waking up over a period of 3 weeks. Collected data were then analyzed with Polar Flow (www.flow.polar.com). Figure 11.12 displays the elite runner's (aged 22 years) tachogram after an overload training period with 24 hours of mountainbike (MTB) training per week (day 7), 14 hours of MTB and 2 hours of running per week (day 14) as well as a recovery period including 7 hours of MTB and 3 hours of running (day 21). According to the training volume, the autonomic nervous system reduces resting HR and increases vagal activity (supine/standing position: HR = 41 per minute/42 per minute, RMSSD = 188 ms/159 ms). The athlete did not develop overtraining but FOR, since the reduction of training volume within the recovery week also decreased vagal modulation to baseline values.

11.6 Optimization of Endurance Training by HRV Monitoring

Long-term performance enhancements require an optimization of the training process. The precondition is a systematic planning of training frequency, intensity, and duration. However, the organism's response to training stimuli is very complex and highly individual, so that training adjustments according to the individual physical and regenerative capacities of the athlete are necessary. The aim of controlling regeneration processes by parameters of HRV is to be able to adequately balance training load and recovery periods in order to elicit optimal adaptations to training and to avoid overreaching. As the autonomic nervous system is mainly responsible for processing stimuli evoked at rest or during exercise, it seems reasonable to assess its activity throughout different training periods and to use this information to control recovery processes. Therefore, Kiviniemi et al. (2007) used an algorithm to prescribe training loads (low or high intensity) in accordance with the current HRV (Figure 11.13). This procedure has proved successful in recreational athletes, but its applicability in competitive sports remains to be evaluated. The algorithm of HRV is based on measurements in supine position. In elite athletes, this model may not allow a sequence of intensive training stimuli, which are necessary to elucidate favorable exercise adaptations.

Several studies of small sample size confirmed performance benefits after quantification of training loads by individual vagal HRV indices. Using a longitudinal design, Kiviniemi et al. (2007, 2010) also found that training prescriptions based on daily HRV assessments allow to individualize and optimize training stimuli in both recreational runners ($n = 30$) and untrained subjects ($n = 48$). Following a baseline period, the authors used HF power (in ln ms² after Kiviniemi et al. 2007) or the SD1 value of the Poincaré plot (after Kiviniemi et al. 2010) to determine whether training has to be adjusted. Whereas an increase or no change of HRV resulted in high-intensity training, a decrease or decreasing trend (2 days) of HRV indices led to the prescription of no or low-intensity training.

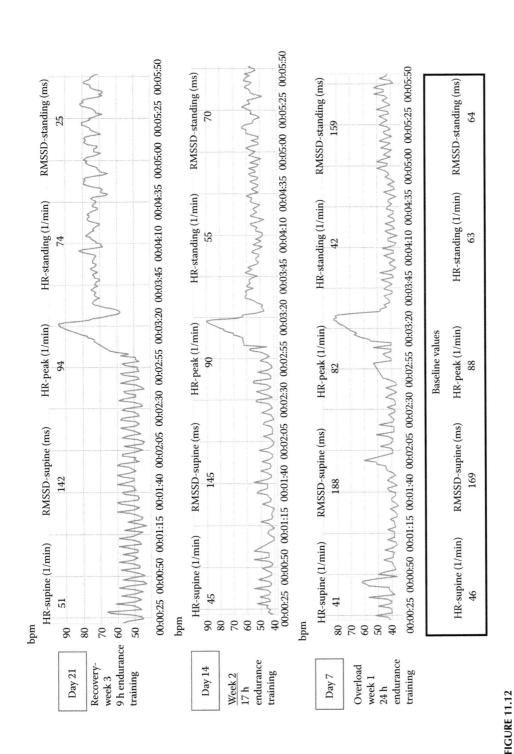

FIGURE 11.12

Tachogram of orthostatic stress tests (Polar V800, Polar Flow) after high-volume training (panel A, Day 7), intensified training with reduced volume (panel B, Day 14), and recovery (panel C, Day 21).

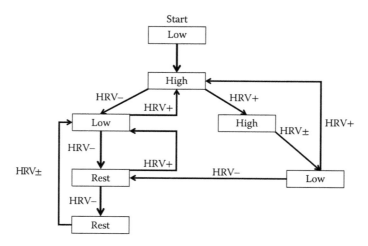

FIGURE 11.13
Algorithm of HRV-guided training prescription. The boxes are labeled with training load (High, Low, or Rest), and decisions are based on changes in HRV. (Adapted from Kiviniemi, M. A. et al., *Eur J Appl Physiol.*, 101, 743–751, 2007.)

Exercise guided by daily HRV measurements elicited greater improvements in maximal power output (+6%–8%) than predefined training (Kiviniemi et al. 2007). The authors also found that HRV-guided training allows the achievement of significant performance improvements with lower training loads (Kiviniemi et al. 2010).

Another approach for the control of individual recovery processes is based on the assessment of an individual baseline. For this purpose, different methods are discussed next. First, it is recommended to measure vagal HRV indices (RMMSD, SD1, and HF) daily over 1–2 weeks of recovery training. Alternatively, session-to-session means of HRV indices can be calculated. This moving average is analyzed in relation to the current daily measure of HRV and allows the interpretation of the recovery state. However, it is still unclear how much the values can deviate from the moving average, before an adjustment of training loads is necessary. For the assessment of the individual baseline, it is not recommended to use this method during an overload period. Following this measurement of baseline values, the athlete can start the scheduled training program. Regular assessments are used to track HRV changes in relation to baseline values. This allows the coach to intervene and adjust the individual training scheme in order to provoke favorable adaptations. However, day-to-day changes of HRV have to be interpreted with caution and should not be used as basis for training adjustments.

Plews et al. (2012, 2013) found that HRV values averaged over 1 week provide a superior representation of training-induced changes than HRV values taken on a single day. In trained athletes, HRV values averaged over 3 days and 7 days both provide accurate information on the training state. In contrast, recreationally athletes need at least 5 days of averaging, because their day-to-day variations in Ln RMSSD values are high (Plews et al. 2012). However, there is some uncertainty about when the deviation of HRV from baseline indicates a need for training adjustment. In this respect, Buchheit (2014) recommend to consider HRV changes greater than the smallest worthwhile change (SWC) to be meaningful. Generally a third of within-athlete variation is determined as SWC, while coefficients of variation of 0.9, 1.6, and 2.5 count as moderate, large, and very large changes

(Hopkins et al. 2009). This formula cannot be transferred to every athlete, because the appropriate magnitude of SWC is very complex and highly depends on the training context. For more information on its determination, the reader may be referred to the review by Buchheit (2014). Another approach for the detection of meaningful HRV changes to justify training adjustments is proposed by Kiviniemi et al. (2007). The authors used the difference between the standard deviation of the 10-day HF power and the 10-day average HF power as daily reference value, which moves day by day over the training period. When the daily value is lower than the reference value for two successive days, HF power is defined as decreased. At this point, the coach is expected to intervene and adjust training load.

The definition and standardization of thresholds, which indicate a need to change the training load, are challenging and require further research. Nevertheless, changes of HRV indices allow determining when the athlete should perform low- or high-intensity training (Figure 11.14). Increases in vagal-related HRV during peak volume-based training loads may be interpreted as positive adaption to training and reductions as a result of the taper are potentially a sign of readiness to perform (Plews et al. 2014). When training adaptations are monitored via HRV, it is necessary to consider the athlete's individual training phase. For example, strong fatigue can be tolerated during the preparation period, as there is sufficient time for recovery. In contrast, HRV changes occurring during the competition period require the coach to quickly adjust the training load.

Our own studies have shown that not only trained athletes, but also recreational runners benefit from training guided by HRV measurements. A HRV-based program included in portable training computers significantly improved maximal oxygen uptake and velocity at the individual anaerobic threshold (Hottenrott et al. 2014). Despite the progression of exercise intensity, no mood disturbances occurred over the intervention period. However, the monitoring of the training status should not be restricted to HRV measurements as this cannot inform on all aspects of wellness, fatigue, and performance. Buchheit (2014) therefore recommends the use of HRV assessments in combination with

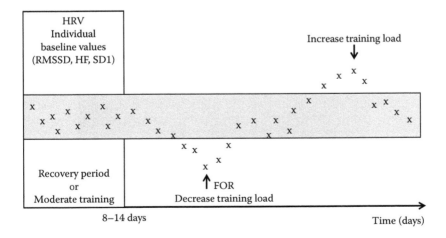

FIGURE 11.14
Schematic representation of changes in vagal HRV indices in relation to baseline (8–14 days; regenerative/moderate training) over the training period (daily assessments of RMSSD, HF power, SD1).

daily training logs, psychometric questionnaires, and noninvasive, cost-effective performance tests.

Moreover, activities of daily living and sleep patterns should be considered when HRV in orthostatic tests is interpreted. This can easily be realized by continous measurement of HR and HRV by HR monitors, such as the V800 (Figure 11.15).

In conclusion, HRV index RMSSD is a sensitive parameter, which allows the detection of changes in autonomic regulation elicited by endurance training. Ideally, data for analysis should be recorded with a standardized measurement at rest (over a period of at least 5 minutes) shortly after awakening. For the differentiation of FOR from NFOR, we recommend to use the orthostatic test, because it may be considered as an adequate tool for assessing both states. During training periods of high-volume or high-intensity, daily HRV measurements are advised to adjust training loads based on the athlete's individual functional state. For training periods of moderate intensity, weekly HRV assessments are suggested to provide sufficient information on exercise-related stress. In competitive sports, HRV should be measured regularly throughout the year to control the athlete's response to different training stimuli, allowing the assessment of individual recovery profiles. Whereas more frequent measurements are recommended in the transition and competitive phase of endurance training, a few weekly HRV assessments may be sufficient during the preparatory phase.

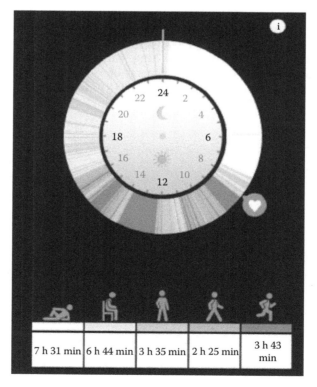

FIGURE 11.15
Sleep, rest, and activity of the runner on the seventh day (see Figure 11.12) of training (Polar V800).

11.7 Summary

In exercise physiology, HRV analysis is considered a useful noninvasive tool for assessing autonomic modulation of heart rate (HR) during rest, exercise, and recovery. Additionally, HRV is being investigated as a descriptive and diagnostic tool for monitoring individual adaptations to short- and long-term training regimens as well as for the detection of overreaching and overtraining phenomena. At first, this chapter describes evident baseline changes in HRV due to endurance training referring to both cross-sectional and longitudinal studies. Afterwards, typical changes in HRV variables during exercise and recovery are presented, and it is shown how these changes are related to training load, exercise capacity, and/or training status, respectively. In this context, data on dose–response relations between exercise training and HRV improvement are reviewed and present analysis methods for HRV-derived threshold detection are shown. Additionally, potentials and constraints of the most frequently used time-domain, frequency-domain, and nonlinear methods are mentioned. Finally, recent perspectives of HRV indices as a tool for prevention of overreaching and overtraining as well as for individual day-to-day training monitoring are critically discussed.

References

Ackel-D'Elia, C., R. L. Vancini, A. Castelo, V. L. Nouailhetas, and A. C. Silva. 2010. Absence of the predisposing factors and signs and symptoms usually associated with overreaching and overtraining in physical fitness centers. *Clinics* 65(11):1161–1166. doi: 10.1590/s1807-59322010001100019.

Al Haddad, H., P. B. Laursen, S. Ahmaidi, and M. Buchheit. 2009. Nocturnal heart rate variability following supramaximal intermittent exercise. *Int J Sports Physiol Perform* 4(4):435–447.

Al Haddad, H., P. B. Laursen, S. Ahmaidi, and M. Buchheit. 2010. Influence of cold water face immersion on post-exercise parasympathetic reactivation. *Eur J Appl Physiol* 108(3):599–606.

Anosov, O., A. Patzak, Y. Kononovich, and P. B. Persson. 2000. High-frequency oscillations of the heart rate during ramp load reflect the human anaerobic threshold. *Eur J Appl Physiol* 83(4–5):388–394.

Arai, Y., J. P. Saul, P. Albrecht, L. H. Hartley, L. S. Lilly, R. J. Cohen, and W. S. Colucci. 1989. Modulation of cardiac autonomic activity during and immediately after exercise. *Am J Physiol* 256(1 Pt 2):H132–141.

Bernardi, L., F. Keller, M. Sanders, P. S. Reddy, B. Griffith, F. Meno, and M. R. Pinsky. 1989. Respiratory sinus arrhythmia in the denervated human heart. *J Appl Physiol* 67(4):1447–1455.

Bernardi, L., C. Passino, R. Roberts, and O. Appenzeller. 1997. Acute and persistent effects of a 46-kilometer wilderness trail run at altitude: Cardiovascular autonomic modulation and baroreflexes. *Cardiovasc Res* 34(2):273–280.

Bernardi, L., F. Salvucci, R. Suardi, P. L. Solda, A. Calciati, S. Perlini, C. Falcone, and L. Ricciardi. 1990. Evidence for an intrinsic mechanism regulating heart rate variability in the transplanted and the intact heart during submaximal dynamic exercise? *Cardiovasc Res* 24(12):969–981.

Blain, G., O. Meste, and S. Bermon. 2005. Influences of breathing patterns on respiratory sinus arrhythmia in humans during exercise. *Am J Physiol Heart Circ Physiol* 288(2):H887–895.

Bonaduce, D., M. Petretta, V. Cavallaro, C. Apicella, A. Ianniciello, M. Romano, R. Breglio, and F. Marciano. 1998. Intensive training and cardiac autonomic control in high level athletes. *Med Sci Sports Exerc* 30(5):691–696.

Borresen, J. and M. I. Lambert. 2008. Autonomic control of heart rate during and after exercise: Measurements and implications for monitoring training status. *Sports Med* 38(8):633–646.

Bosquet, L., F.-X. Gamelin, and S. Berthoin. 2007. Is aerobic endurance a determinant of cardiac auto-nomic regulation? *Eur J Appl Physiol* 100(3):363–369.

Boutcher, S. H. and P. Stein. 1995. Association between heart rate variability and training response in sedentary middle-aged men. *Eur J Appl Physiol Occup Physiol* 70(1):75–80.

Buchheit, M. 2014. Monitoring training status with HR measures: Do all roads lead to Rome? *Front Physiol* 5:73. doi: 10.3389/fphys.2014.00073.

Buchheit, M. and C. Gindre. 2006. Cardiac parasympathetic regulation: Respective associations with cardiorespiratory fitness and training load. *Am J Physiol Heart Circ Physiol* 291(1):H451–458.

Buchheit, M., P. B. Laursen, H. Al Haddad, and S. Ahmaidi. 2009. Exercise-induced plasma volume expansion and post-exercise parasympathetic reactivation. *Eur J Appl Physiol* 105(3):471–481.

Budgett, R. 1998. Fatigue and underperformance in athletes: The overtraining syndrome. *Br J Sports Med* 32(2):107–110.

Camann, H. and J. Michel. 2002. How to avoid misinterpretation of heart rate variability power spec-tra? *Comput Methods Programs Biomed* 68(1):15–23.

Carter, J. B., E. W. Banister, and A. P. Blaber. 2003. The effect of age and gender on heart rate variability after endurance training. *Med Sci Sports Exerc* 35(8):1333–1340.

Casadei, B., S. Cochrane, J. Johnston, J. Conway, and P. Sleight. 1995. Pitfalls in the interpretation of spectral analysis of the heart rate variability during exercise in humans. *Acta Physiol Scand* 153(2):125–131.

Casties, J. F., D. Mottet, and D. Le Gallais. 2006. Non-linear analyses of heart rate variability during heavy exercise and recovery in cyclists. *Int J Sports Med* 27(10):780–785.

Cole, C. R., E. H. Blackstone, F. J. Pashkow, C. E. Snader, and M. S. Lauer. 1999. Heart-rate recovery immediately after exercise as a predictor of mortality. *N Engl J Med* 341(18):1351–1357.

Coote, J. H. 2010. Recovery of heart rate following intense dynamic exercise. *Exp Physiol* 95(3): 431–440.

Cornelissen, V. A., B. Verheyden, A. E. Aubert, and R. H. Fagard. 2010. Effects of aerobic training intensity on resting, exercise and post-exercise blood pressure, heart rate and heart-rate vari-ability. *J Hum Hypertens* 24(3):175–182.

Cornolo, J, J. V. Brugniaux, J.-L. Macarlupu, C. Privat, F. Leon-Velarde, and J.-P. Richalet. 2005. Auto-nomic adaptations in andean trained participants to a 4220-m altitude marathon. *Med Sci Sports Exerc* 37(12):2148–2153.

Cottin, F., F. Durbin, and Y. Papelier. 2004. Heart rate variability during cycloergometric exercise or judo wrestling eliciting the same heart rate level. *Eur J Appl Physiol* 91(2–3):177–184.

Cottin, F., P. M. Lepretre, P. Lopes, Y. Papelier, C. Medigue, and V. Billat. 2006. Assessment of venti-latory thresholds from heart rate variability in well-trained subjects during cycling. *Int J Sports Med* 27(12):959–967.

Cottin, F., C. Medigue, P. Lopes, P. M. Lepretre, R. Heubert, and V. Billat. 2007. Ventilatory thresh-olds assessment from heart rate variability during an incremental exhaustive running test. *Int J Sports Med* 28(4):287–294.

De Meersman, R. E. 1993. Heart rate variability and aerobic fitness. *Am Heart J* 125(3):726–731.

Earnest, C. P., R. Jurca, T. S. Church, J. L. Chicharro, J. Hoyos, and A. Lucia. 2004. Relation between physical exertion and heart rate variability characteristics in professional cyclists during the Tour of Spain. *Br J Sports Med* 38(5):568–575. doi: 10.1136/bjsm.2003.005140.

Fagard, R. H., K. Pardaens, and J. A. Staessen. 1999. Influence of demographic, anthropometric and lifestyle characteristics on heart rate and its variability in the population. *J Hypertens* 17(11):1589–1599.

Forte, R., G. De Vito, and F. Figura. 2003. Effects of dynamic resistance training on heart rate variabil-ity in healthy older women. *Eur J Appl Physiol* 89(1):85–89.

Fraga, R, F. G. Franco, F. Roveda, L. N. J. de Matos, A. M. F. W. Braga, M. U. P. B. Rondon, D. R. Rotta, P. C. Brum, A. C. P. Barretto, H. R. Middlekauff, and C. E. Negrao. 2007. Exercise training reduces sympathetic nerve activity in heart failure patients treated with carvedilol. *Eur J Heart Failure* 9(6–7):630–636. doi: 10.1016/j.ejheart.2007.03.003.

Gladwell, V. F., G. R. H. Sandercock, and S. L. Birch. 2010. Cardiac vagal activity following three intensities of exercise in humans. *Clin Physiol Funct Imaging* 30(1):17–22.

Goldberger, J. J., F. K. Le, M. Lahiri, P. J. Kannankeril, J. Ng, and A. H. Kadish. 2006. Assessment of parasympathetic reactivation after exercise. *Am J Physiol Heart Circ Physiol* 290(6):H2446–2452.

Goldsmith, R. L., J. T. Bigger, Jr., R. C. Steinman, and J. L. Fleiss. 1992. Comparison of 24-hour parasympathetic activity in endurance-trained and untrained young men. *J Am Coll Cardiol* 20(3):552–558.

Hagerman, I., M. Berglund, M. Lorin, J. Nowak, and C. Sylven. 1996. Chaos-related deterministic regulation of heart rate variability in time- and frequency domains: Effects of autonomic blockade and exercise. *Cardiovasc Res* 31(3):410–418.

Hautala, A. J., A. M. Kiviniemi, and M. P. Tulppo. 2009. Individual responses to aerobic exercise: The role of the autonomic nervous system. *Neurosci Biobehav Rev* 33(2):107–115.

Hautala, A. J., T. H. Makikallio, T. Seppanen, H. V. Huikuri, and M. P. Tulppo. 2003. Short-term correlation properties of R-R interval dynamics at different exercise intensity levels. *Clin Physiol Funct Imaging* 23(4):215–223.

Hautala, A., M. P. Tulppo, T. H. Makikallio, R. Laukkanen, S. Nissila, and H. V. Huikuri. 2001. Changes in cardiac autonomic regulation after prolonged maximal exercise. *Clin Physiol* 21(2):238–245.

Hoos, O. 2010. *Dynamics and Complexity of Heart Rate Regulation in Endurance Exercise*. Marburg: Philipps-Universität Marburg. Habilitationsschrift.

Hopkins, W. G., S. W. Marshall, A. M. Batterham, and J. Hanin. 2009. Progressive statistics for studies in sports medicine and exercise science. *Med Sci Sports Exerc* 41(1):3–13. doi: 10.1249/MSS. 0b013e31818cb278.

Horsten, M., M. Ericson, A. Perski, S. P. Wamala, K. Schenck-Gustafsson, and K. Orth-Gomer. 1999. Psychosocial factors and heart rate variability in healthy women. *Psychosom Med* 61(1):49–57.

Hottenrott, K. 2007. *Training with the Herat Rate Monitor*. Oxford: Meyer & Meyer Sport (UK).

Hottenrott, K. and T. Gronwald. 2014. Bedeutung der Herzfrequenzvariabilität für die Regenerationssteuerung. *Leistungssport* 5:9–13.

Hottenrott, K. and T. Haubold. 2006. *Individuelle Beanspruchungskontrolle mit der Herzfrequenzvariabilität bei über 40-jährigen Radsportlern*. In K. Hottenrott (ed.), Herzfrequenzvariabilität: Methoden und Anwendungen in Sport und Medizin (260–274). Hamburg: Czwalina.

Hottenrott, K., O. Hoos, and H. D. Esperer. 2006. Herzfrequenzvariabilitat und Sport. *Herz* 31(6): 544–552.

Hottenrott, K., S. Ludyga, T. Gronwald, and S. Schulze. 2014. Effects of an individualized and time based training program on physical fitness and mood states in recreational endurance runners. *Am J Sports Sci* 2(5):131. doi: 10.11648/j.ajss.20140205.15.

Iellamo, F., J. M. Legramante, F. Pigozzi, A. Spataro, G. Norbiato, D. Lucini, and M. Pagani. 2002. Conversion from vagal to sympathetic predominance with strenuous training in high-performance world class athletes. *Circulation* 105(23):2719–2724.

Iellamo, F. 2001. Neural mechanisms of cardiovascular regulation during exercise. *Auton Neurosci* 90(1–2):66–75.

Iellamo, F., P. Pizzinelli, M. Massaro, G. Raimondi, G. Peruzzi, and J. M. Legramante. 1999. Muscle metaboreflex contribution to sinus node regulation during static exercise: Insights from spectral analysis of heart rate variability. *Circulation* 100(1):27–32.

Ivanov, P. Ch., L. A. Nunes Amaral, A. L. Goldberger, and H. E. Stanley. 1998. Stochastic feedback and the regulation of biological rhythms. *Europhys Lett* 43(4):363–368.

Iwasaki, K.-I., R. Zhang, J. H. Zuckerman, and B. D. Levine. 2003. Dose-response relationship of the cardiovascular adaptation to endurance training in healthy adults: How much training for what benefit? *J Appl Physiol* 95(4):1575–1583.

James, D. V. B., A. J. Barnes, P. Lopes, and D. M. Wood. 2002. Heart rate variability: Response following a single bout of interval training. *Int J Sports Med* 23(4):247–251.

Javorka, M., I. Zila, T. Balharek, and K. Javorka. 2002. Heart rate recovery after exercise: Relations to heart rate variability and complexity. *Braz J Med Biol Res* 35(8):991–1000.

Kaikkonen, P., E. Hynynen, T. Mann, H. Rusko, and A. Nummela. 2010. Can HRV be used to evaluate training load in constant load exercises? *Eur J Appl Physiol* 108(3):435–442.

Kaikkonen, P., A. Nummela, and H. Rusko. 2007. Heart rate variability dynamics during early recovery after different endurance exercises. *Eur J Appl Physiol* 102(1):79–86.

Kaikkonen, P., H. Rusko, and K. Martinmäki. 2008. Post-exercise heart rate variability of endurance athletes after different high-intensity exercise interventions. *Scand J Med Sci Sports* 18(4): 511–519.

Kannankeril, P. J., and J. J. Goldberger. 2002. Parasympathetic effects on cardiac electrophysiology during exercise and recovery. *Am J Physiol Heart Circ Physiol* 282(6):H2091–2098.

Kannankeril, P. J., F. K. Le, A. H. Kadish, and J. J. Goldberger. 2004. Parasympathetic effects on heart rate recovery after exercise. *J Investig Med* 52(6):394–401.

Karapetian, G. K., H. J. Engels, and R. J. Gretebeck. 2008. Use of heart rate variability to estimate LT and VT. *Int J Sports Med* 29(8):652–657.

Karasik, R., N. Sapir, Y. Ashkenazy, P. Ch Ivanov, I. Dvir, P. Lavie, and S. Havlin. 2002. Correlation differences in heartbeat fluctuations during rest and exercise. *Phys Rev E Stat Nonlin Soft Matter Phys* 66(6 Pt 1):062902.

Karavirta, L., M. P. Tulppo, D. E. Laaksonen, K. Nyman, R. T. Laukkanen, H. Kinnunen, A. Hakkinen, and K. Hakkinen. 2009. Heart rate dynamics after combined endurance and strength training in older men. *Med Sci Sports Exerc* 41(7):1436–1443.

Kiviniemi, A. M., A. J. Hautala, H. Kinnunen, and M. P. Tulppo. 2007. Endurance training guided individually by daily heart rate variability measurements. *Eur J Appl Physiol* 101(6):743–751. doi: 10.1007/s00421-007-0552-2.

Kiviniemi, A. M., A. J. Hautala, H. Kinnunen, J. Nissila, P. Virtanen, J. Karjalainen, and M. P. Tulppo. 2010. Daily exercise prescription on the basis of HR variability among men and women. *Med Sci Sports Exerc* 42(7):1355–1363.

Kiviniemi, A. M., A. J. Hautala, T. Seppanen, T. H. Makikallio, H. V. Huikuri, and M. P. Tulppo. 2004. Saturation of high-frequency oscillations of R-R intervals in healthy subjects and patients after acute myocardial infarction during ambulatory conditions. *Am J Physiol Heart Circ Physiol* 287(5):H1921–1927.

Laukkanen, R. M. T., S. Maijanen, and M. P. Tulppo. 1998. Determination of heart rates for training using polar smartedge heart rate monitor. *Med Science Sports Exerc* 30(5):1430.

Laukkanen, R. M. T. and P. Virtanen. 1998. Heart rate monitors: State of the art. *J Sports Sci* 16:53–57.

Le Meur, Y., A. Pichon, K. Schaal, L. Schmitt, J. Louis, J. Gueneron, P. P. Vidal, and C. Hausswirth. 2013. Evidence of parasympathetic hyperactivity in functionally overreached athletes. *Med Sci Sports Exerc* 45(11):2061–2071. doi: 10.1097/MSS.0b013e3182980125.

Lehmann, M. J., W. Lormes, A. Opitz-Gress, J. M. Steinacker, N. Netzer, C. Foster, and U. Gastmann. 1997. Training and overtraining: An overview and experimental results in endurance sports. *J Sports Med Phys Fitness* 37(1):7–17.

Leicht, A. S., G. D. Allen, and A. J. Hoey. 2003. Influence of intensive cycling training on heart rate variability during rest and exercise. *Can J Appl Physiol* 28(6):898–909.

Levy, W. C., M. D. Cerqueira, G. D. Harp, K. A. Johannessen, I. B. Abrass, R. S. Schwartz, and J. R. Stratton. 1998. Effect of endurance exercise training on heart rate variability at rest in healthy young and older men. *Am J Cardiol* 82(10):1236–1241.

Lewis, M. J. and A. L. Short. 2007. Sample entropy of electrocardiographic RR and QT time-series data during rest and exercise. *Physiol Meas* 28(6):731–744.

Lewis, M. J. and A. L. Short. 2010. Exercise and cardiac regulation: What can electrocardiographic time series tell us? *Scand J Med Sci Sports* 20(6):794–804.

Madden, K. M., W. C. Levy, and J. K. Stratton. 2006. Exercise training and heart rate variability in older adult female subjects. *Clin Invest Med* 29(1):20–28.

Malik, M. and A. J. Camm. 1993. Components of heart rate variability—What they really mean and what we really measure. *Am J Cardiol* 72(11):821–822.

Martinelli, F. S., M. P. T. Chacon-Mikahil, L. E. B. Martins, E. C. Lima-Filho, R. Golfetti, M. A. Paschoal, and L. Gallo-Junior. 2005. Heart rate variability in athletes and nonathletes at rest and during head-up tilt. *Braz J Med Biol Res* 38(4):639–647.

Martinmäki, K., K. Hakkinen, J. Mikkola, and H. Rusko. 2008. Effect of low-dose endurance training on heart rate variability at rest and during an incremental maximal exercise test. *Eur J Appl Physiol* 104(3):541–548.

Martinmäki, K. and H. Rusko. 2008. Time-frequency analysis of heart rate variability during immediate recovery from low and high intensity exercise. *Eur J Appl Physiol* 102(3):353–360.

Meeusen, R., M. Duclos, C. Foster, A. Fry, M. Gleeson, D. Nieman, J. Raglin, G. Rietjens, J. Steinacker, and A. Urhausen. 2013. Prevention, diagnosis, and treatment of the overtraining syndrome: Joint consensus statement of the European College of Sport Science and the American College of Sports Medicine. *Med Sci Sports Exerc* 45(1):186–205. doi: 10.1249/MSS.0b013e318279a10a.

Melanson, E. L. 2000. Resting heart rate variability in men varying in habitual physical activity. *Med Sci Sports Exerc* 32(11):1894–1901.

Melanson, E. L. and P. S. Freedson. 2001. The effect of endurance training on resting heart rate variability in sedentary adult males. *Eur J Appl Physiol* 85(5):442–449.

Mourot, L., M. Bouhaddi, S. Perrey, J.-D. Rouillon, and J. Regnard. 2004. Quantitative poincare plot analysis of heart rate variability: Effect of endurance training. *Eur J Appl Physiol* 91(1):79–87.

Mourot, L., M. Bouhaddi, N. Tordi, J.-D. Rouillon, and J. Regnard. 2004. Short- and long-term effects of a single bout of exercise on heart rate variability: Comparison between constant and interval training exercises. *Eur J Appl Physiol* 92(4–5):508–517.

Mourot, L., N. Tordi, M. Bouhaddi, D. Teffaha, C. Monpere, and J. Regnard. 2012. Heart rate variability to assess ventilatory thresholds: Reliable in cardiac disease? *Eur J Prev Cardiol* 19(6):1272–1280. doi: 10.1177/1741826711423115.

Mueller, P. J. 2007. Exercise training and sympathetic nervous system activity: Evidence for physical activity dependent neural plasticity. *Clin Exp Pharmacol Physiol* 34(4):377–384. doi: 10.1111/j.1440-1681.2007.04590.x.

Murrell, C., L. Wilson, J. D. Cotter, S. Lucas, S. Ogoh, K. George, and P. N. Ainslie. 2007. Alterations in autonomic function and cerebral hemodynamics to orthostatic challenge following a mountain marathon. *J Appl Physiol* 103(1):88–96.

Ng, J., S. Sundaram, A. H. Kadish, and J. J. Goldberger. 2009. Autonomic effects on the spectral analysis of heart rate variability after exercise. *Am J Physiol Heart Circ Physiol* 297(4):H1421–1428.

Niewiadomski, W., A. Gasiorowska, B. Krauss, A. Mroz, and G. Cybulski. 2007. Suppression of heart rate variability after supramaximal exertion. *Clin Physiol Funct Imaging* 27(5):309–319.

Okazaki, K., K. Iwasaki, A. Prasad, M. D. Palmer, E. R. Martini, Q. Fu, A. Arbab-Zadeh, R. Zhang, and B. D. Levine. 2005. Dose-response relationship of endurance training for autonomic circulatory control in healthy seniors. *J Appl Physiol* 99(3):1041–1049.

Parekh, A. and C. Matthew Lee. 2005. Heart rate variability after isocaloric exercise bouts of different intensities. *Med Sci Sports Exerc* 37(4):599–605.

Perini, R., N. Fisher, A. Veicsteinas, and D. R. Pendergast. 2002. Aerobic training and cardiovascular responses at rest and during exercise in older men and women. *Med Sci Sports Exerc* 34(4):700–708.

Perini, R., S. Milesi, N. M. Fisher, D. R. Pendergast, and A. Veicsteinas. 2000. Heart rate variability during dynamic exercise in elderly males and females. *Eur J Appl Physiol* 82(1–2):8–15.

Perini, R., C. Orizio, G. Baselli, S. Cerutti, and A. Veicsteinas. 1990. The influence of exercise intensity on the power spectrum of heart rate variability. *Eur J Appl Physiol Occup Physiol* 61(1–2):143–148.

Pichot, V., T. Busso, F. Roche, M. Garet, F. Costes, D. Duverney, J.-R. Lacour, and J.-C. Barthelemy. 2002. Autonomic adaptations to intensive and overload training periods: A laboratory study. *Med Sci Sports Exerc* 34(10):1660–1666.

Platisa, M. M. and V. Gal. 2008. Correlation properties of heartbeat dynamics. *Eur Biophys J* 37(7):1247–1252.

Platisa, M. M., S. Mazic, Z. Nestorovic, and V. Gal. 2008. Complexity of heartbeat interval series in young healthy trained and untrained men. *Physiol Meas* 29(4):439–450.

Plews, D. J., P. B. Laursen, A. E. Kilding, and M. Buchheit. 2012. Heart rate variability in elite triathletes, is variation in variability the key to effective training? A case comparison. *Eur J Appl Physiol* 112(11):3729–3741.

Plews, D. J., P. B. Laursen, Y. Le Meur, C. Hausswirth, A. E. Kilding, and M. Buchheit. 2014. Monitoring training with heart rate-variability: How much compliance is needed for valid assessment? *Int J Sports Physiol Perform* 9(5):783–790. doi: 10.1123/ijspp.2013-0455.

Plews, D. J., P. B. Laursen, J. Stanley, A. E. Kilding, and M. Buchheit. 2013. Training adaptation and heart rate variability in elite endurance athletes: Opening the door to effective monitoring. *Sports Med* 43(9):773–781. doi: 10.1007/s40279-013-0071-8.

Quinart, S., L. Mourot, V. Negre, M. L. Simon-Rigaud, M. Nicolet-Guenat, A. M. Bertrand, N. Meneveau, and F. Mougin. 2014. Ventilatory thresholds determined from HRV: Comparison of 2 methods in obese adolescents. *Int J Sports Med* 35(3):203–208. doi: 10.1055/s-0033-1345172.

Rennie, K. L., H. Hemingway, M. Kumari, E. Brunner, M. Malik, and M. Marmot. 2003. Effects of moderate and vigorous physical activity on heart rate variability in a British study of civil servants. *Am J Epidemiol* 158(2):135–143.

Robinson, B. F., S. E. Epstein, G. D. Beiser, and E. Braunwald. 1966. Control of heart rate by the autonomic nervous system. Studies in man on the interrelation between baroreceptor mechanisms and exercise. *Circ Res* 19(2):400–411.

Roose, J., W. R. de Vries, S. L. Schmikli, F. J. G. Backx, and L. J. P. van Doornen. 2009. Evaluation and opportunities in overtraining approaches. *Res Q Exerc Sport* 80(4):756–764. doi: 10.1080/02701367.2009.10599617.

Rosenblueth, A. and F. A. Simeone. 1934. The interrelations of vagal and accelerator effects on the cardiac rate. *Am J Physiol* 110(1):42–55.

Sacknoff, D. M., G. W. Gleim, N. Stachenfeld, and N. L. Coplan. 1994. Effect of athletic training on heart rate variability. *Am Heart J* 127(5):1275–1278.

Sandercock, G. R. H. and D. A. Brodie. 2006. The use of heart rate variability measures to assess autonomic control during exercise. *Scand J Med Sci Sports* 16(5):302–313.

Sandercock, G. R. H., P. D. Bromley, and D. A. Brodie. 2005. Effects of exercise on heart rate variability: Inferences from meta-analysis. *Med Sci Sports Exerc* 37(3):433–439.

Schmitt, L., J. Regnard, M. Desmarets, F. Mauny, L. Mourot, J.-P. Fouillot, N. Coulmy, and G. Millet. 2013. Fatigue shifts and scatters heart rate variability in elite endurance athletes. *PLOS ONE* 8(8):e71588. doi: 10.1371/journal.pone.0071588.

Seiler, S., O. Haugen, and E. Kuffel. 2007. Autonomic recovery after exercise in trained athletes: Intensity and duration effects. *Med Sci Sports Exerc* 39(8):1366–1373.

Shephard, R. J. 2001. Chronic fatigue syndrome. *Sports Med.* 31(3):167–194. doi: 10.2165/00007256-200131030-00003.

Stanley, J., J. M. Peake, and M. Buchheit. 2013. Cardiac parasympathetic reactivation following exercise: Implications for training prescription. *Sports Med* 43(12):1259–1277. doi: 10.1007/s40279-013-0083-4.

Stein, R., C. M. Medeiros, G. A. Rosito, L. I. Zimerman, and J. P. Ribeiro. 2002. Intrinsic sinus and atrioventricular node electrophysiologic adaptations in endurance athletes. *J Am Coll Cardiol* 39(6):1033–1038.

Stewart, J. M., M. S. Medow, J. L. Glover, and L. D. Montgomery. 2006. Persistent splanchnic hyperemia during upright tilt in postural tachycardia syndrome. *Am J Physiol Heart Cir Physiol* 290(2):H665–673. doi: 10.1152/ajpheart.00784.2005.

Sztajzel, J., G. Atchou, R. Adamec, B. de, and A. Luna. 2006. Effects of extreme endurance running on cardiac autonomic nervous modulation in healthy trained subjects. *Am J Cardiol* 97(2):276–278.

Sztajzel, J., M. Jung, K. Sievert, B. De, and A. Luna. 2008. Cardiac autonomic profile in different sports disciplines during all-day activity. *J Sports Med Phys Fitness* 48(4):495–501.

Takahashi, T., A. Okada, J. Hayano, and T. Tamura. 2002. Influence of cool-down exercise on autonomic control of heart rate during recovery from dynamic exercise. *Front Med Biol Eng* 11(4):249–259.

Takahashi, T., A. Okada, T. Saitoh, J. Hayano, and Y. Miyamoto. 2000. Difference in human cardiovascular response between upright and supine recovery from upright cycle exercise. *Eur J Appl Physiol* 81(3):233–239.

Task Force. 1996. Task Force of the European Society of Cardiology and the North American Society of Pacing and Electrophysiology: Heart rate variability: Standards of measurement, physiological interpretation and clinical use. *Circulation* 93(5):1043–1065.

Taylor, J. A., J. Hayano, and D. R. Seals. 1995. Lesser vagal withdrawal during isometric exercise with age. *J Appl Physiol* 79(3):805–811.

Terziotti, P., F. Schena, G. Gulli, and A. Cevese. 2001. Post-exercise recovery of autonomic cardiovascular control: A study by spectrum and cross-spectrum analysis in humans. *Eur J Appl Physiol* 84(3):187–194.

Tulppo, M. P., A. J. Hautala, T. H. Makikallio, R. T. Laukkanen, S. Nissila, R. L. Hughson, and H. V. Huikuri. 2003. Effects of aerobic training on heart rate dynamics in sedentary subjects. *J Appl Physiol* 95(1):364–372.

Tulppo, M. P., T. H. Makikallio, T. Seppanen, R. T. Laukkanen, and H. V. Huikuri. 1998. Vagal modulation of heart rate during exercise: Effects of age and physical fitness. *Am J Physiol* 274(2 Pt 2): H424–429.

Tulppo, M. P., T. H. Makikallio, T. E. Takala, T. Seppanen, and H. V. Huikuri. 1996. Quantitative beat-to-beat analysis of heart rate dynamics during exercise. *Am J Physiol* 271(1 Pt 2):H244–252.

Uusitalo, A. L. 2001. Overtraining: Making a difficult diagnosis and implementing targeted treatment. *Phys Sportsmed* 29(5):35–50.

Uusitalo, A. L. T., T. Laitinen, S. B. Vaisanen, E. Lansimies, and R. Rauramaa. 2004. Physical training and heart rate and blood pressure variability: A 5-yr randomized trial. *Am J Physiol Heart Circ Physiol* 286(5):H1821–1826.

Wasserman, K., B. J. Whipp, S. N. Koyal, and W. L. Beaver. 1973. Anaerobic threshold and respiratory gas exchange during exercise. *J Appl Physiol* 35:236–243.

Weippert, M., K. Behrens, A. Rieger, R. Stoll, and S. Kreuzfeld. 2013. Heart rate variability and blood pressure during dynamic and static exercise at similar heart rate levels. *PLOS ONE* 8(12):e83690. doi: 10.1371/journal.pone.0083690.

Williamson, J. W. 2010. The relevance of central command for the neural cardiovascular control of exercise. *Exp Physiol* 95 (11):1043–1048.

Yamamoto, K., M. Miyachi, T. Saitoh, A. Yoshioka, and S. Onodera. 2001. Effects of endurance training on resting and post-exercise cardiac autonomic control. *Med Sci Sports Exerc* 33 (9):1496–1502.

12

Monitoring Patients during Neurorehabilitation Following Central or Peripheral Nervous System Injury: Dynamic Difficulty Adaptation

Herbert F. Jelinek, David J. Cornforth, Alexander Koenig, Robert Riener,
Chandan Karmakar, Md. Hasan Imam, Ahsan H. Khandoker, Marimuthu Palaniswami,
and Mario Minichiello

CONTENTS

12.1 Introduction

Brain injuries including stroke often require extensive cognitive and physical rehabilitation. Active mental engagement and a positive emotional state are prerequisites for optimal learning in the rehabilitation of stroke patients. Stroke often affects aspects of gait requiring balance and gait therapy using robot-assisted devices. Ideal cognitive and physical training conditions are an important prerequisite to obtain optimal robot-assisted therapeutic outcomes. Key factors for successful therapy include design of the rehabilitation task, attention to stress, and the psychological state of patients during robot-assisted gait therapy. Although the latter is difficult to gauge in real time, patient stress or anxiety can be inferred from heart rate variability (HRV). This chapter examines the design of robot-assisted therapy and the effect on HRV of increasing task difficulty. Learning to use a robot-assisted device for walking is influenced by the level of motivation or stress experienced by patients. If patients are overchallenged, they may withdraw and have difficulty learning the task. Psychological tests cannot be conducted while patients are strapped into the robot-assisted devices and hence alternative measures need to be considered to obtain information in real time on cognitive and psychological function. The regulation of heart rate by the autonomic nervous system is characterized by reciprocal connections to the cortex and deeper cerebral hemisphere (subcortical) structures and thus measures of HRV can be used as an indicator of cognitive involvement. Using our new method, we process the psychological state data in real time. We introduce HRV analysis as a first step toward real-time, auto-adaptive gait training with management of subject engagement. Our method has the potential to improve rehabilitation results by optimally challenging the patient at all stages of neurorehabilitation.

Adaptation to a task has been shown to be associated with acute stress response depending on the nature and difficulty of the task (McEwen 2007). The biological basis for task-induced stress is outlined by the cognitive-relational theory of stress, coping, and emotions. The theory emphasizes the continuous interaction between the person's resources and their perception of the environment. This reciprocal interaction therefore plays a central role in neurorehabilitation where the environmental stressor may stay constant for some time as is the case in gait rehabilitation but the patients' perception of the task, motivation, coping mechanisms, and physical capacity of the patients' abilities may be continuously changing (Lazarus and Folkman 1987). As such, functional change depends on the patients' sense of control. The engagement with the task and the motivation is linked to patients' coping mechanisms. If the patients perceive the task to be manageable, of benefit, and within the constraints of their self-perceived limitation then the engagement with the task is enhanced (Maddux 1995). HRV is a function of higher cortical, subcortical, and brainstem output; the lower spinal cord (past T2) is not involved in heart rate regulation.

12.2 Neurobiology of Stroke and Stroke Rehabilitation

Cardiovascular diseases, genetic vascular abnormalities, infectious diseases, trauma, anoxia, and other conditions can result in central or peripheral nervous system injury. Central or peripheral nervous system injury such as stroke, traumatic brain injury (TBI), spinal cord injury (SCI), Guillain–Barré syndrome (GBS), or cerebral palsy (CP) can result in physical impairments requiring rehabilitation (Roberts 1970a,b). Stroke results in injury to the brain and often in sensory and/or motor impairments including paralysis on one side of the body (hemiplegia), as well as changes in metabolic regulation by the endocrine system and autonomic nervous system (Crandall and Wilson 2015; Han et al. 2015; Takahashi et al. 2015). This effect is due to connectivity patterns emanating from cortical areas and interacting with the amygdala and hypothalamus located in the cerebral hemispheres and brainstem, where the output from autonomic nervous system fibers is regulated (Liberini et al. 1994; Liutkiene et al. 2007). Importantly, there are also retrograde pathways from peripheral receptors in the blood vessels and heart that reach subcortical and cortical areas (Viltart et al. 2003; Cao et al. 2004).

The goal of rehabilitation is to reduce motor-related impairments, increase participation in activities of daily living, and improve quality of life. Spontaneous recovery of motor skills from stroke plateaus at about 3 months depending on location and level of impairment (Stinear and Byblow 2014). Rehabilitation-based improvements beyond spontaneous recovery have been demonstrated in poststroke patients inspiring research and application of long-term therapies. Ideal training conditions and level of rehabilitation have yet to be established for various rehabilitation programs especially in the diverse area of stroke rehabilitation and robot-assisted device implementation. A particularly difficult part of rehabilitation assessment is obtaining an indicator of active mental engagement, which is important for successful outcomes.

The majority of patients in stroke rehabilitation suffer from diffuse and complex comorbidities including but not limited to cardiovascular disease. Stroke patients exhibit different performance in cognitive and mental activities depending on the location and severity of the neurological impairment and task requirements. For example, stroke patients often respond better to implicit rather than explicit task conditions. That is, explicit strategies are often overridden by the motor planning system, which implements implicit adaptation independent of the type task or location of lesion (Boyd and Winstein 2006; Mazzoni and Krakauer 2006). In addition stroke patients are frequently prescribed a medication regimen to address the underlying cardiovascular disease, depression, or anxiety (Paolucci 2008; Law et al. 2009). Injury to the cortex, cerebral hemispheres, or brainstem causes specific characteristic changes in cognitive function and affects the autonomic nervous system. The response to exercise and mental exertion is characterized by a type of push-pull model where cortical and subcortical activity models peripheral responses and autonomic function and peripheral and autonomic responses affect cortical and subcortical function (Thayer et al. 2012; Porges 2001).

12.3 Stroke and the Autonomic Nervous System

Many studies have investigated the statistics of HRV (Ivanov et al. 1999; Pagani et al. 1986, 1995b; Pincus and Goldberger 1994; Stein et al. 2005; Struzik et al. 2004; Teich et al. 2001; TFESC 1996; Tulppo and Huikuri 2004; Valenza et al. 2012; Wessel et al. 2000a,b; Yamamoto and Hughson 1991). HRV can help identify persons at risk for adverse cardiac events (Huikuri et al. 1993; Lombardi et al. 2001; Makimattila et al. 2000; Lake et al. 2002). HRV can also be instrumental in identifying emotional response (Lane et al. 2009; McCraty et al. 1995; Quintana et al. 2012). Recently, HRV and heart rate asymmetry (HRA) have also been used to identify mental engagement during tasks (Koenig et al. 2011a,b; Jelinek et al. 2011a,b). In stroke patients, the impaired autonomic nervous system modulation is characterized by an increase in sympathetic output, which leads to a lower HRV (Lakusic et al. 2003, 2005). Although the magnitude of HRV is influenced by differences in underlying illness or injury or a result of therapies including medications, HRV reflects adaptation of the organism to physical, cognitive, and emotional conditions (Thayer et al. 2009).

HRV recorded as time or frequency measures or as the complexity of the displayed rhythm can be determined from electrocardiogram (ECG) recordings of varying length. Measures of complexity of the heart rate include fractal analysis, detrended fluctuation analysis, diverse entropy measures, measures derived from the Poincaré plot, and symbolic dynamics (Abásolo et al. 2006; Costa et al. 2002; Peng et al. 1995; Acharya et al. 2006; Voss et al. 2009; Tulppo et al. 1996; Higuchi 1998; Huikuri et al. 2003). Several novel HRV features have been developed by our laboratory including the tone–entropy, complex correlation measure, asymmetry index, and multilag Poincaré analysis (Karmakar et al. 2009; Karmakar et al. 2011; Khandoker et al. 2009b). HRV can also act as a physiological proxy measurement tool that measures cognitive and emotional engagement and has been shown to respond to mental and physical stress (Andreassi 2007; Thayer et al. 2009; Matthews et al. 2012; de la Cruz Torres et al. 2008; Delaney and Brodie 2000).

12.4 Design of the Rehabilitation Task

The use of technology in stroke rehabilitation raises many questions around the design and the user experience. How will older people, who may never have used a computer or played video games, interact with such new modes of health delivery using such technologies? What are the elements of the design of a rehabilitation task that will define the user experience to encourage participation? Learning and exercise can be exceptionally challenging for stroke patients (Jelinek et al. 2011b). It is important for rehabilitation and exercise to be safe, but also to provide a positive experience for the patient. For example, Bailenson argues that designing an avatar that represents the positive aspects of a player in immersive virtual reality "transformed self-esteem and social self-perception" (Lanier 2010).

To address the future needs of the applied health sector such as is the case for neurological rehabilitation, home programs, and eMonitoring, where extensive information technology (IT) and virtual reality-based therapies are found, it is essential that design works more closely with IT (Minichiello 2012). The use of experiential graphic design (XGD), which involves the orchestration of moving images, animation, games, graphics, big data imaging, and typography will be applied to solve difficult problems, in particular complex health problems known as "wicked problems." This is a term first used by Rittel and Webber to frame difficult challenges in social policy and planning (Rittel and Webber 1984). However, wicked problems have also arisen in domains where complexity and diversity exist such as health and well-being. Addressing these issues will require a combination of design and technology working in collaboration. This has been referred to as "supra-functionality" (McDonagh et al. 2002). Increasingly, these aims are being addressed through combining traditional approaches with XGD. This involves the use of digital technologies and design thinking applied in developing and enhancing systems that present dynamic content through motion graphics and make possible rich interactions between users and information, in real or virtual spaces.

This will be further advanced by the application of human-centered design to investigate the relationship between the patient in relation to the interface of products or experience. Using a range of approaches including digital services, lifestyle modeling, visualization, and illustration of data and scientific phenomena using codesign and empathetic design strategies. Empathetic design is the key to the future effectiveness of health systems. While a great deal of the past has been focused on clinical practices led by health workers, it is clear that the future requires a different approach with a combination of clinical thinking and human-centered empathetic design that will enable more self-management of health. This approach is concerned with understanding the needs of the user in developing an empathetic design, product, or experience (Krznaric 2014). By combining design practice and investigative design methodologies with IT, positive experiences can be enhanced using integrated biofeedback such as continuous HRV monitoring to change the landscape of virtual reality.

Selection for rehabilitation should thus identify patients that would benefit most in terms of their neurological impairment and retraining improved functionality with a suitable training protocol. In addition, measures that can inform the clinician of any risk for the individual, such as a sluggish or rapid response to abrupt changes or specific challenges (cognitive, emotional, and exercise) would improve safety for the patient. Driven gait orthosis (DGO)-based neurorehabilitation technology such as the Lokomat (Hocoma, Switzerland) is an exoskeleton used for gait and locomotion training. The Lokomat is designed to assist patients with lower limb movement and provide body weight support. The speed of the system can be kept constant and cadence adjusted to suit the patient.

12.5 The Virtual Environmental Task

The virtual environmental task (VET), which sets the exercise or gait and balance requirements, can be viewed on monitors with auditory information projected from speakers. The VET tasks chosen for the current Lokomat robot-assisted neurorehabilitation required simultaneous mechanical adjustment by changing the walking direction to collect items presented along a path and cognitive processing using a computer mouse button to negotiate over barrels that were rolled toward the patient along the virtual path shown on the monitor. Points were obtained or lost for successfully negotiating the path and picking up items or failing to complete the task (Koenig et al. 2011b). VET difficulty was specific for each participant and initially determined during a practice session using the self-assessment manikin (SAM) questionnaire (Bradley and Lang 1994). Three levels of difficulty were applied consisting of an underchallenged, optimally challenged, and overchallenged task condition. SAM was used to verify that the three conditions in the VR tasks equated with the three motivational stages (boredom, excitement, and overstressed). The underchallenged condition allowed the participant to collect and jump all items. For the appropriately challenged condition patients were expected to complete 80%–90% of the assigned task and for the overchallenged condition less than 10%. Each condition lasted 5 minutes.

12.6 Physiological Recordings

The different levels of mental engagement were also estimated by recording of ECG traces and determining HRV. The ECG was measured using a lead-II configuration at 512 samples/sec. R wave peaks were determined using the algorithm first suggested by Tomkins (Hamilton and Tompkins 1986). Interbeat variation and complexity was determined from the ECG by time-domain, frequency-domain, and nonlinear methods (Khandoker et al. 2009a; Oida et al. 1999; Osipova et al. 2010). All signal processing was performed using MATLAB® 2008 (The Mathworks, Natick, MA, USA, www.mathworks.com).

12.7 Cognitive Engagement

In rehabilitation, the measurement of interest is a measurement that reveals information about the condition of the patient and how the patient responds to the rehabilitation tasks and environment. In this situation, information about healthy participants might be used to help understand how a person differs in their adaptation to an increasing physical and mental task difficulty level. Since direct measures of brain activity are not possible while undertaking robot-assisted tasks and psychological questionnaires need to be completed at completion of the task, HRV measures can be used to directly obtain information on how participants adapt to a task level over time (Thayer et al. 2012; Quintana et al. 2012; Schubert et al. 2009; Alm 2004; Porges 1995; Pagani et al. 1991). This is an important component of neurophysiological and neuropsychological rehabilitation as the adaptive phase of mental and physical exertion provides more accurate information on the capacity of the system, which is hidden in part when the system reaches steady state.

12.8 Adaptation to Task Difficulty

To obtain an indication of whether the HRV can identify changes in motivation associated with the difficulty of task, seven healthy participants (mean age 24.1 ± 2.0 years) with no neurological and physiological impairment were enrolled in a study to investigate adaptation to task difficulty using HRV as a surrogate for mental engagement, applying time and frequency domain as well as Poincaré plot-derived features (Jelinek et al. 2011b). From the 5-minute recording for each task difficulty, the steady state was set as being the last minute of each recording and the adaptation to the task as the difference between the last minute of the current condition and the first minute of the following condition (Koenig et al. 2011b). In this study, Poincaré plot-derived features were of main interest to identify temporal characteristics of HRV. The complex correlation method (CCM) was first proposed by Karmakar and colleagues based on the Poincaré plot description of plotting consecutive points of RR interval time series (i.e., lag-1 plot) to address the lack of temporal information available from the standard descriptors of the Poincaré plot (Karmakar et al. 2011). The standard descriptors, SD1 and SD2, represent the distribution of signal in two-dimensional space and carries only information of width and length. CCM describes the variability in the temporal attributes of the point-to-point variation inherent in the signal rather than a gross description of the Poincaré plot.

If the Poincaré plot is composed of N points, then the temporal variation of the plot is composed of all overlapping three-point windows and can be calculated as

$$\text{CCM}(m) = \frac{1}{C_n(N-2)} \sum_{i=1}^{N-2} \|A(i)\| \tag{12.1}$$

where m represents lag of Poincaré plot, $A(i)$ represents area of the ith triangle, and C_n is the normalizing constant, defined as $C_n = \pi \times \text{SD1} \times \text{SD2}$, which represents the area of the fitted ellipse over Poincaré plot at lag m. The length of the major and minor axes of the ellipse are 2SD1 and 2SD2, where SD1 and SD2 are the dispersion perpendicular to the line of identity (minor axis) and along the line of identity (major axis), respectively. Details on the mathematical formulation of CCM are reported in our previous study (Karmakar et al. 2009).

An increase in the CCM value most likely indicates an increase in parasympathetic activity, especially if other features including RMSSD or SD1 are also increased. Only SD1 and CCM differentiated between the level of difficulty in terms of adaptation, suggesting a rapid response by the parasympathetic nervous system (PNS) to task difficulty from standing to walking and transition from the underchallenged to appropriate challenged task level (Figure 12.1). The PNS output is regulated centrally from the prefrontal cortex via the brainstem and therefore both SD1 and CCM, which provide information on HRV, provide information on the level of cortical engagement. That is, a change in cortical responsiveness

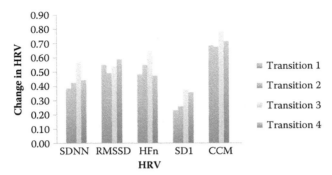

FIGURE 12.1
Gradient of changes of different HRV parameters. SDNN, standard deviation of RR intervals; RMSSD, square root of the mean squared differences of successive normal RR intervals; HFn, normalized high-frequency power; SD1, Poincaré short-time correlation parameter; CCM, complex correlation measure of Poincaré plot; Transition 1, standing to walking; Transition 2, walking to underchallenged; Transition 3, underchallenged to challenged; Transition 4, challenged to overchallenged. Transitions between standing to walking and underchallenged to challenged show significant difference at $p < .05$.

and engagement, as is expected when novel tasks are presented to a subject, will change parasympathetic output and HRV.

The advantages of using a Poincaré plot and its SD1 measure and CCM is that these variables are robust against nonstationarity, and against the effects of respiration and ectopic beats on the ECG signal (Karmakar et al. 2010, 2011). Parasympathetic input to the HRV signal decreases when physical exercise is undertaken or an external or internal stressor is present. Stress decreases function in certain parts of the cortex linked to parasympathetic function (Broadbent 1971; Kim et al. 2006). The decrease in parasympathetic input leads to sympathetic dominance and a decrease in HRV (Srinivasan et al. 2006). We found that the level of challenge is important in how the patient or participant responds to the task and possibly reflects mental engagement as a function of stress, which in turn is reflected by changes in HRV. Standing to walking and underchallenged to challenged transitions brought about the largest change in HRV. Initial conditions of inactivity prior to the exercise session might be partially responsible for the large adaptation observed in the standing to walking transition. Similarly, the transition from underchallenged to challenged increases motivation and cortical activity and therefore the HRV. Further the level of adaptation dropped for challenged to overchallenged for both SD1 and CCM features as described above and back toward the walking to underchallenged transition level. This may be due to the increased physical or cognitive stress associated with the overchallenged condition, both of which would result in a parasympathetic withdrawal and therefore a lower HRV.

From a corticocardiac reciprocal connectivity perspective, we propose that HRV is linked to cortical as well as brainstem modulation with the prefrontal cortex having an inhibitory influence on brainstem nuclei, which in turn inhibits parasympathetic output and therefore the level of HRV (Porges 2007; Thayer and Lane 2009). The decrease in SD1 and CCM when the overchallenged condition commenced indicates a withdrawal of the frontal cortex and emotional positive output. Therefore, the inhibitory output to the brainstem is reduced leading to an increased inhibition of the parasympathetic output and therefore a balance toward sympathetic drive and a decrease in HRV as the polyvagal theory has suggested (Porges 2007).

12.9 HRV Asymmetry Response to Task Difficulty

A different perspective on adaptation to a task and level of mental engagement can be obtained by inspecting HRA. HRV is the net outcome of sympathetic (sympathetic nervous system [SNS]) and parasympathetic (PNS) input to the heart. While SNS input increases heart rate and decreases HRV, PNS lowers the heart rate and increases HRV. Physiologically, there is always some variability in the heart rate, due to the imbalance in SNS and PNS activity levels. The speed at which the heart rate increases or decreases is variable, which implies that the periods of increasing or decreasing RR interval are also not equal. As a result, HRA, which reflects the rate at which HR changes, should be a common phenomenon present in the healthy heart, which is reported by Piskorski and Guzik (2007) and Porta et al. (2008).

The HRA index proposed by Karmakar differs from previous implementations by defining asymmetry from a geometrical point of view by considering a pattern rather than single points of the Poincaré plot (previously used by Guzik et al. [2007] to categorize a point either as increasing, decreasing, or stable with respect to the previous point and it captured HRA). Using Shannon entropy to determine HRA, the RR intervals are determined from the ECG and transformed into the percentage index (PI) and entropy is then determined from the PI probability distribution by using Shannon's formula (Oida et al. 1999; Khandoker et al. 2010). Acceleration of the heart can be expressed as a plus difference and deceleration as a minus difference by separating the PI distributions into two components. HRA can then be calculated from the entropy of the positive and negative differences of PI time series as shown in the following:

$$\text{HRA} = \frac{\text{Entropy of the positive difference part of the PI time series}}{\text{Total entropy of PI time series}}$$

The entropy is defined on the PI probability distribution by using Shannon's formula:

$$- \sum_n p(i)\log_2 p(i) \tag{12.2}$$

where $p(i)$ is the probability that $PI(n)$ has a value in the range $I < PI(n) < i+1$, with i an integer. The entropy evaluates total acceleration–deceleration activities.

No significant difference between the small group of control and stroke patients was observed for any of the experimental task difficulties. However, the data do indicate the difference in autonomic nervous system modulation between the stroke and control participants with respect to task difficulty (Figure 12.2).

In Figure 12.2, values greater than 0.5 indicate sympathetic influence and acceleration of the heart rate, whereas values below 0.5 indicate parasympathetic influence and slowing of the heart rate. HRA is a function of the level of sympathetic and parasympathetic input, which changes when physical exercise is undertaken or an external or internal stressor is present (Kim et al. 2006; Srinivasan et al. 2006). The pilot results shown here are interesting as at the resting stage stroke patients had a slightly increased sympathetic tone. Sympathetic activity is increased with increased stress, which may be due to inappropriate anticipation of the robot-assisted tasks ahead. Control subjects had a slightly greater parasympathetic output as would be expected at rest (Amarenco et al. 2010). The change in task condition from standing to optimal challenged task difficulty led to a steady increase

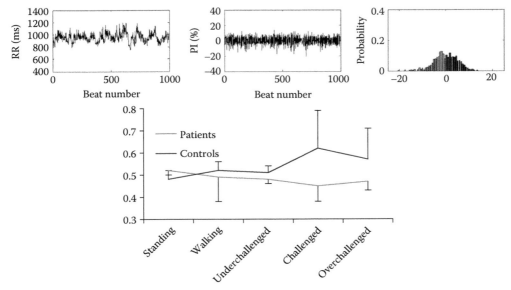

FIGURE 12.2
Change in the pattern of HRA.

in parasympathetic predominance in the stroke patients suggesting a possible decreased motivation in contrast to the controls, who showed an increased sympathetic activity with increases in task difficulty (Figure 12.2). Task preparation has been suggested to be associated with attention or engagement, which may indicate that stroke patients required a greater preparation response, that is, greater prefrontal cortical activation that leads to an inhibition of the subcortical sympathoexcitation (Thayer and Lane 2009). The augmentation of parasympathetic activity in the poststroke patients can also lead to bradycardia or asystole and sudden cardiac death (Olshansky et al. 2008). When working with stroke patients and assessing task difficulty effectiveness by applying HRV analysis, the location of the stroke plays an important part and may have influenced the results reported above.

12.10 Stroke Location

We used a 1-minute recording either at the end of the 5-minute task period, which represented the steady state or the first minute after the task was changed to determine adaptation. Stroke patients were divided into subgroups to represent the site of the lesion as cortical, subcortical including and spinal cord as well as including encephalitis-related lesions. Entropy was used as a HRV tool to measure the level of task engagement by patients with stroke and controls during Lokomat robot-assisted gait rehabilitation coupled with a virtual reality task setting (Koenig et al. 2011b). Recent results indicate significant differences in the adaptation response between poststroke patient groups depending on the challenge difficulty (Jelinek et al. 2014). The opposite responses in cortical stroke and subcortical stroke patients was striking, indicating that cortical stroke patients may be more stressed due to any change in condition and therefore display a large sympathetic surge not seen in the other groups, although spinal and subcortical patient groups had a large reduction in entropy. This reduction in HRV in the patient group may indicate a lack of engagement on the task and differs to the control group.

Similarly, adaptation to task condition differed in the patient groups when the change was from appropriately challenged to overchallenged. The control group showed decrease in entropy and therefore an increase in sympathetic activity. However, the cortical stroke group had a lower entropy, indicating that this group may be indeed overchallenged and not able to respond to the task. In both the subcortical and spinal cord groups HRV entropy response was more than double that of the control group, which indicates that this group is extremely challenged.

Our results indicate that HRV entropy is a suitable measure to characterize post-stroke rehabilitation adaptation to varying challenges in robot-assisted neurorehabilitation. Seven healthy subjects (mean age 24.1 ± 2.0 years) with no neurological and physiological impairment, three right middle cerebral artery stroke patients (mean age 60.3 ± 8.6), three subcortical patients (mean age 42.6 ± 20.1), and three spinal cord patients (mean age 52.6 ± 29.6) participated in the study. Two patients in the cortical group and one in the subcortical group were on beta-blocker medication. Time post infarct ranged from 1 month to 21 months.

Results for entropy with respect to adapting from the underchallenged condition to an appropriately challenged condition indicated that entropy in stroke patients increased, indicating a sympathetic surge, while in spinal cord and subcortical stroke, entropy decreased over the 1-minute adaption period following the change in condition. The control group showed no real change in entropy (Table 12.1).

Adaptation response from the appropriate challenged condition to overchallenged showed that the cortical stroke patients had the least decrease in HRV entropy and therefore the least increase in heart rate accelerations. The subcortical stroke group had the largest decrease in HRV entropy and therefore the most increased sympathetic activity. The response of both the subcortical stroke and spinal cord groups was larger than the control group (Table 12.1).

Significant differences were found between the groups comparing the underchallenged to appropriately challenged condition ($p = .026$) and also for the change between the appropriately challenged to overchallenged condition ($p = .027$).

Substantial differences between the patient groups were observed for age and also for time since incident. The cortical stroke patients were the oldest, whereas the subcortical stroke patients were younger. However, in the spinal cord group, one patient was 19 years old compared to the other two patients (64 and 75 years). The cortical stroke patients had the least time since the incident (4 ± 2.7 months); the spinal cord group had approximately double that time (8.1 ± 11 months), and the subcortical group the longest time since the incident (15.1 ± 19 months).

TABLE 12.1

Heart Rate Asymmetry at Different Stages

Stage Transition	Cortical Stroke	Subcortical Stroke	Spinal Cord	Control
S3–S4	0.27 ± 0.6	0.57 ± 0.34	0.45 ± 0.1	0.04 ± 0.05
S4–S5	0.13 ± 0.1	0.4 ± 0.2	0.37 ± 0.1	0.18 ± 0.05

S3, underchallenged; S4, appropriately challenged; S5, overchallenged.

12.11 Discussion

Robot-assisted training is an important component of neural rehabilitation and requires motivation and mental engagement for optimal task execution. In a previous report, we showed that healthy subjects differ in their steady-state outcome to different levels of physical–mental stimulation tasks as measured by HRV, respiration rate, and skin conductance level when steady state was reached for each of the three levels of challenge (Koenig et al. 2011b).

Cortical responsiveness and engagement, as indicated by the level of HRV, is an important component in any rehabilitation exercise and possibly more difficult in poststroke patients where adaptation to the task is an important attribute that translates into the extent of motivation. Stipulating a corticocardiac axis allows the inference that changes in HRV reflect cortical arousal and motivation to a task. Adaptation to task difficulty is clearly a reflection of mental engagement and identifiable by HRV analysis as shown in control subjects, where SD1 and CCM both increased significantly from rest only while transitioning from an underchallenged condition to an appropriately challenged condition. Appropriate cortical activity is an important component of neurophysiological and neuropsychological rehabilitation as the adaptive phase of mental and physical exertion when a novel task is presented provides more accurate information on the capacity of the system, which is hidden in part when the system reaches steady state. The advantages of using a Poincaré plot and its SD1 measure and CCM is that these variables are robust against the nonstationarity, respiration, and ectopics of the ECG signal (Karmakar et al. 2010, 2011).

Importantly, we found that the level of challenge is important in how HRV changes and reflects possible cortical activity. Standing to walking and underchallenged to challenged transitions brought about the largest cortical response. Initial conditions of inactivity prior to the exercise session might be partially responsible for the large adaptation observed in the standing to walking transition. Similarly the transition from underchallenged to challenged increases motivation and cortical activity and therefore the HRV. Further, the level of adaptation dropped for challenged to overchallenged for both SD1 and CCM back toward the walking to underchallenged transition level. This may be due to physical or cognitive stress, both of which would result in a parasympathetic withdrawal and therefore a lower HRV. HRV is linked to cortical as well as brainstem modulation with the prefrontal cortex having an inhibitory influence on brainstem nuclei, which in turn inhibits parasympathetic output and therefore the level of HRV (Thayer and Lane 2009). The decrease in SD1 and CCM when the overchallenged condition commenced indicates a withdrawal of the frontal cortex and emotional positive output. Therefore, the inhibitory output to the brainstem is reduced leading to increased inhibition of the parasympathetic output and therefore a balance toward sympathetic drive and a decrease in HRV.

References

Abásolo, D., R. Hornero, C. Gómez, M. García, and M. López. 2006. Analysis of EEG background activity in Alzheimer's disease patients with Lempel-Ziv complexity and central tendency measure. *Med Eng Phys* 28(4):315–322.

Acharya, U.R., K.P. Joseph, N. Kannathal, C.M. Lim, and J.S. Suri. 2006. Heart rate variability: A review. *Med Bio Eng Comput* 44:1031–1051.

Alm, P.A. 2004. Stuttering, emotions, and heart rate during anticipatory anxiety: A critical review. *J Fluency Disord* 29(2):123–133. doi: 10.1016/j.jfludis.2004.02.001.

Amarenco, P., L.B. Goldstein, H. Sillesen, O. Benavente, R.M. Zweifler, A. Callahan, M.G. Hennerici, J.A. Zivin, K.M.A. Welch, and on behalf of the SPARCL Investigators. 2010. Coronary heart disease risk in patients with stroke or transient ischemic attack and no known coronary heart disease. Findings from the Stroke Prevention by Aggressive Reduction in Cholesterol Levels (SPARCL) trial. *Stroke* 41:426–430. doi: 10.1161/strokeaha.109.564781.

Andreassi, J.L. 2007. *Psychophysiology: Human Behavior and Physiological Response*. 5th ed. London, Mahwah: Lawrence Erlbaum Associates.

Boyd, L.A. and C.J. Winstein. 2006. Explicit information interferes with implicit motor learning of both continuous and discrete movement tasks after stroke. *J Neurol Phys Therapy* 30(2):46–57. doi: 10.1097/01.NPT.0000282566.48050.9b.

Bradley, M.M. and P.J. Lang. 1994. Measuring emotion: The self-assessment manikin and the semantic differential. *J Behav Ther Exp Psychiatry* 25(1):49–59. doi: 10.1016/0005-7916(94)90063-9.

Broadbent, D.E. 1971. *Decision and Stress*. London: Academic Press.

Cao, W.H., W. Fan, and S.F. Morrison. 2004. Medullary pathways mediating specific sympathetic responses to activation of dorsomedial hypothalamus. *Neuroscience* 126(1):229–240. doi: 10.1016/j.neuroscience.2004.03.013.

Costa, M., A.L. Goldberger, and C-K. Peng. 2002. Multiscale entropy analysis of complex physiologic time series. *Phys Rev Lett* 89(6). doi: 10.1103/PhysRevLett.89.068102.

Crandall, C.G. and T.E. Wilson. 2015. Human cardiovascular responses to passive heat stress. *Compr Physiol* 5(1):17–43. doi: 10.1002/cphy.c140015.

de la Cruz Torres, B., C.L. Lopez, and J. Naranjo Orellana. 2008. Analysis of heart rate variability at rest and during aerobic exercise: A study in healthy people and cardiac patients. *Br J Sports Med* 42(9):715–720. doi: 10.1136/bjsm.2007.043646.

Delaney, J.P.A. and D.A. Brodie. 2000. Effects of short-term psychological stress on the time and frequency domains of heart-rate variability. *Percept Mot Skills* 91(2):515–524.

Guzik, P., J. Piskorski, T. Krauze, A. Schneider, K.H. Wesseling, and H. Wykretowicz. 2007. Correlations between the Poincaré plot and conventional heart rate variability parameters assessed during paced breathing. *J Physiol Sci* 57(1):63–71. doi: 10.2170/physiolsci.RP005506.

Hamilton, P.S. and W.J. Tompkins. 1986. Quantitative investigation of QRS detection rules using the MIT/BIH arrhythmia database. *IEEE Trans Biomed Eng* 33(12):1157–1165.

Han, B.H., M.L. Zhou, A.W. Johnson, I. Singh, F. Liao, A.K. Vellimana, J.W. Nelson, E.Milner, J.R. Cirrito, J. Basak, M. Yoo, H.H. Dietrich, D.M. Holtzman, and G.J. Zipfel. 2015. Contribution of reactive oxygen species to cerebral amyloid angiopathy, vasomotor dysfunction, and microhemorrhage in aged Tg2576 mice. *Proc Natl Acad Sci U S A* 112(8):E881–890. doi: 10.1073/pnas.1414930112.

Higuchi, T. 1998. Approach to an irregular time series on the basis of fractal theory. *Physica D* 31(2):277–283.

Huikuri, H.V., T.H. Mäkikallio, and J. Perkiömäki. 2003. Measurement of heart rate variability by methods based on nonlinear dynamics. *J Electrocardiol* 36 (Suppl 1):95–99.

Huikuri, H.V., J.O. Valkama, K.E. Airaksinen, T. Seppänen, K.M. Kessler, J.T. Takkunen, and R.J. Myerburg. 1993. Frequency domain measures of heart rate variability before the onset of nonsustained and sustained ventricular tachycardia in patients with coronary artery disease. *Circulation* 87(4):1220–1228.

Ivanov, P., L.A.N. Amaral, A.L. Goldberger, S. Havlin, M. Rosenblum, Z.R. Struzik, and H. Eugene Stanley. 1999. Multifractality in human heartbeat dynamics. *Nature* 399:461–465.

Jelinek, H.F., K.G. August, M.H. Imam, A.H. Khandoker, K. Khalaf, A. Koenig, R. Riener, and M. Palaniswami. 2014. Influence of stroke location on heart rate variability in robot-assistive neurorehabilitation. 2nd Middle East Conference on Biomedical Engineering, Doha, Qatar, Feb. 17–20, 2014.

Jelinek, H.F., K.G. August, M.H. Imam, A.H. Khandoker, A. Koenig, and R. Riener. 2011a. Cortical response to psycho-physiological changes in auto-adaptive robot assisted gait training. *Conf Proc IEEE Eng Med Biol Soc* 2011:7409–7412. doi: 10.1109/iembs.2011.6091725.

Jelinek, H.F., K. August, A. Khandoker, H.M. Issam, A. Koenig, and R. Riener. 2011b. Heart rate asymmetry in post stroke patients. Computers in Cardiology, Hangzhou, China.

Karmakar, C.K., A. Khandoker, J. Gubbi, and M. Palaniswami. 2009. Complex correlation measure: A novel desciptor for Poincaré plot. *Biomedical Eng Online* 8(17). http://www.biomedical-engineering-online.com/content/8/1/17.

Karmakar, C.K., A.H. Khandoker, J. Gubbi, and M. Palaniswami. 2011. Defining asymmetry in heart rate variability signals using a Poincare plot. *Physiol Meas* 30:1227–1240. doi: 10.1088/0967-3334/30/11/007.

Karmakar, C., A. Khandoker, and M. Palaniswami. 2010. Heart rate asymmetry in altered parasympathetic nervous system activity. Computers in Cardiology, Belfast, Ireland.

Karmakar, C., A. Khandoker, A. Voss, and M. Palaniswami. 2011. Sensitivity of temporal heart rate variability in Poincare plot to changes in parasympathetic nervous system activity. *Biomed Eng Online* 10(1):17.

Khandoker, A.H., H.F. Jelinek, T. Moritani, and M. Palaniswami. 2010. Association of cardiac autonomic neuropathy with alteration of sympatho-vagal balance through heart rate variability analysis. *Med Eng Phys* 32(2):161–167. doi: 10.1016/j.medengphy.2009.11.005.

Khandoker, A.H., H.F. Jelinek, and M. Palaniswami. 2009a. Cardiac autonomic neuropathy associated alteration of sympatho-vagal balance through the tone entropy analysis of heart periods. In *Computing in Cardiology: 2009 36th Annual Computers in Cardiology Conference*, edited by A. Murray, 373–375. New York, NY: IEEE.

Khandoker, A., H.F. Jelinek, and M. Palaniswami. 2009b. Identifying diabetic patients with cardiac autonomic neuropathy by heart rate variability. *Biomed Eng Online* 8(3). doi: 10.1186/1475-925X-8-3.

Kim, D.H., L.A. Lipsitz, L. Ferrucci, R. Varadhan, J.M. Guralnik, M.C. Carlson, L.A. Fleisher, L.P. Fried, and P.H.M. Chaves. 2006. Association between reduced heart rate variability and cognitive impairment in older disabled women in the community: Women's Health and Aging Study I. *J Am Geriatr Soc* 54(11):1751–1757. doi: 10.1111/j.1532-5415.2006.00940.x.

Koenig, A., X. Omlin, J. Bergmann, L. Zimmerli, M. Bolliger, F. Muller, and R. Riener. 2011a. Controlling patient participation during robot-assisted gait training. *J Neuroeng Rehabil* 8(1):14.

Koenig, A., X. Omlin, L. Zimmerli, M. Sapa, C. Krewer, M. Bolliger, F. Mueller, and R. Riener. 2011b. Psychological state estimation from physiological recordings during robot assisted gait rehabilitation. *J Rehabil Res Dev* 48:4–14.

Krznaric, R. 2014. *Empathy: A Handbook for Revolution*. London: Random House.

Lake, D.E., J.S. Richman, M.P. Griffin, and J.R. Moorman. 2002. Sample entropy analysis of neonatal heart rate variability. *Am J Physiol Regul Integr Comp Physiol* 283(3):R789–797. doi: 10.1152/ajpregu.00069.2002.

Lakusic, N., D. Mahovic, and T. Babic. 2005. Gradual recovery of impaired cardiac autonomic balance within first six months after ischemic cerebral stroke. *Acta Neurol Belg* 105(1):39–42.

Lakusic, N., D. Mahovic, T. Babic, and D. Sporis. 2003. Changes in autonomic control of heart rate after ischemic cerebral stroke. *Acta Med Croatica* 57(4):269–273.

Lane, R.D., K. McRae, E.M. Reiman, K. Chen, G.L. Ahern, and J.F. Thayer. 2009. Neural correlates of heart rate variability during emotion. *Neuroimage* 44:213–222.

Lanier, J. 2010. *You Are Not a Gadget: A Manifesto*. New York, NY: Random House.

Law, M.R., J.K. Morris, and N.J. Wald. 2009. Use of blood pressure lowering drugs in the prevention of cardiovascular disease: Meta-analysis of 147 randomised trials in the context of expectations from prospective epidemiological studies. *BMJ* 338:b1665. doi: 10.1136/bmj.b1665.

Lazarus, R.S. and S. Folkman. 1987. Transactional theory and research on emotions and coping. *Eur J Personality* 1:141–170.

Liberini, P., E.P. Pioro, D. Maysinger, and A.C. Cuello. 1994. Neocortical infarction in subhuman primates leads to restricted morphological damage of the cholinergic neurons in the nucleus basalis of Meynert. *Brain Res* 648(1):1–8.

Liutkiene, G., R. Stropus, A. Dabuzinskiene, and M. Pilmane. 2007. Structural changes of the human superior cervical ganglion following ischemic stroke. *Medicina (Kaunas)* 43(5):390–398.

Lombardi, F, T.H. Mäkikallio, R.J. Myerburg, and H.V. Huikuri. 2001. Sudden cardiac death: Role of HRV to identify patients at risk. *Cardiovasc Res* 50:210–217.

Maddux, J., ed. 1995. *Self-Efficacy, Adaptation, and Adjustment: Theory, Research, and Application.* New York, NY: Plenum Press.

Makimattila, S, A. Schlenzka, M. Mäntysaari, R. Bergholm, P. Summanen, P. Saar, H. Erkkila, and H. Yki-Jarvinen. 2000. Predictors of abnormal cardiovascular autonomic function measured by frequency domain analysis of heart rate variability and conventional tests in patients with type 1 diabetes. *Diabetes Care* 23(11):1686–1693.

Matthews, S., H. Jelinek, S. Vafaeiafraz, and C. S. McLachlan. 2012. Heart rate stability and decreased parasympathetic heart rate variability in healthy young adults during perceived stress. *Int J Cardiol* 156(3):337–338. doi: 10.1016/j.ijcard.2012.02.004.

Mazzoni, P. and J.W. Krakauer. 2006. An implicit plan overrides an explicit strategy during visuomotor adaptation. *J Neurosci* 26(14):3642–3645. doi: 10.1523/jneurosci.5317-05.2006.

McCraty, R., M. Atkinson, W.A. Tiller, G. Rein, and A.D. Watkins. 1995. The effects of emotions on short-term power spectrum analysis of heart rate variability. *Am J Cardiol* 76(14):1089–1093.

McDonagh, D., A. Bruseburg, and C. Haslam. 2002. Visual evaluation: Exploring users' emotional relationships with products. *Appl Ergon* 33(3):237–246.

McEwen, B.S. 2007. Physiology and neurobiology of stress and adaptation: Central role of the brain. *Physiol Rev* 87(3):873–904. doi: 10.1152/physrev.00041.2006.

Minichiello, M.A. 2012. Drawing for visual communication. Design Research Society Bangkok, Thailand.

Oida, E., T. Kannagi, T. Moritani, and Y. Yamori. 1999. Aging alteration of cardiac vagosympathetic balance assessed through the tone-entropy analysis. *J Gerontol A Biol Sci Med Sci* 54(5):M219–M224. doi: 10.1093/gerona/54.5.M219.

Olshansky, B., H.N. Sabbah, P. J. Hauptman, and W.S. Colucci. 2008. Parasympathetic nervous system and heart failure. *Circulation* 118(8):863–871. doi: 10.1161/circulationaha.107.760405.

Osipova, M.A., V.V. Arkov, and A.G. Tonevitsky. 2010. Modulation of alpha-rhythm and autonomic status of human by color photostimulation. *Bull Exp Biol Med* 149(6):759–762.

Pagani, M., S. Guzzetti, G. Sandrone, E. Piccaluga, F. Lombardi, S. Cerutti, and A. Malliani. 1986. Power spectral analysis as a clinical tool. In *Neural Mechanisms and Cardiovascular Disease*, edited by B. Lown, Malliani, A., and Prosdocimi, M, 265–270. Padova: Liviana Press.

Pagani, M., G. Mazzuero, A. Ferrari, D. Liberati, S. Cerutti, and D. Vaitl. 1991. Sympathovagal interaction during mental stress: A study using spectral analysis of heart rate variability in healthy control subjects and patients with a prior myocardial infarction. *Circulation* 83(4 Suppl 2):43–51.

Paolucci, S. 2008. Epidemiology and treatment of post-stroke depression. *Neuropsychiatr Dis Treat* 4(1):145–154.

Peng, C.K., S. Havlin, H.E. Stanley, and A.L. Goldberger. 1995. Quantification of scaling exponents and crossover phenomena in nonstationary heartbeat time series. *Chaos* 5(1):82–87. doi: 10.1063/1.166141.

Pincus, S.M. and A.L. Goldberger. 1994. Physiological time-series analysis: What does regularity quantify? *Am J Physiol Heart Circ Physiol* 266(4):H1643–1656.

Piskorski, J. and P. Guzik. 2007. Geometry of the Poincare plot of RR intervals and its asymmetry in healthy hearts. *Physiol Meas* 28:287–300.

Porges, S.W. 1995. Cardiac vagal tone—A physiological index of stress. *Neurosci Biobehav Rev* 19(2):225–233.

Porges, S.W. 2001. The polyvagal theory: Phylogenetic substrates of a social nervous system. *Int J Psychophysiol* 42:123–146.

Porges, S.W. 2007. The polyvagal theory. *Biol Psychiatr* 74(2):116–143.

Porta, A., K.R. Casali, A.G. Casali, T. Gnecchi-Ruscone, E. Tovaldini, N. Montano, S. Lange, D. Geue, D. Cysarz, and P.V. Leeuwen. 2008. Temporal asymmetries of short-term heart period variability are linked to autonomic regulation. *Am J Physiol—Regul Integr Comp Physiol* 295:R550557.

Quintana, D.S., A.J. Guastella, T. Outhred, I.B. Hickie, and A.H. Kemp. 2012. Heart rate variability is associated with emotion recognition: Direct evidence for a relationship between the autonomic nervous system and social cognition. *Int J Psychophysiol* 86(2):168–172. doi: 10.1016/j.ijpsycho.2012.08.012.

Rittel, H. and M. Webber. 1984. Dilemmas in a general theory of planning. In *Developments in Design Methodology*, edited by N. Cross, 135–144. Cichester: Wiley & Sons.

Roberts, A.H. 1970a. Neurological complications of systemic diseases. I. *Br Med J* 1(5687):33–35.

Roberts, A.H. 1970b. Neurological complications of systemic diseases. II. *Br Med J* 1(5688):95–97.

Schubert, C., M. Lambertz, R.A. Nelesen, W. Bardwell, J.-B. Choid, and J.E. Dimsdaleb. 2009. Effects of stress on heart rate complexity—A comparison between short-term and chronic stress. *Biol Psychol* 80(3):325–332.

Srinivasan, K., M. Vaz, and S. Sucharita. 2006. A study of stress and autonomic nervous function in first year undergraduate medical students. *Indian J Physiol Pharmacol* 50(3):257–264.

Stein, P.K., P.P. Domitrovich, H.V. Huikuri, and R.E. Kleiger. 2005. Traditional and nonlinear heart rate variability are each independently associated with mortality after myocardial infarction. *J Cardiovasc Electrophysiol* 16(1):13–20.

Stinear, C.M. and W.D. Byblow. 2014. Predicting and accelerating motor recovery after stroke. *Curr Opin Neurol* 27(6):624–630. doi: 10.1097/wco.0000000000000153.

Struzik, Z.R., J. Hayano, S. Sakata, S. Kwak, and Y. Yamamoto. 2004. 1/f scaling in heartrate requires antagonistic autonomic control. *Phys Rev E* 70:050901(R).

Takahashi, C., H.E. Hinson, and I.J. Baguley. 2015. Autonomic dysfunction syndromes after acute brain injury. *Handb Clin Neurol* 128:539–551. doi: 10.1016/b978-0-444-63521-1.00034-0.

Teich, M.C., S.B. Lowen, B.M. Jost, and K. Vibe-Rheymer, eds. 2001. Heart rate variability: Measures and models. In *Nonlinear Biomedical Signal Processing, Dynamic Analysis and Modeling*, edited by M. Akay, Vol. 2. New York, NY: IEEE Press.

TFESC. 1996. Special report: Heart rate variability standards of measurement, physiological interpretation, and clinical use. *Circulation* 93(5):1043–1065.

Thayer, J.F., F. Åhs, M. Fredrikson, J.J. Sollers III, and T.D Wager. 2012. A meta-analysis of heart rate variability and neuroimaging studies: Implications for heart rate variability as a marker of stress and health. *Neurosci Biobehav Rev* 36:747–756.

Thayer, J.F., A.L. Hansen, E. Saus-Rose, and B.H. Johnsen. 2009. Heart rate variability, prefrontal neural function, and cognitive performance: The neurovisceral integration perspective on self-regulation, adaptation and health. *Ann Behav Med* 37:141–153. doi: 10.1007/s12160-009-9101-z.

Thayer, J.F. and R.D. Lane. 2009. Claude Bernard and the heart-brain connection: Further elaboration of a model of neurovisceral integration. *Neurosci Biobehav Rev* 33(2):81–88. doi: 10.1016/j.neubiorev.2008.08.004.

Tulppo, M. and H.V. Huikuri. 2004. Origin and significance of heart rate variability. *J Am Coll Cardiol* 43(12):2278–2280. doi: 10.1016/j.jacc.2004.03.034.

Tulppo, M.P., T.H. Mäkikallio, T.E. Takala, and T. Seppänen. 1996. Quantitative beat-to-beat analysis of heart rate dynamics during exercise. *Am J Physiol* 271:H244–H252.

Valenza, G., P. Allegrini, A. Lanata, and E.P. Scilingo. 2012. Dominant Lyapunov exponent and approximate entropy in heart rate variability during emotional visual elicitation. *Front Neuroeng* 5:3.

Viltart, O., O. Mullier, F. Bernet, P. Poulain, S. Ba-M'Hamed, and H. Sequeira. 2003. Motor cortical control of cardiovascular bulbar neurones projecting to spinal autonomic areas. *J Neurosci Res* 73(1):122–135. doi: 10.1002/jnr.10598.

Voss, A., S. Schulz, R. Schroeder, M. Baumert, and P. Caminal. 2009. Methods derived from nonlinear dynamics for analysing heart rate variability. *Philos Trans A Math Phys Eng Sci* 367(1887):277–296. doi: 10.1098/rsta.2008.0232.

Wessel, N., A. Schumann, A. Schirdewan, A. Voss, and J. Kurths. 2000a. Entropy measures in heart rate variability data. *Lect Notes Comput Sci* 1933:78–87.

Wessel, N., A. Voss, H. Malberg, C. Ziehmann, H.U. Voss, A. Schirdewan, U. Meyerfeldt, and J. Kurths. 2000b. Nonlinear analysis of complex phenomena in cardiological data. *Herzschrittmacher Ther Elektrophysiol* 11:159–173.

Yamamoto, Y. and R.L. Hughson. 1991. Coarse-graining spectral analysis: New method for studying heart rate variability. *J Appl Physiol* 71(3):1143–1150.

13

Heart Rate Variability as a Useful Parameter in Assessment of Cardiac Rehabilitation Outcome

Hosen Kiat, Tom Collins, and Herbert F. Jelinek

CONTENTS

13.1 Introduction

This chapter discusses heart rate variability (HRV) analysis as a tool to identify improvement in cardiac function following cardiac rehabilitation (CR). Two main themes are discussed. The use of the Borg Relative Perceived Exertion (RPE) scale and the 6-minute walk test (6MWT) are reviewed as tools for setting an appropriate level of exercise intensity and quantifying the effectiveness of CR, respectively. Cardiac functional changes using HRV are compared following CR and either coronary artery bypass grafting (CABG) or percutaneous coronary angioplasty intervention (PCI) when exercise intensity was based on the more traditional assessment for setting exercise intensity using maximal oxygen uptake (VO_2 max).

13.2 Cardiovascular Disease and CR Programs

Cardiovascular disease (CVD) remains the most significant health issue in Australia and worldwide (Australian Institute of Health and Welfare 2004; Wang et al. 2012). CR programs were developed as a means of slowing CVD progression and the associated health burden (Taylor et al. 2004). The ability of CR interventions to directly reduce the incidence of mortality in those with CVD has been widely documented (Giannuzzi et al. 2003; Leon et al. 2005; Taylor et al. 2004). Recently, Suaya et al. (2009) found a consistent reduction in the mortality over 5 years of patients who enrolled into CR program compared to the same number of patients matched in their pathology, demographics, and clinical profile, but who did not attend CR. The reduction in mortality and the long-term survival benefit continued for the duration of the study (Suaya et al. 2009). Improved cardiac functionality is a likely outcome linked to participation in these rehabilitation programs and the clinical effect of attending CR is similar or greater than that provided by statins, or antihypertensive medications (Hansen et al. 2005).

CR programs involve a formal exercise component, with or without additional education, counseling, and home-exercising. Exercise intensity in these programs is prescribed on the basis of formal testing conducted on entry into the program using either heart rate or oxygen volume measures such as maximum VO_2 (VO_2 max), or using the more subjective Borg RPE scale. In addition, CR effectiveness can be similarly assessed by VO_2 max but also by a 6MWT or HRV.

As such HRV can provide valuable prognostic information regarding the stability of the cardiovascular system and effectiveness of CR programs (TFESC 1996). Reduced HRV is associated with abnormal or insufficient adaptability of the autonomic nervous system (ANS) to internal and external environmental stressors, implying the presence of a physiological malfunction and increased risk of adverse cardiac events (Kleiger et al. 1987; Quintana et al. 1997; Weber et al. 1999). HRV analysis has further shown that CR programs using formal exercise testing have the ability to reduce the likelihood of lethal arrhythmias and sudden cardiac death (SCD) in those with cardiac disease (Malfatto et al. 1998; Iellamo et al. 2000; Stahle et al. 1999).

13.3 Heart Rate Variability

HRV has traditionally been measured by linear methods in the time and frequency domain. Time-domain measures are based on simple statistical methods, either derived from the heart rate or the differences between them (RR intervals) (Tapanainen 2003). It has been shown that specific physiological processes contribute differently to individual components of the HRV spectrum (e.g., high frequency [HF] reflects parasympathetic activity while low frequency (LF) is mediated by primarily sympathetic activity) (Akselrod et al. 1981; Agelink et al. 2001; De Jong and Randal 2005). While these methods have been used successfully, research has shown further prognostic information is available that cannot be examined using linear analyses and is based on linear methods. Complex fluctuations occurring on multiple time scales, treated as uninformative noise by linear analyses and the nonstationarity inherent in biological time signals, are now understood to be indicative of an adaptable system responding to unpredictable stimuli and stress (Goldberger et al. 2002). A loss of this complexity indicates a decrease in the functional responsiveness of the system, making it more vulnerable to abrupt changes and arrhythmia (Goldberger 1997). A large body of literature now clearly demonstrates the advantages of nonlinear analyses, which includes fractal analysis and entropy measures, in fully examining cardiovascular stability (Carney 1997; Huikuri et al. 1994; Tulppo et al. 2005; Vikman et al. 1999; Cornforth et al. 2015; Perkiömäki 2011; Sassi et al. 2009; Goldberger et al. 2002; Kobayashi and Musha 1982; Peng et al. 1995; Gao et al. 2013; Pena et al. 2009; Voss et al. 2009; Stein et al. 2008; Kiyono et al. 2006; Teich et al. 2001; Ivanov et al. 1999).

Measures of HRV illustrate the changes in heart rate over time, which is a function of the intrinsic modulation by the sinoatrial node and the contribution of the ANS to cardiac rhythm and is a valid marker of cardiac autonomic tone.

In the clinical setting, the apparent regularity of a healthy heartbeat is commonly termed "regular sinus rhythm" (Peng et al. 1995). However, in healthy subjects, there is considerable variability in the duration of the beat-to-beat interval (RR interval), due to the competing influences of the sympathetic and parasympathetic branches of the ANS as well as other factors, including the endocrine system. It is suggested that to maintain health, this physiological control mechanism and the ensuing beat-to-beat interval must be able to vary over a wide range to provide flexible adaptation (Bassingthwaighte et al. 1994). Essentially, higher values of HRV seen in healthy subjects are indicative of greater fluctuation and an adaptable system responding to various influences necessary to maintain a physiologically healthy heart rhythm. By the same token, HRV is most often decreased (although increases can also be observed that are deemed pathological) in those with cardiac pathology as a result of decreased parasympathetic activity, increased sympathetic activity, or a combination of both (Frenneaux 2007). Patients with diabetes mellitus, heart failure, postmyocardial infarction, and uncomplicated coronary artery disease all have significant reductions in HRV, placing these individuals at an increased risk of ventricular fibrillation and SCD (Migliaro et al. 2003; Nolan et al. 1998; Tapanainen 2003; Wennerblom et al. 2000). A significant number of studies have now validated the use of HRV analysis as an independent predictor of mortality in patients with CVD (Bigger et al. 1992; Zuanetti et al. 1996; Evrengul et al. 2006; Huikuri et al. 2001; Lake et al. 2002). When compared with other cardiovascular risk factors, HRV has proven to be superior in its ability to predict mortality (Nolan et al. 1998; Tsuji et al. 1996). Findings from these studies have led to the widespread acceptance of the negative prognostic implications of a reduced HRV and spurred a growing interest into modifications that may alter autonomic balance in a favorable direction. CR programs offer this possibility.

13.4 HRV, Exercise, and CR

The benefits of exercise for both the primary and secondary reduction of cardiovascular-related mortality have been extensively documented (Warburton et al. 2006; Murphy et al. 2007; McCauley 2007; Smidt et al. 2005; Houde and Melillo 2002). Improvements in body composition, enhanced lipid lipoprotein profiles, improved autonomic tone, improved glucose control and insulin sensitivity, reduced blood pressure, improved coronary blood flow, and enhanced endothelial function following exercise training undoubtedly contribute to the higher levels of health demonstrated in active individuals (American College of Cardiology, American Heart Association, and European Society of Cardiology 2006; Warburton et al. 2006).

Given the association between ANS dysfunction and SCD, the capacity of exercise to shift this balance in a favorable direction has been investigated (Lahiri et al. 2008). A large number of studies have shown that exercise training increases HRV in athletes, sedentary individuals, and patients with CVD (Rennie et al. 2003; Iellamo et al. 2000; Malfatto et al. 1996, 1998; Stahle et al. 1999; La Rovere et al. 1992; Coats et al. 1992; Kouidi et al. 2002; Deligiannis et al. 2015; Karjalainen et al. 2015; Neves et al. 2011; Hautala et al. 2004; Tulppo et al. 2003). These increases in HRV reflect an enhancement of autonomic tone, which is known to increase the threshold for ventricular fibrillation and decrease the risk of cardiac mortality (Deligiannis 1994). Therefore, the favorable alteration in autonomic tone may be the most significant benefit to be gained from exercise training in patients with preexisting cardiac conditions (Jelinek et al. 2013).

La Rovere et al. (1992) first examined the impact of a structured in-hospital physical training program in 22 patients following a recent myocardial infarction. Participants in this study trained at 75% of their anaerobic threshold in the first week, which progressed to 95% in their fourth week. Researchers did not stipulate the frequency of exercise sessions per week. Physical training caused an increase in HRV measured by time- and frequency-domain analyses, indicating improved autonomic balance in this population (La Rovere et al. 1992).

Malfatto et al. (1996) also found a favorable shift in autonomic balance in postmyocardial infarction patients following exercise based on results of HRV analysis. The population sample in this study was comparable to that in La Rovere et al. (1992) with respect to age (mean was 47 and 52, respectively, both studies excluding those aged > 70 years) and gender (22 males, 0 female and 28 males, 2 females). Exercise training in this study was also highly monitored, requiring participants to train for 1 hour at 80% of their maximal heart rate, 5 days per week for the 8-week program (Malfatto et al. 1996). Similar to the findings of La Rovere et al., linear analyses highlighted a persistent increase in parasympathetic tone on completion of the CR program. Using the same exercise protocol and HRV measures in a similar population sample as their earlier study, Malfatto et al. further examined the factors that may alter autonomic balance with their investigation into the interaction between CR and beta-blocker therapy. They concluded that both therapies resulted in a favorable shift in autonomic balance toward an increased parasympathetic tone (Malfatto et al. 1998).

An Australian study compared the HRV responses between in-hospital CR (4 days per week for 6 weeks) and a home-walking program (Leitch et al. 1997). The CR group trained for 30 minutes in the first week, progressing to 60 minutes by the third week, at 70% of maximum heart rate. Participants of CR were provided with the same home-walking program as the walking group. All measures of cardiac autonomic function (linear HRV analysis and baroreflex testing) improved in both the home-based and hospital-based programs.

Stahle et al. (1999) investigated the impact of CR on HRV in an elderly population sample (over 65 years, 81 males, and 20 females) following an acute coronary event. Participants were randomly assigned to either 3 months of supervised exercise training performed 3 times per week or a control group. On the training days, the CR group trained at 85% of their maximal heart rate (determined from maximal exercise test) for 50 minutes. Researchers used linear HRV analyses to demonstrate that improvements in HRV following exercise training are possible in an older population with cardiac disease (Stahle et al. 1999).

It has also been shown that short periods of rehabilitation with intense exercise regimes have a beneficial impact on cardiovascular function. Oya et al. demonstrated improvements in autonomic after just 2 weeks of exercise training, commencing 1 week after myocardial infarction. Participants in this study trained twice daily for 30 minutes at the anaerobic threshold level to achieve improvements in linear HRV parameters (Oya et al. 1999). A similar exercise protocol (2 weeks of training at 85% of maximum heart rate, 6 days per week) demonstrated improved cardiac autonomic function in a male population following CABG using linear HRV analysis and baroreflex sensitivity tests (Iellamo et al. 2000).

Other studies have shown no effect on both linear and nonlinear HRV measures despite improvements in exercise capacity (Duru et al. 2000; Oliveira et al. 2014). The discrepancies between the results of different studies have raised important methodological issues when assessing the effect of CR and HRV changes. These include controlling breathing frequency, lifestyle factors, and dietary habits, all of which may influence HRV analysis. Other factors such as time following the myocardial infarct, whether PCI or CABG was the intervention, and how long since the intervention that CR was commenced needs to be further investigated. Long-term recovery of the ANS activity and cardiac function is another important consideration. Following CABG and a 2-week CR program (consisting of 30-minute cycling twice daily) commenced 1-week postsurgery, an improvement in HRV, exercise capacity, and significantly decreased plasma norepinephrine levels was observed in the training group. However, parasympathetic function (HF power) did not improve until 3 months after the intervention (Takeyama et al. 2000) and did not reach the age-matched normal value even 1 year after surgery (Table 13.1). A comparison of HRV outcomes following either CABG or PCI and CR follows in the next section.

13.4.1 CR Following CABG or PCI

Many reported studies have not differentiated between CR effectiveness following CABG and PCI, which are known to have different postintervention recovery profiles. Cardiac function and rhythm following CABG or PCI differ with parasympathetic function reduced in patients early following PCI and returning to preintervention level quicker, whereas cardiac rhythm may remain suboptimal up to several years in post-CABG patients (Wennerblom et al. 2000; Cygankiewicz et al. 2004; Wu et al. 2005; Laitio et al. 2007; Janowska-Kulińska et al. 2009). However, data evaluating the impact of CR on HRV in outpatients after CABG are limited (Iellamo et al. 2000; Baumert et al. 2011). Overall return to near normal sinus cardiac rhythm measured by HRV is not as pronounced in patients with greater than one affected target vessel and/or with other comorbidities, regardless of cardiac intervention (Tseng et al. 1996; Birand et al. 1998; Wennerblom et al. 2000; Kanadasi et al. 2002). Following elective coronary angiography, decreased HRV is a reliable and independent predictor of mortality in patients without prior myocardial infarction (Compostella et al. 2017).

TABLE 13.1

Investigations into the Effect of Cardiac Rehabilitation on HRV

Study	Duration	Frequency of Training	Participant Age (mean)	Sex M/F	HRV Effects
La Rovere et al. (1992)	4 weeks	Not specified	47 ± 6 years	22/0	Improved
Malfatto et al. (1996)	8 weeks	5 days/week	54 ± 7 years	28/2	Improved
Leitch et al. (1997)	6 weeks	4 days/week	57 ± 1 years	39/10	No change
Malfatto et al. (1998)	8 weeks	5 days/week	40–66 years	47/6	Improved
Oya et al. (1999)	2 weeks	2× daily 7 days/week	59 ± 6 years	26/2	Improved
Stahle et al. (1999)	3 months	3 days/week	71 ± 4 years	81/20	Improved
Iellamo et al. (2000)	2 weeks	2× daily 6 days/week	58 ± 7 years	86/0	Improved
Takeyama et al. (2000)	2 weeks	2× daily 7 days/week	58.8 ± 6 years	13/0	Improved
Duru et al. (2000)	8 weeks	2× daily 7 days/week	56 ± 5 years	12/0	Limited improvement
Jelinek et al. (2013)	6 weeks	3 days/week	63.7 ± 9.4 years	31/7	CABG improved, PCI no change
Oliveira et al. (2014)	8 weeks	3 days/week	56 ± 10 years	19/28	No change

A recent study investigated the impact on HRV of a short-term, 6-week CR applied to post-CABG and post-PCI during an outpatient CR program and how this compared to current measures of exercise capacity using the 6MWT and cardiorespiratory function (VO_2 max). In this study, participants were recruited at the same time post-CABG and post-PCI and attended the CR program three times per week over a 6-week period. Each participant was given an individualized exercise program consisting of aerobic exercise and was encouraged to maintain a low to moderate intensity throughout exercise sessions.

Participants were also advised to complete a home-walking program, as recommended by the National Heart Foundation, to achieve 30 minutes of moderate intensity physical activity on most or all days of the week. Sixteen participants entered the program following CABG and 22 following PCI. Clinically significant improvements in exercise capacity were observed in both groups. The CR program led to no significant changes in the HRV indices in the PCI group. However, a significant increase was seen for standard deviation of NN (SDNN), LF, and HF in the CABG group similar to previous findings (Iellamo et al. 2000). This study did not show that CR improved the parasympathetic tone and autonomic balance following PCI, contrary to previous findings (Lucini et al. 2002; Tsai et al. 2006). The study was however based on low-intensity interval exercise training, which may account for the difference in HRV outcome. Therefore, CR may have a greater effect in patients with more advanced cardiac dysfunction necessitating CABG. Physiologically, the CABG group had lower HF power at baseline compared to the PCI group and thus for HRV to return to a preintervention or preclinical level a greater improvement in HF power following CR may have been possible (Jelinek et al. 2013). In addition, the extent of improvements in HRV, as reported by Munk et al. and others, may be a function of exercise intensity and duration of the program (Munk et al. 2009; Tsai et al. 2006).

Following PCI, it has been shown that HRV indices decrease, in particular parasympathetic-related measures such as HF power (Airaksinen et al. 1993; Wennerblom et al. 2000; Kanadasi et al. 2002). The results of some studies indicated that this drop in HRV is accompanied by increased sympathetic tone but recovers quickly (Tseng et al. 1996; Bonnemeier et al. 2000). Moreover, a variable reaction was also observed, that is, a decrease in some patients and an increase in others depending on time to reperfusion (Szydlo et al. 1998; Bonnemeier et al. 2000). A difference in the findings between the CABG and PCI groups might have resulted from either the extent of collateral circulation being present or the number of occluded arteries. However, collateral circulation produces only slight improvement in myocardial perfusion following PCI, contrary to the subjects without collateral circulation presenting a sudden change in myocardial perfusion, with previous results confirming these findings, as a group with CABG having three or more vessels obstructed showed more improvement compared to the PCI group (Berry et al. 2007).

13.5 The Borg RPE as a Measure of Exercise Capacity

Formal exercise prescription in CR is based on the findings of either a maximal or submaximal exercise test. Results from these tests are used to ensure that participants maintained the required percentage of their maximal heart rate or VO_2 max throughout the program.

However, there is debateable relevance of this current worldwide practice outside of major CR facilities. The exercise regimes employed by many of the studies reported here from major metropolitan rehabilitation programs have been tightly controlled, prescribing and monitoring training intensity according to the findings of an initial graded exercise test (such as VO_2 max testing). Using these methods allows CR providers to choose a targeted training intensity to elicit desired training responses and provide a mechanism for more accurate selection of training intensity. However, completing the initial graded exercise test is an expensive and potentially onerous task for CR providers to undertake and patients to perform. Therefore, an increasing number of CR providers are moving away from programs based on formal exercise testing to those based on the more subjective Borg RPE scale (Joo et al. 2004; Whaley et al. 1997; Borg 1982). An increasing number of CR programs are now prescribing training intensity using the Borg RPE scale. This scale is a more viable option in CR in local centers as it does not require expensive equipment and lengthy testing procedures, and is unaffected by medications that commonly alter heart rate responses to exercise (Joo et al. 2004; Whaley et al. 1997). The Borg RPE consists of a vertical scale from 6 to 20 with corresponding verbal expressions of progressively increasing sensation intensity (Borg 1982; Mador et al. 1995; Fletcher et al. 1996; Hansen et al. 2005). Participants of CR programs are most commonly advised to exercise at a level of 12–13/20 ("somewhat hard") on this scale, which approximates 55%–69% of maximal heart rate (Fletcher et al. 2001; Pollock et al. 1998; National Heart Foundation of Australia and Australian Cardiac Rehabilitation Association 2004). Studies have shown training with the RPE scale produces equivalent responses to measures of heart rate, VO_2 max, and lactate threshold (Chen et al. 2002, Dunbar et al. 1996, Kang et al. 2003, Potteiger and Evans 1995). The RPE scale has therefore been readily adopted under the assumption that subsequent health outcomes would also be comparable. However, it is important to consider whether equivalent physiological outcomes (i.e., an improved cardiac autonomic balance) can be expected following participation in a CR exercise programs using the Borg RPE scale. While studies have shown that there are no differences between the two approaches in terms of their ability to improve modifiable risk factors and improve exercise capacity (Ilarraza et al. 2004; McConnel et al. 1998), data evaluating the clinical applicability of HRV using the Borg RPE are limited.

In the study by Jelinek et al. (2014), the CR program was conducted over a 6-week period. HRV and 6MWT measures were collected at the start and again following completion of the program (Jelinek et al. 2014). Inclusion criteria for the study were in accordance with the inclusion criteria for the CR program at the Albury Base Hospital located in rural Southeast Australia. This program receives referrals from inpatient settings following acute events and revascularization procedures, or direct referrals from general practitioners and specialists. No exclusions were made on the basis of age, gender, or cardiac condition with the aim of increasing the generalizability and external validity of findings. Participants were however excluded if they were unable to complete the CR program within the 6-week period or could not participate fully in the designated exercise program. A total of 22 participants agreed to take part in the study, 15 of whom were used for the final analysis. HRV values were gathered from a group of age-matched controls without known cardiac disease. Each participant was given an individualized exercise program devised by a physiotherapist according to individual physical capabilities. In accordance with recommendations of the National Heart Foundation of Australia (NHF), all participants were encouraged to maintain a low to moderate intensity, or between 10 and 13/20 on the Borg RPE scale throughout the exercise sessions. In addition, participants were prescribed a home-walking program to achieve 30 minutes of moderate intensity physical activity on most or all days of the week. Compliance with the home-walking program was assessed through self-report, using an exercise diary. A 20-minute 12-lead electrocardiogram (ECG) recording (CardioPerfect, Welsh Allyn, Australia) was obtained and frequency-domain measures such as LF and HF power determined. The 6MWT was conducted twice on the initial assessment to allow for a learning effect in accordance with the American Thoracic Society Guidelines. Chi-square analysis was used to allow for grouping of HRV data into positive change, negative change, and no change in HRV and 6MWT. Positive change was considered as > 10% move toward the group norm, negative change was considered as > 10% away from the expected group norm, and no change was considered < 10% change in either direction. Pre- and posttest results were available for 6MWT from 13 patients and for 15 patients for HRV analysis. Significant differences were seen for LF, HF, and the LF/HF ratio and indicated an improvement in autonomic balance. The current HRV improvements seen based on a RPE scale assessment are in line with previous research with exercise intensity prescribed from a graded maximal exercise test (Iellamo et al. 2000; Leitch et al. 1997; Malfatto et al. 1996, 2002; Oya et al. 1999; Stahle et al. 2010).

13.6 Medication Use in CR

Although medications are known to affect HRV, it is unlikely that they have a dominant effect on results of the current study (Kleiger et al. 1991; Kontopoulos et al. 1996; Sandrone et al. 1994; Malfatto et al. 1998). The most recent of these investigations by Malfatto et al. examined the combined effect of medication and CR on HRV (Malfatto et al. 1998). The HRV of patients who were in CR in addition to taking beta-blockers continued to increase with physical training, indicating a favorable interaction between the two therapies. One finding particularly relevant to HRV analysis was the observation that the percent shift in patients participating in CR in addition to taking beta-blockers was not significantly different from those that were participating in CR alone. Therefore, it can be suggested that those patients taking beta-blockers would most likely experience a similar increase in HRV compared to baseline levels (while these may be higher) to those who are not taking beta-blockers.

13.7 Conclusion

CR interventions are now routine management for patients with CVD as a preventative measure or following cardiac intervention. A large amount of research has shown that exercise programs are capable of inducing both peripheral and cardiopulmonary adaptations that improve health outcomes. These results indicate that CR has the potential to improve cardiac function soon after cardiac intervention. Furthermore, recent research using linear HRV analysis has highlighted that HRV is a valuable parameter to assess effectiveness of more traditional CR programs based on VO_2 max or programs based on the Borg RPE scale.

Acknowledgment

The authors wish to acknowledge the contribution of Jackie Huang, who undertook the data collection.

References

Agelink, M.W., R. Malessa, B. Baumann, T. Majewski, F. Akila, T. Zeit, and D. Ziegler. 2001. Standardized tests of heart rate variability: Normal ranges obtained from 309 healthy humans, and effects of age, gender and heart rate. *Clinical Autonomic Research* 11:99–108.

Airaksinen, K.E., M.J. Ikaheimo, H.V. Huikuri, M.K. Linnaluoto, and J.T. Takkunen. 1993. Responses of heart rate variability to coronary occlusion during coronary angioplasty. *American Journal of Cardiology* 72(14):1026–1030.

Akselrod, S., G. Gordon, F.A. Ubel, D.C. Shannon, A.C. Barger, and R.J. Cohen. 1981. Power spectrum analysis of heart rate fluctuation: A quantitative probe of beat-to-beat cardiovascular control. *Science* 213:220–222.

American College of Cardiology, American Heart Association, and European Society of Cardiology. 2006. Guidelines for management of patients with ventricular arrhythmias and the prevention of sudden cardiac death: A report of the American College of Cardiology/American Heart Association Task Force and the European Society of Cardiology Committee for Practice Guidelines. *Journal of American College of Cardiology* 48:247–346.

Australian Institute of Health and Welfare. 2004. *Heart, Stroke and Vascular Diseases—Australian Facts 2004*. Canberra: AIHW and National Heart Foundation of Australia.

Bassingthwaighte, J.B., L.S. Liebovitch, and B.J. West. 1994. *Fractal Physiology*. New York, NY: Oxford University Press.

Baumert M., M. P. Schlaich, E. Nalivaiko, E. Lambert, C. I. D. M. Sari, Kaye, et al. 2011. Relation between QT interval variability and cardiac sympathetic activity in hypertension. *American Journal of Physiology - Heart and Circulatory Physiology* 300: H1412–H1417. doi: 10.1152/ajpheart.01184.2010.

Berry, C., K.P. Balachandran, P.L. L'Allier, J. Lespérance, R. Bonan, and K.G. Oldroyd. 2007. Importance of collateral circulation in coronary heart disease. *European Heart Journal* 28(3):278.

Bigger, J.T., J.L. Fleiss, R.C. Steinman, L.M. Rolnitzky, R.E. Kleiger, and J.N. Rottman. 1992. Frequency domain measures of heart period variability and mortality after myocardial infarction. *Circulation* 85:164–171.

Birand, A., G.Z. Kudaiberdieva, T.A. Batyraliev, F. Akgul, and S. Saliu. 1998. Relationship between components of heart rate variability and doppler echocardiographic indices of left ventricular systolic performance in patients with coronary artery disease. *International Journal of Angiology* 7(3):244–248.

Bonnemeier, H., F. Hartmannm, U.K.H. Wiegland, C. Irmer, T. Kurz, R. Tölg, H.A. Katus, and Richardt G. 2000. Heart rate variability in patients with acute myocardial infarction undergoing primary coronary angioplasty. *American Journal of Cardiology* 85:815–820.

Borg, G. 1982. Psychophysical bases of perceived exertion. *Medical Science and Sports Exercise* 14:377–381.

Carney, S. 1997. 24-hour blood pressure monitoring: What are the benefits. *Australian Prescriber* 20:18–20.

Chen, M.J., X. Fan, and S.T. Moe. 2002. Criterion-related validity of the Borg ratings of perceived exertion scale in healthy individuals: A meta-analysis. *Journal of Sports Sciences* 20(11):873–899.

Coats, A., S. Adamopoulos, A. Radaelli, A. McCance, T.E. Meyer, L. Bernardi, P.L. Solda, P. Davey, O. Ormerod, C. Forfar, J. Conway, and P. Sleight. 1992. Controlled trial of physical training in chronic heart failure: Exercise performance, hemodynamics, ventilation and autonomic function. *Circulation* 85:2119–2131.

Compostella L., N. Lakusic, C. Compostella, L.V.S. Truong, S. Iliceto, and F. Bellotto. 2017. Does heart rate variability correlate with long-term prognosis in myocardial infarction patients treated by early revascularization? *World Journal of Cardiology* 9(1):27–38. doi: 10.4330/wjc.v9.i1.27.

Cornforth, D., H.F. Jelinek, and M. Tarvainen. 2015. A comparison of nonlinear measures for the detection of cardiac autonomic neuropathy from heart rate variability. *Entropy* 17(3): 1425–1440.

Cygankiewicz, I., J.K. Wranicz, H. Bolinska, J. Zaslonka, R. Jaszewski, and W. Zareba. 2004. Influence of coronary artery bypass grafting on heart rate turbulence parameters. *The American Journal of Cardiology* 94(2):186–189. doi: 10.1016/j.amjcard.2004.03.059.

De Jong, M.M., and D.C. Randal. 2005. Heart rate variability analysis in the assessment of autonomic function in heart failure. *Journal of Cardiovascular Nursing* 20(3):186–195.

Deligiannis, A.P. 1994. The effects of exercise training on cardiac autonomic nervous activity. *Sports Cardiology.* http://www.fac.org.ar/tcvc/llave/c243/deligian.PDF.

Dunbar, C.C., M.I. Kalinski, and R.J. Robertson. 1996. A new method for prescribing exercise: Three-point ratings of perceived exertion. *Perceptual and Motor Skills* 82(1):139–146.

Duru, F., R. Candinas, G. Dziekan, U. Goebbels, J. Myers, and P. Dubach. 2000. Effect of exercise training on heart rate variability in patients with new-onset left ventricular dysfunction after myocardial infarction. *American Heart Journal* 140(1):157–161. doi: 10.1067/mhj.2000.106606.

Evrengul, H., H. Tanriverdi, S. Kose, B. Amasyali, A. Kilic, T. Celik, and H. Turhan. 2006. The relationship between heart rate recovery and heart rate variability in coronary artery disease. *A.N.E.* 11(2):154–162.

Fletcher, G.F., G. Balady, S.N. Blair, J. Blumenthal, C. Caspersen, B. Chaitman, S. Epstein, E.S. Sivarajan Froelicher, V.F. Froelicher, I.L. Pina, and M.L. Pollock. 1996. Statement on exercise: Benefits and recommendations for physical activity programs for all Americans. A statement for health professionals by the Committee on Exercise and Cardiac Rehabilitation of the Council on Clinical Cardiology, American Heart Association. *Circulation* 94:857–862.

Fletcher, G.F., G.J. Balady, E.A. Amsterdam, B. Chaitman, R. Eckel, J. Fleg, V.F. Froelicher, A.S. Leon, I.L. Pina, R. Rodney, D. Simons-Morton, M.A. Williams, and T. Bazzarre. 2001. AHA scientific statement: Exercise standards for testing and training. A statement for healthcare professionals from the American Heart Association. *Circulation* 104(14):1694–1740.

Frenneaux, M.P. 2007. Autonomic changes in patients with heart failure and in post-myocardial infarction patients. *Heart* 90:1248–1255.

Gao, J., B.M. Gurbaxani, J. Hu, K.J. Heilman, V.A. Emauele, G.F. Lewis, M. Davila, E.R. Unger, and J.M. Lin. 2013. Multiscale analysis of heart rate variability in nonstationary environments. *Frontiers in Physiology* 4. doi: 10.3389/fphys.2013.00119.

Giannuzzi, P., A. Mezzani, H. Saner, H. Björnstad, P. Fioretti, M. Mendes, A. Cohen-Solal, L. Dugmore, R. Hambrecht, and I. Hellemans. 2003. Physical activity for primary and secondary prevention. Position paper of the Working Group on Cardiac Rehabilitation and Exercise Physiology of the European Society of Cardiology. *European Journal of Cardiovascular Prevention & Rehabilitation* 10(5):319.

Goldberger, A.L. 1997. Fractal variability versus pathologic periodicity: Complexity loss and stereotypy in disease. *Perspectives in Biology and Medicine* 40(4):543–561.

Goldberger, A.L., L.A. Amaral, J.M Hausdorff, P.C. Ivanov, C.K. Peng, and H.E. Stanley. 2002. Fractal dynamics in physiology: Alterations with disease and aging. *PNAS* 99:2456–2472.

Hansen, D., P. Dendale, J. Berger, and R. Meeusen. 2005. Rehabilitation in patients: What do we know about training modalities. *Sports Medicine* 35(12):1063–1084.

Hautala, A.J., T.H. Mäkikallio, A. Kiviniemi, R.T. Laukkanen, S. Nissilä, H.V. Huikuri, and M.P. Tulppo. 2004. Heart rate dynamics after controlled training followed by home-based exercise program. *European Journal of Applied Physiology* 92:289–297. doi: 10.1007/s00421-004-1077-6.

Houde, S.C., and K.D. Melillo. 2002. Cardiovascular health and physical activity in older adults: An integrative review of research methodology and results. *Journal of Advanced Nursing* 38(3): 219–234.

Huikuri, H.V., A. Castellanos, and R.J. Myerburg. 2001. Sudden death due to cardiac arrhythmias. *New England Journal of Medicine* 345(20):1473–1482. doi: doi:10.1056/NEJMra000650.

Huikuri, H.V., M.J. Niemela, S. Ojala, A. Rantala, M.J. Ikaheimo, and K.E. Airaksinen. 1994. Circadian rhythms of frequency domain measures of heart rate variability in healthy subjects and patients with coronary artery disease. Effects of arousal and upright posture. *Circulation* 90(1): 121–126.

Iellamo, F., J.M. Legramante, M. Massaro, G. Raimondi, and A. Galante. 2000. Effects of a residential exercise training on baroreflex sensitivity and heart rate variability in patients with coronary artery disease: A randomized, controlled study. *Circulation* 102(21):2588.

Ilarraza, H., K. Myers, W. Kottman, H. Rickli, and P. Dubach. 2004. An evaluation of training responses using self-regulation in a residential rehabilitation program. *Journal of Cardiopulmonary Rehabilitation* 24(1):27–33.

Ivanov, P., L.A. Amaral, A.L. Goldberger, S. Havlin, M. Rosenblum, Z.R. Struzik, and H. Eugene Stanley. 1999. Multifractality in human heartbeat dynamics. *Nature* 399:461–465.

Janowska-Kulińska, A., K. Torzyńska, A. Markiewicz-Grochowalska, A. Sowińska, M. Majewski, O. Jerzykowska, K. Pawlak-Buś, L. Kramer, J. Moczko, and T. Siminiak. 2009. Changes in heart rate variability caused by coronary angioplasty depend on the localisation of coronary lesions. *Kardiologia Polska* 67:130–138.

Jelinek, H.F., T. Collins, M.E. Smith, and H. Kiat. 2014. Assessment of a cardiac rehabilitation program based on the Borg RPE Scale and six-minute walk test. *International Journal of Cardiology and Angiology* 2(2):109–117.

Jelinek, H.F, Z. Huang, A.H. Khandoker, D. Chang, and H. Kiat. 2013. Cardiac rehabilitation outcomes following a 6-week program of PCI and CABG Patients. *Frontiers in Physiology* 4. doi: 10.3389/fphys.2013.00302.

Joo, K.C., P.H. Brubaker, A. MacDougall, A.M. Saikin, J.H. Ross, and M.H. Whaley. 2004. Exercise prescription using resting heart rate plus 20 or perceived exertion in cardiac rehabilitation. *Journal of Cardiopulmonary Rehabilitation* 24:178–186.

Kanadasi, M., G. Kudaiberdieva, and A. Birand. 2002. Effect of the final coronary arterial diameter after coronary angioplasty on heart rate variability responses. *Annals of Noninvasive Electrocardiology* 7(2):106–113.

Kang, J., J.R. Hoffman, H. Walker, E.C. Chaloupka, and A.C. Utter. 2003. Regulating intensity using perceived exertion during extended exercise periods. *European Journal of Applied Physiology* 89(5):475–482.

Karjalainen, J.J., A.M. Kiviniemi, A.J. Hautala, O.P. Piira, E.S. Lepojärvi, J.S. Perkiömäki, M.J. Junttila, H.V. Huikuri, and M.P. Tulppo. 2015. Effects of physical activity and exercise training on cardiovascular risk in coronary artery disease patients with and without type 2 diabetes. *Diabetes Care*. doi: 10.2337/dc14-2216.

Kiviniemi, A.M, A.J Hautala, J. Karjalainen, O.P. Piira, S. Lepojärvi, O. Ukkola, H.V. Huikuri, and M.P. Tulppo. 2015. Acute post-exercise change in blood pressure and exercise training response in patients with coronary artery disease. *Frontiers in Physiology* 5. doi: 10.3389/fphys.2014.00526.

Kiyono K., Z.R. Struzik, N. Aoyagi, Y. Yamamoto. 2006. Multiscale probability density function analysis: Non-Gaussian and scale-invariant fluctuations of healthy human heart rate. *IEEE Transactions on Bio-medical Engineering* 53(1):95–102. doi: 10.1109/tbme.2005.859804.

Kleiger, R.E., J.T. Bigger, M.S. Bosner, M.K. Chung, J.R. Cook, L.M. Rolnitzky, R. Steinman, and J.L. Fleiss. 1991. Stability over time of variables measuring heart rate variability in normal subjects. *American Journal of Cardiology* 68(6):626–630.

Kleiger, R.E., J.P. Miller, J.T. Bigger Jr., and A.J. Moss. 1987. Decreased heart rate variability and its association with increased mortality after acute myocardial infarction. *American Journal of Cardiology* 59(4):256–262.

Kobayashi, M., and T. Musha. 1982. 1/f fluctuation of heart beat period. *IEEE Transactions Biomedical Engineering* 29:456–457.

Kontopoulos, A.G., V.G. Athyros, A.A. Papageorgiou, G.V. Papadopoulos, M.J. Avramidis, and H. Boudoulas. 1996. Effect of quinapril or metoprolol on heart rate variability in post-myocardial infarction patients. *American journal of cardiology* 77(4):242–246.

Kouidi, E., K. Haritonidis, N. Koutlianos, and A. Deligiannis. 2002. Effects of athletic training on heart rate variability triangular index. *Clinical Physiology and Functional Imaging* 22(4):279–284. doi: 10.1046/j.1475-097X.2002.00431.x.

La Rovere, M.T. 2010. Heart rate and arrhythmic risk: Old markers never die. *Europace* 12(2):155–157. doi: 10.1093/europace/eup437.

La Rovere, M.T., A. Mortara, G. Sandrone, and F. Lombardi. 1992. Autonomic nervous system adaptations to short-term exercise training. *Chest* 101:299–303.

Lahiri, M.K., P.J. Kannankeril, and J.J. Goldberger. 2008. Assessment of autonomic function in cardiovascular disease: Physiological basis and prognostic implications. *Journal of the American College of Cardiology* 51(18):1725–1733. doi: 10.1016/j.jacc.2008.01.038.

Laitio, T., J. Jalonen, T. Kuusela, and H. Scheinin. 2007. The role of heart rate variability in risk stratification for adverse postoperative cardiac events. *Anesthesia and Analgesia* 105(6):1548–1560. doi: 10.1213/01.ane.0000287654.49358.3a.

Lake, D.E., J.S. Richman, M.P. Griffin, and J.R. Moorman. 2002. Sample entropy analysis of neonatal heart rate variability. *American Journal of Physiology Regulatory Integrative Comparative Physiology* 283(3):R789–97. doi: 10.1152/ajpregu.00069.2002.

Leitch, J.W., R.P. Newling, M. Basta, K. Inder, K. Dear, and P.J. Fletcher. 1997. Randomized trial of a hospital-based exercise training program after acute myocardial infarction: Cardiac autonomic effects. *Journal of the American College of Cardiology* 29(6):1263–1268.

Leon, A.S., B.A. Franklin, F. Costa, G.J. Balady, K.A. Berra, K.J. Stewart, P.D. Thompson, M.A. Williams, and M.S. Lauer. 2005. Cardiac rehabilitation and secondary prevention of coronary heart disease. *Circulation* 111:369–376.

Lucini, D., R.V. Milani, G. Costantino, C.J. Lavie, A. Porta, and M. Pagani. 2002. Effects of cardiac rehabilitation and exercise training on autonomic regulation in patients with coronary artery disease. *American Heart Journal* 143(6):977–983.

Mador, J., A. Rodis, and U. Magakang. 1995. Reproducibility of Borg scale measurements or dyspnea during exercise in patients with COPD. *Chest* 107(6):1590–1597.

Malfatto, G., G. Branzi, B. Riva, L. Sala, G. Leonetti, and M. Facchini. 2002. Recovery of cardiac autonomic responsiveness with low-intensity physical training in patients with chronic heart failure. *European Journal of Heart Failure* 4(2):159–166.

Malfatto, G., M. Facchini, R. Bragato, G. Branzi, L. Sala, and G. Leonetti. 1996. Short and long term effects of exercise training on the tonic autonomic modulation of heart rate variability after myocardial infarction. *European Heart Journal* 17(4):532.

Malfatto, G., F. Facchini, F. Sala, G. Branzi, R. Bragato, and G. Leonetti. 1998. Effects of cardiac rehabilitation and beta-blocker therapy on heart rate variability after first acute myocardial infarction. *American Journal of Cardiology* 81:834–840.

McCauley, K.M. 2007. Modifying women's risk for cardiovascular disease: Systematic review. *Journal of Obstetric, Gynecologic, and Neonatal Nursing* 36(2):116–124.

McConnel, T., T.A. Klinger, J.K. Gardner, C.A. Laubach, C.E. Herman, and C.A. Hauck. 1998. Cardiac rehabilitation without exercise tests for post-myocardial infarction and post-bypass surgery patients. *Journal of Cardiopulmonary Rehabilitation* 18(6):458–463.

Migliaro, E.R., R. Canetti, P. Contreras, and M. Hakas. 2003. Heart rate variability: Short-term studies are as useful as holter to differentiate diabetic patients from healthy subjects. *Annals of Noninvasive Electrocardiology* 8:313–320.

Munk, P.S., N. Butt, and A.I. Larsen. 2009. High-intensity interval exercise training improves heart rate variability in patients following percutaneous coronary intervention for angina pectoris. *International Heart Journal* 145(2):312–314.

Murphy, M.H., A.M. Nevil, E.M. Murtagh, and R.L. Holder. 2007. The effect of walking on fitness, fatness and resting blood pressure: A meta-analysis of randomised, controlled trials. *Preventive Medicine* 44(5):377–385.

National Heart Foundation of Australia and Australian Cardiac Rehabilitation Association. 2004. Recommended framework for Cardiac Rehabilitation '04. https://heartfoundation.org.au/.

Neves, V.R., A.M. Kiviniemi, A.J. Hautala, J. Karjalainen, O.P. Piira, A.M. Catai, T.H. Mäkikallio, H.V. Huikuri, and M.P. Tulppo. 2011. Heart rate dynamics after exercise in cardiac patients with and without type 2 diabetes. *Frontiers in Physiology* 2. doi: 10.3389/fphys.2011.00057.

Nolan, J., P.D. Batin, R. Andrews, S.J. Lindsay, P. Brooksby, M. Mullen, W. Baig, A.D. Flapan, A. Cowley, R.J. Prescott, J.M. Neilson, and K.A. Fox. 1998. Prospective study of heart rate variability and mortality in chronic heart failure: Results of the United Kingdom heart failure evaluation and assessment of risk trial (UK-heart). *Circulation* 98(15):1510–1516.

Oliveira, N.L., F. Ribeiro, M. Teixeira, L. Campos, A.J. Alves, G. Silva, and J. Oliveira. 2014. Effect of 8-week exercise-based cardiac rehabilitation on cardiac autonomic function: A randomized controlled trial in myocardial infarction patients. *Am Heart J* 167(5):753–761.e3. doi: 10.1016/j.ahj.2014.02.001.

Oya, M., H. Itoh, K. Kato, K. Tanabe, and M. Murayama. 1999. Effects of exercise training on the recovery of the autonomic nervous system and exercise capacity after acute myocardial infarction. *Japanese Circulation Journal* 63:843–848.

Pena, M.A., J.C. Echeverria, M.T. Garcia, and R. Gonzalez-Camarena. 2009. Applying fractal analysis to short sets of heart rate variability data. *Medical Biological Engineering Computing* 47(7):709–717. doi: 10.1007/s11517-009-0436-1.

Peng, C.K., S. Havlin, H.E. Stanley, and A.L. Goldberger. 1995. Quantification of scaling exponents and crossover phenomena in nonstationary heartbeat time series. *Chaos* 5(1):82–87.

Perkiömäki, J. 2011. Heart rate variability and nonlinear dynamics in risk stratification. *Frontiers in Physiology* 2. doi: 10.3389/fphys.2011.00081.

Pollock, M.L., G.A. Gaesser, J. Butcher, J.P. Despres, R.K. Dishman, B.A. Franklin, and C.E. Garber. 1998. ACSM position stand: The recommended quantity and quality of exercise for developing and maintaining cardiorespiratory and muscular fitness, and flexibility in healthy adults. *Medicine and Science in Sports and Exercise* 30(6):975–991.

Potteiger, J.A., and B.W. Evans. 1995. Using heart rate and ratings of perceived exertion to monitor intensity in runners. *Journal of Sports Medicine and Physical Fitness* 35(3):181–186.

Quintana, M., N. Storck, L.E. Lindblad, K. Lindvall, and M. Ericson. 1997. Heart rate variability as a means of assessing prognosis after acute myocardial infarction. *European Heart Journal* 18(5):789.

Rennie, K.L., H. Hemingway, M. Kumari, E. Brunner, M. Malik, and M. Marmot. 2003. Effects of moderate and vigorous physical activity on heart rate variability in a British study of civil servants. *American Journal of Epidemiology* 158(2):135–143.

Sandrone, G., A. Mortara, D. Torzillo, M.T. La Rovere, A. Malliani, and F. Lombardi. 1994. Effects of beta blockers (Atenolol or Metoprol) on heart rate variability after acute myocardial infarction. *American Journal of Cardiology* 74:340–345.

Sassi, R., M.G. Signorini, and S. Cerutti. 2009. Multifractality and heart rate variability. *Chaos* 19(2). doi: http://dx.doi.org/10.1063/1.3152223.

Smidt, N., H.C. de Vet, L.M. Bouter, and J. Dekker. 2005. Effectiveness of exercise therapy: A best-evidence summary of systematic reviews. *Australian Journal of Physiotherapy* 51(2):71–85.

Stahle, A., R. Nordlander, and L. Bergfeldt. 1999. Aerobic group training improves exercise capacity and heart rate variability in elderly patients with a recent coronary event. *European Heart Journal* 20:1638–1646.

Stein, P. K., J.I. Barzilay, P.H. Chaves, S.Q. Mistretta, P.P. Domitrovich, J.S. Gottdiener, M.W. Rich, and R.E. Kleiger. 2008. Novel measures of heart rate variability predict cardiovascular mortality in older adults independent of traditional cardiovascular risk factors: The Cardiovascular Health Study (CHS). *Journal of Cardiovascular Electrophysiology* 19(11):1169–1174. doi: 10.1111/j.1540-8167.2008.01232.x.

Suaya, J.A., W.B. Stason, P.A. Ades, S.L.T. Normand, and D.S. Shepard. 2009. Cardiac rehabilitation and survival in older coronary patients. *Journal of the American College of Cardiology* 54(1):25–33.

Szydlo, K., M. Trusz-Gluza, J. Drzewiecki, I. Wozniak-Skowerska, and J. Szczogiel. 1998. Correlation of heart rate variability parameters and QT interval in patients after PTCA of infarct related coronary artery as an indicator of improved autonomic regulation. *Pacing and Clinical Electrophysiology* 21(11 Pt 2):2407–2410.

Takeyama, J., H. Itoh, M. Kato, A. Koike, K. Aoki, F.L. Tai, H. Watanabe, M. Nagayama, and T. Katagiri. 2000. Effects of physical training on the recovery of the autonomic nervous activity during exercise after coronary artery bypass grafting—Effects of physical training after CABG. *Japanese Circulation Journal* 64(11):809–813. doi: 10.1253/jcj.64.809.

Tapanainen, J. 2003. Non-invasive predictors of mortality after acute myocardial infarction. PhD Thesis. ISBN 951-42-7011-8. http://herkules.oulu.fi/isbn9514270118/.

Taylor, R.S., A. Brown, S. Ebrahim, J. Jolliffe, H. Noorani, K. Rees, B. Skidmore, J.A. Stone, D.R. Thompson, and N. Oldridge. 2004. Exercise-based rehabilitation for patients with coronary heart disease: Systematic review and meta-analysis of randomized controlled trials. *American Journal of Medicine* 116(10):682–692.

Teich, M.C., S.B. Lowen, B.M. Jost, and K. Vibe-Rheymer, eds. 2001. Heart rate variability: Measures and models. Edited by M. Akay. Vol. II, *Nonlinear Biomedical Signal Processing, Dynamic Analysis and Modeling*. New York, NY: IEEE Press.

TFESC. 1996. Special report: Heart rate variability standards of measurement, physiological interpretation, and clinical use. *Circulation* 93(5):1043–1065.

Tsai, M.W., W.C. Chie, T.B.J. Kuo, M.F. Chen, J.P. Liu, T.H.H. Chen, and Y.T. Wu. 2006. Effects of exercise training on heart rate variability after coronary angioplasty. *Physical Therapy* 86(5):626.

Tseng, C.D., T.L. Wang, J.L. Lin, K.L. Hsu, F.T. Chiang, and Y.Z. Tseng. 1996. The cause-effect relationship of sympathovagal activity and the outcome of percutaneous transluminal coronary angioplasty. *Japanese Heart Journal* 37(4):455–462.

Tsuji, H., M.G. Larson, F.J. Venditti, E.S. Manders, J.C. Evans, C.L. Feldman, and D. Levy. 1996. Impact of reduced heart rate variability on risk for cardiac events: The Framingham Heart Study. *Circulation* 94(11):2850–2855.

Tulppo, M.P., A.J. Hautala, T.H. Mäkikallio, R.T. Laukkanen, S. Nissilä, R.L. Hughson, and H.V. Huikuri. 2003. Effects of aerobic training on heart rate dynamics in sedentary subjects. *Journal of Applied Physiology* 95(1):364–372. doi: 10.1152/japplphysiol.00751.2002.

Tulppo, M.P., A.M. Kiviniemi, A.J. Hautala, M. Kallio, T. Seppänen, Timo H. Mäkikallio, and H.V. Huikuri. 2005. Physiological background of loss of fractal heart rate dynamics. *Circulation* 112:314–319.

Vikman, S., T.H. Makikiallio, S. Yli-Mayry, S. Pikkujamsa, AM. Koivisto, P. Reinikainen, K.E. Airaksinen, and H.V. Huikuri. 1999. Altered complexity and correlation properties of R-R interval dynamics before the onset of spontaneous onset of paroxysmal atrial fibrillation. *Circulation* 100:2097–2084.

Voss, A., S. Schulz, R. Schroeder, M. Baumert, and P. Caminal. 2009. Methods derived from nonlinear dynamics for analysing heart rate variability. *Philosophical Transactions of the Royal Society A: Mathematical, Physical and Engineering Sciences* 367(1887):277–296. doi: 10.1098/rsta.2008.0232.

Wang, H., L. Dwyer-Lindgren, K.T. Lofgren, J.K. Rajaratnam, J.R. Marcus, A. Levin-Rector, C.E. Levitz, A.D. Lopez, and C.J.L. Murray. 2012. Age-specific and sex-specific mortality in 187 countries, 1970–2010: A systematic analysis for the Global Burden of Disease Study 2010. *The Lancet* 380(9859):2071–2094. doi: http://dx.doi.org/10.1016/S0140-6736(12)61719-X.

Warburton, D.E., C. Whitney Nicol, and S.S. Bredin. 2006. Health benefits of physical activity: The evidence. *Canadian Medical Association Journal* 174(6):801–809.

Weber, F., H. Schneider, T. Von Arnim, and W. Urbaszek. 1999. Heart rate variability and ischaemia in patients with coronary heart disease and stable angina pectoris. *European Heart Journal* 20(1):38.

Wennerblom, B., L. Lurje, J. Solem, H. Tygesen, M. Udén, R. Vahisalo, and Å. Hjalmarson. 2000. Reduced heart rate variability in ischemic heart disease is only partially caused by ischemia. *Cardiology* 94(3):146–151.

Whaley, M., P.H. Brubaker, L.A. Kaminsky, and C.R. Miller. 1997. Validity of rating of perceived exertion during graded exercise testing in apparently health adults and cardiac patients. *Journal of Cardiopulmonary Rehabilitation* 17(4):261–267.

Wu, Z.K, S. Vikman, J. Laurikka, E. Pehkonen, T. Iivainen, H.V. Huikuri, and M.R. Tarkka. 2005. Nonlinear heart rate variability in CABG patients and the preconditioning effect. *European Journal of Cardio-Thoracic Surgery* 28(1):109–113. doi: 10.1016/j.ejcts.2005.03.011.

Zuanetti, G., J.M. Neilson, R. Latini, E. Santoro, A.P. Maggioni, and D.J. Ewing. 1996. Prognostic significance of heart rate variability in post-myocardial infarction patients in the fibrolytic era. *Circulation* 94:432–436.

14

Acquired Brain Injury Rehabilitation: What Can HRV Tell You?

Ian J. Baguley and Melissa T. Nott

CONTENTS

14.1 Introduction

While much of the heart's function is semiautonomous, the central nervous system (CNS) exerts a high degree of control over heart rate (HR) via multiple centers located throughout the CNS. The relative influence of these centers produces beat-to-beat variability that can be quantified via heart rate variability (HRV) assessment. HRV changes have long been recognized in health and disease, at rest and during exercise. However, research into how direct damage to the CNS centers that drive HRV modifies central HR control is relatively underinvestigated. This chapter presents a brief overview of how the CNS modulates HR control, before discussing how various forms of acquired brain injury (ABI) may impact upon these systems. Finally, the clinical significance of HRV in patients with ABI will be discussed, with examples of how HRV can be used to investigate aspects of injury and treatment following ABI.

14.2 Structural Considerations

The heart has two intrinsic drivers of HR, the atrioventricular (AV) and sinoatrial (SA) nodes, connected by a myelinated nerve tract known as the bundle of His. In the normal heart, the AV node has an intrinsic rate of around 40 beats per minute (bpm), and in conditions such as complete heart block, the ventricles adopt this slow rate of contraction. Where the SA node and bundle of His are intact, the higher intrinsic rate of the SA node (60–80 bpm at rest) drives the rate of ventricular contraction.

Various noncardiac structures modify the firing rate of the SA node, many of which originate in the brain stem. Moving higher in the CNS, these brainstem centers receive inputs from the hypothalamus, usually considered the main control center of the autonomic nervous system (ANS; Guyton and Hall 2006). However, the hypothalamus receives inputs from multiple higher centers, such as the thalami, and the insula and prefrontal cortices (Takahashi et al. 2015). The fine detail of the innervation of these higher centers remains uncertain, but animal studies and some human research (Barron et al. 1994; Oppenheimer 2006, 2007; Rincon et al. 2008) point toward the right posterior insula region regulating sympathetic outflow, while the left posterior insula modulates parasympathetic outflow. Additionally, cardiac control will be influenced by the adrenal glands (regulating cardiac rate, contractility, and peripheral vascular tone). Control of these various structures necessitates complex though often poorly characterized feedback loops. Taken together, these various structures form part of what has been labeled the central autonomic nervous system (CAN; Benarroch 1997).

14.3 Acquired Brain Injury

Brain injuries are most usually classified according to their etiology. The first subdivision for brain injuries derives from their time of onset, with congenital brain injuries occurring before birth and ABIs accounting for all other forms of postpartum injury. Within ABI, two broad classes are recognized: traumatic and nontraumatic. The category of nontraumatic ABI is extremely eclectic, including etiologies such as infections, tumors, metabolic conditions, and various degenerative conditions (e.g., multiple sclerosis and dementia) (Entwistle and Newby 2013), along with environmental and other toxins. Among the most common nontraumatic ABI are cerebrovascular accidents (CVAs), otherwise known as stroke. Ischemic stroke follows blockage of the cerebral arterial supply by thrombus or plaque. Ischemic strokes are typically focal in nature and usually defined by clinical manifestations of large vessel syndromes specific to cerebrovascular territories (Eckerle and Southerland 2013). In contrast, hemorrhagic stroke, or intracerebral hemorrhage (ICH), refers to spontaneous bleeding into the brain parenchyma, often in the context of chronic hypertension or aneurysmal rupture, and accounts for about 5%–15% of acute strokes in Western countries (Kramer 2013). Hemorrhagic stroke can co-occur with subarachnoid hemorrhage (SAH), where bleeding occurs into the cerebrospinal fluid.

In contrast, traumatic brain injuries (TBIs) occur when external mechanical force is applied to the brain. TBI can be divided into blunt (closed) or penetrating (open) injuries. Blunt TBI is more common in incidence, typically occurring after following motor vehicle accidents, assaults, and falls, while penetrating injuries are usually associated with gunshot wounds or bladed weapons (Baron and Jallo 2007). Depending on their severity, these injuries produce a complex mixture of diffuse and focal lesions, with transient or permanent neurological dysfunction (Khan et al. 2003). TBI lesions are further classified by their pathological and morphological properties. Cerebral contusions can occur anywhere within the brain; however, they are most common in the frontal and temporal lobes of the brain adjacent to bony surfaces of the skull base. These injuries are likely to produce focal injury to both cortical and subcortical ANS control mechanisms.

Traumatic SAH can also occur in the interhemispheric fissure or the basilar cisterns and can result in hydrocephalus (Graham 1996). Diffuse axonal or shear injury (DAI) is an additional pathological term referring to microscopic axonal damage occurring as a result of rotational forces. The extent and depth of DAI tends to be proportional to the energy expended on the brain, with more force resulting in deeper lesions (Khan et al. 2003). In this way, milder injuries lead to relative disconnection between intra- and interhemispheric white matter tracts. Deeper lesions adversely affect periventricular regions, the reticular activating system, and the brainstem. However, only the worst 5% of DAI cases are estimated to be visible on conventional computed tomography (CT) scanning, meaning that the extent of DAI can only be inferred from the clinical situation, for example, prolonged depressed consciousness (Baron and Jallo 2007), prolonged posttraumatic amnesia (Khan et al. 2003), and slowed speed of processing (Felmingham et al. 2004).

14.4 The CAN and Structural Damage

The impact of the structural damage resulting from ABI can be difficult to predict, particularly with regard to the ANS. While structural lesions should be determinants of the autonomic consequences of ABI, a number of practical limitations exist. First, injury patterns vary considerably from one individual to the next. Structural investigations such as CT and magnetic resonance imaging (MRI) provide macroscopic information regarding the injury that does not necessarily inform the observer what residual function exists in the area of damage. In routine scanning, it is not possible to differentiate between infarcted tissue and the ischemic penumbra. In this situation, the infarcted area cannot recover, whereas a variable proportion of the penumbra may be salvageable with appropriate medical intervention. Finally, DAI is often unobservable on scanning, meaning that apparently intact neurons may be effectively deafferentated from their afferent and/or efferent connections. The integrity of ANS responses immediately following TBI is therefore likely to depend on a range of parameters including the overall severity of the injury, the relative contribution of diffuse, focal, and/or hypoxic injury from the primary injury, and the extent of secondary postinjury brain damage.

Second, while many of the hypothalamic and brainstem nuclei that contribute to the CAN have been identified, the location and function of other areas are poorly understood. The clearest example of this is the ongoing debate surrounding the effect of the insular cortices (discussed previously). This limited understanding of anatomical pathways further limits the clinical usefulness of these CT/MRI investigations in this context. In addition to these limitations, there can be considerable interindividual variability in the details of CNS morphology.

For these reasons, there is uncertainty how a particular structural lesion may impact upon the ability of the CAN to control the ANS. In clinical contexts, therefore, it is prudent to presume that any autonomic abnormalities present are occurring on the basis of current illness rather than structural abnormalities. Therefore, it has been suggested that the impact of "autonomic dysfunction after acute brain injury is an underrecognized, yet important source of complications following a variety of neurologic injuries" (Hinson and Sheth 2012, p. 139).

14.5 Structure versus Function

Another limitation with interpreting the effect of structural lesions on the ANS is that autonomic control is a dynamic process, and its responses will be phasically affected by other physiological stressors such as sepsis, reduced blood volume, pain, and anxiety. Even if our knowledge of the CAN was comprehensive, the complicated feedback loops between stressors may produce unpredictable effects on function. Therefore, to better understand the impact of ABI on the ANS, it is preferable to use a dynamic measure that can assess the ANS's response to the prevailing homeostatic milieu.

One such measure of the state of play in the ANS is HRV. HRV data can be used to approximate the relative contributions of the sympathetic and parasympathetic arms of the ANS. While HRV itself is not completely understood, reduced HRV is a common feature of elevated catecholamines, indicative of heightened physiological stress (Van Ravenswaaij-Arts et al. 1993). Under control situations, there is a moderately strong relationship between HR and HRV ($r^2 = 0.5$) (Huikuri et al. 1990). In disease states, reduced HRV power is partly a general indicator of the severity of disease, but it is also partly a consequence of increased HR.

14.6 Cardiac Consequences from ABI

In the clinical context of ABI, epidemiological studies, animal studies, and retrospective data all suggest that brain injury can be associated with cardiac dysfunction syndromes. The extent of this clinical awareness differs for different etiologies, with greater awareness of the role of the ANS in diseases showing an acute onset and those tending to have more extreme symptomatology rather than slow, degenerative diseases.

In nontraumatic ABI, for example, the Northern Manhattan Study (NOMAS) followed 655 poststroke patients, finding 6.7% of patients suffered fatal cardiac events. In this data, patients with left parietal lobe infarction were at a fourfold increased risk of cardiac death (Rincon et al. 2008). Associations between frontal, temporal, or insular stroke and fatal cardiac events were not evident. A direct mechanism for how ischemic stroke increases the near-term risk for cardiac mortality has yet to be identified (Prosser et al. 2007).

There is some evidence that ischemic strokes involving the insular cortices show greater cardiac autonomic dysregulation. Oppenheimer et al. (1996) showed that acute *left* insular stroke increased basal cardiac sympathetic tone and was associated with a reduced HRV. Later work by Oppenheimer (2006) identified that injuries adjacent to the *right* circuminsular cortex have led to loss of inhibition. As circumstantial support, Sander et al. (2001) found insular lesions (and those with increased norepinephrine levels) were associated with worse patient outcomes, as measured by modified Rankin scores and Barthel indices. More recently, Gao et al. (2014) highlighted that both insular cortices affect sympathetic tone, with the suggestion that right-sided injuries were slightly more likely to produce sympathetic overactivity. This has been interpreted as suggesting that the inhibition of sympathetic outflow is greater from the left compared to the right insular cortex. However, other studies do not support these findings, for example, Barron et al. found that the HRV (measured by the R-R interval) was reduced regardless of stroke laterality (Barron et al. 1994).

The situation for nontraumatic SAH is somewhat different. There is considerable research evidence for an excessive, monophasic increase in sympathetic drive postbleed (Hinson and Sheth 2012). Various causes have been postulated including that the rapid increase in intracranial pressure (ICP) associated with the onset of bleeding (Masuda et al. 2002), free blood within and around the brain occurring (Hinson and Sheth 2012) or discrete hypothalamic (Reynolds 1963; Doshi and Neil-Dwyer 1977) or medullary lesions (Ochiai et al. 2001) producing the hypersympathetic drive. The presence of this hypersympathetic drive is associated with a recognized increase in mortality (Hamill et al. 1987).

In most cases of acute TBI, ANS control of HR is disrupted in proportion to the degree of neurologic insult (Goldstein et al. 1998). Focal injuries such as contusions or ICHs carry the potential to produce localized damage to ANS control centers; for example, focal injury to the hypothalamus or brainstem would be particularly likely to affect mid-level CAN reflex centers. In contrast, DAI has the capacity to produce a relative differentiation between mid-level ANS control centers and mechanisms higher in the CAN hierarchy. This "disconnection" could hypothetically reduce integration of more complex homeostatic mechanisms. Severe hypoxic injuries may have a preferential effect on grey matter, therefore making it relatively more likely to damage neuronal clusters rather than axonal connections (Guo et al. 2011; Baguley and Nott 2013).

Considered in overview, the impact that ABI will exert on ANS responsivity will be the cumulative result of damage to the CAN, the integrity of multiple feedback loops, and threats to physiological homeostasis resulting from the injury. Rather than radiology, the severity of ANS dysfunction is best inferred from monitoring physiological parameters in the intensive care unit (ICU).

14.7 HRV and ABI

While HR is immediately interpretable at the bedside, it is a relatively crude tool. Additional information can be obtained through HRV, but its use in neuroscience and medicine has been questioned (Benarroch 2007; Thayer et al. 2009). Methods for collecting HRV information benefit from being noninvasive, with high benefit/cost ratio. HRV measures can be obtained with minimal cost and labor, producing accurate recordings and information on the autonomic system functional condition or response, albeit indirectly. Objective HRV data are obtainable in the absence of the patient's collaboration (as in cases of minimally responsive patients with severe ABI), whenever sophisticated experimental designs and data recording procedures are impracticable (e.g., in the intensive care unit), and when observation needs to be noninvasive or when long-term observation is necessary (Riganello et al. 2012). HRV can be obtained in real time or as a post hoc analysis, and can be reviewed over long periods of time, producing a robust response across numerous forms of stimuli including physical (e.g., touch, movement, or nociception), medical (e.g., the effect of propofol or other treatments in the ICU), or psychological (e.g., response to voice). Furthermore, HRV analysis becomes more powerful if the data are time-linked to these stimuli to produce a dynamic snapshot of the individual's ANS response to stimuli.

In patients with TBI, reduced HRV power is associated with episodes of increased ICP and decreased cerebral perfusion pressure, along with increased mortality and disability (Mowery et al. 2008). These HRV changes may precede changes in ICP, and both increases in ICP and cardiac uncoupling (low HRV) predict mortality (Mazzeo et al. 2011). Many investigative research studies involving patients with ABI assume that HRV remains static, in that if it is "bad" at one point then it will stay bad. Some researchers have suggested that low power on HRV or high LF/HF ratios are indicative of a poor outcome, or indeed of brain death (Marthol et al. 2010).

14.8 Paroxysmal Sympathetic Hyperactivity and HRV

As a general rule, the greater the cumulative damage to cerebral ANS pathways, the cruder and less coordinated the ANS response to homeostatic challenge is likely to be (Baguley and Nott 2013). Therefore, it is common for the sympathetic drive of patients with severe TBI to be elevated. This is particularly true in the condition known as paroxysmal sympathetic hyperactivity (PSH). Clinically, PSH presents with episodic increases in HR, respiratory rate, temperature, sweating, and blood pressure, often associated with overactive and uncontrolled muscle movements (spasticity, posturing, and dystonia).

PSH has been defined in a recent international consensus statement as the *"syndrome, recognized in a subgroup of survivors of severe acquired brain injury, of simultaneous, paroxysmal transient increases in sympathetic [elevated heart rate, blood pressure, respiratory rate, temperature, sweating] and motor [posturing] activity"* (Baguley et al. 2014, p. 1516). This term has been adopted to replace the 31 eponyms that have previously existed in the literature including dysautonomia, paroxysmal autonomic instability with dystonia (PAID), "sympathetic storms," and so on. In a recent review (Perkes et al. 2010), 349 cases of PSH were identified, with the most common etiologies being TBI (79.4%), hypoxic brain injury (9.7%), and stroke (5.4%). However, there are also case reports of PSH following many other etiologies.

Of all of the physiological parameters that are affected by PSH, data have confirmed that changes in HR are the most prolonged (Baguley et al. 1999; Hughes and Rabinstein 2014). The effect of PSH on HR can be seen in Figure 14.1, which presents the mean maximum data for 35 patients with and without PSH over the first 28 days post brain injury. There was no discernible group differences until the withdrawal of sedation around day 5. At this point, maximum HRs are significantly greater in the PSH cohort than in the non-PSH cohort who were matched for age, sex, and injury severity. This difference became more evident during the later days of the study period. Group HR differences were persistent and are easy to measure, suggesting that HR could represent a robust marker of the status of the disorder.

In contrast to the *monophasic* hypersympathetic state observed in SAH, PSH often follows a prolonged, *polyphasic* course. Furthermore, the observed "paroxysms" fluctuate in an unpredictable manner, with a single individual showing marked variation in episode timing, severity, and duration of elevated sympathetic tone. This is observed in the 24-hour Holter monitor data of two individuals with PSH (Figure 14.2). In the upper panel,

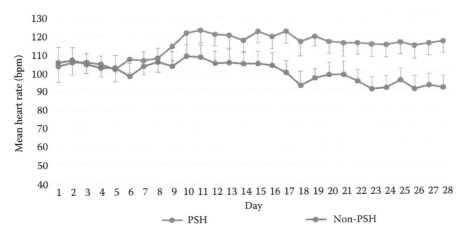

FIGURE 14.1
Mean daily heart rate during initial 4 weeks post traumatic brain injury (TBI) comparing TBI patients with and without paroxysmal sympathetic hyperactivity (PSH).

paroxysms are easily defined, with the individual's baseline HR consistent with someone lying in bed. When the intermittent paroxysms occur, HR rises 60 bpm above this level for around an hour before showing an initially rapid fall followed by a slower reduction back to baseline. In contrast, the lower panel presents a patient where normal resting HR is rarely reached. In this individual's recording, it is much harder to differentiate where paroxysms start and end. The maximum HR of both individuals was similar (145 and 142, respectively); however, this value alone does not convey the complexity of each patient's cardiac control across the entire day.

However, describing the course of the disorder cannot be undertaken using maximum HR as a sole variable. Early data examining HRV in adults with PSH confirmed this conjecture. In a study of 16 patients with severe TBI (half with PSH and half without) (Baguley et al. 2006), 5 minutes of electrocardiogram (ECG) data were processed to determine spectral power across three bands: very low frequency (VLF), low frequency (LF: 0.04–0.15 Hz), and high frequency (HF: 0.15–0.4 Hz). The latter two bands are considered to equate to sympathetic and parasympathetic cardiac influences. The resulting data were compared to 16 healthy matched controls. As seen in Figure 14.3, the relative proportion of power in the three bands was different in each group, with the two TBI groups showing reduced LF and HF power, and the PSH patients showing significantly less power in these bands than non-PSH TBI patients.

14.9 Stimulus Dependent Data

Another limitation in the field of PSH research has been the relative uncertainty regarding diagnosis. By its very nature, patients with high temperatures, tachycardia, and tachypnea following an ABI are presumed to have sepsis or another immediate medical illness. As a

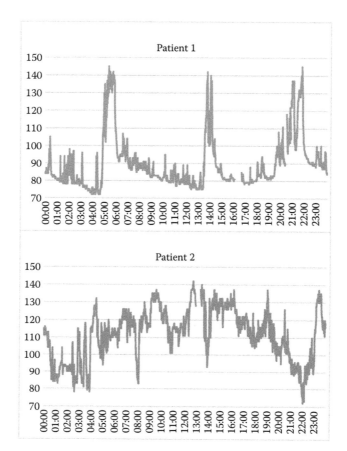

FIGURE 14.2
Heart rate variations (HRVs) over a 24-hour period collected via Holter monitor.

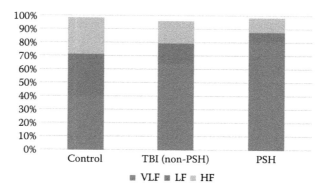

FIGURE 14.3
Relative proportion of very low frequency (VLF), low frequency (LF), and high frequency (HF) power between clinical groups.

result, the diagnosis of PSH has been one of exclusion, and as such, requires a high index of suspicion from the clinician (Perkes et al. 2010). However, group-level data analysis for HR or HRV did not assist in determining whether an individual was displaying PSH or not. Furthermore, developing an understanding of the pathophysiology of the condition has been difficult as the paroxysmal nature of the condition has made it hard to measure the efficacy of medical intervention.

It had been suggested by multiple authors that a central feature of PSH is an exaggerated responsiveness to what should be minimally nociceptive stimuli. Case reports of multiple stimuli including bathing, turning, endotracheal suctioning, passive movement and muscle stretching, constipation or urinary retention, and emotional and environmental stimuli such as noise have been reported to provoke paroxysms of hypersympathetic drive (summarized in Baguley 2008).

To confirm whether the observed sympathetic hyperactivity was stimulus dependent, an approach was adopted from psychological research, namely event-related data evaluation. In this paradigm, data before and after a stimulus is recorded, allowing for the effect of the stimulus on the particular parameter to be gauged. This has been undertaken in many fields including choice reaction time tasks and interpretation of electroencephalogram (EEG) changes in response to target versus nontarget auditory tones (event-related potentials). This allows each subject to act as his or her own control, reducing the impact of the marked intersubject variability (seen in Figure 14.2). It is important in this paradigm to standardize the stimulus as much as possible to allow between-subject comparison to be undertaken.

As it relates to this topic, Figure 14.4 provides an example of event-related HRV. This figure provides data from a spectral analysis of pre-/postdata performed via fast Fourier transform of resampled data via a Welch window with 50% overlap. Using standard cutoffs to differentiate the sympathetically mediated LF and parasympathetic HF components, the prestimulus LF and HF peaks are easily seen. Following application of the stimulus, there is an increase in the power in the LF band, alongside a reduction in HF power. In this individual, the LF/HF ratio increased markedly following stimulus application, consistent

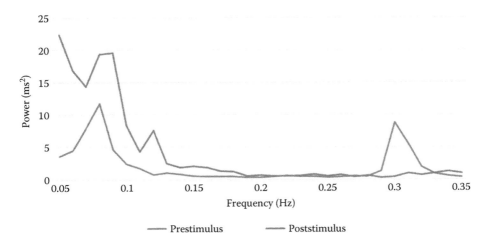

FIGURE 14.4
Spectral analysis of a subject with PSH pre- and poststimulus.

with sympathetic efflux and reduced parasympathetic activation. It was reasoned that by applying standardized stimulus across different clinical groups, event-related HRV may have the capacity to distinguish whether neurological cardiac control is disordered in a target population.

In order to evaluate this hypothesis, 79 consecutive patients with severe TBI were recruited from an intensive care setting in the first few days postinjury (Baguley et al. 2009b). Of this group, a subset of 27 patients were assessed prior to and following suctioning of their tracheostomy tube. This routine nursing care task provided a semistandardized, mildly nociceptive stimulus. Subjects were then divided into three groups; those without symptoms of PSH ($n = 11$) were taken as a control group. Subjects with PSH were divided into two groups based on the duration of sympathetic hyperactivity into short ($n = 10$) and long ($n = 6$) duration PSH (defined as sympathetic features lasting less than or greater than 14 days). These data are displayed in Figure 14.5. Assessing HR responses for 100 beats before and after the stimulus commencement of suctioning found a 2%, 8%, and 16% increase in HR for the subsequent 100 beats for the TBI control, PSH short, and PSH long groups, respectively.

HRV spectral analysis of individuals in this study suggested CNS cardiac control differences in the way each group responded to the stimulus (Figure 14.6). In this figure, spectral analysis of 5 minutes of HR data was performed immediately prior to and poststimulus. Resting HRs were equivalent at the baseline (y axis); however, HR significantly increased postsuctioning in the autonomically aroused groups (PSH short and PSH long). In contrast, between-group differences were evident in LF/HF ratio *both prior to and after* suctioning. In particular, there was a graded sympathetic response to the stimulus by group, with the long-duration PSH group demonstrating greater LF/HF ratios both pre- and poststimulus.

This combined HR/HRV data provided the first empirical evidence that the pathophysiology of PSH included an overresponsivity to external stimuli, at least in the first few weeks postinjury. It had previously been hypothesized that there was an uncoupling of LF/HF ratio and HR in acute brain injury, with worse injury producing greater uncoupling (Goldstein et al. 1998). However, there were no significant differences in injury severity

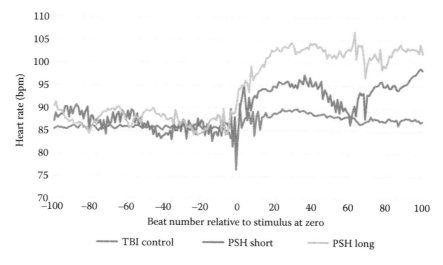

FIGURE 14.5
Heart rate response to stimulus by clinical group.

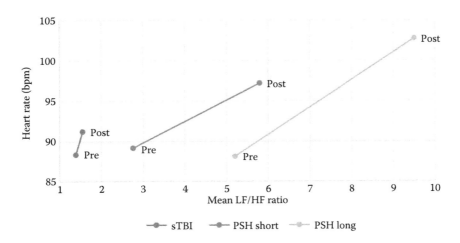

FIGURE 14.6
Mean LF/HF ratio and heart rate pre- and poststimulus by clinical group. Note: connecting points are added for demonstration purposes only and do not imply that extra data were available.

markers between groups to explain the greater sympathetic activation in the PSH groups. Further, the colinearity of PSH and non-PSH response patterns suggested an underlying physiological process in each group, potentially linked to a participant's individual degree of stimulus overresponsivity.

Although subject numbers are small (a perennial problem in PSH research) (Perkes et al. 2010), the data are consistent with the suggestion that a neurological process underlies PSH. There are distinct similarities between the overresponsiveness to stimuli seen in PSH and to allodynia, a well-understood physiological process whereby nonnociceptive sensations are perceived as painful. In everyday life, many people will have experienced the allodynia accompanying sunburn, where light touch becomes painful.

Combined with other research, these observations led to an integrative model, the excitatory:inhibitory ratio (EIR) model, being proposed to provide a common pathophysiology for a variety of syndromes exhibiting sympathetic hyperactivity (Baguley 2008). This model proposes, in part, that the hypersympathetic drive results from maladaptive plasticity at the spinal cord level. This hyperactivity is most severe in the early postacute period, progressively settling over time with the recovery of supraspinal inhibition. This model was tested in a second event-related HRV study involving 26 survivors of ABI (approximately 5 years postinjury) with muscle spasticity requiring medical intervention (Baguley et al. 2009a). These 26 adults with ABI were examined via subgroup analysis: 15 participants with a history of severe TBI (seven with PSH and eight without PSH) were contrasted against a group of 11 people with a history of stroke. These participants formed the three groups: the PSH TBI group, the non-PSH TBI group, and the non-PSH ABI group. This study again employed a semistandardized stimulus, in this case, injection of Botulinum toxin A as part of spasticity management. HRV data were collected for all subjects in 5-minute intervals preceding, during, and following the intramuscular injections (Figure 14.7).

As shown in the figure, there were no significant between-group differences in LF/HF ratio before or after the stimulus. However, the PSH group displayed a very strong and significant hypersympathetic response to the stimulus when compared to both other groups.

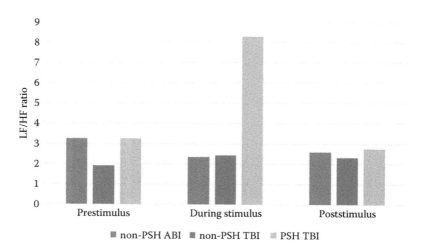

FIGURE 14.7
Mean LH/HF ratio pre-, during, and poststimulus by clinical group.

This finding supports the EIR model's hypothesis that the "allodynic" tendency becomes hardwired into the spinal cord; however, its severity reduces over time due to the recovery of descending inhibition.

14.10 HRV and Medical Intervention

14.10.1 Medication Trials: $n = 1$ and Small Case Series

As another component of the event-related HRV "proof of concept" process, HR and HRV data have been used for preliminary investigation of medication trials. A number of pharmacological treatments have been promoted for use in PSH (Baguley 2008); however, there has been a lack of empirical evidence regarding their efficacy. To date, "best practice" has been guided by anecdotal case reports and small case series (Perkes et al. 2010). The main limiting factors for efficacy trials have been outlined earlier: small subject numbers and the marked inter- and intrasubject variability in the severity, duration, and frequency of paroxysms in PSH. As a consequence, it is hard to objectively state whether an observed treatment response is due to the intervention or merely to a change in other drivers of the condition. For this reason, HRV was used in a number of $n = 1$ trials to determine if measurement of cardiac parameters could gauge treatment efficacy. Two drugs with strong anecdotal evidence for efficacy in treating PSH were trialed, namely intrathecal baclofen (ITB) and gabapentin.

14.10.2 Intrathecal Baclofen

Baclofen is a GABA B analog medication that decreases spasticity through its action on inhibitory interneurons in the spinal cord. Oral baclofen has limited efficacy due to its

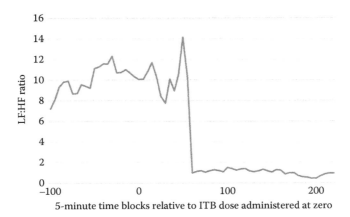

FIGURE 14.8
LF/HF ratio response to intrathecal baclofen trial.

inability to penetrate the blood–brain barrier. In cases of severe spasticity, baclofen can be injected directly into the cerebrospinal fluid of the spinal cord, thereby bypassing the blood–brain barrier. Injected in this way, ITB is said to have maximal effect around 90–180 minutes postinjection. A single bolus produces a direct pharmacological effect for approximately 24 hours.

To investigate the utility of ITB, 5-minute HRV data were extracted from Holter monitor data over a 2-day period centered on a 50 mcg bolus of ITB. Clinically, ITB was being trialed for severe spasticity in a patient with coincident acute PSH. For the duration of the data collection period, the patient was nursed supine in bed. This represented an opportunity to see what effect ITB had on HRV in this context. As can be seen in Figure 14.8, LF/HF ratio altered dramatically around 4 hours postbolus and this response persisted for more than 10 hours, until the time the Holter monitor was removed.

14.10.3 Gabapentin

The molecular structure of gabapentin is that of a GABA analog, but the medication produces selective inhibition of the $\alpha 2 \delta$ auxiliary subunit of voltage-sensitive Ca^{2+} channels in the CNS. The exact mechanism of action of gabapentin remains unknown. Gabapentin was first reported to have efficacy in treating PSH in a 2007 case series (Baguley et al. 2007); however, further investigation has yet to be published. Using a similar approach to that outlined above, another patient with PSH following ABI was given a single 300 mg capsule of gabapentin. Blocks of 5-minute LF/HF ratio data are shown in Figure 14.9, with the pregabapentin phase in light gray and postgabapentin phase in dark gray. As displayed, mean LF/HF ratio for the 24-hour period before and after gabapentin halved in this patient, and the degree of variability decreased substantially.

While not conclusive evidence, these results suggest that HRV analysis may provide a worthwhile approach in trying to identify which medications are the most useful in treating the condition, and may also provide further insights into the pathophysiology of PSH.

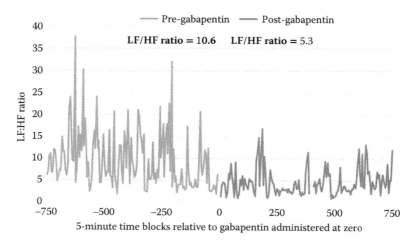

FIGURE 14.9
LF/HF ratio response to gabapentin trial.

14.11 Conclusion

HR control can be severely affected by ABI, with the consequences partially determined by the etiology of the ABI. Analysis of HRV provides a robust and dynamic way of interpreting CNS control of the heart, and event-related HRV shows a good deal of promise as a means of establishing treatment efficacy and understanding the underlying pathophysiology of some specific conditions in this context.

References

Baguley, I. J. (2008a). Autonomic complications following central nervous system injury. *Seminars in Neurology* **28**(5): 716–725.

Baguley, I. J. (2008b). The excitatory:inhibitory ratio model (EIR model): An integrative explanation of acute autonomic overactivity syndromes. *Medical Hypotheses* **70**(1): 26–35.

Baguley, I. J., R. E. Heriseanu, K. L. Felmingham, and I. D. Cameron (2006). Dysautonomia and heart rate variability following severe traumatic brain injury. *Brain Injury* **20**(4): 437–444.

Baguley, I. J., R. E. Heriseanu, J. A. Gurka, A. Nordenbo, and I. D. Cameron (2007). Gabapentin in the management of dysautonomia following severe traumatic brain injury: A case series. *Journal of Neurology, Neurosurgery and Psychiatry* **78**(5): 539–541.

Baguley, I. J., R. E. Heriseanu, M. T. Nott, J. Chapman, and J. Sandanam (2009a). Dysautonomia after severe traumatic brain injury: Evidence of persisting overresponsiveness to afferent stimuli. *American Journal of Physical Medicine and Rehabilitation* **88**(8): 615–622.

Baguley, I. J., J. L. Nicholls, K. L. Felmingham, J. Crook, J. A. Gurka, and L. D. Wade (1999). Dysautonomia after traumatic brain injury: A forgotten syndrome? *Journal of Neurology, Neurosurgery and Psychiatry* **67**(1): 39–43.

Baguley, I. J. and M. T. Nott (2013). Autonomic dysfunction. *Brain Injury Medicine*. N. D. Zasler, D. I. Katz, R. D. Zafonte et al. (eds.). New York, NY: Demos Medical Publishers.

Baguley, I. J., M. T. Nott, S. Slewa-Younan, R. E. Heriseanu, and I. E. Perkes (2009b). Diagnosing dysautonomia after acute traumatic brain injury: Evidence for overresponsiveness to afferent stimuli. *Archives of Physical Medicine and Rehabilitation* **90**(4): 580–586.

Baguley, I. J., I. E. Perkes, J. F. Fernandez-Ortega, A. A. Rabinstein, G. Dolce, and H. T. Hendricks (2014). Paroxysmal sympathetic hyperactivity after acquired brain injury: Consensus on conceptual definition, nomenclature, and diagnostic criteria. *Journal of Neurotrauma* **31**(17): 1515–1520.

Baron, E. M. and J. I. Jallo (2007). TBI: Pathology, pathophysiology, acute care and surgical management, critical care principles, and outcomes. *Brain Injury Medicine*. N. D. Zasler, D. I. Katz, and R. D. Zafonte (eds.). New York, NY: Demos Medical Publishing.

Barron, S. A., Z. Rogovski, and J. Hemli (1994). Autonomic consequences of cerebral hemisphere infarction. *Stroke* **25**(1): 113.

Benarroch, E. E. (1997). *Central Autonomic Network: Functional Organization and Clinical Correlations*. New York, NY: Futura Publishing Company.

Benarroch, E. E. (2007). The autonomic nervous system: Basic anatomy and physiology. *CONTINUUM: Lifelong Learning in Neurology* **13**(6, Autonomic Disorders): 13–32.

Doshi, R. and G. Neil-Dwyer (1977). Hypothalamic and myocardial lesions after subarachnoid haemorrhage. *Journal of Neurology, Neurosurgery and Psychiatry* **40**(8): 821–826.

Eckerle, B. J. and A. M. Southerland (2013). Bedside evaluation of the acute stroke patient. *Stroke*. K. M. Barrett and J. F. Meschia (eds.). West Sussex: Wiley-Blackwell. pp. 13–34.

Entwistle, H. and G. Newby (2013). The very basic basics: Definitions, prevalence and consequences. *Practical Neuropsychological Rehabilitation in Acquired Brain Injury: A Guide for Working Clinicians*. G. Newby, R. Coetzer, A. Daisley, and S. Weatherhead (eds.). London: Karnac Books. pp. 30–37.

Felmingham, K. L., I. J. Baguley, and A. M. Green (2004). Effects of diffuse axonal injury on speed of information processing following severe traumatic brain injury. *Neuropsychology* **18**(3): 564–571.

Gao, B., J. A. Pollock, and H. E. Hinson (2014). Paroxysmal sympathetic hyperactivity in hemispheric intraparenchymal hemorrhage. *Annals of Clinical and Translational Neurology* **1**(3): 215–219.

Goldstein, B., D. Toweill, S. Lai, K. Sonnenthal, and B. Kimberly (1998). Uncoupling of the autonomic and cardiovascular systems in acute brain injury. *The American Journal of Physiology—Regulatory, Integrative and Comparative Physiology* **275**(4): R1287–R1292.

Graham, D. I. (1996). Neuropathology of head injury. *Neurotrauma*. R. Narayan, J. Wilberger and J. Povlishock (eds.). New York, NY: McGraw Hill. pp. 43–59.

Guo, M.-F., J.-Z. Yu, and C.-G. Ma (2011). Mechanisms related to neuron injury and death in cerebral hypoxic ischaemia. *Folia Neuropathologica* **49**(2): 78.

Guyton, A. C. and J. E. Hall (2006). The autonomic nervous system and the adrenal medulla. *Textbook of Medical Physiology*. A. C. Guyton and J. E. Hall (eds.). Philadelphia, PA: Saunders.

Hamill, R. W., P. D. Woolf, J. V. McDonald, L. A. Lee, and M. Kelly (1987). Catecholamines predict outcome in traumatic brain injury. *Annals of Neurology* **21**(5): 438–443.

Hinson, H. E. and K. N. Sheth (2012). Manifestations of the hyperadrenergic state after acute brain injury. *Current Opinion in Critical Care* **18**(2): 139–145.

Hughes, J. D. and A. A. Rabinstein (2014). Early diagnosis of paroxysmal sympathetic hyperactivity in the ICU. *Neurocrit Care* **20**(3): 454–459.

Huikuri, H. V., K. M. Kessler, E. Terracall, A. Castellanos, M. K. Linnaluoto, and R. J. Myerburg (1990). Reproducibility and circadian rhythm of heart rate variability in healthy subjects. *The American Journal of Cardiology* **65**(5): 391–393.

Khan, F., I. J. Baguley, and I. D. Cameron (2003). Rehabilitation after traumatic brain injury. *Medical Journal of Australia* **178**(6): 290–295.

Kramer, A. H. (2013). Treatment of hemorrhagic stroke. *Stroke*. K. M. Barrett and J. F. Meschia (eds.). West Sussex: Wiley-Blackwell. pp. 106–135.

Marthol, H., T. Intravooth, J. Bardutzky, P. De Fina, S. Schwab, and M. J. Hilz (2010). Sympathetic cardiovascular hyperactivity precedes brain death. *Clinical Autonomic Research* **20**(6): 363–369.

Masuda, T., A. Matsunaga, S. Obuchi, Y. Shiba, S. Shimizu, K. Sato, N. Matsuyama, T. Shimohama, T. Izumi, and S.-I. Yamamoto (2002). Sympathetic nervous activity and myocardial damage immediately after subarachnoid hemorrhage in a unique animal model. *Stroke* 33(6): 1671–1676.

Mazzeo, A. T., E. La Monaca, R. Di Leo, G. Vita, and L. B. Santamaria (2011). Heart rate variability: A diagnostic and prognostic tool in anesthesia and intensive care. *Acta Anaesthesiologica Scandinavica* 55(7): 797–811.

Mowery, N. T., P. R. Norris, W. Riordan, J. M. Jenkins, A. E. Williams, and J. A. Morris Jr. (2008). Cardiac uncoupling and heart rate variability are associated with intracranial hypertension and mortality: A study of 145 trauma patients with continuous monitoring. *The Journal of Trauma* 65(3): 621–627.

Ochiai, H., Y. Yamakawa, and E. Kubota (2001). Deformation of the ventrolateral medulla oblongata by subarachnoid hemorrhage from ruptured vertebral artery aneurysms causes neurogenic pulmonary edema. *Neurologia Medico-Chirurgica* 41(11): 529–534.

Oppenheimer, S. (2006). Cerebrogenic cardiac arrhythmias: Cortical lateralization and clinical significance. *Clinical Autonomic Research* 16(1): 6–11.

Oppenheimer, S. (2007). Cortical control of the heart. *Cleveland Clinic Journal of Medicine* 74: 27.

Oppenheimer, S. M., G. Kedem, and W. M. Martin (1996). Left-insular cortex lesions perturb cardiac autonomic tone in humans. *Clinical Autonomic Research* 6(3): 131–140.

Perkes, I., I. J. Baguley, M. T. Nott, and D. K. Menon (2010). A review of paroxysmal sympathetic hyperactivity after acquired brain injury. *Annals of Neurology* 68(2): 126–135.

Prosser, J., L. MacGregor, K. R. Lees, H.-C. Diener, W. Hacke, and S. Davis (2007). Predictors of early cardiac morbidity and mortality after ischemic stroke. *Stroke* 38(8): 2295.

Reynolds, R. W. (1963). Pulmonary edema as a consequence of hypothalamic lesions in rats. *Science* 141(3584): 930–932.

Riganello, F., G. Dolce, and W. G. Sannita (2012). Heart rate variability and the central autonomic network in the severe disorder of consciousness. *Journal of Rehabilitation Medicine* 44(6): 495–501.

Rincon, F., M. Dhamoon, Y. Moon, M. C. Paik, B. Boden-Albala, S. Homma, M. R. Di Tullio, R. L. Sacco, and M. S. V. Elkind (2008). Stroke location and association with fatal cardiac outcomes: Northern Manhattan study (NOMAS). *Stroke* 39(9): 2425–2431.

Sander, D., K. Winbeck, J. Klingelhöfer, T. Etgen, and B. Conrad (2001). Prognostic relevance of pathological sympathetic activation after acute thromboembolic stroke. *Neurology* 57(5): 833–838.

Takahashi, C., H. E. Hinson, and I. J. Baguley (2015). Autonomic dysfunction syndromes after acute brain injury. *Handbook of Clinical Neurology*, 3rd Series. A. Salazar and J. Grafman (eds). United Kingdom: Elsevier.

Thayer, J. F., A. L. Hansen, E. Saus-Rose, and B. H. Johnsen (2009). Heart rate variability, prefrontal neural function, and cognitive performance: The neurovisceral integration perspective on self-regulation, adaptation, and health. *Annals of Behavioral Medicine* 37(2): 141–153.

Van Ravenswaaij-Arts, C. M. A., L. A. A. Kollee, J. C. W. Hopman, G. B. A. Stoelinga, and H. P. Van Geijn (1993). Heart rate variability. *Annals of Internal Medicine* 118(6): 436–447.

15

Heart Rate Variability in Psychiatric Disorders, Methodological Considerations, and Recommendations for Future Research

A. H. Kemp and D. S. Quintana

CONTENTS

15.1 Introduction

Research on heart rate variability (HRV) has been conducted for more than four decades, and the increasing interest in this complex psychophysiological phenomenon continues unabated. A PubMed search for the phrase "heart rate variability" on March 30, 2015, revealed 12,208 "hits," and results by year reveals an increasing number of studies since the 1980s (see Figure 15.1). Reasons for this increasing research interest in HRV likely reflect a combination of factors including relatively noninvasive data collection, low cost, a solid theoretical framework linking the high-frequency (HF) component of HRV (in particular) to parasympathetic (vagal) nervous system function and broad implications for well-being and morbidity. This chapter contains a focused review of this literature in regards to psychiatric disorders in adults, highlights a variety of methodological issues facing researchers in this field, and provides some recommendations for future studies in this exciting area of research at the intersection of psychology, psychiatry, and cardiology.

HRV indexes activity in the vagus nerve, the primary nerve in the parasympathetic nervous system. Given its critical role in both mental and physical health (Kemp and Quintana 2013), it is perhaps the most important nerve in the human body. A variety of measures in the time, frequency, and nonlinear domains can be extracted from HRV analysis. While HRV measures predominantly reflect vagal function, different measures of HRV index distinct physiological mechanisms. For instance, HF HRV (0.15–0.4 Hz) reflects respiratory processes, low-frequency HRV (LF HRV, 0.04–0.15 Hz) indexes blood pressure control mechanisms and vasomotor tone, while very low frequency HRV (VLF HRV, 0.0033–0.04 Hz) is driven by thermoregulation and kidney functioning (Reyes et al. 2013). The standard deviation of NN intervals (SDNN) is a commonly reported time-domain measure,

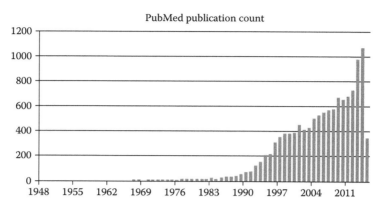

FIGURE 15.1
PubMed publication count on the phrase "heart rate variability."

reflecting all cyclic components responsible for variability. SDNN extracted from long-term recordings (usually 24 hours) is a robust predictor of adverse cardiovascular events and mortality (Hillebrand et al. 2013; Huikuri and Stein 2013). Commonly reported measures of HRV from short-term recordings (2–15 minutes) include the root mean square of successive differences (RMSSD) and HF HRV. While RMSSD—a time-domain measure—and HF HRV are highly correlated, the former is less affected by changes in breathing frequency (Penttilä et al. 2001; Saboul et al. 2013), highlighting the utility of this measure during ambulatory studies, and in patient populations such as those with an anxiety disorder. Another commonly reported measure of vagal function is respiratory sinus arrhythmia (RSA), a measure that combines heart rate with respiration data, and like HF HRV reflects the ebb and flow of heart rate associated with respiration. There has also been much research interest in nonlinear measures of HRV, which assess qualitative properties rather than the magnitude of heart rate dynamics, although their physiological basis is less clear.

Vagal function is often indexed by resting-state HRV from short-term recordings; it is psychophysiological marker that reflects an individual's *capacity* to flexibly respond to an environmental stressor (Friedman and Thayer 1998; Kashdan and Rottenberg 2010; Kemp et al. 2012a). The psychological construct of "flexibility" is a fundamental component of health (Kashdan and Rottenberg 2010), and HRV may provide a psychophysiological foundation for such flexibility (Friedman and Thayer 1998; Kashdan and Rottenberg 2010). Vagal dysfunction—which may be indexed by chronic reductions in resting-state HRV—plays an important role in psychiatric illness, both as a causal factor and as an outcome of the illness itself. Vagal nerve outflow and connections with other cranial nerves contribute to the capacity for social engagement, impairment of which is a core characteristic of the psychiatric disorders (Porges 2011; Quintana et al. 2013a). Vagal dysfunction manifests as flattened affect, poor eye gaze, attenuated facial expressions, lack of prosody, and hyperacusis (Porges 2011). Chronic reductions in HRV are also associated with perseverative cognition (Verkuil et al. 2010), a pathogenic psychophysiological state associated with worry and rumination that may have a "wear and tear" effect on the human body. HRV may therefore provide a structural link between mental and physical health.

There is now a significant body of theoretical and experimental evidence for *an important regulatory role of vagal function over a variety of allostatic systems* including inflammatory processes (Huston and Tracey 2010), the hypothalamic–pituitary–adrenal (HPA) axis

(Porges 2011), and glucose metabolism (Pocai et al. 2005; Wang et al. 2008; see also Thayer and Sternberg 2006a). Allostasis is a term that describes multisystemic adaptations to maintain homeostasis, allowing the body to cope with environmental challenges (McEwen 1998). Vagal dysfunction will therefore lead to overstimulation of these allostatic systems, a condition that has been labeled "allostatic load" (McEwen 1998), increasing risk for medical morbidity (McEwen 2012). Chronic reductions in HRV may therefore provide an early marker of ill health in psychiatric patients without comorbid medical illness that precedes other more established risk factors for medical illness.

We now turn our attention to prior studies that have sought to determine the impact of a variety of psychiatric disorders on HRV in adult populations, many of which have been conducted in our own laboratory.

15.2 HRV in Psychiatric Disorders

The association between psychiatric disorders—particularly the mood and anxiety disorders—and HRV has attracted much research attention. Debate has focused in particular on whether HRV is reduced in the mood and anxiety disorders or whether HRV reductions are driven primarily by medications for these conditions (Kemp 2011, 2012; Kemp et al. 2011a,b; Licht et al. 2011a,b; Brunoni et al. 2012). Our meta-analyses on resting-state HRV in major depressive disorder (MDD) (Kemp et al. 2010), anxiety disorders (Chalmers et al. 2014), and alcohol dependence (Quintana et al. 2013b) sought to draw objective conclusions from a contradictory body of evidence, demonstrating robust, small-to-moderate reductions in HRV. Meta-analysis is an important quantitative technique that allows researchers to draw conclusions from contradictory findings reported by individual studies, which may themselves be affected by low study power. Meta-analysis overcomes this limitation by drawing conclusions on the basis of summary statistics calculated from multiple individual studies.

The meta-analysis on patients with MDD (Kemp et al. 2010) was conducted to determine whether otherwise healthy and unmedicated depressed patients display reductions across a variety of time-domain, frequency-domain, and nonlinear domain measures of HRV. This was important because cardiovascular disease (CVD) may have led to overestimation of the association between depression and resting-state HRV in prior studies. An earlier study (Licht et al. 2008) based on the large Netherlands Study of Depression and Anxiety (NESDA) cohort ($n = 2373$) had also concluded that lowered HRV in depression was mainly driven by the effect of antidepressants. Supporting the hypotheses of the more recent study (Kemp et al. 2010), MDD patients ($n = 673$) displayed lower HRV relative to healthy controls ($n = 407$), effect sizes ranging from small (based on time- and frequency-domain HRV measures) to large (nonlinear measures), highlighting the utility of nonlinear HRV measures. Depression severity was also negatively correlated with HRV ($r = -0.35, p < .001$). Tricyclic antidepressants—but not other classes of antidepressants—were also associated with substantial HRV reductions, findings associated with a large effect size over and above the effects observed in unmedicated patients.

The meta-analysis on anxiety disorders (Chalmers et al. 2014) was conducted on a total of 2,086 patients and 2,294 controls. Like the meta-analysis conducted on MDD, this study was conducted because prior studies had reported inconsistent findings, again highlighting the need for objective meta-analysis. An earlier study, again on the NESDA cohort

($n = 2,095$), had concluded that while HRV was reduced in the anxiety disorders, that findings were again primarily driven by the effects of antidepressant medications. In the more recent meta-analysis (Chalmers et al. 2014), anxiety disorders were characterized by lower HRV (based on HF HRV and time-domain measures), findings associated with a small-to-moderate effect size. Importantly, medication use and medical comorbidity did not impact on these findings. Further inspection of specific disorders indicated that patients with panic disorder ($n = 447$), posttraumatic stress disorder ($n = 192$), generalized anxiety disorder ($n = 68$) and social anxiety disorder ($n = 90$) all displayed moderate reductions in HF HRV, relative to controls. Patients with specific phobias ($n = 61$) also displayed reductions in time-domain measures of HRV, although these findings were associated with a small effect size. Only obsessive-compulsive disorder was not associated with significant reductions in HRV, null findings that may have been due to a relatively small sample size ($n = 40$). Unfortunately, no meta-analysis was able to be conducted on specific treatments of anxiety disorders due to the small number of studies investigating this issue, highlighting the need for further research in this area.

It is important to realize that MDD and anxiety are frequently comorbid conditions: MDD has high comorbidities with the whole range of anxiety disorders (Goldberg and Fawcett 2012). Correlations range from 0.62 for generalized anxiety disorder, to 0.52 for agoraphobia and social phobia, to 0.48 for panic disorder, and to 0.42 for obsessive compulsive disorder (Goldberg and Fawcett 2012). The close relationship between MDD and generalized anxiety disorder, in particular, is thought to relate to shared symptoms—especially negative affect—and genetic risk factors (Goldberg and Fawcett 2012). Recent studies have demonstrated that patients with generalized anxiety disorder, in particular, may display the most robust reductions in HRV (Kemp et al. 2012b, 2014). These findings may relate to patients inability to disengage from threat detection, even in the absence of any real threat (Thayer and Lane 2000; Kemp et al. 2012b). This behavioral characteristic may be underpinned by prolonged prefrontal inactivity, disinhibition of the central nucleus of the amygdala, and activation of medullary cardioacceleratory circuits (Thayer et al. 2009; Kemp et al. 2012b).

The mood and anxiety disorders themselves are often comorbid with alcohol dependence (e.g. Merikangas et al. 1998), a condition that has also been associated with a body of contradictory evidence. A large study on 2,947 participants from the NESDA cohort (Boschloo et al. 2011) had reported that alcohol use, but not its dependence, is associated with dysregulation of the HPA axis and the autonomic nervous system. Critically, however, heavy drinkers only displayed an increased heart rate, but no decreases in HRV, as measured by RSA. The more recent meta-analysis on patients with alcohol dependence ($n = 177$) (Quintana et al. 2013b) observed a lowered HRV in this patient group (relative to nondependent individuals, $n = 216$), a finding associated with a medium effect size. Interestingly, inclusion of the data reported by Boschloo et al. (2011) did not change the conclusions drawn in the meta-analysis (Quintana et al. 2013b). Furthermore, findings were not dependent on comorbid psychiatric disorders. It is possible that lowered HRV in alcohol dependence may underpin some of the behavioral features of the disorder including social dysfunction (Monnot et al. 2001) and impulse control (Ingjaldsson et al. 2003). Meta-analytic findings may also help to explain reported epidemiological findings of increased risk of CVD in alcohol-dependent patients (Corrao et al. 2000).

In addition to findings based on meta-analysis (e.g. Kemp et al. 2010; Quintana et al. 2013a; Chalmers et al. 2014), other work has reported reduced vagal function in multiple, independent cohorts of patients with the mood and anxiety disorders (Kemp et al. 2012b,

2014; Alvares et al. 2013; Brunoni et al. 2013). In the largest independent cohort to date ($n = 15,105$), use of antidepressant medications was associated with substantial decreases in HRV (Kemp et al. 2014). Only generalized anxiety disorder was observed to display robust, albeit small, reductions in vagal activity after controlling for multiple confounding variables, including medication use. This work used propensity score matching procedures, a technique that involves estimating the difference between groups after accounting for the covariates that predict group membership. This technique has several advantages over traditional analytical techniques such as analysis of covariance (ANCOVA) and multiple regression analysis including reduced bias by accounting for the effects of covariates without reference to the outcome variable (HRV) and the opportunity to analyze data with some of the advantages of a randomized controlled design (McCaffrey et al. 2013). Although participants with comorbid depression and anxiety disorders were not observed to display lowered HRV, it is important to bear in mind that many of the factors that adversely affect HRV were controlled for in that study. As the mood and anxiety disorders are known to raise metabolic and cardiovascular risk (Nemeroff and Goldschmidt-Clermont 2012), comprehensive cardiovascular risk reduction strategies in such patients are needed to minimize subsequent morbidity and mortality.

Interestingly, studies have also observed HRV reductions during remission (Kemp et al. 2010; Braeken et al. 2013; Brunoni et al. 2013; Chang et al. 2013) from the disorder. These findings suggest that vagal impairment may actually persist despite successful treatment, perhaps providing a psychophysiological mechanism for the observation that asymptomatic individuals are more vulnerable to future episodes, a phenomenon known as "kindling" (Post 1992). Persistently lowered HRV may, in part, relate to the impacts of medications including antidepressants (Kemp et al. 2010, 2014; Licht et al. 2010) and medications with anticholinergic effects (often prescribed for hypertension and CVD). Further study on the impact of nonpharmacological therapies will have major public health significance.

While medication may contribute to persistent HRV reductions when previously ill patients are well, it was recently demonstrated that unmedicated women ($n = 22$) with a history of anxiety disorders also display decreases in HRV (Braeken et al. 2013). These findings indicate that HRV reductions may be revealed in patients with prior psychiatric illness (in this case anxiety), even in unmedicated individuals. Extending this idea, another study (on MDD, $n = 93$ following treatment) by Brunoni et al. (2013) argued that HRV reductions may be a trait marker of the disorder. This study demonstrated that HRV did not change following treatment with either a nonpharmacological (transcranial direct current stimulation) or pharmacological (sertraline) intervention, nor was HRV observed to increase with clinical response to either treatment. Another study however on unmedicated individuals with a diagnosis of MDD earlier in life ($n = 470$) (Chang et al. 2013) observed that while HRV resolved in patients with fully remitted MDD, autonomic dysregulation was observed in those remitted patients with a history of suicidal ideation ($n = 237$).

In summary, a variety of psychiatric disorders—including the mood and anxiety disorders, and alcohol dependence—display impairment in vagal function. Further study is needed to determine whether particular disorders display greater reductions than others, and the pathways by which these reductions contribute to physical ill health. While decreases in HRV are generally indicative of autonomic dysfunction (Thayer et al. 2010), higher values may also reflect an unhealthy, highly irregular heart rate pattern in cardiac patients (Huikuri and Stein 2013). We now turn our attention to some of the methodological considerations facing researchers using HRV in their research activities.

15.3 Methodological Considerations

Drawing definitive conclusions on the basis of the reported evidence has been made difficult by a variety of methodological factors, which need to be considered in future research. A recent study (Moon et al. 2013) that attempted to compare multiple psychiatric disorders including schizophrenia, bipolar disorder, posttraumatic disorder, and MDD on resting-state measures of HRV in the time domain, frequency domain, and nonlinear domain provides a case in point. This study observed robust decreases in patients with bipolar disorder across a variety of HRV measures. Significant reductions in HF HRV were also observed in schizophrenia, posttraumatic stress disorder, and MDD relative to controls. While HRV reductions were observed, Moon et al. (2013) were unable to discriminate among the disorders. A major limitation of this study however was that these patient groups were being treated with a variety of medications, which may impact on HRV (Kemp et al. 2010, 2014; Licht et al. 2010). While it is difficult (and often unethical) to withdraw patients from their medication, it has been the subject of significant debate as to whether different psychiatric disorders display lowered HRV over and above their medications, as discussed in the previous section. Another limitation of this study (Moon et al. 2013) related to group differences on age, a major confounding variable (Voss et al. 2012), which again makes it difficult to draw robust conclusions from this study.

In fact, a variety of sociodemographic factors including age, sex, and ethnicity all impact on HRV. It is well established that HRV decreases with increasing age (O'Brien et al. 1986; Umetani et al. 1998; Antelmi et al. 2004; Voss et al. 2012), a consequence of modifications of the cardiovascular system with aging including a loss of sinoatrial pacemaker cells, loss of vagal function, and an uncoupling of respiratory activity from vagal outflow (Ferrari 2002; Voss et al. 2015). In one of the first studies to investigate this issue on a relatively large sample of healthy participants ($n = 310$) (O'Brien et al. 1986), a statistically significant negative correlation was reported between age and a variety of nonstandard, short-term measures of HRV across a variety of procedures including rest, a single deep breath, the Valsalva maneuver, and standing. More recent studies have confirmed these initial findings using standardized measures of HRV (Umetani et al. 1998; Antelmi et al. 2004; Zulfiqar et al. 2010; Voss et al. 2012 2015). These more recent studies have also expanded their focus to sex differences on HRV and their interaction with age (Umetani et al. 1998; Antelmi et al. 2004; Voss et al. 2015).

A study on 260 healthy individuals aged from 10 to 99 years (Umetani et al. 1998) reported that all measures of HRV extracted from 24-hour long recordings decreased with age. The mean of the standard deviations of all normal sinus RR intervals for all 5-minute segments (SDNN index) decreased linearly with aging ($r = -0.63$) < reaching 46% of baseline (as defined by values collected from participants in their second decade) by the tenth decade. The RMSSD HRV measure decreased rapidly, reaching 47% of baseline by the sixth decade and then stabilized (quadratic pattern, $r = -0.62$). The authors of this study highlighted that age-related declines in HRV make it difficult to distinguish low HRV due to disease from that due to normal aging. This insight has important implications for the investigation of HRV differences between patients with psychiatric illness in the elderly, as the aging process may actually ameliorate any depression-specific differences on HRV. Indeed, no significant differences have been observed in recent studies on HRV measures in elderly patients with depression (O'Regan et al. 2014; Licht et al. 2015).

Although the impact of sex is less than that of age (Voss et al. 2015), these differences may still have important implications for interpreting the findings from studies on psychiatric illness. For instance, research has demonstrated that depressed males may display lower HRV (as measured by time- and frequency-domain measures), while depressed females may display higher HRV relative to their nondepressed counterparts (Thayer et al. 1998). The authors of this study in fact highlighted that sex may be a possible explanation for the contradictory findings that had been reported in the literature up until that time. It is notable however that this study (Thayer et al. 1998) was conducted on a relatively young, healthy, and nonclinical population (college students, mean age = 20.37 years). Two recent studies (Voss et al. 2012, 2015) focused on HRV measures extracted from 5-minute electrocardiogram (ECG) recordings collected under resting conditions in a supine position. While prior studies have often drawn conclusions based on 24-hour ambulatory ECG recordings, reliable and valid measures of HRV may also be obtained from shorter recordings under standardized and controlled conditions (Anonymous 1996). These recent studies (Voss et al. 2012, 2015) provide reference values for a variety of linear and nonlinear indices from 1906 healthy subjects ranging from 25 to 74 years. Findings support previous observations of decreased HRV with increasing age (Voss et al. 2012). Age-dependent reductions were particularly apparent across the younger age groups 25–34, 35–44, and 45–54, highlighting the importance of age in younger samples in particular. The major age-related difference was observed between participants aged 33–44 versus 45–54 years (Voss et al. 2015). Although women were observed to display a higher complexity of heartbeat generation in younger ages than men, these effects disappeared with an age older than 55 years, a finding the authors speculated may relate to hormonal restructuring caused by menopause.

Robust ethnicity effects were recently reported in a meta-analysis of 17 studies published between 1995 and 2013 (Hill et al. 2015), which demonstrated that HRV is higher in African Americans (Blacks) than European Americans (Whites). Increased HRV in African Americans represents a paradox because these individuals are also characterized by a high prevalence of cardiovascular morbidity and mortality (Sharma et al. 2004; Mensah et al. 2005). These findings highlight the importance of controlling for ethnicity (and/or race) when considering effects of psychiatric illness and their treatments on HRV. The practice of using ethnicity and race as a distinguishing feature of populations to improve diagnostic or therapeutic efforts is a common practice in medicine, albeit a controversial one (Cho 2006; Cohn 2006). There is no scientific support for the use of race as a marker of genetic susceptibility (see Kaplan and Bennett 2003 for discussion), and responses for the same person may actually change over time, a characteristic that may represent shifts in self-identification (Fish 2000; Travassos and Williams 2004). It is clear however that while race is a social construct, it is one with biological consequences (Travassos and Williams 2004). The observed differences on HRV are likely due to a variety of factors including gene–environment interactions and psychosocial issues such as discrimination, on which further study is required.

Major health indicators including smoking and levels of physical activity should also be considered in HRV studies. A study (Felber et al. 2007) on 1,218 nonsmokers, aged 50 years and above, reported a 15% reduction in total power, LF power, LF/HF ratio, and ultralow frequency power of HRV—as measured through 24-hour ambulatory ECG recordings—in participants exposed to environmental tobacco smoke at home or at work for more than 2 hours per day ($n = 80$) compared to those not exposed ($n = 1034$). Importantly, this study demonstrated that results from HRV collected during the sleep period were similar to the results from the 24-hour measures, indicating that findings were not merely acute responses. Smoking is even associated with HRV decreases in depressed patients ($n = 77$) (Harte et al. 2013), a particularly striking finding considering that depressed patients are already characterized by low HRV, as discussed above. This study (Harte et al. 2013) reported that depressed smokers ($n = 34$) display decreased HRV including HF HRV and RSA relative to depressed nonsmokers ($n = 43$), even after controlling for demographic and medical characteristics and medication use (Harte et al. 2013). In another recent study by the same authors ($n = 62$) (Harte and Meston 2014), smoking cessation ($n = 20$) in successful quitters was associated with increases in HRV at follow-up, 4 weeks after patch discontinuation. By contrast, HRV indices among unsuccessful quitters were generally unchanged across time.

Physical activity also has strong effects over vagal function, such that physically active individuals display increased variability during the resting state (as reviewed by Carter et al. 2003; Thayer et al. 2010). One of the first studies reported that fit individuals ($n = 18$)—from a group of university students aged 17–25 years—display greater vagal control of the heart relative to low-fit individuals ($n = 16$), as determined by time- and frequency-domain measures of HRV, even after controlling for body mass index (BMI) (Rossy and Thayer 1998). The findings were observed across all tasks including a resting baseline demonstrating the robustness of these findings. A more recent study on the Whitehall II cohort ($n = 3,328$) of older civil servants aged 45–68 years (Rennie et al. 2003) demonstrated that moderate and vigorous activity is associated with higher HRV during a 5-minute resting-state, and these findings remained significant after adjustment for smoking and alcohol intake. Activity levels in this study were determined by a questionnaire that allows for a metabolic equivalent (MET) value to be determined, such that 1 MET corresponds to the metabolic energy expended lying quietly (equivalent to 1 kcal per kilogram of body weight per hour). Vigorous activity was defined as greater than or equal to 5 MET hours per week (Rennie et al. 2003). Another randomized-controlled study on sedentary young adults ($n = 149$, mean age 30 years) reported that 12 weeks of aerobic conditioning, but not strength training, enhances autonomic control of the heart, as determined by decreases in heart rate (3.49 beats per minute) and increases in HF HRV during 10 minutes of quiet rest (Sloan et al. 2009). These authors further reported that 4 weeks of deconditioning following the training period led to these measures returning to pretraining levels.

One of the most commonly reported indices of HRV is the HF power component, which reflects parasympathetic (vagal) contributions that are strongly coupled with respiration. While some researchers have argued that respiration must be controlled in HRV studies by having participants breathe at the same rate, others have argued that this is an artificial control that may confound the visceral–medullary feedback system and shift respiratory parameters (Porges 2011). A more appropriate solution may be the application of autoregressive techniques rather than fast-Fourier transform (FFT), which determines an empirically appropriate breathing frequency for each participant (Kay and Marple 1981; Zisner and Beauchaine 2014). We further suggest that researchers should consider reporting on multiple measures of HRV to provide a more comprehensive and robust picture of change with task or differences between groups. In this regard, RMSSD is less affected by changes in breathing frequency (Penttilä et al. 2001).

Analytical issues are another issue that HRV researchers need to consider. Psychopathological studies have often controlled for confounding factors using ANCOVA, yet this statistical technique is not appropriate when participants have not been randomly allocated to a group (Miller and Chapman 2001), an issue that we have discussed previously in regards to HRV (Kemp et al. 2011a,b). The reason for this is that quasi-experimental designs are subject to what is known as the "Lord's" or "Simpson's" paradox, a phenomenon in which "the association between two variables may be reversed, diminished or enhanced when another variable is statistically controlled" (Tu et al. 2008). One approach to address this issue controls for potentially confounding factors using propensity score matching (Kemp et al. 2014), which accounts for the effects of covariates before examining differences between groups on the outcome variable (HRV). While the technique of propensity score matching has been applied to other areas of research (and epidemiology in particular), our recent study (Kemp et al. 2014) was the first to apply this technique to the study of the impacts of psychiatric illness and antidepressant medications on HRV. Another potential explanation for the contradictory findings reported in the literature may be the choice to restrict the reporting of measures to time- and frequency-based domains. The reported effect sizes relating to the association between the mood disorders and common comorbid conditions and measures of HRV in these domains are typically small. By contrast, findings based on nonlinear measures of HRV—in MDD at least (Kemp et al. 2010)—are associated with larger effects, suggesting that nonlinear measures of HRV may be more sensitive to alterations in patients with MDD. As HRV may reflect nonlinear mechanisms involved in cardiovascular regulation (Kaplan et al. 1991; Goldberger 1996), HRV alterations may go undetected if researchers focus solely on conventional measures. Unfortunately, there is a lack of understanding as to what these nonlinear measures may actually signify (Tan et al. 2009), unlike the solid theoretical foundation for HF HRV, which relates specifically to the action of the vagus (Akselrod et al. 1981; Kamath and Fallen 1992).

In summary, these many methodological considerations highlight the importance of examining the association between psychiatric disorders and HRV using a variety of different strategies including meta-analysis (e.g. Kemp et al. 2010; Chalmers et al. 2014), propensity score matching (e.g. Kemp et al. 2014), and replication in multiple independent samples (e.g. Kemp et al. 2012b; Alvares et al. 2013; Brunoni et al. 2013). Interested readers are referred to several published reviews (Montano et al. 2009; Quintana and Heathers 2014) for further discussion of methodological considerations relating to HRV research. We now turn our attention to some of the questions that will keep researchers occupied in the years to come.

15.4 Future Directions

Research to date has largely focused on whether there is an effect, rather than when, or how, an effect appears. This focus may, in part, have led to some of the contradictory and discrepant findings reported in the literature, and subsequent debate, especially when focusing on time- and frequency-domain measures of HRV. For instance, a study involving 22-hour ambulatory monitoring (Schwerdtfeger and Friedrich-Mai 2009) demonstrated that while depression is associated with reduced time-domain HRV (RMSSD) when participants are alone, social interactions (with partner, family, or friends) may ameliorate this effect. These findings are important as laboratory-based recordings involve social interaction with experimenters, which may inadvertently ameliorate differences between depressed participants and controls. Social connectedness is associated with increased HRV (Kok and Fredrickson 2010), and Porges' polyvagal theory (Porges 2011) provides a theoretical basis for such findings, which may also be apparent in psychiatric populations, particularly depressed individuals. It is possible however that examination of group differences under multiple conditions including resting state, stressor, and recovery from stressor may elucidate more robust effects in psychiatric disorders, and especially MDD.

Researchers also need to give consideration to what might moderate HRV reductions in order to better clarify the conditions under which effects may or may not be observed. It is possible, for instance, that the effect sizes of the disorders are larger than have been reported, but that they have been suppressed by not taking into consideration particular moderating factors. In addition to the above example in regards to social engagement, certain clinical characteristics may also moderate observed findings. For example, specific subtypes of depression (e.g., melancholia) or symptoms of a depressive episode or the anxiety disorders (e.g., somatic symptoms) may have stronger effects on vagal activity. This particular issue was examined in a recently published report, with findings indicating that patients with melancholia display more robust reductions in resting-state HRV, relative to controls, than those patients without melancholic symptoms (Kemp et al. 2014).

Another potential moderator that should be investigated in studies on psychiatric disorders is the impact of ethnic differences. As noted above, recent work has demonstrated large ethnicity effects on HRV demonstrating that African Americans have higher HRV than individuals with a white European background (Hill et al. 2015). Curiously, African Americans also have higher mortality rates from coronary heart disease and stroke (Keenan and Shaw 2011), a surprising finding considering that increased HRV is usually associated with reduced, not increased, risk for CVD, a phenomenon the authors (Hill et al. 2015) labeled as a cardiovascular "conundrum." These findings highlight a need for further research to better understand the moderating and mediating mechanisms underpinning not only decreases in HRV in psychiatric disorders, but also in the downstream causal pathways leading to increased morbidity and mortality in the context of established risk markers such as hypertension, diabetes, abnormal cholesterol, and modifiable factors including smoking, physical activity, and obesity.

In regards to the causal pathways from psychiatric illness to morbidity and mortality, researchers still need to determine what might be major mediators of downstream adverse effects (i.e., physical disease and mortality) in otherwise healthy patients with psychiatric illness. Research methodologists argue that "we better understand some phenomenon when we can answer not only whether X affects Y, but also how X exerts its effect on Y, and when X affects Y and when it does not." (Hayes 2013). In this regard, "the how question relates to the underlying psychological, cognitive, or biological process that causally links X to Y, whereas the 'when' question pertains to the boundary conditions of the causal association" (Hayes 2013) Researchers need to move beyond questions like "is there an effect?" to questions such as "when do effects appear?" (moderation), "how do effects arise?" (mediation), and "how strong are these effects?" (effect size) (Cumming 2012; Hayes 2013). In doing so, researchers will gain better understanding of the causal pathways involved and clarify whether, how, and when these effects (HRV reductions) lead to morbidity and mortality. Longitudinal studies also play an important role in finding the right answers to these questions.

Another important question relates to the effects of different types of treatment—particularly nonpharmacological treatments—on HRV, and how to ameliorate the adverse effects of antidepressant medications (Licht et al. 2010; Kemp et al. 2014). Even the most commonly prescribed class of antidepressants, the selective serotonin reuptake inhibitors (SSRIs), appear to have adverse effects on HRV (Licht et al. 2010; but see Kemp et al. 2011a). These considerations have important implications for future research on HRV in psychiatry and psychology, raising the question as to whether regular physical activity—a health behavior with powerful beneficial effects on the autonomic nervous system—is able to increase HRV in participants using antidepressant medications. Given that antidepressant drugs alone do not seem to protect patients from CVD (Whang et al. 2009; Hamer et al.

2011; Kemp et al. 2015), longitudinal studies are needed to evaluate the impact of exercise in patients receiving long-term antidepressant treatment.

In summary, while researchers have generated a significant body of research on which our understanding of the relationship between HRV and adult psychiatric disorders, has improved, much research on causal pathways among HRV, psychiatric disorders, and cardiovascular risks remains to be done.

15.5 Conclusions

Previous studies investigating the association between psychiatric disorders have largely been correlational in nature. Therefore, it remains unclear whether psychiatric disorders adversely affect HRV or whether reductions in HRV precede the manifestation of the disorder. We suggest here that the relationship between mood and HRV is a bidirectional one. Higher baseline levels of HRV are associated with increased positive emotions and social connectedness over a 9-week period (Kok and Fredrickson 2010). Importantly, this study also showed that increases in positive emotions and connectedness predicted increases in HRV, independent of baseline levels. The authors concluded that results supported "an upward spiral relationship of reciprocal causality" such that HRV and psychological well-being reciprocally and prospectively predict each other. We suggest that this reciprocal relationship may work similarly in those experiencing psychiatric disorders such that negative emotions will also reciprocally and prospectively predict each other in a "downward" spiral relationship.

The vagus nerve clearly plays an important role in the psychiatric disorders. Through its interconnections with other cranial nerves, it underpins a host of symptoms such as flattened facial affect and lack of prosody (Porges 2011). A poorly functioning cholinergic anti-inflammatory reflex (Tracey 2002)—underpinned by the vagus—contributes to the chronic low-grade inflammation that is characteristic of depression and other psychiatric disorders (Berk et al. 2013), subsequently contributing to physical ill-health over the longer term. As the vagus nerve plays a critical role in the regulation of inflammatory processes (Tracey 2002) and other allostatic systems (Thayer and Sternberg 2006b), vagal function—indexed by HRV—is an important factor underpinning individual differences in morbidity and mortality from a host of conditions and disorders.

References

Akselrod, S, D Gordon, FA Ubel, DC Shannon, AC Berger, and RJ Cohen. 1981. Power spectrum analysis of heart rate fluctuation: A quantitative probe of beat-to-beat cardiovascular control. *Science (New York, NY)* 213 (4504): 220–222.

Alvares, GA, DS Quintana, AH Kemp, A Van Zwieten, BW Balleine, IB Hickie, and AJ Guastella. 2013. Reduced heart rate variability in social anxiety disorder: Associations with gender and symptom severity. Edited by L Fontenelle. *PLOS ONE* 8 (7): e70468. doi:10.1371/journal.pone.0070468.

Anonymous. 1996. Heart rate variability: Standards of measurement, physiological interpretation and clinical use. Task Force of the European Society of Cardiology and the North American Society of Pacing and Electrophysiology. *Circulation* 93: 1043–1065.

Antelmi, I, RS de Paula, AR Shinzato, CA Peres, AJ Mansur, and CJ Grupi. 2004. Influence of age, gender, body mass index, and functional capacity on heart rate variability in a cohort of subjects without heart disease. *American Journal of Cardiology* 93 (3): 381–85. doi:10.1016/j.amjcard.2003.09.065.

Berk, M, LJ Williams, FN Jacka, AO Neil, JA Pasco, S Moylan, NB Allen, AL Stuart, AC Hayley, ML Bryne, and M Maes. 2013. So depression is an inflammatory disease, but where does the inflammation come from? *BMC Medicine* 11 (1): 1–1. doi:10.1186/1741-7015-11-200.

Boschloo, L, N Vogelzangs, CM Licht, SA Vreeburg, JH Smit, W van den Brink, DJ Veltman, EJ de Geus, Aartjan TF Beekman, and BW Penninx. 2011. Heavy alcohol use, rather than alcohol dependence, is associated with dysregulation of the hypothalamic-pituitary-adrenal axis and the autonomic nervous system. *Drug and Alcohol Dependence* 116 (1–3): 170–176. doi:10.1016/j.drugalcdep.2010.12.006.

Braeken, MA, AH Kemp, T Outhred, RA Otte, GJ Monsieur, A Jones, and BR Van den Bergh. 2013. Pregnant mothers with resolved anxiety disorders and their offspring have reduced heart rate variability: Implications for the health of children. Edited by James Coyne. *PLOS ONE* 8 (12): e83186. doi:10.1371/journal.pone.0083186.

Brunoni, AR, AH Kemp, EM Dantas, AC Goulart, MA Nunes, PS Boggio, JG Mill, PA Lotufo, F Fregni, and IM Benseñor. 2013. Heart rate variability is a trait marker of major depressive disorder: Evidence from the sertraline vs. electric current therapy to treat depression clinical study. *International Journal of Neuropsychopharmacology* 16 (9): 1937–1949. doi:10.1017/S1461145713000497.

Brunoni, AR, PA Lotufo, and IM Benseñor. 2012. Are antidepressants good for the soul but bad for the matter? Using noninvasive brain stimulation to detangle depression/antidepressants effects on heart rate variability and cardiovascular risk. *Biological Psychiatry* 71 (7): e27–28; author reply e29–30. doi:10.1016/j.biopsych.2011.08.026.

Carter, JB, EW Banister, and AP Blaber. 2003. Effect of endurance exercise on autonomic control of heart rate. *Sports Medicine (Auckland, NZ)* 33 (1): 33–46 doi: 10.2165/00007256-200333010-00003.

Chalmers, JA, DS Quintana, MJ Abbott, and AH Kemp. 2014. Anxiety disorders are associated with reduced heart rate variability: A meta-analysis. *Frontiers in Psychiatry/Frontiers Research Foundation* 5: 80. doi:10.3389/fpsyt.2014.00080.

Chang, HA, CC Chang, CL Chen, T Kuo, RB Lu, and S Huang. 2013. Heart rate variability in patients with fully remitted major depressive disorder. *Acta Neuropsychiatrica* 25(1): 33–42. doi:10.1111/j.1601-5215.2012.00658.x.

Cho, MK. 2006. Racial and ethnic categories in biomedical research: There is no baby in the bathwater. *Journal of Law, Medicine and Ethics: A Journal of the American Society of Law, Medicine and Ethics* 34 (3): 497–499, 479.

Cohn, JN. 2006. The use of race and ethnicity in medicine: Lessons from the African-American heart failure trial. *Journal of Law, Medicine and Ethics: A Journal of the American Society of Law, Medicine and Ethics* 34 (3): 552–554, 480.

Corrao, G, L Rubbiati, V Bagnardi, A Zambon, and K Poikolainen. 2000. Alcohol and coronary heart disease: A meta-analysis. *Addiction* 95 (10): 1505–1523.

Cumming, G. 2012. *Understanding The New Statistics: Effect Sizes, Confidence Intervals, and Meta-Analysis*. New York: Routledge.

Felber DD, J Schwartz, C Schindler, JM Gaspoz, JC Barthélémy, JM Tschopp, F Roche, A von Eckardstein, O Brändli, P Leuenberger, DR Gold, U Ackermann-Liebrich; SAPALDIA Team. 2007. Effects of passive smoking on heart rate variability, heart rate and blood pressure: An observational study. *International Journal of Epidemiology* 36 (4): 834–840. Oxford University Press. doi:10.1093/ije/dym031.

Ferrari, AU. 2002. Modifications of the cardiovascular system with aging. *American Journal of Geriatric Cardiology* 11 (1): 30–33.

Fish, JM. 2000. What anthropology can do for psychology: Facing physics envy, ethnocentrism, and a belief in 'Race'. *American Anthropologist* 102 (3): 552–563. doi:10.1525/aa.2000.102.3.552.

Friedman, BH, and J Thayer. 1998. Anxiety and autonomic flexibility: A cardiovascular approach. *Biological Psychology* 49 (3): 303–323. doi:10.1016/S0301-0511(98)00051-9.

Goldberg, D and J Fawcett. 2012. The importance of anxiety in both major depression and bipolar disorder. *Depression and Anxiety* 29 (6): 471–478. doi:10.1002/da.21939.

Goldberger, AL. 1996. Non-linear dynamics for clinicians: Chaos theory, fractals, and complexity at the bedside. *Lancet* 347 (9011): 1312–1314.

Hamer, M, GD Batty, A Seldenrijk, and M Kivimaki. 2011. Antidepressant medication use and future risk of cardiovascular disease: The Scottish health survey. *European Heart Journal* 32 (4): 437–442. doi:10.1093/eurheartj/ehq438.

Harte, CB, GI Liverant, DM Sloan, and BW Kamholz. 2013. Association between smoking and heart rate variability among individuals with depression. *Annals of Behavioral* 46 (1) :73–80 doi: 10.1007/s12160-013-9476-8.

Harte, CB and CM Meston. 2014. Effects of smoking cessation on heart rate variability among long-term male smokers. *International Journal of Behavioral Medicine* 21 (2): 302–309. doi:10.1007/s12529-013-9295-0.

Hayes, AF. 2013. *Introduction to Mediation, Moderation and Conditional Process Analysis* (pp. 1–527). New York: The Guildford Press.

Hill, LK, DD Hu, J Koenig, JJ Sollers, G Kapuku, X Wang, H Snieder, and J Thayer. 2015. Ethnic differences in resting heart rate variability: A systematic review and meta-analysis. *Psychosomatic Medicine* 77 (1): 16–25. doi:10.1097/PSY.0000000000000133.

Hillebrand, S, KB Gast, R de Mutsert, CA Swenne, JW Jukema, S Middeldorp, FR Rosendaal, and OM Dekkers. 2013. Heart rate variability and first cardiovascular event in populations without known cardiovascular disease: Meta-analysis and dose-response meta-regression. *Europace: European Pacing, Arrhythmias, and Cardiac Electrophysiology: Journal of the Working Groups on Cardiac Pacing, Arrhythmias, and Cardiac Cellular Electrophysiology of the European Society of Cardiology* 15 (5): 742–749. doi:10.1093/europace/eus341.

Huikuri, HV and PK Stein. 2013. Heart rate variability in risk stratification of cardiac patients. *Progress in Cardiovascular Diseases* 56 (2): 153–159. doi:10.1016/j.pcad.2013.07.003.

Huston, JM and KJ Tracey. 2010. The pulse of inflammation: Heart rate variability, the cholinergic anti-inflammatory pathway and implications for therapy. *Journal of Internal Medicine* 269 (1): 45–53. doi:10.1111/j.1365-2796.2010.02321.x.

Ingjaldsson, JT, JC Laberg, and J Thayer. 2003. Reduced heart rate variability in chronic alcohol abuse: Relationship with negative mood, chronic thought suppression, and compulsive drinking. *Biological Psychiatry* 54 (12): 1427–1436.

Kamath, MV and EL Fallen. 1992. Power spectral analysis of heart rate variability: A noninvasive signature of cardiac autonomic function. *Critical Reviews in Biomedical Engineering* 21 (3): 245–311.

Kaplan, DT, MI Furman, SM Pincus, SM Ryan, LA Lipsitz, and AL Goldberger. 1991. Aging and the complexity of cardiovascular dynamics. *Biophysical Journal* 59 (4): 945–949. doi:10.1016/S0006-3495(91)82309-8.

Kaplan, JB and T Bennett. 2003. Use of race and ethnicity in biomedical publication. *Journal of the American Medical Association* 289 (20): 2709–2716. doi:10.1001/jama.289.20.2709.

Kashdan, T and J Rottenberg. 2010. Psychological flexibility as a fundamental aspect of health. *Clinical Psychology Review* 30 (7): 865–878. doi:10.1016/j.cpr.2010.03.001.

Kay, SM and SL Marple Jr. 1981. Spectrum analysis—A modern perspective. *Proceedings of the IEEE*, 69: 1380–1419.

Keenan, NL and KM Shaw. 2011. Coronary heart disease and stroke deaths — United States, 2006. *MMWR Surveillance Summaries* 60: 62–66.

Kemp, AH. 2011. Depression, antidepressant treatment and the cardiovascular system. *Acta Neuropsychiatrica* 23 (2): 82–83. doi:10.1111/j.1601-5215.2011.00535.x.

Kemp, AH. 2012. Reply to: Are antidepressants good for the soul but bad for the matter? Using noninvasive brain stimulation to detangle depression/antidepressants effects on heart rate variability and cardiovascular risk. *Biological Psychiatry* 71 (7): e29–e30. doi:10.1016/j.biopsych.2011.11.002.

Kemp, AH, AR Brunoni, MS Bittencourt, MA Nunes, IM Benseñor, and PA Lotufo. 2015. The association between antidepressant medications and coronary heart disease in Brazil: A cross-sectional analysis on the Brazilian longitudinal study of adult health (ELSA-Brazil). *Frontiers in Public Health* 3: 9. doi:10.3389/fpubh.2015.00009.

Kemp, AH, AR Brunoni, IS Santos, MA Nunes, EM Dantas, R Carvalho de Figueiredo, AC Pereira, AL Ribeiro, JG Mill, RV Andreão, JF Thayer, IM Benseñor, PA Lotufo. 2014. Effects of depression, anxiety, comorbidity, and antidepressants on resting-state heart rate and its variability: An ELSA-Brasil cohort baseline study. *American Journal of Psychiatry* 171(12): 1328–1334. doi:10.1176/appi.ajp.2014.13121605.

Kemp, AH and DS Quintana. 2013. The relationship between mental and physical health: Insights from the study of heart rate variability. *International Journal of Psychophysiology: Official Journal of the International Organization of Psychophysiology* 89 (3): 288–296. doi:10.1016/j.ijpsycho.2013.06.018.

Kemp, AH, DS Quintana, KL Felmingham, S Matthews, and HF Jelinek. 2012b. Depression, comorbid anxiety disorders, and heart rate variability in physically healthy, unmedicated patients: Implications for cardiovascular risk. Edited by Kenji Hashimoto. *PLOS ONE* 7 (2): e30777. doi:10.1371/journal.pone.0030777.t002.

Kemp, AH, DS Quintana, and MA Gray. 2011b. Is heart rate variability reduced in depression without cardiovascular disease? *Biological Psychiatry* 69 (4): e3–e4. doi:10.1016/j.biopsych.2010.07.030.

Kemp, AH, DS Quintana, MA Gray, KL Felmingham, K Brown, and JM Gatt. 2010. Impact of depression and antidepressant treatment on heart rate variability: A review and meta-analysis. *Biological Psychiatry* 67 (11): 1067–1074. doi:10.1016/j.biopsych.2009.12.012.

Kemp, AH, DS Quintana, and GS Malhi. 2011a. Effects of serotonin reuptake inhibitors on heart rate variability: Methodological issues, medical comorbidity, and clinical relevance. *Biological Psychiatry* 69 (8): e25–26; author reply e27–28. doi:10.1016/j.biopsych.2010.10.035.

Kemp, AH, DS Quintana, RL Kuhnert, K Griffiths, IB Hickie, and AJ Guastella. 2012a. Oxytocin increases heart rate variability in humans at rest: Implications for social approach-related motivation and capacity for social engagement. Edited by Kenji Hashimoto. *PLOS ONE* 7 (8): e44014. doi:10.1371/journal.pone.0044014.

Kemp, AH, DS Quintana, CR Quinn, P Hopkinson, and AW Harris. 2014. Major depressive disorder with melancholia displays robust alterations in resting state heart rate and its variability: Implications for future morbidity and mortality. *Frontiers in Psychology* 5: 1387. doi:10.3389/fpsyg.2014.01387.

Kok, BE and BL Fredrickson. 2010. Upward spirals of the heart: Autonomic flexibility, as indexed by vagal tone, reciprocally and prospectively predicts positive emotions and social connectedness. *Biological Psychology* 85 (3): 432–436. doi:10.1016/j.biopsycho.2010.09.005.

Licht, CM, EJ de Geus, R van Dyck, and BW Penninx. 2010. Longitudinal evidence for unfavorable effects of antidepressants on heart rate variability. *Biological Psychiatry* 68 (9): 861–868. doi:10.1016/j.biopsych.2010.06.032.

Licht, CM, EJC de Geus, FG Zitman, WJG Hoogendijk, R van Dyck, and BWJH Penninx. 2008. Association between major depressive disorder and heart rate variability in the Netherlands Study of Depression and Anxiety (NESDA). *Archives of General Psychiatry*, 65(12): 1358–1367. http://doi.org/10.1001/archpsyc.65.12.1358

Licht, CM, P Naarding, BW Penninx, RC van der Mast, EJ de Geus, and H Comijs. 2015. The association between depressive disorder and cardiac autonomic control in adults 60 years and older. *Psychosomatic Medicine* 77(3), 279–291. doi:10.1097/PSY.0000000000000165.

Licht, CM, BW Penninx, and EJ de Geus. 2011a. Reply to: Effects of serotonin reuptake inhibitors on heart rate variability: Methodological issues, medical comorbidity, and clinical relevance. *BPS*, March, 1–2. doi:10.1016/j.biopsych.2010.12.039.

Licht, CM, BW Penninx, and EJ de Geus. 2011b. To include or not to include? A response to the meta-analysis of heart rate variability and depression. *Biological Psychiatry* 69 (4): e1; author reply e3–4. doi:10.1016/j.biopsych.2010.06.034.

McCaffrey, DF, BA Griffin, D Almirall, ME Slaughter, R Ramchand, and LF Burgette. 2013. A tutorial on propensity score estimation for multiple treatments using generalized boosted models. *Statistics in Medicine* 32 (19): 3388–3414. doi:10.1002/sim.5753.

McEwen, BS. 1998. Stress, adaptation, and disease: Allostasis and allostatic load. *Annals of the New York Academy of Sciences* 840 (1): 33–44. Blackwell Publishing Ltd. doi:10.1111/j.1749-6632.1998.tb09546.x.

McEwen, BS. 2012. Brain on stress: How the social environment gets under the skin. *Proceedings of the National Academy of Sciences* 109 Suppl 2 (October): 17180–17185. doi:10.1073/pnas.1121254109.

Mensah, GA, AH Mokdad, ES Ford, KJ Greenlund, and JB Croft. 2005. State of disparities in cardiovascular health in the United States. *Circulation* 111 (10): 1233–1241. Lippincott Williams & Wilkins. doi:10.1161/01.CIR.0000158136.76824.04.

Merikangas, KR, RL Mehta, BE Molnar, EE Walters, JD Swendsen, S Aguilar-Gaziola, R Bijl, G Borges, JJ Caraveo-Anduaga, DJ DeWit, B Kolody, WA Vega, HU Wittchen, RC Kessler 1998. Comorbidity of substance use disorders with mood and anxiety disorders: Results of the international consortium in psychiatric epidemiology. *Addictive Behaviors* 23 (6): 893–907.

Miller, GA, and JP Chapman. 2001. Misunderstanding analysis of covariance. *Journal of Abnormal Psychology* 110 (1): 40–48.

Monnot, M, S Nixon, W Lovallo, and E Ross. 2001. Altered emotional perception in alcoholics: Deficits in affective prosody comprehension. *Alcoholism: Clinical and Experimental Research* 25 (3): 362–369.

Montano, N, A Porta, C Cogliati, G Costantino, E Tobaldini, KR Casali, and F Iellamo. 2009. Heart rate variability explored in the frequency domain: A tool to investigate the link between heart and behavior. *Neuroscience and Biobehavioral Reviews* 33 (2): 71–80. doi:10.1016/j.neubiorev.2008.07.006.

Moon, E, SH Lee, DH Kim, and B Hwang. 2013. Comparative study of heart rate variability in patients with schizophrenia, bipolar disorder, post-traumatic stress disorder, or major depressive disorder. *Clinical Psychopharmacology and Neuroscience: The Official Scientific Journal of the Korean College of Neuropsychopharmacology* 11 (3): 137–143. doi:10.9758/cpn.2013.11.3.137.

Nemeroff, CB and PJ Goldschmidt-Clermont. 2012. Heartache and heartbreak—The link between depression and cardiovascular disease. *Nature Publishing Group* 9 (9): 526–539. doi:10.1038/nrcardio.2012.91.

O'Brien, IA, P O'Hare, and RJ Corrall. 1986. Heart rate variability in healthy subjects: Effect of age and the derivation of normal ranges for tests of autonomic function. *Heart (British Cardiac Society)* 55 (4): 348–354. doi:10.1136/hrt.55.4.348.

O'Regan, C, RA Kenny, H Cronin, C Finucane, and PM Kearney. 2014. Antidepressants strongly influence the relationship between depression and heart rate variability: Findings from the Irish longitudinal study on ageing (TILDA). *Psychological Medicine* 1–14. doi:10.1017/S0033291714001767.

Penttilä, J, A Helminen, T Jartti, T Kuusela, HV Huikuri, MP Tulppo, R Coffeng, and H Scheinin. 2001. Time domain, geometrical and frequency domain analysis of cardiac vagal outflow: Effects of various respiratory patterns. *Clinical Physiology* 21 (3): 365–376. doi:10.1046/j.1365-2281.2001.00337.x.

Pocai, A, S Obici, GJ Schwartz, and L Rossetti. 2005. A brain-liver circuit regulates glucose homeostasis. *Cell Metabolism* 1 (1): 53–61. doi:10.1016/j.cmet.2004.11.001.

Porges, SW. 2011. *The Polyvagal Theory: Neurophysiological Foundations of Emotions, Attachment, Communication, and Self-Regulation.* 1st ed. New York, NY: W. W. Norton & Company.

Post, RM. 1992. Transduction of psychosocial stress into the neurobiology of recurrent affective disorder. *American Journal of Psychiatry* 149 (8): 999–1010.

Quintana, DS and JA Heathers. 2014. Considerations in the assessment of heart rate variability in biobehavioral research. *Emotion Science* 5 (July): 1–10. doi:10.3389/fpsyg.2014.00805.

Quintana, DS, AH Kemp, GA Alvares, and AJ Guastella. 2013. A role for autonomic cardiac control in the effects of oxytocin on social behavior and psychiatric illness. *Frontiers in Neuroscience* 7: 48. doi:10.3389/fnins.2013.00048.

Quintana, DS, IS McGregor, AJ Guastella, GS Malhi, and AH Kemp. 2013. A meta-analysis on the impact of alcohol dependence on short-term resting-state heart rate variability: Implications for cardiovascular risk. *Alcoholism: Clinical and Experimental Research* 37 Suppl 1 (January): E23–E29. doi:10.1111/j.1530-0277.2012.01913.x.

Rennie, KL, H Hemingway, M Kumari, E Brunner, M Malik, and M Marmot. 2003. Effects of moderate and vigorous physical activity on heart rate variability in a British study of civil servants. *American Journal of Epidemiology* 158 (2): 135–143.

Reyes Del Paso, GA, W Langewitz, LJM Mulder, A Roon, and S Duschek. 2013. The utility of low frequency heart rate variability as an index of sympathetic cardiac tone: A review with emphasis on a reanalysis of previous studies. *Psychophysiology* 50 (5): 477–487. doi:10.1111/psyp.12027.

Rossy, LA and J Thayer. 1998. Fitness and gender-related differences in heart period variability. *Psychosomatic Medicine* 60 (6): 773–781.

Saboul, D, V Pialoux, and C Hautier. 2013. The impact of breathing on HRV measurements: Implications for the longitudinal follow-up of athletes. *European Journal of Sport Science* 13 (5): 534–42. doi:10.1080/17461391.2013.767947.

Schwerdtfeger, A and P Friedrich-Mai. 2009. Social interaction moderates the relationship between depressive mood and heart rate variability: Evidence from an ambulatory monitoring study. *Health Psychology* 28 (4): 501–509. doi:10.1037/a0014664.

Sharma, S, AM Malarcher, WH Giles, and G Myers. 2004. Racial, ethnic and socioeconomic disparities in the clustering of cardiovascular disease risk factors. *Ethnicity and Disease* 14 (1): 43–48.

Sloan, RP, PA Shapiro, RE DeMeersman, E Bagiella, EN Brondolo, PS McKinley, I Slavov, Y Fang, and MM Myers. 2009. The effect of aerobic training and cardiac autonomic regulation in young adults. *American Journal of Public Health* 99 (5): 921–928. doi:10.2105/AJPH.2007.133165.

Tan, CO, MA Cohen, DL Eckberg, and JA Taylor. 2009. Fractal properties of human heart period variability: Physiological and methodological implications. *Journal of Physiology* 587 (Pt 15): 3929–41. doi:10.1113/jphysiol.2009.169219.

Thayer, J, AL Hansen, E Saus-Rose, and BH Johnsen. 2009. Heart rate variability, prefrontal neural function, and cognitive performance: The neurovisceral integration perspective on self-regulation, adaptation, and health. *Annals of Behavioral Medicine* 37 (2): 141–153. doi:10.1007/s12160-009-9101-z.

Thayer, J and RD Lane. 2000. A model of neurovisceral integration in emotion regulation and dysregulation *Journal of Affective Disorders* 61 (3): 201–216.

Thayer, J, M Smith, LA Rossy, JJ Sollers, and BH Friedman. 1998. Heart period variability and depressive symptoms: Gender differences. *Biological Psychiatry* 44 (4): 304–306.

Thayer, J and E Sternberg. 2006a. Beyond heart rate variability: Vagal regulation of allostatic systems. *Annals of the New York Academy of Sciences* 1088 (1): 361–372. doi:10.1196/annals.1366.014.

Thayer, J and E Sternberg. 2006b. Beyond heart rate variability: Vagal regulation of allostatic systems. *Annals of the New York Academy of Sciences* 1088 (November): 361–372. doi:10.1196/annals.1366.014.

Thayer, J, SS Yamamoto, and JF Brosschot. 2010. The relationship of autonomic imbalance, heart rate variability and cardiovascular disease risk factors. *International Journal of Cardiology* 141 (2): 122–131. doi:10.1016/j.ijcard.2009.09.543.

Tracey, KJ. 2002. The inflammatory reflex. *Nature* 420 (6917): 853–859. doi:10.1038/nature01321.

Travassos, C, and DR Williams. 2004. The concept and measurement of race and their relationship to public health: A review focused on Brazil and the United States. *Cadernos De Saúde Pública* 20 (3): 660–678.

Tu, YK, D Gunnell, and MS Gilthorpe. 2008. Simpson's paradox, Lord's paradox, and suppression effects are the same phenomenon—The reversal paradox. *Emerging Themes in Epidemiology* 5 (1): 2. doi:10.1186/1742-7622-5-2.

Umetani, K, DH Singer, R McCraty, and M Atkinson. 1998. Twenty-four hour time domain heart rate variability and heart rate: Relations to age and gender over nine decades. *Journal of the American College of Cardiology* 31 (3): 593–601.

Verkuil, B, J Brosschot, W Gebhardt, and J Thayer. 2010. When worries make you sick: A review of perseverative cognition, the default stress response and somatic health. *Journal of Experimental Psychopathology* 1 (1): 87–118. doi:10.5127/jep.009110.

Voss, A, A Heitmann, R Schroeder, A Peters, and S Perz. 2012. Short-term heart rate variability—Age dependence in healthy subjects. *Physiological Measurement* 33 (8): 1289–1311. doi:10.1088/0967-3334/33/8/1289.

Voss, A, R Schroeder, A Heitmann, A Peters, and S Perz. 2015. Short-term heart rate variability—Influence of gender and age in healthy subjects. Edited by Adrian V. Hernandez. *PLOS ONE* 10 (3): e0118308. doi:10.1371/journal.pone.0118308.

Wang, PY, L Caspi, CK Lam, M Chari, X Li, and PE Light. 2008. Upper intestinal lipids trigger a gut–brain–liver axis to regulate glucose production. *Nature* 52(7190), 1012–1016.

Whang, W, LD Kubzansky, I Kawachi, KM Rexrode, CH Kroenke, RJ Glynn, H Garan, and CM Albert. 2009. Depression and risk of sudden cardiac death and coronary heart disease in women. *Journal of the American College of Cardiology* 53 (11): 950–958. doi:10.1016/j.jacc.2008.10.060.

Zisner, AR and TP Beauchaine. 2014. Psychophysiological methods and developmental psychopathology. In *Developmental Psychopathology* (pp. 832–884), D Cicchetti (ed.). Hoboken NJ: Wiley.

Zulfiqar, U, DA Jurivich, W Gao, and DH Singer. 2010. Relation of high heart rate variability to healthy longevity. *American Journal of Cardiology* 105 (8): 1181–1185. doi:10.1016/j.amjcard.2009.12.022.

16

Cardiac Autonomic Dysfunction in Patients with Schizophrenia and Their Healthy Relatives

Karl-Jürgen Bär, Steffen Schulz, and Andreas Voss

CONTENTS

16.1 Background

A large body of evidence has documented shortened life expectancy in patients with schizophrenia (Osby et al. 2000; Rasanen et al. 2005; Colton and Manderscheid 2006; Bushe et al. 2010). It has been assumed that suicides, accidents, and cardiovascular disorders are the main reasons for the excess of premature and sudden deaths among patients with schizophrenia (Colton and Manderscheid 2006; Loas et al. 2008; Bushe et al. 2010; Manu et al. 2011). In patients treated with antipsychotics, research has shown evidence that the incidence-rate ratio of sudden cardiac death (SCD) was doubled in individuals receiving first- or second-generation antipsychotics in the last month of life (Ray et al. 2009). The dose-dependent effect of antipsychotics on myocardial cell repolarization was assumed to lead to torsades de pointes, arrhythmias, and finally to ventricular fibrillation and SCD. In this line of evidence, a recent study reporting autopsy findings in inpatients with schizophrenia showed that cardiovascular disorders were the most common cause of death (Ifteni et al. 2014). Thus, schizophrenia may represent a disorder with a specific cardiac vulnerability to SCD (Beary et al. 2012). This assumption is supported by a recent study by Mothi et al. (2015) showing that cardiovascular and metabolic dysfunction is increased in healthy first-degree relatives of patients. This is very suggestive of an overlapping genetic background of cardiac/metabolic conditions and psychotic disorders.

SCD happens when a malignant arrhythmia is triggered by an acute cardiac event (e.g., acute myocardial ischemia, platelet activation, or neuroendocrine variations) on the basis of a diseased myocardium (e.g., postnecrotic scar or hypertrophy). In addition to coronary artery disease or diseases of the myocardium, cardiac electrophysiological abnormalities might predispose to the development of ventricular fibrillation. This is especially important after acute myocardial infarction (AMI). Physicians found that various indices of heart rate variability (HRV) are of predictive value for the outcome of patients after AMI. Subsequently, these measures were transferred to other patient populations. Abnormalities were found for patients suffering from depression, anxiety disorders, alcohol dependence, and, in particular, patients suffering from schizophrenia (Koschke et al. 2009; Herbsleb et al. 2014; Yeragani et al. 2007; Agelink et al. 2002; Bär et al. 2006a; Jochum et al. 2011; Schulz et al. 2010). The main difference, however, is the significance of these values. After AMI, the risk prediction of HRV values for SCD is defined by a measurable endpoint (death). In contrast, the exact meaning of reduced HRV measures in mental disorders is more difficult to define, since patients live with the disease and altered cardiac autonomic function for many years. Therefore, the definite influence of profound autonomic dysfunction in patients with schizophrenia for reduced life expectancy needs to be shown in long-term prospective studies.

16.2 Heart Rate Variability

The term HRV refers to a number of measures of different types. In general, nearly all HRV measures reflect mainly vagal (parasympathetic) modulation at the level of the heart. HRV is the physiological phenomenon of variation in the time interval between heartbeats and it is determined by measuring the variation in the beat-to-beat (BBI) interval. Although HRV measures can be obtained quite easily nowadays, there are numerous pitfalls. Autonomic indices depend very much on circadian rhythms, the duration and measurement procedure, the environment, and artefact management. Time-domain and frequency-domain measures are most often used. In general, if time-domain measures (e.g., root mean square successive difference [RMSSD]) are extremely low, true autonomic dysfunction can be assumed. Frequency-domain measures (e.g., high frequency [HF], low frequency [LF], and very low frequency [VLF]) are very susceptible to artefacts and quantify the amount of variance in heart rate at different underlying frequencies. Again, extremely low values of HF are associated with a lack of autonomic vagal modulation of heart rate.

Besides linear HRV parameters describing the variance of BBI intervals, nonlinear complexity measures have been developed to describe the regularity of heart rate time series. The application of these analyses has led to a higher sensitivity for detecting autonomic dysfunction (Baumert et al. 2004; Hoyer et al. 2006), patients at risk for sudden death (Voss et al. 1996), and survivors of myocardial infarction (Voss et al. 1998). A high complexity of biosignals reflects diverse influences of different regulatory systems. In the case of BBI interval, these are, among others, neuronal (autonomic nervous system), hormonal (e.g., cortisol, atrial naturetic peptide [ANP]), and myocardium inherent mechanisms (Yeragani and Sree Hari Rao 2006). Overall, up to a certain point, the more irregular and complex heart rate series are the more adaptive and stable is the underlying system. Such complexity is only in part reflected in measures of classical moment statistics such as means and standard errors (e.g., time-domain or frequency-domain measures), which mainly describe the fluctuation of the biosignal (Goldberger et al. 2002). However, classical parameters do not contain sufficient information on the regularity pattern of these fluctuations. For example, a sine curve might have the same mean and standard error as a very irregularly shaped curve, which is why nonlinear measures are required to detect these differences in system complexity.

16.3 Heart Rates of Unmedicated Patients Suffering from Schizophrenia

"Taking the pulse" has always been the first point of contact between physicians and the patient. It has recently been suggested that the heart rate corresponds to the rate of energy needed by the body. A reduction in heart rate of 10 beats per minute a day saves 5 kg of adenosine triphosphate (ATP). Furthermore, an increase in heart rate of 5 beats per minute corresponds to a significant increase in atherosclerosis progression. Animal and human studies show that life expectancy is closely related to the medium heart rate. Increased resting heart rate has been shown to be a risk factor for reduced life expectancy in both the general population (Jensen et al. 2013b; Greenland et al. 1999) and in populations with cardiovascular diseases (Diaz et al. 2005; Jensen et al. 2013a).

In 1899, Kraepelin described extensive autonomic alterations in patients with schizophrenia, including increased heart rates, altered pupillary function, increased sweating and salivation as well as temperature changes (Kraepelin 1899). Most of these described signs suggest increased sympathetic output, decreased parasympathetic modulation, or both. For a long time, psychiatrists attributed increased heart rates in patients with schizophrenia to antipsychotic treatment. This assumption is only correct to some extent. Treatment with clozapine, for instance, is associated with reduced vagal function and increased heart rates (Agelink et al. 2001; Zahn and Pickar 1993; Iwamoto et al. 2012). However, several studies have reported increased heart rates in first episode and unmedicated patients (Zahn and Pickar 1993; Bär et al. 2005; Chang et al. 2013; Schulz et al. 2013c). In a pooled analysis, we found that among 119 unmedicated patients the heart rate at rest was increased by about 10 beats per minute in over 40% of patients and by about 20 beats per minute in 25% of patients (unpublished data). It is important to understand that antipsychotic drugs might increase heart rates due to anticholinergic side effects even further (Mujica-Parodi et al. 2005). Here, a dose-dependent increase has been described (Iwamoto et al. 2012). However, other authors have found improved autonomic function after the introduction of antipsychotic treatment, possibly due to changes in clinical presentation (Chang et al. 2010) or only minor effects of treatment on cardiac autonomic function (Hempel et al. 2009).

Investigations in healthy first-degree relatives of patients displayed similarly increased heart rates, although less pronounced (Bär et al. 2010, 2012; Abhishekh et al. 2014; Berger et al. 2010; Jauregui et al. 2011). Comparable to other findings such as structural brain changes in healthy relatives of patients with schizophrenia (Oertel-Knochel et al. 2012), autonomic dysfunction seems to have a genetic basis. A summary of investigations of autonomic domains in patients and their healthy relatives is shown in Figure 16.1.

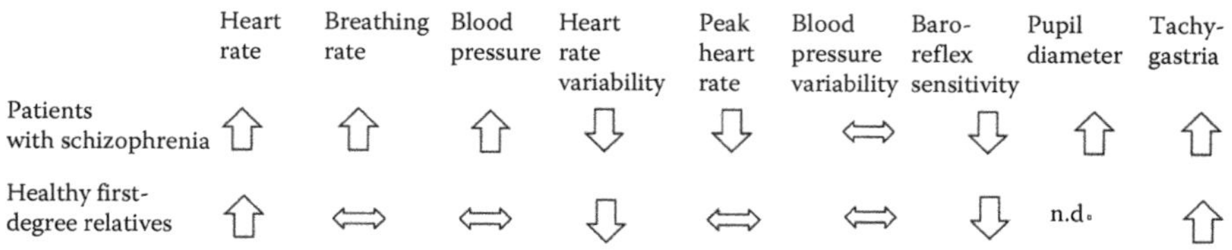

	Heart rate	Breathing rate	Blood pressure	Heart rate variability	Peak heart rate	Blood pressure variability	Baro-reflex sensitivity	Pupil diameter	Tachy-gastria
Patients with schizophrenia	⇧	⇧	⇧	⇩	⇩	⇔	⇩	⇧	⇧
Healthy first-degree relatives	⇧	⇔	⇔	⇩	⇔	⇔	⇩	n.d.	⇧

FIGURE 16.1

The figure shows investigated autonomic domains in patients with schizophrenia and their healthy first-degree relatives. Arrows specify increased or reduced values in comparison to controls. Peak heart rates indicate heart rates during vigorous exercises. Tachygastria is a sympathetic parameter obtained in the electrogastrogram.

16.4 Time- and Frequency-Domain Parameters of HRV in Patients with Schizophrenia

As described above, HRV is the BBI oscillation of RR intervals over time. It is the result of complex regulatory mechanisms through which the autonomic nervous system influences heart rate and keeps cardiovascular parameters within physiological health ranges.

Both time-domain and frequency-domain parameters of HRV show reduced efferent vagal activity in unmedicated patients (Bär et al. 2005; Berger et al. 2010; Boettger et al. 2006; Henry et al. 2010; Malaspina et al. 1997; Mujica-Parodi et al. 2005; Chang et al. 2009; Schulz et al. 2015a). Results were obtained by short-time measurements (5 and 30 minutes) as well as by 24-hour Holter electrocardiogram (ECG) measurements. Reduced HRV cannot be explained by increased heart rates alone, nor is it solely related to sympathetic modulation.

16.5 Complexity Measures of Heart Rate in Patients with Schizophrenia

A concept that is closely connected to that of variability is complexity. It is important to realize that complexity is different from variability, and there is no simple definition for it. A time series might show high variability and very low complexity. "Simple" time series are readily understood, and can be described concisely as having low information content or low complexity. Conversely, complex series are not easy to understand completely; they are full of unforeseeable shifting and require lengthy descriptions, making their information content high. Complex signals produced by healthy organisms might have dynamic properties such as nonlinearity (the relationships among components are not additive, so small perturbations can cause large effects) or nonstationarity (statistical properties of the system's output change with time). Thus, high complexity describes to a certain degree healthy physiological properties, while low complexity describes reduced influence of various regulatory circuits. Vice versa, the more irregular and complex heart rate series are to a limit, the more adaptive and stable is the underlying system. Since no single measure is sufficient to capture the properties of the most complex signals, different complexity measures are needed. For heart rate in patients with schizophrenia, researchers have mainly used compression entropy (Baumert et al. 2004; Ziv and Lempel 1977), measures of symbolic dynamics (Kurths et al. 1995; Voss et al. 1996), and approximate entropy (Pincus 1991).

Similarly to variability parameters, various recent studies have described reduced complexity of heart rate dynamics in patients with schizophrenia (Bär et al. 2007b, 2008b; Boettger et al. 2006; Moon et al. 2013; Mujica-Parodi et al. 2005; Jindal et al. 2009; Schulz et al. 2015a). The reduction in complexity indicates that in patients with schizophrenia, the heart rate cannot adapt to different requirements arising from posture or exertion and the heart is at higher risk of developing arrhythmias. In addition, one can speculate that reduced regulatory influence from the vagal system might contribute to reduced complexity. It is a method-inherent problem that complexity measures cannot be attributed to one single physiological system.

16.6 Baroreflex Sensitivity

The evaluation of baroreflex sensitivity (BRS) is an established tool for the assessment of autonomic control of the cardiovascular system. The baroreflex or baroreceptor reflex is one of the body's homeostatic mechanisms to maintain blood pressure at nearly constant levels. The baroreflex provides a negative feedback loop in which an elevated blood pressure reflexively causes the heart rate to decrease. In contrast, diminished blood pressure reduces baroreflex activation and causes heart rate to increase. A reduction in baroreflex control of heart rate has been reported in hypertension, coronary artery disease, myocardial infarction, and heart failure (Eckberg and Sleight 1992). There are various methods to assess BRS. For patients with schizophrenia, the noninvasive sequence method is used (Bertinieri et al. 1985). Here, spontaneous sequences of at least three consecutive beats are analyzed when an increased systolic blood pressure (SBP) of at least 1 mmHg causes an increased BBI interval of at least 5 ms (bradycardic sequence) or a decreased SBP causes a decreased BBI interval (tachycardic sequence). For each sequence, the regression between the three SBP values and three BBI values is calculated and the slope (tachycardic slope: tslope; bradycardic slope: bslope) of the regression line is used as an index of BRS.

Studies in unmedicated patients with schizophrenia show significantly reduced tachycardic and bradycardic slopes (Bär et al. 2007a, 2008a, 2010; Schulz et al. 2013c). Thus, the fine-tuning of blood pressure and heart rate is severely impaired among acute psychotic patients. Interestingly, blood pressure values and blood pressure variability (BPV) are only marginally altered in these patients (Bär et al. 2006b). Interestingly this is in contrast to findings in depressed patients. Here, the nonlinear dynamics of BPV considerably improves the detection of autonomic dysfunction in depressed patients in comparison to linear measures from HRV and BPV. Specifically, complexity indices from BPV seem to mirror major depressive disorders–related autonomic dysfunction more sensitively than those from HRV (Schulz et al. 2010).

We have therefore concluded that the primary change in psychotic (or schizophrenic) patients is observed in the heart rate domain. To explain putative mechanisms for reduced BRS in patients, it is important to realize that powerful negative feedback loops between heart rate and blood pressure can be inhibited to allow the organism to adjust to demanding environmental stress (inhibition of baroreflex vagal bradycardia [BVB]). Thus, BRS has been shown to decrease during specific cognitive demands, such as basic arithmetic operations (Reyes del Paso et al. 2004) or physical activity (Nosaka 1996). Thus, this might imply that the decrease of efferent vagal activity and the inhibition of BVB in acute schizophrenia are actually caused by stress due to psychotic experiences or the psychosis itself, a process that allows the organism under physiological conditions to adjust to demanding environmental stress.

16.7 Patients' Breathing Rates

During acute episodes, a putative relation between breathing rates and symptom severity was described in patients with schizophrenia 80 years ago (Peupelmann et al. 2009a,b; Wittkower 1934; Paterson 1935; Bär et al. 2012). The German Psychiatrist Wittkower described the breathing rate in psychotic patients to be faster and more regular. In our analysis, we found that a fast breathing rate is the dominant feature in unmedicated patients and that it is accompanied by some shallowness of breathing. We also found more variability within the breathing pattern (Bär et al. 2012; Schulz et al. 2015b). Applying complexity measures (symbolic dynamics, sample entropy, and compression entropy), we found significantly increased complexity in respiratory variability. We hypothesize that the varying cardiorespiratory regulation possibly contributes to the increased risk for cardiac mortality rates in schizophrenia (Schulz et al. 2015a). However, the minute ventilation is not altered in patients. Interestingly, when healthy subjects breathe in the modus of patients, we observed increased heart rates and reduced variability (Bär et al. 2012). Healthy relatives of patients do not show changes within their breathing pattern (Bär et al. 2012). We speculate that the breathing pattern is closely associated with symptoms during acute episodes, while the HRV pattern seems to be a trait marker. Of course, it is impossible to disentangle breathing and HRV completely because of their close interrelationship.

The changes within the cardiorespiratory system in schizophrenia seem to be disease-inherent characteristics and might reflect arousals during the psychosis stage in acutely ill schizophrenic patients. Relatives are obviously not in the same emotional and psychotic state as their diseased schizophrenic relatives. Therefore, it seems to be more evident that the alterations of cardiorespiratory system found in schizophrenia are closely connected to emotions such as sadness, happiness, anxiety, and fear that appear during this disease (Schulz et al. 2015b).

16.8 Cardiovascular and Cardiorespiratory Coupling

In recent years, it became of great importance in different fields of science to understand how regulatory systems interact with each other (directly or indirectly, causally or non-causally). Therefore, especially in the medical field, several methods for analyzing couplings in biological systems have been developed to quantify the physiological regulatory mechanisms, especially of the cardiovascular and cardiorespiratory systems, with the aim to gain insights into the interaction between regulatory mechanisms in healthy and diseased persons (Schulz and Voss 2014). The couplings within and between the cardiovascular and cardiorespiratory systems very likely interact with each other in a linear and nonlinear way. Interactions within the cardiovascular system can be described as closed loops with feed-forward (FF) and feedback (FB) mechanisms. On the one hand, blood pressure changes detected by baroreceptors lead to changes in heart rate through the arterial baroreflex control loop, and on the other hand, heart rate variations affect blood pressure via the Windkessel function (Cohen and Taylor 2002). Interactions within the cardiorespiratory system are commonly described as the respiratory sinus arrhythmia (RSA), the rhythmic fluctuation of cardiac cycle intervals (RR interval) in relation to respiration (Schulz et al. 2013a).

Recent advances in nonlinear dynamics and information theory have allowed the multivariate study of information transfer between time series. Here, several concepts are available based on Granger causality, nonlinear prediction, entropies, symbolization, and phase synchronization that are able to characterize these linear and nonlinear couplings (Schulz et al. 2013a; Schulz and Voss 2014).

For schizophrenia, there are only a few studies that have investigated cardiovascular and cardiorespiratory couplings in patients with schizophrenia and their relatives.

For cardiovascular coupling, studies (Bär et al. 2007a; Schulz et al. 2012a, 2013a,c) found an impaired baroreflex-mediated coupling pattern of cardiovascular regulation in patients in comparison to healthy subjects, which was further reinforced by anticholinergic effects of antipsychotic drugs, which might be interpreted as a decreased vagal modulation in schizophrenia.

For cardiorespiratory couplings, these studies (Bär et al. 2012; Peupelmann et al. 2009; Schulz et al. 2012a,b, 2015; Schulz et al. 2013, 2015) revealed commonly significantly altered respiratory regulation (variability and dynamics) and a reduced cardiorespiratory coupling for patients with schizophrenia but not for their healthy first-degree relatives. Schulz et al. (2015b) applied the high-resolution joint symbolic dynamics (HRJSD) approach and found altered heart rate pattern, respiratory pattern, and cardiorespiratory coupling in patients with schizophrenia and only marginal changes for their healthy first-degree relatives in comparison to healthy subjects. We speculate that these findings might be based on decreased vagal activity within the brainstem, altered or suppressed interaction of the brainstem and higher regulatory centers, or panic- and anxiety-related changes in the brainstem due to acute psychosis in those patients. Patients suffering from schizophrenia revealed cardiorespiratory coupling patterns, which were characterized as less predominant but more widely distributed in comparison to healthy subjects, indicating a decreased cardiorespiratory coupling in schizophrenia. In addition, Schulz et al. (2015a) found by means of normalized short-time partial-directed coherence (NSTPDC) a clear bidirectional coupling, with a driver–responder relationship from respiration (driver) to heart rate (responder) accompanied by reduced coupling strength in schizophrenic patients, confirming the results of a restricted RSA modulation in schizophrenia (Figure 16.2). Moreover, a slight driver–responder relationship from heart rate (driver) to respiration (responder) could also be recognized in patients.

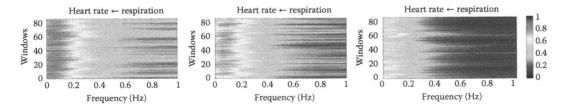

FIGURE 16.2
Normalized short-time partial-directed coherence (NSTPDC) plots for cardiorespiratory coupling analyses for (left) healthy subjects, (middle) healthy first-degree relatives, and (right) schizophrenic patients. The arrow on the top indicates the causal coupling direction from respiration to heart rate (heart rate ← respiration). Coupling strength ranges from dark blue (no coupling, 0) to dark red (maximum coupling, 1).

16.9 Exercise and Autonomic Function

Cardiorespiratory fitness is a strong and independent mortality predictor for humans (Myers et al. 2002). Therefore, it is important to investigate fitness in patients with schizophrenia, since it might be one approach for modifying the increased cardiac mortality risk associated with the disease. Overall, reduced physical fitness is a commonly reported trait among patients with schizophrenia that can be improved by means of physical interventional studies (Herbsleb et al. 2014; Falkai et al. 2013; Pajonk et al. 2010). Ostermann et al. (2013) investigated autonomic function during physical exercise. Interestingly, they showed increased breathing rates and reduced vagal modulation during the entire test. However, heart rates were only initially increased in comparison to controls. The authors reported that reduced vagal function during the exercise test correlated with the inflammatory response after exercise as assessed by tumor necrosis factor-alpha (TNF-α) levels. This result touches on a further important relationship between vagal modulation and inflammatory response (Boeckxstaens 2013). Most interestingly, Bär (2015) showed that chronotropic incompetence (CI), which is a strong predictor for cardiovascular mortality, is reported in about 60% of patients with schizophrenia taking regular medication. CI is defined as the inability of the heart to increase its rate commensurate with increased activity or demand. It has been established as a predictor of cardiovascular events and all-cause mortality (Lauer et al. 1999). Most interestingly, the authors describe similarly a lack of catecholamine increase and a close correlation between CI and the duration of disease. Thus, future studies need to investigate the cardiovascular benefit which patients might gain due to different types of exercise to reduce their potential cardiovascular risk profile (Herbsleb et al. 2014).

16.10 Psychopathology and Autonomic Function

Autonomic dysfunction is most likely the consequence of long-lasting stressful experiences associated with the psychotic state, in addition to a genetic underlying predisposition to autonomic dysfunction as observed in relatives of patients. Therefore, the notion of a relation between the severity of the disease assessed by the global assessment of functioning scale (GAF) and autonomic dysfunction is not surprising (Fujibayashi et al. 2009). However, it is rather interesting that autonomic dysfunction seems to be somehow related to the degree and amount of delusional states found in patients (Bär et al. 2005, 2007a,b, 2008a). A clear relation to negative symptoms was less often observed (Boettger et al. 2006). Altogether, there is no simple and linear relation between the severity of a current episode and the degree of autonomic dysfunction but some relation to the delusional state.

16.11 Future Perspectives

There are three important areas for future research in patients with schizophrenia. First of all, studies need to investigate the definite relation between the degree of autonomic dysfunction and the potential risk of cardiovascular events for these patients. At a minimum, schizophrenic patients at increased risk should be identified. Second, the brain activations underlying autonomic dysfunction need to be assessed to elucidate pathophysiological mechanisms. Third, psychiatric research is focused mainly on mental aspects of the disease, thereby neglecting obvious physical health needs of patients with schizophrenia. Here, a joint effort is needed to design interventional strategies in everyday clinical settings to improve physical health and quality of life of our patients.

References

Abhishekh, H. A., N. C. Kumar, J. Thirthalli, H. Chandrashekar, B. N. Gangadhar, and T. N. Sathyaprabha. 2014. Prolonged reaction to mental arithmetic stress in first-degree relatives of schizophrenia patients. *Clin Schizophr Relat Psychoses* 8 (3):137–42. doi: 10.3371/CSRP. ABKU.022213.

Agelink, M. W., C. Boz, H. Ullrich, and J. Andrich. 2002. Relationship between major depression and heart rate variability. Clinical consequences and implications for antidepressive treatment. *Psychiatry Res* 113 (1–2):139–49. doi: S0165178102002251 [pii].

Agelink, M. W., T. Majewski, C. Wurthmann, K. Lukas, H. Ullrich, T. Linka, and E. Klieser. 2001. Effects of newer atypical antipsychotics on autonomic neurocardiac function: A comparison between amisulpride, olanzapine, sertindole, and clozapine. *J Clin Psychopharmacol* 21 (1): 8–13.

Bär, K. J. 2015. Cardiac autonomic dysfunction in patients with schizophrenia and their healthy relatives - A small review. *Front Neurol* 6:139. doi: 10.3389/fneur.2015.00139.

Bär, K. J., S. Berger, M. Metzner, M. K. Boettger, S. Schulz, C. T. Ramachandraiah, J. Terhaar, A. Voss, V. K. Yeragani, and H. Sauer. 2010. Autonomic dysfunction in unaffected first-degree relatives of patients suffering from schizophrenia. *Schizophr Bull* 36 (5):1050–8. doi: 10.1093/schbul/sbp024.

Bär, K. J., M. K. Boettger, S. Berger, V. Baier, H. Sauer, V. K. Yeragani, and A. Voss. 2007a. Decreased baroreflex sensitivity in acute schizophrenia. *J Appl Physiol (1985)* 102 (3):1051–6. doi: 10.1152/japplphysiol.00811.2006.

Bär, K. J., M. K. Boettger, S. Boettger, M. Groteluschen, R. Neubauer, T. Jochum, V. Baier, H. Sauer, and A. Voss. 2006a. Reduced baroreflex sensitivity in acute alcohol withdrawal syndrome and in abstained alcoholics. *Drug Alcohol Depend* 85 (1):66–74. doi: 10.1016/j.drugalcdep.2006.03.014.

Bär, K. J., M. K. Boettger, M. Koschke, S. Schulz, P. Chokka, V. K. Yeragani, and A. Voss. 2007b. Nonlinear complexity measures of heart rate variability in acute schizophrenia. *Clin Neurophysiol* 118 (9):2009–15. doi: 10.1016/j.clinph.2007.06.012.

Bär, K. J., M. K. Boettger, S. Schulz, C. Harzendorf, M. W. Agelink, V. K. Yeragani, P. Chokka, and A. Voss. 2008a. The interaction between pupil function and cardiovascular regulation in patients with acute schizophrenia. *Clin Neurophysiol* 119 (10):2209–13. doi: 10.1016/j.clinph.2008.06.012.

Bär, K. J., M. K. Boettger, and A. Voss. 2006b. Differences between heart rate and blood pressure variability in schizophrenia. *Biomed Tech (Berl)* 51 (4):237–9. doi: 10.1515/BMT.2006.045.

Bär, K. J., M. Koschke, S. Berger, S. Schulz, M. Tancer, A. Voss, and V. K. Yeragani. 2008b. Influence of olanzapine on QT variability and complexity measures of heart rate in patients with schizophrenia. *J Clin Psychopharmacol* 28 (6):694–8. doi: 10.1097/JCP.0b013e31818a6d25.

Bär, K. J., A. Letzsch, T. Jochum, G. Wagner, W. Greiner, and H. Sauer. 2005. Loss of efferent vagal activity in acute schizophrenia. *J Psychiatr Res* 39 (5):519–27. doi: 10.1016/j.jpsychires. 2004.12.007.

Bär, K. J., T. Rachow, S. Schulz, K. Bassarab, S. Haufe, S. Berger, K. Koch, and A. Voss. 2012. The phrenic component of acute schizophrenia—A name and its physiological reality. *PLOS ONE* 7 (3):e33459. doi: 10.1371/journal.pone.0033459.

Baumert, M., V. Baier, J. Haueisen, N. Wessel, U. Meyerfeldt, A. Schirdewan, and A. Voss. 2004. Forecasting of life threatening arrhythmias using the compression entropy of heart rate. *Methods Inf Med* 43 (2):202–6. doi: 10.1267/METH04020202.

Beary, M., R. Hodgson, and H. J. Wildgust. 2012. A critical review of major mortality risk factors for all-cause mortality in first-episode schizophrenia: Clinical and research implications. *J Psychopharmacol* 26 (5 Suppl):52–61. doi: 10.1177/0269881112440512.

Berger, S., M. K. Boettger, M. Tancer, S. M. Guinjoan, V. K. Yeragani, and K. J. Bar. 2010. Reduced cardio-respiratory coupling indicates suppression of vagal activity in healthy relatives of patients with schizophrenia. *Prog Neuropsychopharmacol Biol Psychiatry* 34 (2):406–11. doi: 10.1016/j.pnpbp.2010.01.009.

Bertinieri, G., M. di Rienzo, A. Cavallazzi, A. U. Ferrari, A. Pedotti, and G. Mancia. 1985. A new approach to analysis of the arterial baroreflex. *J Hypertens Suppl* 3 (3):S79–81.

Boeckxstaens, G. 2013. The clinical importance of the anti-inflammatory vagovagal reflex. *Handb Clin Neurol* 117:119–34. doi: 10.1016/B978-0-444-53491-0.00011-0.

Boettger, S., D. Hoyer, K. Falkenhahn, M. Kaatz, V. K. Yeragani, and K. J. Bär. 2006. Altered diurnal autonomic variation and reduced vagal information flow in acute schizophrenia. *Clin Neurophysiol* 117 (12):2715–22. doi: 10.1016/j.clinph.2006.08.009.

Bushe, C. J., M. Taylor, and J. Haukka. 2010. Mortality in schizophrenia: A measurable clinical endpoint. *J Psychopharmacol* 24 (4 Suppl):17–25. doi: 10.1177/1359786810382468.

Chang, H. A., C. C. Chang, N. S. Tzeng, T. B. Kuo, R. B. Lu, and S. Y. Huang. 2013. Cardiac autonomic dysregulation in acute schizophrenia. *Acta Neuropsychiatr* 25 (3):155–64. doi: 10.1111/acn.12014.

Chang, J. S., C. S. Yoo, S. H. Yi, K. H. Hong, Y. S. Lee, H. S. Oh, D. C. Jung, Y. S. Kim, and Y. M. Ahn. 2010. Changes in heart rate dynamics of patients with schizophrenia treated with risperidone. *Prog Neuropsychopharmacol Biol Psychiatry* 34 (6):924–9. doi: 10.1016/j.pnpbp.2010.04.017.

Chang, J. S., C. S. Yoo, S. H. Yi, K. H. Hong, H. S. Oh, J. Y. Hwang, S. G. Kim, Y. M. Ahn, and Y. S. Kim. 2009. Differential pattern of heart rate variability in patients with schizophrenia. *Prog Neuropsychopharmacol Biol Psychiatry* 33 (6):991–5. doi: 10.1016/j.pnpbp.2009.05.004.

Cohen, M. A., and J. A. Taylor. 2002. Short-term cardiovascular oscillations in man: Measuring and modelling the physiologies. *J Physiol* 542 (Pt 3):669–83.

Colton, C. W. and R. W. Manderscheid. 2006. Congruencies in increased mortality rates, years of potential life lost, and causes of death among public mental health clients in eight states. *Prev Chronic Dis* 3 (2):A42.

Diaz, A., M. G. Bourassa, M. C. Guertin, and J. C. Tardif. 2005. Long-term prognostic value of resting heart rate in patients with suspected or proven coronary artery disease. *Eur Heart J* 26 (10):967–74. doi: 10.1093/eurheartj/ehi190.

Eckberg, D. L. and P. Sleight (eds.). 1992. *Human Baroreflexes in Health and Disease*. Oxford: Clarendon Press.

Falkai, P., B. Malchow, T. Wobrock, O. Gruber, A. Schmitt, W. G. Honer, F. G. Pajonk, F. Sun, and T. D. Cannon. 2013. The effect of aerobic exercise on cortical architecture in patients with chronic schizophrenia: A randomized controlled MRI study. *Eur Arch Psychiatry Clin Neurosci* 263 (6):469–73. doi: 10.1007/s00406-012-0383-y.

Fujibayashi, M., T. Matsumoto, I. Kishida, T. Kimura, C. Ishii, N. Ishii, and T. Moritani. 2009. Autonomic nervous system activity and psychiatric severity in schizophrenia. *Psychiatry Clin Neurosci* 63 (4):538–45. doi:10.1111/j.1440-1819.2009.01983.x.

Goldberger, A. L., L. A. Amaral, J. M. Hausdorff, P. Ch. Ivanov, C. K. Peng, and H. E. Stanley. 2002. Fractal dynamics in physiology: Alterations with disease and aging. *Proc Natl Acad Sci U S A* 99 (1 Suppl):2466–72. doi: 10.1073/pnas.012579499.

Greenland, P., M. L. Daviglus, A. R. Dyer, K. Liu, C. F. Huang, J. J. Goldberger, and J. Stamler. 1999. Resting heart rate is a risk factor for cardiovascular and noncardiovascular mortality: The Chicago Heart Association Detection Project in Industry. *Am J Epidemiol* 149 (9):853–62.

Hempel, R. J., J. H. Tulen, N. J. van Beveren, C. H. Roder, and M. W. Hengeveld. 2009. Cardiovascular variability during treatment with haloperidol, olanzapine or risperidone in recent-onset schizophrenia. *J Psychopharmacol* 23 (6):697–707. doi: 10.1177/0269881108091254.

Henry, B. L., A. Minassian, M. P. Paulus, M. A. Geyer, and W. Perry. 2010. Heart rate variability in bipolar mania and schizophrenia. *J Psychiatr Res* 44 (3):168–76. doi: 10.1016/j.jpsychires.2009.07.011.

Herbsleb, M., T. Muhlhaus, and K. J. Bär. 2014. Differential cardiac effects of aerobic interval training versus moderate continuous training in a patient with schizophrenia: A case report. *Front Psychiatry* 5:119. doi: 10.3389/fpsyt.2014.00119.

Hoyer, D., B. Frank, B. Pompe, H. Schmidt, K. Werdan, U. Muller-Werdan, R. Baranowski, J. J. Zebrowski, W. Meissner, U. Kletzin, D. Adler, S. Adler, and R. Blickhan. 2006. Analysis of complex physiological systems by information flow: A time scale-specific complexity assessment. *Biomed Tech (Berl)* 51 (2):41–8. doi: 10.1515/BMT.2006.009.

Ifteni, P., C. U. Correll, V. Burtea, J. M. Kane, and P. Manu. 2014. Sudden unexpected death in schizophrenia: Autopsy findings in psychiatric inpatients. *Schizophr Res* 155 (1–3):72–6. doi: 10.1016/j.schres.2014.03.011.

Iwamoto, Y., C. Kawanishi, I. Kishida, T. Furuno, M. Fujibayashi, C. Ishii, N. Ishii, T. Moritani, M. Taguri, and Y. Hirayasu. 2012. Dose-dependent effect of antipsychotic drugs on autonomic nervous system activity in schizophrenia. *BMC Psychiatry* 12:199. doi: 10.1186/1471-244X-12-199.

Jauregui, O. I., E. Y. Costanzo, D. de Achaval, M. F. Villarreal, E. Chu, M. C. Mora, D. E. Vigo, M. N. Castro, R. C. Leiguarda, K. J. Bar, and S. M. Guinjoan. 2011. Autonomic nervous system activation during social cognition tasks in patients with schizophrenia and their unaffected relatives. *Cogn Behav Neurol* 24 (4):194–203. doi: 10.1097/WNN.0b013e31824007e9.

Jensen, M. T., J. L. Marott, P. Lange, J. Vestbo, P. Schnohr, O. W. Nielsen, J. S. Jensen, and G. B. Jensen. 2013a. Resting heart rate is a predictor of mortality in COPD. *Eur Respir J* 42 (2):341–9. doi: 10.1183/09031936.00072212.

Jensen, M. T., P. Suadicani, H. O. Hein, and F. Gyntelberg. 2013b. Elevated resting heart rate, physical fitness and all-cause mortality: A 16-year follow-up in the Copenhagen Male Study. *Heart* 99 (12):882–7. doi: 10.1136/heartjnl-2012-303375.

Jindal, R. D., M. S. Keshavan, K. Eklund, A. Stevens, D. M. Montrose, and V. K. Yeragani. 2009. Beat-to-beat heart rate and QT interval variability in first episode neuroleptic-naive psychosis. *Schizophr Res* 113 (2–3):176–80. doi: 10.1016/j.schres.2009.06.003.

Jochum, T., M. Weissenfels, A. Seeck, S. Schulz, M. K. Boettger, A. Voss, and K. J. Bär. 2011. Endothelial dysfunction during acute alcohol withdrawal syndrome. *Drug Alcohol Depend* 119 (1–2):113–22. doi: 10.1016/j.drugalcdep.2011.06.002.

Koschke, M., M. K. Boettger, S. Schulz, S. Berger, J. Terhaar, A. Voss, V. K. Yeragani, and K. J. Bar. 2009. Autonomy of autonomic dysfunction in major depression. *Psychosom Med* 71 (8):852–60. doi: 10.1097/PSY.0b013e3181b8bb7a.

Kraepelin, E. 1899. *Psychiatrie. Ein Lehrbuch fur Studierende und Aertze, Psychiatry. A Textbook for Students and Physicians*. Canton, MA: Publishing International.

Kurths, J., A. Voss, P. Saparin, A. Witt, H. J. Kleiner, and N. Wessel. 1995. Quantitative analysis of heart rate variability. *Chaos* 5 (1):88–94. doi: 10.1063/1.166090.

Lauer, M. S., G. S. Francis, P. M. Okin, F. J. Pashkow, C. E. Snader, and T. H. Marwick. 1999. Impaired chronotropic response to exercise stress testing as a predictor of mortality. *JAMA* 281 (6):524–9.

Loas, G., A. Azi, C. Noisette, and V. Yon. 2008. Mortality among chronic schizophrenic patients: A prospective 14-year follow-up study of 150 schizophrenic patients. *Encephale* 34 (1):54–60. doi: 10.1016/j.encep.2007.07.005.

Malaspina, D., G. Bruder, G. W. Dalack, S. Storer, M. Van Kammen, X. Amador, A. Glassman, and J. Gorman. 1997. Diminished cardiac vagal tone in schizophrenia: Associations to brain laterality and age of onset. *Biol Psychiatry* 41 (5):612–7.

Manu, P., J. M. Kane, and C. U. Correll. 2011. Sudden deaths in psychiatric patients. *J Clin Psychiatry* 72 (7):936–41. doi: 10.4088/JCP.10m06244gry.

Moon, E., S. H. Lee, D. H. Kim, and B. Hwang. 2013. Comparative study of heart rate variability in patients with schizophrenia, bipolar disorder, post-traumatic stress disorder, or major depressive disorder. *Clin Psychopharmacol Neurosci* 11 (3):137–43. doi: 10.9758/cpn.2013.11.3.137.

Mothi, S. S., N. Tandon, J. Padmanabhan, I. T. Mathew, B. Clementz, C. Tamminga, G. Pearlson, J. Sweeney, and M. S. Keshavan. 2015. Increased cardiometabolic dysfunction in first-degree relatives of patients with psychotic disorders. *Schizophr Res*. doi: 10.1016/j.schres.2015.03.034.

Mujica-Parodi, L. R., V. Yeragani, and D. Malaspina. 2005. Nonlinear complexity and spectral analyses of heart rate variability in medicated and unmedicated patients with schizophrenia. *Neuropsychobiology* 51 (1):10–5.

Myers, J., M. Prakash, V. Froelicher, D. Do, S. Partington, and J. E. Atwood. 2002. Exercise capacity and mortality among men referred for exercise testing. *N Engl J Med* 346 (11):793–801.

Nosaka, S. 1996. Modifications of arterial baroreflexes: Obligatory roles in cardiovascular regulation in stress and poststress recovery. *Jpn J Physiol* 46 (4):271–88.

Oertel-Knochel, V., C. Knochel, S. Matura, A. Rotarska-Jagiela, J. Magerkurth, D. Prvulovic, C. Haenschel, H. Hampel, and D. E. Linden. 2012. Cortical-basal ganglia imbalance in schizophrenia patients and unaffected first-degree relatives. *Schizophr Res* 138 (2–3):120–7. doi: 10.1016/j.schres.2012.02.029.

Osby, U., N. Correia, L. Brandt, A. Ekbom, and P. Sparen. 2000. Mortality and causes of death in schizophrenia in Stockholm county, Sweden. *Schizophr Res* 45 (1–2):21–8.

Ostermann, S., M. Herbsleb, S. Schulz, L. Donath, S. Berger, D. Eisentrager, T. Siebert, H. J. Muller, C. Puta, A. Voss, H. W. Gabriel, K. Koch, and K. J. Bär. 2013. Exercise reveals the interrelation of physical fitness, inflammatory response, psychopathology, and autonomic function in patients with schizophrenia. *Schizophr Bull* 39 (5):1139–49. doi: 10.1093/schbul/sbs085.

Pajonk, F. G., T. Wobrock, O. Gruber, H. Scherk, D. Berner, I. Kaizl, A. Kierer, S. Muller, M. Oest, T. Meyer, M. Backens, T. Schneider-Axmann, A. E. Thornton, W. G. Honer, and P. Falkai. 2010. Hippocampal plasticity in response to exercise in schizophrenia. *Arch Gen Psychiatry* 67 (2):133–43. doi: 10.1001/archgenpsychiatry.2009.193.

Paterson, A. S. 1935. The respiratory rhythm in normal and psychotic subjects. *Journal of Neurology and Psychopathology* 16 (36):13–18.

Peupelmann, J., M. K. Boettger, C. Ruhland, S. Berger, C. T. Ramachandraiah, V. K. Yeragani, and K. J. Bar. 2009a. Cardio-respiratory coupling indicates suppression of vagal activity in acute schizophrenia. *Schizophr Res* 112 (1–3):153–7. doi: 10.1016/j.schres.2009.03.042.

Peupelmann, J., C. Quick, S. Berger, M. Hocke, M. E. Tancer, V. K. Yeragani, and K. J. Bär. 2009b. Linear and non-linear measures indicate gastric dysmotility in patients suffering from acute schizophrenia. *Prog Neuropsychopharmacol Biol Psychiatry* 33 (7):1236–40.

Pincus, S. M. 1991. Approximate entropy as a measure of system complexity. *Proc Natl Acad Sci U S A* 88 (6):2297–301.

Rasanen, S., H. Hakko, K. Viilo, V. B. Meyer-Rochow, and J. Moring. 2005. Avoidable mortality in long-stay psychiatric patients of Northern Finland. *Nord J Psychiatry* 59 (2):103–8. doi: 10.1080/08039480510022909.

Ray, W. A., C. P. Chung, K. T. Murray, K. Hall, and C. M. Stein. 2009. Atypical antipsychotic drugs and the risk of sudden cardiac death. *N Engl J Med* 360 (3):225–35. doi: 10.1056/NEJMoa0806994.

Reyes del Paso, G. A., I. Gonzalez, and J. A. Hernandez. 2004. Baroreceptor sensitivity and effectiveness varies differentially as a function of cognitive-attentional demands. *Biol Psychol* 67 (3):385–95. doi: 10.1016/j.biopsycho.2004.02.001.

Schulz, S., F. C. Adochiei, I. R. Edu, R. Schroeder, H. Costin, K. J. Bär, and A. Voss. 2013a. Cardiovascular and cardiorespiratory coupling analyses: A review. *Philos Trans A Math Phys Eng Sci* 371 (1997):20120191. doi: 10.1098/rsta.2012.0191.

Schulz, S., K. J. Bär, and A. Voss. 2012a. Cardiovascular and cardiorespiratory coupling in unmedicated schizophrenic patients in comparison to healthy subjects. *Conference Proceeding IEEE Engineering in Medicine and Biology Society*, San Diego, CA, USA, 28 Aug.–1 Sept. 2012

Schulz, S., K. J. Bär, and A. Voss. 2012b. Respiratory variability and cardiorespiratory coupling analyses in patients suffering from schizophrenia and their healthy first-degree relatives. *Biomed Tech (Berl)* 57 (1 Suppl):1044. doi: 10.1515/bmt-2012-4336.

Schulz, S., K. J. Bär, and A. Voss. 2015a. Analyses of heart rate, respiration and cardiorespiratory coupling in patients with schizophrenia. *Entropy* 17 (2):483–501.

Schulz, S., J. Haueisen, K. J. Bär, and V. Andreas. 2015b. High-resolution joint symbolic analysis to enhance classification of the cardiorespiratory system in patients with schizophrenia and their relatives. *Philos Trans A Math Phys Eng Sci* 373 (2034). doi: 10.1098/rsta.2014.0098.

Schulz, S., J. Haueisen, K. J. Bär, and A. Voss. 2013b. Quantification of cardiorespiratory coupling in acute schizophrenia applying high resolution joint symbolic dynamics. *Computing in Cardiology Conference (CinC)*, Zaragoza, Spain, 22–25 Sept. 2013.

Schulz, S., M. Koschke, K. J. Bär, and A. Voss. 2010. The altered complexity of cardiovascular regulation in depressed patients. *Physiol Meas* 31 (3):303–21. doi: 10.1088/0967-3334/31/3/003.

Schulz, S., N. Tupaika, S. Berger, J. Haueisen, K. J. Bär, and A. Voss. 2013c. Cardiovascular coupling analysis with high-resolution joint symbolic dynamics in patients suffering from acute schizophrenia. *Physiol Meas* 34 (8):883–901. doi: 10.1088/0967-3334/34/8/883.

Schulz, S., and A. Voss. 2014. Cardiovascular and cardiorespiratory coupling analysis—State of the art and future perspectives. *Cardiovascular Oscillations (ESGCO), 2014 8th Conference of the European Study Group on*, Trento, 25–28 May 2014.

Voss, A., K. Hnatkova, N. Wessel, J. Kurths, A. Sander, A. Schirdewan, A. J. Camm, and M. Malik. 1998. Multiparametric analysis of heart rate variability used for risk stratification among survivors of acute myocardial infarction. *Pacing Clin Electrophysiol* 21 (1 Pt 2):186–92.

Voss, A., J. Kurths, H. J. Kleiner, A. Witt, N. Wessel, P. Saparin, K. J. Osterziel, R. Schurath, and R. Dietz. 1996. The application of methods of non-linear dynamics for the improved and predictive recognition of patients threatened by sudden cardiac death. *Cardiovasc Res* 31 (3):419–33.

Wittkower, E. 1934. Further studies in the respiration of psychotic patient. *British Journal of Psychiatry* 80:692–704.

Yeragani, V. K., R. Pohl, K. J. Bar, P. Chokka, and M. Tancer. 2007. Exaggerated beat-to-beat R amplitude variability in patients with panic disorder after intravenous isoproterenol. *Neuropsychobiology* 55 (3–4):213–8. doi: 10.1159/000108380.

Yeragani, V. K. and V. Sree Hari Rao. 2006. Patterns of oscillatory behavior in different human systems: A special reference to psychiatry and techniques to quantify such patterns. *Bipolar Disord* 8 (5 Pt 1):421–2. doi: 10.1111/j.1399-5618.2006.00377.x.

Zahn, T. P. and D. Pickar. 1993. Autonomic effects of clozapine in schizophrenia: Comparison with placebo and fluphenazine. *Biol Psychiatry* 34 (1–2):3–12. doi: 0006-3223(93)90250-H [pii].

Ziv, J. and A. Lempel. 1977. Universal algorithm for sequential data compression. *IEEE Trans Inf Ther* 20:337–43.

.

17

Fetal Heart Rate Variability

Faezeh Marzbanrad, Yoshitaka Kimura, Marimuthu Palaniswami,
and Ahsan H. Khandoker

CONTENTS

17.1 Introduction

Early identification of fetal risks is a field of increasing interest and significance in most societies. A large body of research advocates various fetal assessment techniques to evaluate antepartum fetal risks. Such risks indicate the need for intervention that may reduce the risk of intrauterine death [1–3]. The risks include uteroplacental insufficiency, hypoxia, or fetal abnormalities. Antenatal fetal assessment may particularly have an impact for some maternal- or pregnancy-related conditions associated with increased perinatal morbidity and mortality, which are summarized in Table 17.1 [4].

Fetal assessment is not only necessary for high-risk pregnancies, but also recommended for all pregnancies in general, since it has been demonstrated that low-risk pregnancies have a larger contribution in perinatal mortality than high-risk pregnancies [8].

Conventional techniques of fetal assessment include fetal movement counting, amniotic fluid volume (AFV) test, sonographic assessment and biophysical profile (BPP), contraction stress test (CST), nonstress test (NST), vibroacoustic stimulation (VAS), Doppler velocimetry, and integrated methods [1–3,9,10]. Fetal circulation is one of the main concerns in fetal assessment and is of crucial importance, especially since the evaluation of the heart action may give more useful information about the fetus during pregnancy [3]. Heart rate (HR) provides reliable evaluation of the autonomic nervous system (ANS) function, which

TABLE 17.1

Maternal, Fetal, and Pregnancy-Related Conditions Which Are Indications for Fetal Surveillance

Maternal Conditions	Fetal- and Pregnancy-Related Conditions
Antiphospholipid syndrome	Pregnancy-induced hypertension/preeclampsia
Hypertensive disorders	Insulin-requiring gestational diabetes
Hyperthyroidism	Decreased fetal movements
Hemoglobinopathies	Multiple gestation (with significant growth discrepancy)
Cyanotic heart disease	Intrauterine growth restriction (IUGR)
Systemic lupus erythematosus	Small for gestational age (SGA) fetus
Chronic renal disease	Post-term pregnancies (> 294days)
Prepregnancy diabetes	Isoimmunization (moderate to severe)
Advanced maternal age	Previous fetal demise (unexpected/recurrent)
Morbid obesity	Preterm prelabor rupture of membranes (PPROM) with oligohydramnios
	Polyhydramnios
	Chronic abruption

Source: Modified from the table in G. Ramanathan and S. Arulkumaran, *Obstetrics and Gynecology for Postgraduates*, 1; P. Steer and P. Danielian, *High Risk Pregnancy Management Options*, 1999; R. Liston et al., *Journal of Obstetrics and Gynaecology Canada*, 29(9 Suppl 4), S3–56, 2007; A. T. Bianco et al., *Obstetrics & Gynecology*, 91(1), 97–102, 1998; R. Von Kries et al., *European Journal of Pediatrics*, 156(12), 963–967, 1997.

regulates the heartbeat dynamics. Therefore, fetal heart rate (FHR) monitoring is commonly used to assess fetal well-being and can also provide information about the development of fetal ANS.

Based on a study in 1978, around 99.8% of fetal movements that last for more than 3 seconds are associated with FHR accelerations [11]. Therefore, monitoring of FHR using the NST has become popular for fetal assessment since then. Movement of the fetus with no acidosis and no neurological depression shows intermittent FHR acceleration [11]. FHR deceleration is another parameter that is associated with an abnormal status of the pregnancy, especially when followed by a womb contraction occurring within a given time period [12,13]. The NST aims to reduce the rate of fetal compromise caused by fetal hypoxia or placental insufficiencies.

FHR monitoring is generally performed by cardiotography (CTG) for which the noninvasive Doppler ultrasound (DUS) transducer is used during a 20-minute test. Additionally, a strain gauge or a tocodynamometer is also used to monitor uterine activity. The NST is defined as reactive if at least two accelerations of more than 15 bpm from the baseline (which is 110–160 bpm) lasting more than 15 seconds occur within the 20-minute test. However, the absence of accelerations may be due to fetal sleep and in that case, the test is extended to 40 minutes [9]. In practice, if the fetus does not show reactivity after 40 minutes, further assessment is performed by the CST or BPP test. VAS can also be used to interrupt fetal sleep and provoke FHR acceleration, which results in a decrease in the test duration and the number of false positive tests due to fetal sleep [14]. Another cause of false-positive results is the gestational age, since 50% of the normal fetuses in 24–28 weeks and 15% of the ones in 28–32 weeks of pregnancy fail to show reactivity in FHR [15,16].

Overall, nonreactive FHR may be associated with prolonged fetal sleep, immaturity of the fetus, ingestion of sedatives by the mother, and cardiac or neurologic anomalies of the fetus. The false-negative rate of this test is quite low at 0.3%, but the false-positive rate is around 50% [17].

Although FHR monitoring has been used as an NST or CST to find accelerations, decelerations, and baseline variability of FHR, it is not enough for a thorough assessment of the fetal state. In particular, the usefulness of these conventional methods for detection of fetal acidemia has been questioned [18]. More advanced quantitative analysis of HR is required to evaluate FHR changes and complexity in the time and frequency domain. For example, the root mean square of successive differences (RMSSD) is a time-domain parameter of FHR variability that is highly correlated with gestational age, and it can be employed to monitor the development of the parasympathetic nervous system during pregnancy [19]. The spectrum analysis of FHR variability provides features to detect intrauterine growth restriction (IUGR) [20–22]. The regularity of R-R interval series can be examined by entropy approaches [23]. Ferrario et al. applied the approximate entropy and the sample entropy (SampEn) to FHR signals to identify fetal sufferance and showed that multiscale entropy (MSE) features can be used to reliably detect the fetal distress associated with the presence of a pathological condition during pregnancy and at birth [23]. A review of the FHR variability analysis methods and their application for evaluating fetal well-being and development is provided in the following sections.

There are several methods that can be used for monitoring FHR noninvasively, including CTG, ultrasound M-mode analysis, fetal electrocardiography (fECG), and magnetocardiography (fMCG) [24]. The advantages and shortcomings of these methods are discussed in the next section.

17.2 FHR Acquisition Techniques

17.2.1 Doppler CTG

FHR monitoring is most commonly performed by CTG for which the noninvasive DUS transducer is used. An ultrasound beam of 1.5 MHz is transmitted and then reflected back from the fetal heart to the transducer. Fetal heart movements (from valves or walls of the heart) cause Doppler frequency shifts of the received signal. FHR estimation is based on the periodicity of the envelope of the received signal. However the complex and changing nature of the DUS signal complicates this task. Therefore the estimated FHR is usually constrained to high and low limits and beat-to-beat FHR variation is also bounded.

Although this is an efficient and effective established method, beat-to-beat HRV is difficult to obtain and usually an averaging process is performed. Another shortcoming is that there is no single well-defined fiducial point in the waveform to identify each heart cycle [24]. Accurate low frequency (LF) domain spectral analysis can be still achieved by DUS, while high frequency (HF) measures needs to be improved [20].

DUS can provide more information about the fetal heart in addition to the FHR. The Doppler shift of the ultrasound beam, which is reflected from moving valves of the fetal heart and collected by the transducer, uncovers the opening and closure of the fetal cardiac valves [25–27]. Using one-dimensional DUS, the timings of cardiac valve motions are estimated and used to evaluate different systolic and diastolic cardiac intervals [27–30].

Obtaining these timings from the DUS signal requires signal processing because they cannot be identified from the raw signal; therefore, signal filtering and decomposition are required.

Early studies in the 1980s proposed noninvasive methods based on band-pass filtering approaches to extract the HF component of the DUS, from which the valve movements were identified manually by experts [25,26,31,32]. There are several challenges involved in identification of valve motion. First, the DUS signal is contaminated by noise and interference from movements of other fetal and maternal organs. The content of the DUS signal is highly variable, and it depends on the respective fetus and transducer orientation [27]. Therefore, several studies suggested applying improved signal processing techniques and powerful processors, such as short-time Fourier transform (STFT), wavelet analysis, and empirical mode decomposition (EMD), to extract the information content of the DUS signal [27,29,30]. Second, manual identification of beat-to-beat opening and closing of valves is time consuming, requires special expertise, and is subject to inter- and intraobserver and visual errors. Therefore, automated methods have been recently developed for identification of valve motions using the DUS signal and fECG as a reference [33–35].

17.2.2 Fetal Electrocardiography

Obtaining noninvasive fECG through the maternal abdomen has been a vast and challenging area of research in engineering and clinical technology over the last decade [36–39]. Noninvasive fECG can be used during pregnancy as early as the 18th week of gestation, while invasive fECG via scalp requires data collection using intrauterine electrodes with direct contact to fetal skin, which requires uterine rupture and generally can be only used during labor [40,41].

In noninvasive fECG, data are collected using a set of electrodes placed on the maternal abdomen. When the signal is obtained by this method, it is weak and has a low signal-to-noise ratio (SNR), because it has to pass several low conductive layers to reach the maternal abdomen surface. fECG is not the only signal recorded, but it is mixed with the maternal ECG and the voltage of fECG (≈ 5–$20\ \mu V$) is quite smaller than the maternal ECG voltage ($\approx 1,000\ \mu V$). It is also contaminated by maternal respiratory, motion artifacts, and uterine contractions. The movement of the fetus itself also causes nonstationarity of the signal and changes in the signals recorded by each electrode. fECG is of a 3D form, but unlike the adult's ECG, the electrodes are not attached to the fetus itself to collect a specific waveform. Different and changeable fetal presentation and lack of a standard lead system on maternal abdomen makes extraction of fECG even more complicated. In brief, the reliable extraction of fECG as a nonlinear and nonstationary 3D signal from a highly complex abdominal mixture corrupted by noise, which is even greater than the signal, requires signal processing. Many different methods have been proposed and used for this purpose, including but not limited to [37,38]:

- Direct fECG analysis: this method is based on peak detection [42] using the raw signal, which is not always possible since it depends on the fetal orientation and age.
- Adaptive filtering techniques: the purpose may be to cancel the maternal ECG or other artifacts or to extract fECG by training an adaptive or matched filter [40,43]. Partition-based weighted sum filters [44], least-square error fittings [45] and Kalman filtering methods [46] are other alternatives. The complication of these methods is that they require a reference, which may be a maternal ECG or a waveform that is

similar to interfering signal, in order to exclude it from the mixture. However in the Kalman filtering approach an arbitrary maternal ECG is used as the reference, which makes it more practical and promising [46].

- Linear decomposition techniques: these approaches are based on single or multichannel decomposition of the collected data, which are assumed to be linear and stationary mixtures of the signals and noises. The applied methods may use time, frequency, or scaling properties of the signals, such as wavelet analysis methods [47,48]; spatial filtering, such as singular value decomposition (SVD) methods [49–51]; using the independence of the mixing components through blind source separation (BSS) techniques [52–54]; or a combination of these approaches [55–57].

Considering the large noise contamination and low signal-to-noise ratio, sole use of BSS is not promising. This method is not stable for this application, as it tends to extract noise rather than the tiny fECG signal [38]. A more stable method is blind source separation with reference (BSSR), which improves BSS methods by adding a learning process with reference signals, which might be periodic signals mimicking the fECG [58]. For example, to find the ECG signal from lead II, the lead-II ECG shape is used as a reference to extract the fECG. Moreover, other reference signals can be found from other fetal heart sources, such as the continuous Doppler signal [38]. The schematic illustration of this method is shown in Figure 17.1.

Using the BSSR method, reliable fECG traces can be extracted and shown to be useful for detecting fetal heart arrhythmia, including premature atrial contractions (PAC), premature ventricular contractions (PVCs), and sick sinus syndrome (SSS) [38]. However, it is still difficult to diagnose complete atrioventricular (AV) block, because of the small size of P waves in some cases. An example of PVC identification from a previous study is shown in

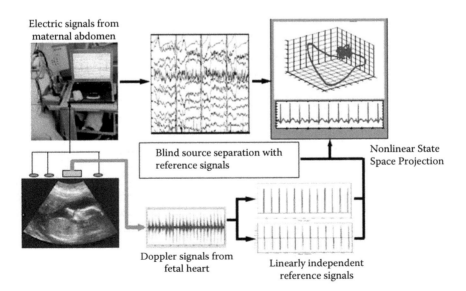

Electric signals from maternal abdomen

Blind source separation with reference signals

Nonlinear State Space Projection

Doppler signals from fetal heart

Linearly independent reference signals

FIGURE 17.1
The schematic diagram of the blind source separation with reference (BSSR) fetal electrocardiography (ECG) extraction system, using Nonlinear State Space Projection (NSSP). (From Y. Kimura et al., *Open Medical Devices Journal*, 4, 7–12, 2012; M. Sato et al., *Biomedical Engineering, IEEE Transactions on*, 54(1), 49–58, 2007.)

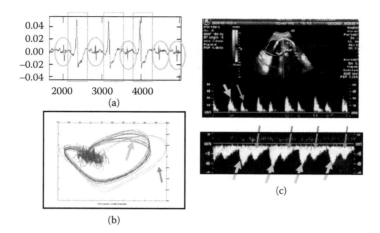

FIGURE 17.2
An example of premature ventricular contractions (PVC) identification. (a) PVC is clearly apparent in red squares, while normal heart electrocardiography (ECG) is shown in green circles in the panel. (b) The vector ECG of this case, with PVC clearly shown as an excursion from normal. (c) In the Doppler velocity waveform of fetal blood flow, a normal ECG (green arrows) corresponds to a normal flow whereas PVC (red arrows) makes a weak blood flow in (c). (From Y. Kimura et al., *Open Medical Devices Journal*, 4, 7–12, 2012.)

Figure 17.2 [38]. Normal heart ECG is shown in the light gray circles, while PVC is marked by dark gray squares. Also as shown in the figure, a normal ECG corresponds to a normal flow in the Doppler velocity waveform, but PVC results in a weak blood flow. The corresponding vector ECG is shown for this case in which PVC is clearly noticeable. The PVC case studied here was recognized at 24 weeks of gestation, and persisted throughout the pregnancy with atrioventricular septal defect (AVSD) as an outcome. This kind of arrhythmia diagnosed during pregnancy can be a marker of congenital heart defects. There are also transient arrhythmia, usually with functional causes from physiological phenomena such as hyperactivation of ion channels in the fetal myocardial cell. Furthermore, ectopic beats, which might be recognized as an important pathologic association, can be detected using fECG.

The main purpose of analyzing fECG is to estimate R peaks and find HR on a beat-to-beat basis. From this, other HRV-related features can be estimated. Beat-to-beat FHRV is precisely coincident for invasively and non-invasively recorded fECG. For example, in a previous study based on data from two pregnant women with singleton pregnancy and gestation age of 38–41 years during the first stage of labor, the indirect fECG extracted by BSSR was compared with invasive fECG. They were found consistent and coincident as shown in Figure 17.3 (correlation coefficient of 0.998 and less than 0.51 bpm bias according to Bland–Altman test) [38].

An earlier study compared HRV measures calculated from fECG and from traditional Doppler CTG, based on 10 subjects between 24 and 38 gestation weeks. An example of results for a 24-week subject is illustrated in Figure 17.4 [38]. The correlation coefficient and Bland–Altman plots were used to evaluate the comparisons. It was found that compared to the DUS method, FHR from fECG provides more details on short-term variability (STV) of HR [38]. STV is shown to be associated with fetal autonomic activity [59] and can be used as an effective tool for fetal assessment.

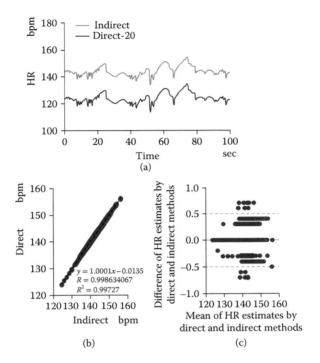

FIGURE 17.3
Accuracy of fetal electrocardiography (fECG) via the maternal abdominal wall. (a) The red graph shows an instantaneous heart rate (HR) tracing pattern of a deceleration calculated from the fECG via the maternal abdomen (indirect). The blue graph shows an instantaneous HR tracing pattern of the deceleration pattern calculated from the scalp electrode fetal ECG (direct). Both HRs are almost completely coincident. (b) A linear correlation between the two HRs. The correlation coefficient was 0.9986. (c) The Bland–Altman plots where a small bias of 0.51 bpm was significant. The minimum value for the limits of agreement was −0.51 bpm and the maximum was +0.51 bpm wherein 95% intervals of the points lie within ±1bpm. (From Y. Kimura et al., *Open Medical Devices Journal*, 4, 7–12, 2012.)

A more accurate estimation of fECG waveform with more details of P wave and T waves as well as accurate QRS complex will provide additional features such as ST-segment analysis. Different factors have influence on the fECG waveform, including hypoxia, ion channel activity of myocardial cells, autonomic nervous activity, and congenital heart defects. For example, the ST-segment waveform of fECG is changed in case of hypoxia [38,60] and the QT interval can be used to detect long QT (LQT) syndrome, which carries a high risk for developing life-threatening arrhythmias and sudden cardiac death in children and adults [61]. Figure 17.5 shows an example of the changes in fECG waveform during hypoxia based on previous study. In a previous study, the changes of PR and QT intervals with gestational age were also investigated. These can be used to assess development of the fetus during pregnancy [38]. In that study, fECG was successfully extracted using the method illustrated in Figure 17.1 for 163 out of 179 subjects (91.1%) with singleton pregnancies from 18 to 41 weeks of gestation. Then the terminal point of the T wave and the width of the P wave were calculated from averaged waves formed over 15 seconds of data with Doppler signals as reference. The changes of PR and QT intervals with growing gestation weeks are shown in Figure 17.6 [38,58].

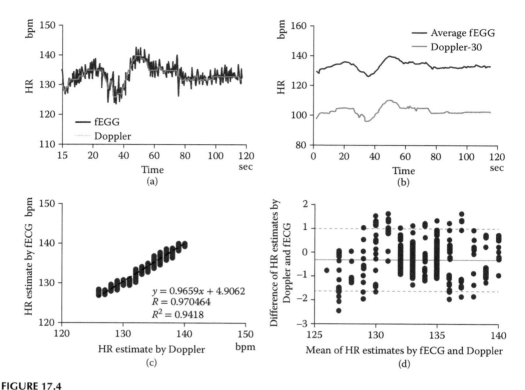

FIGURE 17.4

Comparison of Doppler cardiotocography (CTG) with noninvasive fetal electrocardiography (fECG) extracted by BSSR. (a) One example of comparison between fetal heart rate (FHR) from fECG (blue line) and FHR from traditional Doppler CTG (Doppler, red line) in a singleton fetus at 24 weeks of gestation. The former clearly had more short-term variability (STV) than the latter. (b) The blue line shows the moving average of fECG over each of the 15 time points (3.75 seconds) (average fECG). The red line represents the Doppler −30 bpm line. (c) A linear relationship between the two datasets. The correlation coefficient was 0.970. (d) Bland–Altman plot showing a significant small bias of 1.3 bpm. The minimum value for the limits of agreement was −1.6 bpm and the maximum was +1.0 bpm, wherein 95% intervals of the points lie within ±5 bpm. (From Y. Kimura et al., *Open Medical Devices Journal*, 4, 7–12, 2012.)

Although invasively recorded fECG through the fetal scalp electrodes provides detailed ST segment analysis [62,63], beat-to-beat identification of T waves from noninvasive fECG is more difficult and challenging because of noise and interferences, which contaminate the fECG signal.

17.2.3 Fetal Magnetocardiography

fMCG is the recording of a very weak magnetic field (10^{-12} tesla) generated by the flowing currents in the fetal heart. The superconductive quantum interference device (SQUID) is a very sensitive sensor that is used to record fMCG. Liquid helium has to be used to cool SQUID and the instruments of the fMCG are expensive, large in size, and complex [24,64]. fMCG can be measured as early as the second trimester and unlike the fECG, the effect of the vernix caseosa from the 28th to 32nd weeks of gestation does not affect it.

Examples of the signals recorded by fECG and fMCG, and the averaged waveforms, are illustrated in Figure 17.7. The fECG is the best of 20 channels while the fMCG is

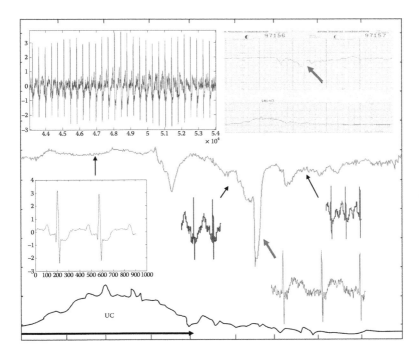

FIGURE 17.5

An example of a fetal electrocardiography (fECG) waveform during hypoxia. The left upper panel shows an 11-second trend of the fECG during uterine contractions (UC). The right upper panel shows the fetal cardiotocogram during a late deceleration. The late deceleration occurred with a uterine contraction. The middle big panel shows an instantaneous heart rate (HR) tracing pattern of this deceleration calculated from the fetal electrocardiogram. The dark gray arrow in this panel indicates an abrupt drop of fetal heart rate (FHR). Such sudden drops could not be detected in traditional Doppler cardiotocograms (dark gray arrow in right upper panel). The left middle small panel shows the averaged fetal electrocardiogram waveforms. ST depressions were clearly noticed. The ST depressions were noted to disappear and the ST elevations were noticed during deceleration. (From Y. Kimura et al., *Open Medical Devices Journal*, 4, 7–12, 2012.)

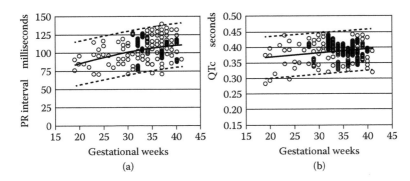

FIGURE 17.6

The standard values of PR intervals (a) and QTc (b) throughout gestation weeks. (From Y. Kimura et al., *Open Medical Devices Journal*, 4, 7–12, 2012; M. Sato et al., *Biomedical Engineering, IEEE Transactions on*, 54(1), 49–58, 2007.)

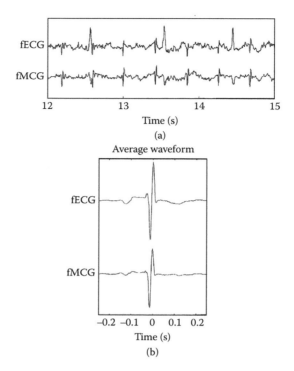

FIGURE 17.7
The traces of fetal ECG and MCG (a), which are simultaneously recorded, as well as the average waveform for one cardiac cycle of fECG and fMCG (b). (Modified from M. Peters et al., *Journal of Perinatal Medicine*, 29(5), 408–416, 2001.)

compromised by the noise due to simultaneous recording of the fECG. This fECG trace is of the best-quality recordings, which is not guaranteed for any recording at any time. However, fMCG provides good-quality waveforms as well as an fECG map on the maternal abdomen by means of a trigger; therefore, fECG can be averaged over that. fMCG can be used as a complement of fECG. The detailed waveforms obtained by this technique can be used for diagnosing the conduction disorders of the fetal heart and arrhythmias. However, during fMCG, the patient is not allowed to move and the duration of the test is usually short, while fECG can be measured at any time and for longer duration with cheaper and easier to handle equipment [24].

17.2.4 Fetal Echocardiography

Fetal echocardiography is the most informative noninvasive technique for fetal cardiac assessment. The four-chamber view of the heart is one of the easiest and most useful views to obtain in fetal echocardiography, by which the position and the size of the heart in the chest and its inner parts, the structure, and the function of the heart are examined. The size and contractility of the ventricles and the appearance of the AV valves are among the features evaluated from the four-chamber view [65]. As an extended basic examination, views of the outflow tracts can be also evaluated, which include the right and left ventricular outflow tracts of the heart. The latter is called the "five-chamber view" and demonstrates the four chambers and the aorta emerging from the left ventricle. The pulmonary artery, which opens to the right ventricle, is illustrated in the right outflow tract view [66]. According to a study of the low-risk population for congenital heart disease (CHD) screening with prospective study design, a sensitivity of 60.3% was obtained using the four-chamber view examination, and the sensitivity of the extended examination was found to be 65.5% [67].

The speed and accuracy of cardiac analysis has been enhanced by the introduction of Doppler color mapping about two decades ago [68]. The presence and direction of the blood flow and the presence of small vessels, as well as the areas of turbulence, can be found and confirmed by means of color doppler.

Pulsed–wave Doppler is recommended for a complete evaluation of the fetal heart, especially in the case of fetal cardiac malformation or compromise. This technique demonstrates the blood-flow velocity through the cardiac valves. Overall, the following aspects of Doppler evaluation are examined: the direction, pattern, and velocity of the flow and measuring volume flow and function.

M-mode echocardiography is less used in fetal cardiac evaluation but has the main following applications: measurement of cardiac structures, estimation of left ventricular function, and evaluation of atrial and ventricular contraction sequence [65]. Although M-mode can provide an estimation of PR intervals and atrial and ventricular coordination, the images are often not easy to read and timings may not be accurate. Moreover, fetal echocardiography is an expensive method and only particular maternal and fetal conditions indicate the need for it. In most cases, primary care physicians or obstetricians cannot appropriately analyze the heart views and only qualified individuals can perform this highly specialized examination [69].

17.2.5 Overview of the Cardiac Monitoring Methods

Table 17.2 shows an overview of the advantages and disadvantages of different heart monitoring techniques. More details are provided in [24].

TABLE 17.2

Overview of Different Methods for FHR Monitoring

Methods	Apparatus	Gestational age	Accuracy	Remarks
Doppler ultrasound	Cheap; easy to handle	20–40 weeks	>95% reliable, FHR short-term variability may not be observable	Can also be used during labor and recorded from 16th week; Valve movements can be detected
Fetal echo-cardigraphy	Expensive, specialized, skilled personnel required	18–40 weeks	90%–95% reliable FHR, anatomy, physiology of heart depends on quality of images; accuracy intervals limited	Cardiac scanning is possible from 11th week by transvaginal probe
fECG	Cheap; easy to handle	20–40 weeks possibly with a dip around 32 weeks	60% reliable in last month, for FHR beat-to-beat accuracy, limited fECG morphology	Can be used during labor, good for long-term ambulatory use
fMCG	Expensive, skilled personnel required	20–40 weeks	Fully reliable, waveforms observable in an averaged signal; accuracy intervals about 5 ms	Measured in 13th week

17.3 FHRV Analysis

FHRV can be analyzed in more detail by different mathematical approaches. In adults, HRV has been extensively investigated for characterizing ANS in controlling HR and general ANS function [70]. Fluctuations of the intervals between normal heartbeats provide information about cardiac autonomic modulation, since they are mediated by autonomic inputs to the sinus node, where the parasympathetic component of the ANS leads to increase in the interbeat intervals and the sympathetic component to a decrease in interbeat intervals. These fluctuations can be quantified by HRV analysis. Different parameters are used for assessment of interbeat interval variability, which range from linear time- and frequency-domain analysis to nonlinear measurements including entropy, fractal, and multiscale analysis. For fetuses, changes in different FHRV parameters with gestational age can be investigated to assess the development of sympathetic and parasympathetic components of fetal ANS. In this section, two main categories of methods, that is, time-domain and the frequency-domain FHRV analysis, are reviewed.

17.3.1 Time-Domain and Complexity Analysis

In time-domain analysis, ectopic beats are usually excluded and normal-to-normal (NN) beats are considered for analysis. This means that RR intervals, which are due to extra systole source and suprabifurcational block-type rhythm changes, are removed. Several time-domain and complexity measurement parameters have been used in previous studies.

17.3.1.1 Linear Time-Domain Analysis

The mean RR interval (mRR) or mean heart rate (mHR) are the simple time-domain measures. It has been found that mRR slightly increases with gestational age but it is not consistent over all subjects [19]. The decrease of FHR is affected by increasing parasympathetic activity compensating the acceleration effect of sympathetic tone [71]. Fetal behavioral states corresponding to quiet sleep, active (REM) sleep, quiet awake, and active awake also affect the HR [72,73]. For example, decrease of mHR (hence increase of mRR) with gestational age is almost significant during the quiet/nonaccelerative sleep state, which shows decreasing basal FHR (Pearson coefficient $r^2 = -0.293$; $p = 0.063$), but not during the active/accelerative sleep state [22].

Changes in vagal function are characterized by changes in HRV. This can be analyzed by the standard deviation (SD) and RMSSD, which are calculated as follows:

$$SDNN = \sqrt{\frac{\sum_{i=1}^{k}(NN_i - \overline{NN})^2}{k-1}} \qquad (17.1)$$

$$RMSSD = \sqrt{\frac{\sum_{i=2}^{k}(NN_i - NN_{i-1})^2}{k-1}} \qquad (17.2)$$

SDNN and RMSSD are the measures of overall variability and STV, respectively, and they can be used to assess sympathovagal balance [74]. Both of these parameters increase with gestational age and this increase is more pronounced for RMSSD. The high correlation of RMSSD (median of Pearson coefficient over subjects: 0.83) can be used as a stable marker for assessing fetal maturation, especially the development of the parasympathetic nervous system [19]. The ratio SDNN/RMSSD is also used as a potential sympathovagal balance marker. During quiet FHR patterns, SDNN/RMSSD decreases with gestational age, more significantly before 32 weeks. After 32 weeks, this ratio is more influenced by RMSSD during the quiet FHR pattern, which indicates parasympathetic dominance in the second half of the third trimester. On the other hand, in the active FHR pattern, mHR increases over basal FHR, SDNN becomes more dominant for SDNN/RMSSD, and SDNN and RMSSD become strongly correlated. The sympathetic dominance in active FHR patterns is characterized by the relationship of mHR, SDNN, and SDNN/RMSSD after 32 weeks [22].

17.3.1.2 Complexity Analysis

The dynamics of the FHR can be further investigated by complexity analysis. The contraction or expansion of the HR represented by a nonlinear dynamics model can be analyzed by the approximate maximal Lyapunov exponent (ApML), while scaling features of the distribution and the expansion properties of the generating dynamics can be described by approximate information dimension (ApD1) and approximate entropy (ApEn) [19]. It is found that ApEn and ApML increase with gestational age, while APD1 does not change significantly, which shows different sensitivity of these parameters to various features of temporal complexity. The increasing complexity with gestational age can be explained by the changing parasympathetic effect during the development of ANS [19].

The ApEn mainly measures the regularity of the signal by investigating the presence of similar patterns in the time series [23]. A lower value of ApEn during labor was found to be associated with poorer outcome [75]. Fetal acidosis and distress might also be associated with lower complexity values measured by ApEn [76]. It was also found in another study that in quiet periods, ApEn is significantly higher ($p < 0.05$) for pathological cases (IUGR and maternal diabetes) compared to normal subjects [21].

SampEn was developed by Richman and Moorman as a modification of ApEn, to overcome some of its imperfections such as lack of consistency in some cases [77]. These two measures can be obtained in the MSE analysis scheme to achieve features as a function of different scales [23,78]. Ferrario et al. have shown by MSE analysis that single-scale entropy analysis is not sufficient for detection of pathological conditions, because they can affect the regularity of the signal at different time scales. They have found that entropy values for fetuses with severe IUGR are significantly lower than nonsevere IUGR and normal fetuses for the scale factors $\tau > 3$ but not significant at scale factor $\tau = 1$ [79].

MSE entropy measures were also found to be higher for normal fetuses at all scale factors compared to the fetuses with antepartum pathological conditions and distress at birth while linear time-domain analysis could not reveal any difference in the same experiment. The reason might be the increase of regularity in pathological cases because of the loss of complexity in the regularity mechanisms [23].

17.3.2 Spectral Analysis

fHRV have been further evaluated by power spectral analysis to assess the ANS function. For this purpose, the power spectral density (PSD) is evaluated at the following frequency ranges: low (LF: 0.03–0.15 Hz), medium (MF: 0.15–0.5 Hz), and high (HF: 0.5–1 HZ) frequency [21]. According to the previous studies, the HF component is linked to fetal breathing movements and more visible during quiet state, while MF and especially LF components are more pronounced during the active state [21,80,81]. Therefore, the respiratory peaks are observable in some short-term traces during the fetal quiet state in the frequency range of 0.7–0.8 Hz [21,80]; they are more apparent in mature fetuses (36 weeks) [81]. Moreover, Karin et al. found a higher level of HRV spectral power for young fetuses (<30 weeks) compared to mature fetuses, with more stable ANS in the last period of pregnancy in both states [80]. However, they used the fast Fourier transform (FFT) for spectral analysis, which is complicated, and as the fetal heart beats change nonlinearly, the effectiveness of that method has not been established [20,82].

Another issue to consider is that FHR fluctuations are not stationary long term in quiet nor active states. Therefore, an earlier study suggested the use of a nonparametric test with the assumption of nonstationarity of the FHR fluctuations and observed stationarity for periods of less than 300 beats [20]. The autoregression method based on 24-cycle stationarity was used for spectral analysis of stable FHR series obtained from DUS [20]. The changes of the low-frequency area (LFA) resulting from integration over the LF range (0.025–0.125 Hz) were found to be well correlated with the changes of fetal blood gas levels. The LFA is associated with the ANS activity related to the sympathetic nerve as the LF component is correlated with neural sympathetic activity [20,21]. The relationship between changes of LFA with gestational age is shown in Figure 17.8, which can be explained by the development of the sympathetic nerve activity. For example, from 26 to 30 weeks of gestation, the development of sympathetic nerves and increase in LFA with gestational age are both rapid, while they are both slow around 32 weeks. Therefore, it is concluded that LFA can be used to assess the development of fetal ANS [20].

Another study suggested to use the LF(0.08–0.2 Hz)/HF(0.7–1.7 Hz) ratio as an index corresponding to sympathovagal balance in the frequency domain [22]. In the quiet state, this ratio was found to be markedly negatively correlated with gestational age (Pearson coefficient $r^2 = -0.360$; $p < 0.01$) for fetuses before 32 weeks of gestation and not noticeable after that. In the active state, however, this ratio has a positive correlation with age ($r^2 = 0.389$; $p < 0.1$) prior to 32 weeks. In the active state, LF/HF is more related to HF, while in the quiet state, it is more related to LF before 32 weeks and after that it becomes related to HF. Overall, prior to 32 weeks, LF/HF indicates a more rapidly progressive parasympathetic

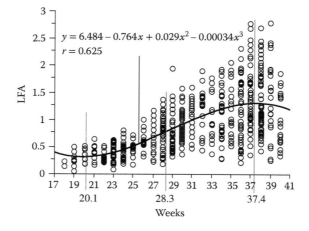

FIGURE 17.8
Alteration of low-frequency area (LFA) of the spectrum of heartbeat fluctuation in normal fetuses during pregnancy. LFA is calculated on the basis of integration of peaks in the low-frequency domain (0.025–0.125 cycles/beat) in the spectrum. Minimum point, reflection point, and maximum point are indicated with arrows. (Modified from From T. Ohta et al., *Fetal Diagnosis and Therapy*, 14(2), 92–97, 1999.)

effect. Furthermore, HF and LF parameters are negatively correlated with mHR in both states, while their ratio is positively correlated with mHR only in the active state [22].

Spectral parameters have been found to be promising for discrimination of pathological subjects from normal ones. Generally, higher spectral power in the LF range and also its ratio $\left(\frac{LF}{MF+HF}\right)$ is ascertained for normal fetuses [21]. In a previous study, LFA was found decreased for IUGR. It was shown that in fetuses with IUGR, LFA was correlated with the concentration of oxygen and the pH level in blood. Overall, LFA was shown to be useful for monitoring fetal well-being.

According to another study, the LF ratio $\frac{LF}{MF+HF}$ for both IUGR and maternal diabetes subjects was significantly different from normal fetuses ($p < 0.05$). The decrease in LF power component for abnormal fetuses is due to the reduction of the contribution of neural sympathetic control [21].

The MF component is mainly related to the fetal movements and maternal breathing effect; its ratio to the total power significantly increased for the fetuses at risk, and can be described as indicating a disturbed quiet status [21].

17.4 Summary

FHR monitoring is a common method of fetal assessment. For this purpose, FHR can be obtained by different techniques, each with some advantages and disadvantages regarding the accuracy, costs, and possible duration of measurement. Furthermore to the conventional techniques such as Doppler CTG, more detailed HRV analysis can provide information about fetal well-being and development of the ANS, which can be obtained using fECG. Linear time-domain measures such as SDNN and RMSSD can be used to assess sympathovagal balance and fetal development. In addition, there are complexity measurement techniques including MSE analysis that have been found to be promising markers to detect severe IUGR and other pathological conditions. FHRV has been further evaluated by power spectral analysis. In particular, the LF component of the PSD can be used to evaluate the development of sympathetic nerve activity and the LF/HF ratio can be used as an index of sympathovagal balance. Despite the current advances, further research is still required for enhancement of FHR acquisition and processing as well as advanced FHRV analysis.

References

1. G. Ramanathan and S. Arulkumaran, Antenatal fetal surveillance, *Obstetrics and Gynecology for Postgraduates*, 1: 63–73, 2009..
2. L. D. Devoe, Antenatal fetal assessment: Contraction stress test, nonstress test, vibroacoustic stimulation, amniotic fluid volume, biophysical profile, and modified biophysical profile—An overview, in *Seminars in Perinatology*, 32, pp. 247–252, Elsevier, 2008.
3. P. Malcus, Antenatal fetal surveillance, *Current Opinion in Obstetrics and Gynecology*, 16(2): 123–128, 2004.
4. P. Steer and P. Danielian, Fetal distress in labour, In: James, DK, Steer, PJ, Weiner, CP, Gonik, B (eds.), *High Risk Pregnancy Management Options*, London: WB Saunders, 1994.

5. R. Liston, D. Sawchuck, and D. Young, Fetal health surveillance: Antepartum and intra-partum consensus guideline, *Journal of Obstetrics and Gynaecology Canada*, 29(9 Suppl 4): S3–56, 2007.

6. A. T. Bianco, S. W. Smilen, Y. Davis, S. Lopez, R. Lapinski, and C. J. Lockwood, Pregnancy outcome and weight gain recommendations for the morbidly obese woman, *Obstetrics and Gynecology*, 91(1): 97–102, 1998.

7. R. Von Kries, R. Kimmerle, J. Schmidt, A. Hachmeister, O. Böhm, and H. Wolf, Pregnancy outcomes in mothers with pregestational diabetes: A population-based study in North Rhine (Germany) from 1988 to 1993, *European Journal of Pediatrics*, 156(12): 963–967, 1997.

8. D. Sim, R. Beattie, and J. Dornan, Evaluation of biophysical fetal assessment in high-risk pregnancy to assess ultrasound parameters suitable for screening in the low-risk population, *Ultrasound in Obstetrics and Gynecology*, 3(1): 11–17, 1993.

9. P. Bobby, Multiple assessment techniques evaluate antepartum fetal risks, *Pediatric Annals*, 32(9): 609, 2003.

10. G. Davies, Medico-Legal Commmittee. Antenatal fetal assessment. SOGC Clinical Practice Guideline, *Jounal of Obstetrics and Gynaecology*, 22(6): 456–62, 2000.

11. I. Timor-Tritsch, L. Dierker, I. Zador, R. Hertz, and M. Rosen, Fetal movements associated with fetal heart rate accelerations and decelerations, *American Journal of Obstetrics and Gynecology*, 131(3): 276, 1978.

12. S. Cerutti, A. L. Goldberger, and Y. Yamamoto, Recent advances in heart rate variability signal processing and interpretation, *Biomedical Engineering, IEEE Transactions on*, 53(1): 1–3, 2006.

13. F. Kovács, C. Horváth, Á. T. Balogh, and G. Hosszú, Fetal phonocardiographypast and future possibilities, *Computer Methods and Programs in Biomedicine*, 104(1): 19–25, 2011.

14. K. Tan and A. Sabapathy, Fetal manipulation for facilitating tests of fetal wellbeing, *Cochrane Database of Systematic Reviews*, 4: 1–11, 2001.

15. J. P. Lavin Jr, M. Miodovnik, and T. P. Barden, Relationship of nonstress test reactivity and gestational age, *Obstetrics and Gynecology*, 63(3): 338–344, 1984.

16. M. L. Druzin, A. Fox, E. Kogut, and C. Carlson, The relationship of the nonstress test to gestational age, *American Journal of Obstetrics and Gynecology*, 153(4): 386–389, 1985.

17. R. D. Eden, F. H. Boehm, and M. Haire, *Assessment and Care of the Fetus: Physiological, Clinical, and Medicolegal Principles*. Norwalk, CT: Appleton & Lange, 1990.

18. L. Pello, S. Rosevear, G. Dawes, M. Moulden, and C. Redman, Computerized fetal heart rate analysis in labor, *Obstetrics and Gynecology*, 78(4): 602–610, 1991.

19. P. Van Leeuwen, S. Lange, H. Bettermann, D. Grönemeyer, and W. Hatzmann, Fetal heart rate variability and complexity in the course of pregnancy, *Early Human Development*, 54(3): 259–269, 1999.

20. T. Ohta, K. Okamura, Y. Kimura, T. Suzuki, T. Watanabe, T. Yasui, N. Yaegashi, and A. Yajima, Alteration in the low-frequency domain in power spectral analysis of fetal heart beat fluctuations, *Fetal Diagnosis and Therapy*, 14(2): 92–97, 1999.

21. M. G. Signorini, G. Magenes, S. Cerutti, and D. Arduini, Linear and nonlinear parameters for the analysisof fetal heart rate signal from cardiotocographic recordings, *IEEE Transactions on Biomedical Engineering*, 50(3): 365–374, 2003.

22. U. Schneider, E. Schleussner, A. Fiedler, S. Jaekel, M. Liehr, J. Haueisen, and D. Hoyer, Fetal heart rate variability reveals differential dynamics in the intrauterine development of the sympathetic and parasympathetic branches of the autonomic nervous system, *Physiological Measurement*, 30(2): 215, 2009.

23. M. Ferrario, M. G. Signorini, G. Magenes, and S. Cerutti, Comparison of entropybased regularity estimators: Application to the fetal heart rate signal for the identification of fetal distress, *IEEE Transactions on Biomedical Engineering*, 53(1): 119–125, 2006.

24. M. Peters, J. Crowe, J. F. Piéri, H. Quartero, B. Hayes-Gill, D. James, J. Stinstra, and S. Shakespeare, Monitoring the fetal heart non-invasively: A review of methods, *Journal of Perinatal Medicine*, 29(5): 408–416, 2001.

25. Y. Murata, J. Chester, and B Martin, Systolic time intervals of the fetal cardiac cycle, *Obstetrics and Gynecology*, 44(2): 224–232, 1974.
26. Y. Murata, C. B. Martin, T. Ikenoue, and P. Lu, Antepartum evaluation of the preejection period of the fetal cardiac cycle, *American Journal of Obstetrics and Gynecology*, 132: 278–284, 1978.
27. S. Shakespeare, J. Crowe, B. Hayes-Gill, K. Bhogal, and D. James, The information content of doppler ultrasound signals from the fetal heart, *Medical and Biological Engineering and Computing*, 39(6): 619–626, 2001.
28. T. Koga, N. Athayde, B. Trudinger, and H. Nakano, A new and simple Doppler method for measurement of fetal cardiac isovolumetric contraction time, *Ultrasound in Obstetrics & Gynecology*, 18(3): 264–267, 2001.
29. A. H. Khandoker, Y. Kimura, T. Ito, N. Sato, K. Okamura, and M. Palaniswami, Antepartum non-invasive evaluation of opening and closing timings of the cardiac valves in fetal cardiac cycle, *Medical and Biological Engineering and Computing*, 47(10): 1075–1082, 2009.
30. F. Marzbanrad, A. Khandoker, K. Funamoto, R. Sugibayashi, M. Endo, C. Velayo, Y. Kimura, and M. Palaniswami, Automated identification of fetal cardiac valve timings, in *Engineering in Medicine and Biology Society, 2013. IEEE-EMBC'13. 35th Annual International Conference of the IEEE*, pp. 3893–3896, IEEE, 2013.
31. M. B. Sampson, Antepartum measurement of the preejection period in high-risk pregnancy, *Obstetrics and Gynecology*, 56(3): 289–290, 1980.
32. L. Organ, A. Bernstein, and P. Hawrylyshyn, The pre-ejection period as an antepartum indicator of fetal well-being, *American Journal of Obstetrics and Gynecology*, 137(7): 810, 1980.
33. F. Marzbanrad, Y. Kimura, K. Funamoto, R. Sugibayashi, M. Endo, T. Ito, M. Palaniswami, and A. H. Khandoker, Automated estimation of fetal cardiac timing events from Doppler ultrasound signal using hybrid models, *IEEE Journal of Biomedical and Health Informatics*, 18(4): 1169–1177, 2014.
34. F. Marzbanrad, Y. Kimura, M. Endo, S. Oshio, K. Funamoto, N. Sato, M. Palaniswami, and A. Khandoker, Model based estimation of aortic and mitral valves opening and closing timings in developing human fetuses, *IEEE Journal of Biomedical and Health Informatics*, 20.1: 240–248, 2016.
35. F. Marzbanrad, A. Khandoker, M. Endo, Y. Kimura, and M. Palaniswami, A multi-dimensional hidden Markov model approach to automated identification of fetal cardiac valve motion, in *Engineering in Medicine and Biology Society (EMBC), 2014 36th Annual International Conference of the IEEE*, pp. 1885–1888, Aug 2014.
36. M. J. Lewis, Review of electromagnetic source investigations of the fetal heart, *Medical Engineering and Physics*, 25(10): 801–810, 2003.
37. R. Sameni and G. D. Clifford, A review of fetal ECG signal processing; issues and promising directions, *The Open Pacing, Electrophysiology and Therapy Journal*, 3: 4, 2010.
38. Y. Kimura, N. Sato, J. Sugawara, C. Velayo, T. Hoshiai, S. Nagase, T. Ito, Y. Onuma, A. Katsumata, K. Okamura, and N Yaegashi, Recent advances in fetal electrocardiography, *Open Medical Devices Journal*, 4: 7–12, 2012.
39. G. D. Clifford, I. Silva, J. Behar, and G. B. Moody, Non-invasive fetal ECG analysis, *Physiological Measurement*, 35(8): 1521, 2014.
40. N. Outram, E. Ifeachor, P. Van Eetvelt, and S. Curnow, Techniques for optimal enhancement and feature extraction of fetal electrocardiogram, *IEE Proceedings—Science, Measurement and Technology*, 142(6): 482–489, 1995.
41. K.-C. Lai and J. J. Shynk, A successive cancellation algorithm for fetal heartrate estimation using an intrauterine ECG signal, *IEEE Transactions on Biomedical Engineering*, 49(9): 943–954, 2002.
42. S. D. Larks, Present status of fetal electrocardiography, *IRE Transactions on Bio-Medical Electronics*, 9(3): 176–180, 1962.
43. B. Widrow, J. R. Glover Jr, J. M. McCool, J. Kaunitz, C. S. Williams, R. H. Hearn, J. R. Zeidler, E. Dong Jr, and R. C. Goodlin, Adaptive noise cancelling: Principles and applications, *Proceedings of the IEEE*, 63(12): 1692–1716, 1975.

44. M. Shao, K. E. Barner, and M. H. Goodman, An interference cancellation algorithm for noninvasive extraction of transabdominal fetal electroencephalogram (TaFEEG), *IEEE Transactions on Biomedical Engineering*, 51(3): 471–483, 2004.
45. S. M. Martens, C. Rabotti, M. Mischi, and R. J. Sluijter, A robust fetal ECG detection method for abdominal recordings, *Physiological Measurement*, 28(4): 373, 2007.
46. R. Sameni, M. B. Shamsollahi, C. Jutten, and G. D. Clifford, A nonlinear Bayesian filtering framework for ECG denoising, *IEEE Transactions on Biomedical Engineering*, 54(12): 2172–2185, 2007.
47. C. Li, C. Zheng, and C. Tai, Detection of ECG characteristic points using wavelet transforms, *IEEE Transactions on Biomedical Engineering*, 42(1): 21–28, 1995.
48. A. Khamene and S. Negahdaripour, A new method for the extraction of fetal ECG from the composite abdominal signal, *IEEE Transactions on Biomedical Engineering*, 47(4): 507–516, 2000.
49. A. Damen and J. Van Der Kam, The use of the singular value decomposition in electrocardiography, *Medical and Biological Engineering and Computing*, 20(4): 473–482, 1982.
50. D. Callaerts, *Signal separation methods based on singular value decomposition and their application to the real-time extraction of the fetal electrocardiogram from cutaneous recordings*, Ph.D. Thesis, K.U.Leuven - E.E. Dept., Dec. 1989
51. P. P. Kanjilal, S. Palit, and G. Saha, Fetal ECG extraction from single-channel maternal ECG using singular value decomposition, *IEEE Transactions on Biomedical Engineering*, 44(1): 51–59, 1997.
52. L. De Lathauwer, B. De Moor, and J. Vandewalle, Fetal electrocardiogram extraction by blind source subspace separation, *IEEE Transactions on Biomedical Engineering*, 47(5): 567–572, 2000.
53. V. Zarzoso, A. Nandi, and E. Bacharakis, Maternal and foetal ECG separation using blind source separation methods, *Mathematical Medicine and Biology*, 14(3): 207–225, 1997.
54. E. Bacharakis, A. Nandi, and V. Zarzoso, Foetal ECG extraction using blind source separation methods, *Signal Processing Division*. University of Srathclyde, 1996.
55. V. Zarzoso, J. Millet-Roig, and A. Nandi, Fetal ECG extraction from maternal skin electrodes using blind source separation and adaptive noise cancellation techniques, in *Computers in Cardiology 2000*, pp. 431–434, IEEE, 2000.
56. V. Vigneron, A. Paraschiv-Ionescu, A. Azancot, O. Sibony, and C. Jutten, Electrocardiogram extraction based on non-stationary ICA and wavelet denoising, in *Proceedings of IEEE in Seventh International Symposium on Signal Processing and its Applications, 2003*, 2: pp. 69–72, 2003.
57. M. G. Jafari and J. A. Chambers, Fetal electrocardiogram extraction by sequential source separation in the wavelet domain, *IEEE Transactions on Biomedical Engineering*, 52(3): 390–400, 2005.
58. M. Sato, Y. Kimura, S. Chida, T. Ito, N. Katayama, K. Okamura, and M. Nakao, A novel extraction method of fetal electrocardiogram from the composite abdominal signal, *IEEE Transactions on Biomedical Engineering*, 54(1): 49–58, 2007.
59. Y. Kimura, K. Okamura, T. Watanabe, J. Murotsuki, T. Suzuki, M. Yano, and A. Yajima, Power spectral analysis for autonomic influences in heart rate and blood pressure variability in fetal lambs, *American Journal of Physiology-Heart and Circulatory Physiology*, 271(4): H1333–H1339, 1996.
60. K. R. Greene and K. G. Rosen, Long-term ST waveform changes in the ovine fetal electrocardiogram: The relationship to spontaneous labour and intrauterine death, *Clinical Physics And Physiological Measurement: An Official Journal of the Hospital Physicists' Association, Deutsche Gesellschaft Für Medizinische Physik and the European Federation of Organisations for Medical Physics*, 10(Suppl B): 33–40, 1989.
61. P. J. Schwartz, M. Periti, and A. Malliani, The long QT syndrome, *American Heart Journal*, 89(3): 378–390, 1975.
62. I. Amer-Wåhlin, C. Hellsten, H. Norén, H. Hagberg, A. Herbst, I. Kjellmer, H. Lilja, C. Lindoff, M. Månsson, L. Mårtensson, P. Olofsson, A. Sundström, and K. Marsál. Cardiotocography only versus cardiotocography plus ST analysis of fetal electrocardiogram for intrapartum fetal monitoring: A Swedish randomised controlled trial, *Lancet*, 358(9281): 534–538, 2001.

63. M. A. Oudijk, A. Kwee, G. H. Visser, S. Blad, E. J. Meijboom, and K. G. Rosén, The effects of intrapartum hypoxia on the fetal QT interval, *BJOG: An International Journal of Obstetrics and Gynaecology*, 111(7): 656–660, 2004.

64. M. Peters, J. Stinstra, S. Van Den Broek, J. Huirne, H. Quartero, H. Ter Brake, and H. Rogalla, On the fetal magnetocardiogram, *Bioelectrochemistry and Bioenergetics*, 47(2): 273–281, 1998.

65. L. D. Allan, A. C. Cook, and I. C. Huggon, *Fetal Echocardiography: A Practical Guide*. Cambridge, UK: Cambridge University Press, 2009.

66. A. Z. Abuhamad and R. Chaoui, *A Practical Guide to Fetal Echocardiography: Normal and Abnormal Hearts*. Philadelphia, PA: Lippincott Williams & Wilkins, 2010.

67. G. Ogge, P. Gaglioti, S. Maccanti, F. Faggiano, and T. Todros, Prenatal screening for congenital heart disease with four-chamber and outflow-tract views: A multicenter study, *Ultrasound in Obstetrics and Gynecology*, 28(6): 779–784, 2006.

68. G. DeVore, J. Horenstein, B. Siassi, and L. Platt, Fetal echocardiography. VII. Doppler color flow mapping: A new technique for the diagnosis of congenital heart disease., *American Journal of Obstetrics and Gynecology*, 156(5): 1054, 1987.

69. L. Caserta, Z. Ruggeri, L. D'Emidio, C. Coco, P. Cignini, A. Girgenti, L. Mangiafico, and C. Giorlandino, Two-dimensional fetal echocardiography: Where we are, *Journal of Prenatal Medicine*, 2(3): 31, 2008.

70. U. R. Acharya, K. P. Joseph, N. Kannathal, C. M. Lim, and J. S. Suri, Heart rate variability: A review, *Medical and Biological Engineering and Computing*, 44(12): 1031–1051, 2006.

71. J. T. Parer, *"Fetal Heart Rate," Maternal-Fetal Medicine*. Philadelphia, PA: WB Saunders, vol. 1266, 1999.

72. J. Nijhuis, H. F. Prechtl, C. J. Martin, and R. Bots, Are there behavioural states in the human fetus? *Early Human Development*, 6(2): 177–195, 1982.

73. J. A. DiPietro, D. M. Hodgson, K. A. Costigan, S. C. Hilton, and T. R. Johnson, Fetal neurobehavioral development, *Child Development*, 67(5): 2553–2567, 1996.

74. U. Schneider, B. Frank, A. Fiedler, C. Kaehler, D. Hoyer, M. Liehr, J. Haueisen, and E. Schleussner, Human fetal heart rate variability-characteristics of autonomic regulation in the third trimester of gestation, *Journal of Perinatal Medicine*, 36(5): 433–441, 2008.

75. G. Dawes, M. Moulden, O. Sheil, and C. Redman, Approximate entropy, a statistic of regularity, applied to fetal heart rate data before and during labor, *Obstetrics and Gynecology*, 80(5): 763–768, 1992.

76. S. M. Pincus and R. R. Viscarello, Approximate entropy: A regularity measure for fetal heart rate analysis, *Obstetrics and Gynecology*, 79(2): 249–255, 1992.

77. J. S. Richman and J. R. Moorman, Physiological time-series analysis using approximate entropy and sample entropy, *American Journal of Physiology-Heart and Circulatory Physiology*, 278(6): H2039–H2049, 2000.

78. M. Costa, A. L. Goldberger, and C.-K. Peng, Multiscale entropy analysis of complex physiologic time series, *Physical Review Letters*, 89(6): 068102, 2002.

79. M. Ferrario, M. G. Signorini, and G. Magenes, Complexity analysis of the fetal heart rate variability: Early identification of severe intrauterine growth-restricted fetuses, *Medical and Biological Engineering and Computing*, 47(9): 911–919, 2009.

80. J. Karin, M. Hirsch, and S. Akselrod, An estimate of fetal autonomic state by spectral analysis of fetal heart rate fluctuations, *Pediatric Research*, 34(2): 134–138, 1993.

81. E. Ferrazzi, G. Pardi, P. L. Setti, M. Rodolfi, S. Civardi, and S. Cerutti, Power spectral analysis of the heart rate of the human fetus at 26 and 36 weeks of gestation, *Clinical Physics and Physiological Measurement*, 10(4B): 57, 1989.

82. D. G. Chaffin, C. C. Goldberg, and K. L. Reed, The dimension of chaos in the fetal heart rate, *American Journal of Obstetrics and Gynecology*, 165(5): 1425–1429, 1991.

18

Heart Rate Variability and Eating Disorders

Jane Russell and Ian Spence

CONTENTS

18.1 Introduction

Eating disorders are life-threatening disorders with a high risk of death. Up to 20% of patients with anorexia nervosa (AN) die prematurely as a result of their illness. While suicide is a major cause of these deaths, a second significant cause is cardiac arrest (American Psychiatric Association 2000). The precise cause of this cardiac arrest is in many cases unexplained and a variety of factors ranging from chronic hypokalemia and chronically low plasma albumin to functional and physical changes in the heart have been implicated (Jauregui-Garrido and Jauregui-Lobera 2012). Disturbances of cardiac function are well documented in patients with AN (Kalager et al. 1978; Casper 1986). These include slower heart rate, lower blood pressure, decreased heart rate variability (HRV), prolonged QT intervals, and physical changes in the heart with accompanying functional changes (Casiero and Frishman 2006). Evidence for a link between the autonomic nervous system and cardiovascular mortality, including sudden cardiac death, has accumulated over the last 50 years (Wolf et al. 1978; Kleiger et al. 1987).

18.2 Autonomic Function in Eating Disorders

Changes in the autonomic function in the cardiovascular system can be assessed from various aspects of the electrocardiogram (ECG). The simplest of these is measurement of QT intervals. Bradycardia is a common observation in AN patients with longer QT and corrected QT intervals (QTc) than in age- and sex-matched controls and regression to the mean with recovery (Cooke and Chambers 1995). Here correction for heart rate was done as it most often is, using Bazett's correction (QTc = QT/sqrtRR), although some controversy exists as to the reliability of this correction in all cases and it can overestimate the number of patients with QT prolongation (Sagie et al. 1993). A meta-analysis of 10 studies, which examined heart rate and alterations in QT interval, found that while the QTc intervals tended to be longer in AN patients than in the corresponding controls, these differences did not reach statistical significance (Lesinskiene et al. 2008). QT interval prolongation may not have such good predictive value in recognizing patients who are at particular risk of sudden death (Jauregui-Garrido and Jauregui-Lobera 2012). QT intervals in patients with eating disorders are generally <600 ms, a duration that has been clearly associated with significant risk of sudden death (Jackman et al. 1988). While QT interval duration alone may not have good predictive power, Jáuregui-Garrido suggests that increased QT interval dispersion may be an independent predictor of sudden cardiac death, provided it can be measured with sufficient reliability (Jauregui-Garrido and Jauregui-Lobera 2012).

18.3 HRV in Eating Disorders

A possible alternative method for assessing cardiac health in emergency department (ED) patients is by assessing the patterns of cardiac activity. The fluctuations in the time between heartbeats reflect the convergence of several factors: the intrinsic rhythm of the heart, the input from the sympathetic and parasympathetic nervous systems, their interplay, and the effects of circulating factors. The principal factor is generally thought to be autonomic input and assessment of HRV has been shown to be a useful noninvasive method of assessing cardiovascular autonomic function in a number of clinical conditions (Task Force 1996). Assessment of HRV might therefore provide a useful indicator of cardiovascular risk, particularly of dysrhythmic events in eating-disorder patients. The simplicity of the technique means that it can be included in the evaluation of patients relatively easily. In this brief review, the major conclusions of previous studies will be outlined with some discussion of the problems associated with definition of patient status and some consideration of potential confounding factors. The results of some of our recent studies are discussed later in the text.

18.4 HRV in AN

It is beyond the scope of this discussion to attempt a comprehensive review of the literature on HRV and eating disorders so we have attempted to summarize key observations from published studies, which allow comparison. Problems in comparing these studies include the use of different measures of HRV as well as differences in sample sizes and patient groups. The results of a number of studies on HRV in AN patients where meaningful comparisons were possible are summarized in Table 18.1. The aim is to give an overview of the main findings of each study. The table does contain some simplifications and does not attempt to record all the observations in all the studies. Short-term data is only for supine measurement and data of effects of standing/lying are not included nor are results related to other eating disorder groups unless noted in *Comments*.

18.4.1 Time-Domain Analysis

The limited short-term time-domain data (standard deviation of normal to normal [NN] intervals [SDNN], square root of the mean squared differences of successive NN intervals [RMSSD], and proportion derived by dividing NN50 by the total number of NN intervals [pNN50]) from anorexic patients do not present a clear picture. Increases, decreases, and no changes in time-domain parameters have been reported. The usefulness of these estimates is limited and comparisons of values from recordings of different durations may not be appropriate (Task Force 1996). The data from 24-hour studies present a slightly clearer picture, that is, that there is a general increase in time-domain parameters, which would be consistent with increased parasympathetic modulation. In contrast the study by Melanson et al. obtained opposite results but used the smallest sample (six patients) employed in any study and the results may reflect sampling bias (Melanson et al. 2004).

18.4.2 Frequency-Domain Analysis

Although values for high-frequency (HF) and low-frequency (LF) power in anorexic patients show variations in different studies, the HF/LF ratio was consistently reduced. This would be consistent with reduced HRV and might reasonably arise from either increased sympathetic or reduced parasympathetic modulation of heart rate.

18.4.3 Nonlinear Analysis

Few studies have examined HRV in anorexic patients using nonlinear methods. The reduced values of the scaling exponent, α, from detrended fluctuation analysis in anorexic patients compared to controls is also consistent with reduced HRV.

Mazurek et al. (2011) reviewed the literature on HRV as a measure of cardiac autonomic function in AN. They found conflicting results in the 20 studies of linear and nonlinear measures from short-term and 24-hour monitoring, which they reviewed, although the majority reported parasympathetic/sympathetic imbalance with parasympathetic dominance and decreased sympathetic modulation. Lack of uniformity in the studies, small sample numbers, and many confounding factors led the authors to conclude that at that stage HRV could only be used as a research tool and not a routine predictor for mortality risk.

18.4.4 Eating Disorders and Confounding Factors

Two factors that may complicate the identification of the relationship between AN and changes in HRV are the presence of other psychological factors such as depression and stress, and the use of medication and biological factors related to altered endocrine function. Depression is a common comorbidity in ED patients (Hudson et al. 1987). In patients with a recent myocardial infarction, HRV has been shown to be significantly lower in patients who were depressed as compared to a similar group of patients without

TABLE 18.1

HRV Parameters in Eating Disorders

Study	SDNN	RMSSD	pNN50	LF	HF	LF/HF	TP	α	ApEn	Number of Subjects (Controls)/Comments
Short term										
Bär et al. (2006)		↑				↓				$N = 15$ (C = 15)
Billeci et al. (2015)		↑		↓	↑	↓				$N = 27$ (C = 15)
Bomba et al. (2014)	↑	↑	—	—	↑	↓				$N = 21$ (C = 21)
Casu et al. (2002)				—	↓	—				$N = 13$ (C = 16)
Het et al. (2015)				—	↑	↓				$N = 28$, AN and bulimic not distinguished (C = 26)
Jacoangeli et al. (2013)	↓									$N = 20$ (C = 15)
Kollai et al. (1994)	↓	↓			↓					$N = 11$ (C = 11)
Kreipe et al. (1994)				↓	↓					$N = 8$ (C = 8)
Lachish et al. (2009)				↓	↓	↓				$N = 24$ (C = 19), reductions in LF and HF reversed with refeeding
Melanson et al. (2004)	↓	—	—	—	—	—				$N = 6$ (C = 10)
Murialdo et al. (2007)				↓	—	—	—			$N = 34$ (C = 30), LF also reduced in 16 bulimic patients
Nakai et al. (2015)				—	—	—				$N = 14$ (C = 22)
Palova et al. (2012)				—	↑	↓				$N = 30$ (C = 30)
Rechlin et al. (1998)				↓	—	↓				Only data from acutely anorexic group; $N = 18$ (C = 18)
Vigo et al. (2008)	—	—	—	↓	—	—	—	↓	—	$N = 17$ (C = 19), also examined bulimic patient group ($N = 19$) who showed reduced ApEn
Wu et al. (2004)				↓	↓	↓				$N = 14$ (C = 12)
Ishizawa et al. (2008)					↑	↓	↑	↓		$N = 32$ (C = 37)
24 hour										
Cong et al. (2004)				—	↑	↓				$N = 6$ (C = 11), similar effects on HF and HF/LF ratio in 8 bulimic patients
Dippacher et al. (2014)	↑									$N = 17$ (C = 52)
Galetta et al. (2003)	↑	↑	↑	—	↑	↓				$N = 25$ (C = 25)
Melanson et al. (2004)	↓	↓	↓	↓	↓	—				$N = 6$ (C = 10)
Mont et al. (2003)	↑	↑								$N = 31$, patients served as own controls before and after refeeding
Petretta et al. (1997)	↑	↑	↑	↓	—	↓				$N = 13$ (C = 10)
Platisa et al. (2006)				↓			↓			$N = 17$ (C = 8)
Roche et al. (2004)	↑	↑		↓	↑	↑				$N = 14$ (C = 10)
Yoshida et al. (2006)				↓	↑					$N = 9$, patients served as own controls before and after refeeding

(Continued)

TABLE 18.1 *(Continued)* HRV Parameters in Eating Disorders

Key		Definitions	
↓	Statistically significant reduction relative to controls	SDNN	Standard deviation of all normal to normal (NN) intervals
↑	Statistically significant increase relative to controls	RMSSD	The square root of the mean squared differences of successive NN intervals
–	No difference from controls	pNN50	The proportion derived by dividing NN50 (the number of interval differences of successive NN intervals greater than 50 ms) by the total number of NN intervals
	Blank cell—not examined or not reported	LF	Spectral power in the low-frequency range (0.04–0.15 Hz)
		HF	Spectral power in the high-frequency range (0.15–0.4 Hz)
		LF/HF	Ratio LF/HF
		TP	Total power—variance of all NN intervals in frequency range ≤0.4 Hz
		α	Scaling exponent based on detrended fluctuation analysis. Quantifies short-term fractal correlation properties of NN intervals
		ApEn	Approximate entropy estimates regularity/complexity of NN interval time series

depression (Carney et al. 2000). Stress has been linked to reduced HRV (Chandola et al. 2009) and levels are often high in patients with eating disorders for a variety of reasons. Disturbances of endocrine function in eating disorders are well documented (Warren 2011) and may contribute to alterations of HRV. These include "functional" hypothyroidism and sympathetic downregulation as mechanisms for energy conservation in AN, and the autonomic instability associated with bingeing and purging behaviors in bulimia nervosa (BN) and eating disorder not otherwise specified (EDNOS, now termed otherwise specified eating disorder [OSFED] in DSM-5; see APA [2013]) where body weight is in the normal range or not so far from this. This is in contrast to AN where body weight is such that body mass index (BMI) is less than 18.5, usually with endocrine consequences, and BN where body weight is normal and the patient engages in binge eating behavior at a specified frequency associated with weight-losing behaviors, most commonly purging, although there is a non-purging subtype where exercise is usually the preferred weight-losing behavior. In OSFED, weight is not as low as in AN and the frequency of bingeing and purging behaviors is less than that specified for BN.

18.5 Studies of HRV in Eating-Disorder Patients

Our group has examined HRV in three different cohorts of patients diagnosed with eating disorders, ranging in number from 17 to 35 patients, and compared them to equivalent numbers of age- and gender-matched healthy controls. The majority of patients were female and suffering from AN although in our first study, we looked at the differences in HRV between AN patients and those with other eating disorder diagnoses at normal or relatively normal body weight/BMI (Russell et al. 2010). Later studies have explored the effects of treatment, orthostatic changes, and depression on HRV parameters in AN, the aim being to explore the practical application of this technique to predict medical risk in this patient population.

18.5.1 AN Compared to Normal-Weight Eating-Disorder Patients

The initial study found reduced linear and nonlinear HRV parameters indicating reduced complexity in patients with AN ($N = 17$) and patients of normal body weight ($N = 12$) diagnosed with BN and OSFED. The combined group differed significantly from controls on almost all HRV parameters at the time of admission to a specialized treatment program but not after completion of 6 weeks of treatment. However, there were differences ($p < 0.05$) between the AN group and the normal-weight eating-disorder group at first assessment. Undoubtedly, treatment resulted in weight gain in AN patients and cessation of weight-losing behaviors, primarily restricting, exercising, and purging, in the patient group as a whole and return of HRV to control values.

18.5.2 Nonlinear Parameters and Treatment Effects

One other study examined linear and nonlinear parameters, respectively, in 18 patients with AN compared to 31 controls in the first study and 35 patients and 35 controls before and after treatment (Jelinek et al. 2011). Again differences were no longer significant after treatment but heterogeneity of the patient group attributed to illness duration was seen as a problem and nonlinear measures posited to be more helpful in assessing HRV.

18.5.3 Depression and HRV

Depression comorbidity was the focus of another study involving 30 patients with a mean BMI of 17.9 (AN as defined by DSM-5) and 44 healthy age-matched controls (Jelinek et al. in press). Thirteen patients were clinically diagnosed with depression and 11 of these met diagnostic criteria on the Beck Depression Inventory (BDI) for moderate-to-severe depressive disorder. HRV changes were accentuated in the depressed group particularly using nonlinear parameters and the possibility of increased cardiac risk was inferred. Medication, mainly antidepressant medication of the selective serotonin reuptake inhibitor (SSRI) type, was found to exert no significant effect on HRV.

18.5.4 Orthostatic Change and HRV

Whether cardiac risk can be quantified is explored in another study (Jelinek et al. 2017). Here, it was shown that the differences in HRV between newly admitted AN patients ($N = 35$) and controls ($N = 43$) were enhanced by orthostatic challenge. Vagal predominance and significant sympathovagal changes were identified in the AN group especially with nonlinear measures and with patients moving only from sitting to standing (instead of the more usual lying to standing to obviate patient discomfort and more importantly, major heart rate changes due to cardiac dysregulation).

18.5.5 Summary of Our Findings

The question remains as to whether measurement of HRV is of practical utility in the management of eating disorders and then which parameters, what diagnostic groups, and under what conditions is this of value. AN is the diagnostic group with the highest mortality rate and where clinical decisions concerning restrictive treatment often need to be made. There is more data from our studies and those of other researchers concerning this patient group and demonstrating reduced HRV suggestive of autonomic imbalance in cardiac regulation. Nonlinear parameters in our experience may offer a more integrated measure of the necessary unpredictability or lack thereof in the system conferred by the interplay of parasympathetic and sympathetic influences. Significant depression seems to accentuate the reduction in HRV independent of the effect of medication. Effective treatment in a specialized program returns HRV to control values.

18.5.6 Eating Disorders, HRV, and Medical Risk

Eating-disorder patients in general tend to be quite secretive if not dishonest about their food- and exercise-related behaviors and the extent of these. AN patients, in particular, often have impaired decision making and lack insight into their need for treatment; they frequently falsify their weights so an objective measure of medical risk would be invaluable.

Some physicians insist that eating-disorder patients, no matter how emaciated, are medically stable in 24–48 hours even when the patient is in ED and may have received some intravenous fluids, investigations, little or nothing to eat, and no medical interventions apart from having to desist from exercise and some of their more overt eating-disordered, weight-losing behaviors. The patients' electrolytes and blood count may look normal, particularly in the presence of mild dehydration. Body temperature might not have been measured and orthostatic effects on blood pressure and heart rate are likely not to have been assessed. The patient may have been weighed in street clothes, wearing shoes, and height is frequently not measured at all and "guestimated" by the patient. Blood pressure might be somewhat low and a single ECG may only show bradycardia. Tachycardia in this situation is very worrying as it can indicate covert infection (emaciated patients do not have a pyrexial response), impending heart failure, or refeeding syndrome (particularly where the patient has eaten an excess of high-carbohydrate food in an effort to avoid hospitalization). HRV in the ED situation might be useful in indicating the need for more restrictive treatment or at least a need to keep the patient under closer observation—if only the normal range had been established, which thus far it has not (Mazurak et al. 2011).

18.5.7 Future Directions

A 24-hour Holter monitor reading, even in an asymptomatic anorexic patient, can be particularly alarming and shows runs of sinus tachycardia, periods of bradycardia, and even asystole, nodal, and junctional rhythms, ectopic beats, and runs of supraventricular tachycardias (SVT), which are fortunately mostly benign and self-limited, but cardiac death can occur and may do so in the presence of normal-looking blood tests. The relationship of these transient arrhythmic events to HRV needs to be explored either with a short recording (as described in our studies) immediately before and after or better still at periods throughout the 24-hour Holter monitoring (as has already been examined in some of the studies considered by Mazurak and by those listed in our table). This would not be difficult technically and would permit ascertainment of a more exact relationship of HRV to arrhythmic events to determine whether reduced HRV parameters and which, in particular, are in proximity to arrhythmic and dysrhythmic events. These could result in death under certain circumstances such as hypothermia, sleep, hypoglycemia, "functional" hypothyroidism, depression, anxiety, and eating-disordered behaviors, alone or in combination with each other and emaciation. Improvement and reduction of dysrhythmic events with treatment could also be determined. HRV would thus offer an integrated and objective measure of cardiac risk and benefits of treatment but there still remains much to be done before HRV can become a routine part of clinical practice.

18.6 Conclusion

Eating disorders are serious mental and physical disorders and they are becoming alarmingly prevalent in the Western (and Westernizing) world and a major public health problem. Effective, intensive treatment is becoming increasingly rationed and provision of this to those who most need it is of high priority and often vigorously disputed by various parties. Determination rests in the first instance on medical risk and HRV is a promising technique in this regard, even if more work to determine normal ranges, risk profiles, and the most useful parameters is necessary.

References

American Psychiatric Association. 2000. Practice guidelines for the treatment of patients with eating disorders. *Am J Psych* 157 (suppl):1–39.
APA. 2013. *American Psychiatric Association DSM-5 Diagnostic and Statistical Manual of Mental Disorders*. 5th ed. Washington, DC: American Psychiatric Association.
Bär, K. J., S. Boettger, G. Wagner, C. Wilsdorf, U. J. Gerhard, M. K. Boettger, et al. 2006. Changes of pain perception, autonomic function, and endocrine parameters during treatment of anorectic adolescents. *J Am Acad Child Adolesc Psychiatry* 45:1068–1076.
Billeci, L., G. Tartarisco, E. Brunori, G. Crifaci, S. Scardigli, R. Balocchi, et al. 2015. The role of wearable sensors and wireless technologies for the assessment of heart rate variability in anorexia nervosa. *Eat Weight Disord* 20:23–31. doi: 10.1007/s40519-014-0135-2.
Bomba, M. F. Corbetta, A. Gambera, F. Nicosia, L. Bonini, F. Neri, L. Tremolizzo and R. Nacinovich. 2014. Heart rate variability in adolescents with functional hypothalamic amenorrhea and anorexia nervosa. *Psychiat Res* 215:406–409.
Carney, R.M, K.E Freeland, P.K Stein, J.A Skala, P Hoffman, and A.S Jaffe. 2000. Change in heart rate and heart rate variability during treatment for depression in patients with coronary heart disease. *Psychosomatic Med* 62:639–647.
Casiero, D. and W.H. Frishman. 2006. Cardiovascular complications of eating disorders. *Cardiol Rev* 14 (5):227–231. doi: 10.1097/01.crd.0000216745.96062.7c.
Casper, R.C. 1986. The pathophysiology of anorexia nervosa and bulimia nervosa. *Ann Rev Nutr* 6:299–316.
Casu, M., V. Patrone, M. V. Gianelli, A. Marchegiani, G. Ragni, Murialdo, et al. 2002. Spectral analysis of R-R interval variability by short-term recording in anorexia nervosa. *Eat Weight Disord* 7, 239–243.
Chandola, T., H.A. Alexandros, and M. Kumari. 2009. Psychophysiological biomarkers of workplace stressors. *Neurosci Biobehav Rev* 35 (1):51–57. doi: 10.1016/j.neubiorev.2009.11.005.
Cong, N. D., T.Saikawa, R. Ogawa, M. Hara, N. Takahashi, and T. Sakata, 2004. Reduced 24 hour ambulatory blood pressure and abnormal heart rate variability in patients with dysorexia nervosa. *Heart* 90, 563–564.

Cooke, R.A. and J.B Chambers. 1995. Anorexia nervosa and the heart. *Br J Hosp Med* 54 (7):313–317.

Dippacher S., C. Willaschek and R. Buchhorn 2014, Different nutritional states and autonomic imbalance in childhood. Eur *J Clin Nut* 68:1271–1273. doi:10.1038/ejcn.2014.198.

Galetta, F., F. Franzoni, F. Prattichizzo, M. Rolla, G.Santoro and F.Pentimone. 2003. Heart rate variability and left ventricular diastolic function in anorexia nervosa. *J Adolesc Health* 32: 416–421.

Het, S., S, Vocks, J.M. Wolf, P. Hammelstein, S. Herpertz and O.T. Wolf . 2015. Blunted neuroendocrine stress reactivity in young women with eating disorders. *J Psychosom Res* 78:260–7. doi: 10.1016/j.jpsychores.2014.11.001. Epub 2014 Nov 8.

Hudson, J.I., H.G. Pope, O.G. Cameron, and G. Oliver. 1987. Presentations of depression. In *Depressive Symptoms and other Psychiatric Disorders. Wiley Series in General and Clinical Psychiatry*, pp. 33–66. Oxford, UK: John Wiley and Sons.

Ishizawa, T., K. Yoshiuchi, Y. Takimoto, Y. Yamamoto and A. Akabayashi. 2008. Heart rate and blood pressure variability and baroreflex sensitivity in patients with anorexia nervosa. Psychosom Med 70(6): 695–700.

Jackman, W.M., K.J. Friday, J.L. Anderson, E.M. Aliot, M. Clark, and R. Lazzara. 1988. The long QT syndromes: A critical review, new clinical observations and a unifying hypothesis. *Prog Cardiovasc Dis* 31 (2):115–172.

Jacoangeli F., F.S. Mezzasalma, G. Canto, F. Jacoangeli, C. Colica, A, de Lorenzo et al. 2013. Baroreflex sensitivity and heart rate variability are enhanced in patients with anorexia nervosa. *Int J Cardiol* 162:263–264.

Jauregui-Garrido, B. and I. Jauregui-Lobera. 2012. Sudden death in eating disorders. *Vasc Health Risk Manag* 8:91–98. doi: 10.2147/vhrm.s28652.

Jelinek, H.F., A. Khandoker, D. Quintana, H.M. Issam, and A.H. Kemp. 2011. Complex correlation measure as a sensitive indicator of risk for sudden cardiac death in patients with depression. *Computing in Cardiology*, Hangzhou, China. pp. 809–812.

Jelinek, H.F., D.J. Cornforth, M.P. Tarvainen, I. Spence and J. Russell. Decreased sample entropy to orthostatic challenge in anorexia nervosa. *J Metabolic Syndrome* (in press)

Jelinek, H.F., I. Spence D.J. Cornforth, M.P. Tarvainen, and J. Russell. 2017. Depression and cardiac dysautonomia in eating disorders. *Eat Weight Disord*. doi: 10.1007/s40519-017-0363-3.

Kalager, T., O. Brubakk, and H.H. Bassoe. 1978. Cardiac performance in patients with anorexia nervosa. *Cardiology* 63:1–4.

Kleiger, R.E., J.P. Miller, J.T. Bigger, Jr., and A.J. Moss. 1987. Decreased heart rate variability and its association with increased mortality after acute myocardial infarction. *Am J Cardiol* 59 (4):256–262.

Kollai, M., I. Bonyhay, G. Jokkel and L. Szony. 1994. Cardiac vagal hyperactivity in adolescent anorexia nervosa. *Eur. Heart J* 15: 1113–1118.

Kreipe, R.E., B.Goldstein, D.E. Deking, R.Tipton and M. H. Kempski. 1994. Heart rate power spectrum analysis of autonomic dysfunction in adolescents with anorexia nervosa lnt *J Eat Disord* 16(2): 159–165.

Lachish, M., D. Stein, Z. Kaplan, M. Matar, M. Faigin, I. Korsunski, et al. 2009. Irreversibility of cardiac autonomic dysfunction in female adolescents diagnosed with anorexia nervosa after short- and longterm weight gain. *World J Biol Psychiatry* 10:503–511.

Lesinskiene, S., A. Barkus, N. Ranceva, and A. Dembinskas. 2008. A meta-analysis of heart rate and QT interval alteration in anorexia nervosa. *World J Biol Psychiatry* 9 (2):86–91. doi: 10.1080/15622970701230963.

Mazurak, N., P. Enck, E. Muth, M. Teufel, and S. Zipfel. 2011. Heart rate variability as a measure of cardiac autonomic function in anorexia nervosa: A review of the literature. *Eur Eat Disord Rev* 19:87–99.

Melanson, E.L., W.T. Donahoo, M.J. Krantz, P. Poirier, and P.S. Mehler. 2004. Resting and ambulatory heart rate variability in chronic anorexia nervosa. *Am J Cardiol* 94 (9):1217–1220. doi: 10.1016/j.amjcard.2004.07.103.

Mont L., J. Castro, B. Herreros, C. Paré, M.Azqueta, J.Magrinã, et al. 2003. Reversibility of cardiac abnormalities in adolescents with anorexia nervosa after weight recovery. *J Am Acad Child Adolesc Psychiatry* 42, 808–813.

Murialdo, G., M. Casu, M. Falchero, A. Brugnolo, V. Patrone, P.F. Cerro, P. Ameri, G. L. Andraghetti, F. Briatore, R. Copello, G. Cordera, Rodriguez and A.M. Ferro 2007. Alterations in the autonomic control of heart rate variability in patients with anorexia or bulimia nervosa: Correlations between sympathovagal activity, clinical features, and leptin levels. *J Endocrinol Invest* 30: 356–362.

Nakai, Y,. M. Fujita, K., Nin, S. Noma and S.Teramukai 2015. Relationship between duration of illness and cardiac autonomic nervous activity in anorexia nervosa. *BioPsychoSocial Med* 9:12–16. doi: 10.1186/s13030-015-0032-6.

Palova S.1., J. Havlin and J. Charvat 2012. The association of heart rate variability examined in supine and standing position with ambulatory blood pressure monitoring in anorexia nervosa. *Neuro Endocrinol Lett* 33(2):196–200.

Petretta, M., D. Bonaduce, L. Scalfi, E. de Filippo, F. Marciano, M. L. Migaux, et al. 1997. Heart rate variability as a measure of autonomic nervous system function in anorexia nervosa. *Clin Cardiol* 20: 219–224.

Platisa, M., Z. Nestorovic, S. Damjanovic and V. Gal, 2006. Linear and non-linear heart rate variability measures in chronic and acute phase of anorexia nervosa. *Clin Physiol* 26, 54–60.

Rechlin T., M. Weis, C. Ott, F. Bleichner and P. Joraschky 1998. Alterations of autonomic cardiac control in anorexia nervosa. *Biol Psychiatry* 43:358–363.

Roche, F., M. Kadem, J-C. Barthélémy, M. Garet, F. Costes, V. Pichot, D. Duverney, L. Millot, and B. Estour. 2004. Chronotropic incompetence to exercise separates low body weight from established anorexia nervosa. *Clin Physiol* 24, 270–275.

Russell, J., S. Hijazi, L. Edington, I. Spence, and H.F. Jelinek. 2010. Cardiovascular complications and sudden death associated with eating disorders. *IJCVR* 7 (1). http://www.ispub.com/journal/the_internet_journal_of_cardiovascular_research/current.html. doi: 10.5580/248.

Sagie, A., M.G. Larson, R.J. Goldberg, J.R. Bengtson, and D. Levy. 1993. An improved method for adjusting the QT interval for heart rate (the Framingham Heart Study). *Am J Cardiol* 71:504.

Task Force. 1996. Heart rate variability: Standards of measurement, physiological interpretation and clinical use. Task Force of the European Society of Cardiology and the North American Society of Pacing and Electrophysiology. *Circulation* 93 (5):1043–1065.

Vigo, D.E., Castro, A. Dorpinghaus, H. Weidema, D.P. Cardinali, L.N. Siri, B. Rovira, R.D. Fahrer, M. Nogues, R.C. Leiguarda and S.M. Guinjoan 2008, Nonlinear analysis of heart rate variability in patients with eating disorders. *World J Biol Psychiatry* 9(3): 183–189.

Warren, M.P. 2011. Endocrine manifestations of eating disorders. *J Clin Endocrinol Metab* 96 (2):333–343. doi: 10.1210/jc.2009-2304.

Wolf, M.M., G.A. Varigos, D. Hunt, and J.G. Sloman. 1978. Sinus arrhythmia in acute myocardial infarction. *Med J Aust* 2 (2):52–53.

Wu Y., T. Nozaki, T. Inamitsu, and C. Kubo 2004. Physical and psychological factors influencing heart rate variability in anorexia nervosa. *Eat Weight Disord* 9: 296–299.

Yoshida, N. M., K. Yoshiuchi, H. Kumano, T. Sasaki, and T. Kuboki. 2006. Changes in heart rate with refeeding in anorexia nervosa: A pilot study. *J Psychosom Res*, 61, 571–575.

19

Applying Heart Rate Variability in Clinical Practice Following Acute Myocardial Infarction

Juha S. Perkiömäki and Heikki V. Huikuri

CONTENTS

19.1 Introduction

Among clinical conditions, heart rate (HR) variability, a measure of cardiac autonomic regulation, has been most widely studied in patients who have experienced acute myocardial infarction (AMI). The prognostic significance of several HR variability variables, including classic time- and frequency-domain parameters as well as some nonlinear and newer parameters, has been assessed in post-AMI patients. A selection of the studies is briefly introduced in the present chapter. In these studies, the HR variability parameters have been measured from 24-hour ambulatory Holter recordings or sometimes from shorter term recordings. The shorter term recordings have usually been carried out under controlled conditions in terms of breathing, position, or activity. In some studies, the recordings have been obtained during the hospital stay after AMI, or weeks to months after AMI. The HR variability analyses have almost invariably been done after editing premature depolarizations from the beat-to-beat (RR interval) time series. The values of HR variability parameters are dependent on HR, with values of conventional HR variability variables being more sensitive to HR than the values of newer nonlinear variables. Selection criteria and characteristics of AMI patients, which have been reported in the literature, have varied dramatically. In many studies, HR-uncorrected and in some studies, HR-corrected HR variability values were used. Further the prognostic value of HR variability measurements has been evaluated in post-AMI patients who have had well-preserved left ventricular function, moderately decreased left ventricular function or severely depressed left ventricular function.

In terms of functional class, the post-AMI populations in HR variability studies have varied from asymptomatic/mildly symptomatic to symptomatic. There have also been differences in the use of medications, such as beta-blockers, among the post-AMI populations in HR variability studies. Different studies have also used different endpoints, such as total mortality, cardiac mortality, noncardiac mortality, sudden death, sudden cardiac death, sudden arrhythmic death, resuscitated death, heart failure death, life-threatening ventricular tachyarrhythmias, various nonfatal events, or combinations of different endpoints. Age, gender distribution, and the involvement of other diseases have also varied between different post-AMI populations in HR variability studies. These differences in study populations have led to study results that are not directly comparable, especially with respect to the contribution of the autonomic nervous system.

A vast majority of studies in post-AMI populations have shown that HR variability yields prognostic information indicating that reduced HR variability is associated with increased risk of mortality and adverse events. However, all the abovementioned factors modify the prognostic significance of HR variability variables. Therefore, it is very difficult to exactly generalize the findings to all real-world post-AMI populations. It is even more difficult to extrapolate the findings to an individual post-AMI patient. For these reasons, HR variability is not yet widely applied in practice as a guide for clinical decision making after AMI. The larger the studied post-AMI population, the greater the chance of finding a HR variability parameter as a statistically significant predictor of adverse events. This does not necessarily translate into clinical usefulness for individual post-AMI patients. It is further noteworthy that if a risk indicator is used in an individual patient's risk stratification, there should be a treatment option available that is beneficial particularly to the patient group, which was identified to be at risk. Many beneficial therapies, such as medications, are applied in the treatment of virtually all patients with AMI, if there are no contraindications and there is no need for finding subgroups that are at the greatest risk to start the treatments. The post-AMI patients who have experienced a life-threatening ventricular tachyarrhythmia after an acute phase without a transient cause need an implantable cardioverter-defibrillator (ICD) for secondary prophylactic reasons. The post-AMI patients with severely depressed left ventricular function but without any history of life-threatening ventricular tachyarrhythmias should receive a primary prophylactic ICD (Moss et al. 2002; Bardy et al. 2005). However, the majority of sudden arrhythmic deaths occur in the post-AMI patients with moderately decreased or well-preserved left ventricular function (Huikuri et al. 2001). It would therefore be beneficial to find risk indicators that could predict the risk for sudden arrhythmic death as accurately as possible, especially in patients with preserved left ventricular function, as most of these deaths could be prevented by implanting an ICD for primary prophylactic reasons. There are data to support the concept that HR variability predicts the risk for life-threatening arrhythmic events in post-AMI patients. An example of such data is the results of the Cardiac Arrhythmias and Risk Stratification after Acute Myocardial Infarction (CARISMA) study. In this study, the primary endpoint of ventricular fibrillation or symptomatic sustained ventricular tachycardia was detected using implantable loop recorders in post-AMI patients with left ventricular ejection fraction (LVEF) $\leq 40\%$ measured from 3 to 21 days after AMI with follow-up for 2 years. Several HR variability parameters measured 6 weeks after AMI predicted the primary endpoint (Huikuri et al. 2009, Figure 19.1). After further research and developments, HR variability, particularly when combined with other risk indicators, has the potential to become a useful indicator of the risk for sudden arrhythmic death in post-AMI patients.

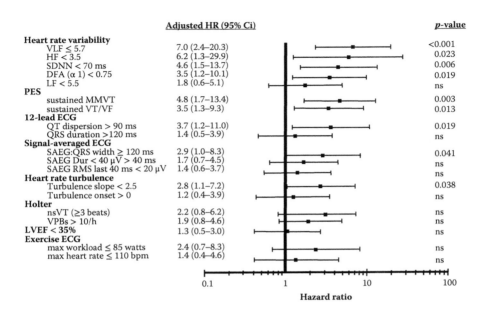

Heart rate variability	Adjusted HR (95% Ci)		*p*-value
VLF ≤ 5.7	7.0 (2.4–20.3)		<0.001
HF < 3.5	6.2 (1.3–29.9)		0.023
SDNN < 70 ms	4.6 (1.5–13.7)		0.006
DFA (α 1) < 0.75	3.5 (1.2–10.1)		0.019
LF < 5.5	1.8 (0.6–5.1)		ns
PES			
sustained MMVT	4.8 (1.7–13.4)		0.003
sustained VT/VF	3.5 (1.3–9.3)		0.013
12-lead ECG			
QT dispersion > 90 ms	3.7 (1.2–11.0)		0.019
QRS duration >120 ms	1.4 (0.5–3.9)		ns
Signal-averaged ECG			
SAEG:QRS width ≥ 120 ms	2.9 (1.0–8.3)		0.041
SAEG Dur < 40 µV > 40 ms	1.7 (0.7–4.5)		ns
SAEG RMS last 40 ms < 20 µV	1.4 (0.6–3.7)		ns
Heart rate turbulence			
Turbulence slope < 2.5	2.8 (1.1–7.2)		0.038
Turbulence onset > 0	1.2 (0.4–3.9)		ns
Holter			
nsVT (≥3 beats)	2.2 (0.8–6.2)		ns
VPBs > 10/h	1.9 (0.8–4.6)		ns
LVEF < 35%	1.3 (0.5–3.0)		ns
Exercise ECG			
max workload ≤ 85 watts	2.4 (0.7–8.3)		ns
max heart rate ≤ 110 bpm	1.4 (0.4–4.6)		ns

Hazard ratio

FIGURE 19.1

Adjusted hazard ratios with 95% confidence intervals (CI) of the variables as predictors of primary endpoint in the CARISMA study (see text). Hazard ratios are calculated from predefined threshold values of continuous variables. Hazard ratios are adjusted for age, prior myocardial infarction, history of congestive heart failure, and diabetes. The variables are listed in descending order starting with the highest hazard ratio for each risk stratification method. DFA (α1), the short-term scaling exponent obtained by the detrended fluctuation analysis technique; HF, high-frequency component of power spectrum; LF, low-frequency component of power spectrum; LVEF, left ventricular ejection fraction; MMVT, monomorphic ventricular tachycardia; nsVT, nonsustained ventricular tachycardia; SDNN, standard deviation of all normal-to-normal intervals; VLF, very-low-frequency component of power spectrum; VPBs, ventricular premature beats; VT/VF, ventricular tachycardia/ventricular fibrillation. (Reproduced from Huikuri HV et al., Eur Heart J., 30, 689–98, 2009. With permission.)

19.2 HR Variability and the Risk for Adverse Events in Post-AMI Patients

19.2.1 Studies Applying Conventional Methods of HR Variability Analysis

There are a huge number of studies that have shown that decreased HR variability is associated with increased risk for mortality and adverse events in post-AMI patients. Some of the studies are introduced here.

Schneider and Costiloe (1965) studied the prognostic significance of HR variability in ischemic heart disease and proposed that decreased HR variability in patients with AMI is associated with a worse prognosis. Wolf et al. (1978) assessed prospectively HR variability from electrocardiographic rhythm strips for 176 patients with AMI. They found that more pronounced sinus arrhythmia was associated with lower in-hospital mortality. The study by Kleiger et al. (1987) can be considered as a cornerstone study in assessing the prognostic significance of HR variability in post-AMI patients. Their study was the first large multicenter trial that showed that reduced HR variability is associated with worse long-term prognosis in post-AMI patients based on HR variability results in 808 post-AMI patients from 24-hour electrocardiographic recordings obtained 11 ± 3 days after AMI.

Approximately 34% of the patients with the standard deviation of all normal-to-normal intervals (SDNN) < 50 ms died after a mean follow-up time of 31 months, in comparison to approximately 12% of patients who had higher values. The patients with SDNN < 50 ms had a 5.3 times higher relative risk of death compared with the patients with SDNN > 100 ms. Reduced HR variability retained its significant prognostic power after adjustments with other risk indicators.

The triangular index of HR variability was analyzed by Cripps et al. (1991) in 177 patients with AMI from 24-hour electrocardiographic recordings, which were obtained a median of 7 days after AMI. The relative risk of sudden death or symptomatic sustained ventricular tachycardia during a median follow-up of 16 months was observed to be seven times greater in patients with an index of < 25 compared with those with an index of ≥ 25. Odemuyiwa et al. (1991) compared HR variability index and LVEF for the prediction of all-cause mortality, arrhythmic events, and sudden death in 385 post-AMI patients. They found that HR variability index worked better than LVEF in predicting postinfarction arrhythmic complications. However, both indexes were equally good predictors of all-cause mortality. In another study, 24-hour ambulatory electrocardiographic recording was obtained between 5 and 11 days after AMI in 477 patients. It was observed that the HR variability index, LVEF, and the frequency of ventricular premature depolarizations in various combinations of these risk indicators more reliably predicted sudden death in patients who were aged under 60 years than in older ones (Odemuyiwa et al. 1992). In a study of 433 survivors of first AMI, the HR variability index was analyzed from 24-hour ambulatory electrocardiographic recordings obtained before discharge from the hospital. It was found that HR variability index independently predicted sudden death and total cardiac mortality only during the first 6 months of follow-up (Odemuyiwa et al. 1994). In a prospective study of 303 post-AMI patients, the HR variability index was independently associated with arrhythmic events during 15±7 months of follow-up (Pedretti et al. 1993).

Bigger et al. (1992) analyzed frequency-domain measures of HR variability from 24-hour electrocardiographic recordings obtained 2 weeks after AMI in 715 patients. They observed that after adjustments for known risk indicators, the total, ultra-low-frequency, and very-low-frequency powers of HR variability remained significant and powerful predictors of mortality. However, low-frequency and high-frequency power had only a moderate association with mortality. The very-low-frequency component of the power spectrum was the only variable, which more strongly predicted arrhythmic death than cardiac or all-cause death. In another study, Bigger et al. (1993) assessed the prognostic value of the frequency-domain parameters of HR variability analyzed from 2 to 15-minute segments of 24-hour electrocardiographic recordings made 11 ± 3 days after AMI in 715 patients. They concluded that the frequency-domain values of HR variability analyzed from short recordings are similar compared with the values analyzed from 24-hour recordings and that they predict all-cause mortality and sudden cardiac death. In a study including 700 consecutive post-AMI patients, the time-domain measure, SDNN, analyzed from 5-minute short-term RR interval data, was found to be a less accurate predictor of 1-year mortality than the HR variability index analyzed from 24-hour period. Nevertheless, it could be used in preselection of high-risk patients (Fei et al. 1996).

Consecutive post-AMI patients ($n = 226$) had 24-hour electrocardiographic recordings on average 83 hours after AMI. Both time- and frequency-domain variables were analyzed from the recordings, and patients were followed up for a mean of 8 months. There was significant difference in the low-frequency component of HR variability between those who died and survivors, but the difference in the high-frequency component was less marked.

Time-domain analysis, such as the standard deviation of averaged normal-to-normal intervals (SDANN), showed also that HR variability was reduced in nonsurvivors compared with survivors. However, there was no significant difference in the percentage of absolute differences between successive RR intervals > 50 ms (pNN50) or the root mean square of successive differences (RMSSD) between the groups (Vaishnav et al. 1994). Overall HR variability, measured by time-domain variables, was found to retain its independent predictive significance for total and cardiovascular mortality in 567 patients with AMI treated with fibrinolysis and followed up for 1000 days (Zuanetti et al. 1996).

Of interest is that the results obtained by comparing the mean RR interval and HR variability analyzed from predischarge Holter recordings in 579 post-AMI patients and LVEF during a 2-year follow-up found that the mean RR interval (HR) and HR variability were stronger predictors of mortality than LVEF (Copie et al. 1996). The prognostic significance of HR variability and baroreflex sensitivity were evaluated in 1284 patients with a recent (<28 days) AMI in the Autonomic Tone and Reflexes After Myocardial Infarction (ATRAMI) trial. Low HR variability (SDNN < 70 ms) analyzed from 24-hour electrocardiographic recordings obtained 15 ± 10 days after the AMI or baroreflex sensitivity predicted cardiac death during 21 ± 8 months of follow-up, further confirming the prognostic value of reduced HR variability in post-AMI patients (La Rovere et al. 1998).

Decreased HR variability has been attributed to both arrhythmic and nonarrhythmic death in post-AMI patients (Hartikainen et al. 1996). It has been suggested that the reduced HR variability is more closely related to the vulnerability of ventricular fibrillation than monomorphic ventricular tachycardia in post-AMI patients (Perkiömäki et al. 1997). However, there has been some contradictory data about the prognostic accuracy of HR variability in post-AMI patients with diabetes. Some studies have suggested that the association between reduced HR variability and mortality is at least as strong in patients with diabetes as in nondiabetic patients (Whang and Bigger 2003), but other studies have suggested that diabetes decreases the association (Stein et al. 2004).

19.2.2 Studies Using Nonlinear Methods of HR Variability and HR Turbulence and Newer Studies

Some studies have suggested that some of the nonlinear parameters of HR variability may be slightly better predictors of mortality in post-AMI patients than the conventional measurements (Bigger et al. 1996; Mäkikallio et al. 1999a; Huikuri et al. 2000). Some of the nonlinear HR variability parameters, such as the short-term scaling exponent obtained by the detrended fluctuation analysis (DFA) technique (Peng et al. 1994, 1995), have some advantages over the traditional HR variability variables as risk indicators: less dependency on HR, less interindividual and intraindividual variation (Pikkujämsä et al. 2001; Perkiömäki et al. 2001c; Maestri et al. 2007), smaller relative changes of individual values over time after AMI (Perkiömäki et al. 2001c), and relatively good comparability of individual values between long-term and short-term electrocardiographic recordings (Perkiömäki et al. 2001b). Mäkikallio et al. (1999a) analyzed the short-term scaling exponent, which describes short-term scaling properties of HR variability (Peng et al. 1994, 1995) in 159 post-AMI patients with LVEF < 35%, who were followed up for 4 years. They found that the short-term scaling exponent was a better predictor of mortality than other HR variability measurements including traditional time- and frequency-domain HR variability indexes. Decreased short-term scaling exponent values have also been associated with vulnerability to ventricular tachycardia (Mäkikallio et al. 1997), ventricular fibrillation

(Mäkikallio et al. 1999b), arrhythmic death, and nonarrhythmic cardiac death (Huikuri et al. 2000) in post-AMI patients. The prognostic value of the short-term scaling exponent has also been shown in post-AMI patients of whom a high proportion were taking beta-blockers (Tapanainen et al. 2002; Jokinen et al. 2003). The short-term scaling exponent has also been observed to predict recurrent nonfatal coronary events (Perkiömäki et al. 2008) and long-term risk for heart failure hospitalization after AMI (Perkiömäki et al. 2010). Decreased values of the short-term scaling exponent have also been shown to be associated with the risk for perpetuating ventricular tachyarrhythmias, but not with risk for self-terminating ventricular tachyarrhythmias in post-AMI patients with moderately decreased LVEF. This suggests that there are differences in modifying factors of these arrhythmias (Perkiömäki et al. 2011).

Bigger et al. (1996) also studied long-term fractal-like scaling characteristics of HR variability from 24-hour electrocardiographic recordings in 715 post-AMI patients. They found that the power-law slope was steeper in post-AMI patients than in healthy subjects and that a steeper power-law slope was a better predictor of all-cause mortality or arrhythmic death than the conventional power spectral measurements in post-AMI patients.

As mentioned in the introduction, the CARISMA study included 312 post-AMI patients with LVEF ≤40% measured 3–21 days after AMI. The primary endpoint of the study was ventricular fibrillation or symptomatic sustained ventricular tachycardia, which were detected using implantable loop recorders. During the follow-up of 2 years, among the studied risk indicators, the measures of HR variability were the strongest predictors of the primary endpoint. Many HR variability parameters, when analyzed from 24-hour electro-cardiographic recordings obtained 6 weeks after the AMI, predicted the primary endpoint after adjustments with clinical characteristics (Figure 19.1). The very-low-frequency component of the power spectrum performed best. The area under the curve from the receiver operator characteristics curve for the very-low-frequency component of the power spectrum in predicting the primary endpoint was 0.73 ± 0.07, $p = 0.002$ (Huikuri et al. 2009).

HR turbulence, a measurement describing the changes of the sinus node–originated RR interval after ventricular premature depolarizations, has been shown to be a strong predictor of mortality in post-AMI patients even after adjustments with general known risk indicators (Schmidt et al. 1999; Barthel et al. 2003; Bauer et al. 2008). Blunted HR turbulence slope has also been observed to be an independent predictor of sudden cardiac death in post-AMI patients (Mäkikallio et al. 2005) in a subgroup analysis, particularly in those with LVEF > 35%, but not in those with LVEF ≤35%. The Risk Estimation Following Infarction Noninvasive Evaluation (REFINE) study included 322 post-AMI patients with LVEF < 50%. When assessed at 10–14 weeks after AMI, impaired HR turbulence plus abnormal T-wave alternans predicted independently the primary outcome of cardiac death or resuscitated cardiac arrest after a median 47 months of follow-up. Reduced HR variability (SDNN) only tended to be an independent predictor of the primary endpoint ($p = 0.066$) in this study (Exner et al. 2007).

19.3 Factors Influencing the Values and Prognostic Significance of HR Variability Measurements in Postinfarction Patients

HR variability values are dependent on HR (Sacha et al. 2013a), with values of nonlinear HR variability measurements being somewhat less dependent than those of the conventional measurements (Pikkujämsä et al. 2001; Perkiömäki et al. 2001c; Maestri et al. 2007). The higher the HR, the lower the HR variability. Some authorities recommend using HR-uncorrected HR variability values. However, in some studies HR-corrected HR variability values are also used. HR has been shown to be a strong predictor of mortality in post-AMI patients (Copie et al. 1996). Increasing the dependence of spectral HR variability indices on HR by a mathematical modification increases the prognostic power of HR variability for cardiac death in post-AMI patients (Sacha et al. 2013b). It is also known that beta-blocker therapy increases HR variability in post-AMI patients (Sandrone et al. 1994; Keeley et al. 1996). However, this increase in the values of HR variability has partly been attributed to the decrease in HR following beta-blocker therapy. Lampert et al. (2003) observed that propranolol therapy increased parasympathetic tone measured by HR variability and improved outcome in post-AMI patients.

It is noteworthy that HR variability parameters are better risk indicators in patients with more preserved left ventricular function (Mäkikallio et al. 2005) or less severe heart failure (Mäkikallio et al. 2001) than in those with more severe left ventricular dysfunction or more advanced heart failure. Furthermore, reduced HR variability is more closely linked to cardiac death in general than sudden arrhythmic death in post-AMI patients with severely decreased left ventricular function (Perkiömäki et al. 2001a; Zareba et al. 2003).

An important observation when using HR variability for predicting outcome following AMI is the timing of HR variability measurement after AMI, as this has a significant influence on its prognostic value. In the CARISMA study, HR variability was a much more stronger predictor of life-threatening ventricular tachyarrhythmias when analyzed from 24-hour electrocardiographic recordings obtained at 6 weeks after the AMI than when analyzed from those obtained at 1 week after the AMI in which case only the short-term scaling exponent determined from DFA significantly predicted the arrhythmias (Huikuri et al. 2009). In the REFINE study, HR variability tended to predict cardiac death or resuscitated cardiac arrest when measured at 10–14 weeks after the AMI; however, it was not associated with this endpoint when measured at 2–4 weeks after the AMI (Exner et al. 2007).

In general, HR variability, regardless of the parameters used, can be considered to yield prognostic information. However, in some studies, some nonlinear methods of HR variability have been observed to be slightly better predictors of mortality in post-AMI patients than the conventional methods (Bigger et al. 1996; Mäkikallio et al. 1999a). Furthermore, some conventional beat-to-beat measures of HR variability, such as the high-frequency power of the power spectrum, pNN50, and RMSSD, have not constantly been shown to be associated with outcome in post-AMI patients (Vaishnav et al. 1994). This may due to common erratic fluctuations of HR in these patients (Huikuri and Stein 2012). When these erratic fluctuations are removed from the analysis, respiratory cycle-related HR variability regains its prognostic power (Peltola et al. 2008). HR variability variables have been found to provide similar or in some studies slightly weaker prognostic information when analyzed from short-term electrocardiographic recordings than when analyzed from 24-hour recordings (Bigger et al. 1993; Fei et al. 1996). The type of editing of the RR interval data also has also significantly different influence on various HR variability variables (Salo et al. 2001). However, premature depolarizations increase the randomness in the short-term scaling exponent and should not necessarily be edited from the analysis (Peltola et al. 2004). Therefore, the type of editing of the RR interval data may modify the prognostic information in HR variability indices.

Age and gender influence the HR dynamics (Lipsitz and Goldberger 1992; Iyengar et al. 1996; Pikkujämsä et al. 1999, 2001). Various medical conditions, such as diabetes, may also modify the prognostic significance of HR variability in post-AMI patients (Whang and

Bigger 2003; Stein et al. 2004). Data on the influence of interventions on HR variability and on its prognostic significance are limited. However, it has been observed that more random HR dynamics after a coronary bypass operation is associated with a more complicated clinical course (Laitio et al. 2000). Pharmacologic, behavioral, and exercise strategies have been shown to increase HR variability in patients with coronary artery disease (Nolan et al. 2008). Thus, although HR variability can be considered as a marker of clinical outcome in post-AMI patients, it has not been established whether the prognosis can be improved by increasing HR variability by interventions.

19.4 HR Variability in Clinical Decision Making in Postinfarction Patients

At the moment, HR variability cannot be recommended for routine clinical use in the individual post-AMI patient's risk stratification. For a HR variability parameter to be useful in guiding the post-AMI patient treatment, it should change the patient's management in a manner that improves outcome. In the Defibrillator in Acute Myocardial Infarction Trial (DINAMIT), patients with AMI at 6–40 days previously, LVEF $\leq 35\%$, and SDNN ≤ 70 ms or HR ≥ 80 beats per minute as assessed by 24-hour Holter recording at least 3 days after the infarction were randomized to have ICD therapy or no ICD therapy. There was no difference in the primary endpoint of all-cause mortality between the treatment groups during the 30 ± 13 months of follow-up. Although there was a reduction in the rate of arrhythmic deaths, there was an increase in the rate of nonarrhythmic deaths in those who were treated by ICD therapy (Hohnloser et al. 2004; Dorian et al. 2010). These findings are in alignment with the previous observations, which have shown that reduced HR variability is associated with the risk for cardiac death in general, but not specifically with the risk for arrhythmic death in post-AMI patients with severely decreased left ventricular function (Perkiömäki et al. 2001a; Zareba et al. 2003). Nevertheless, when the information included in HR variability is combined with information in repolarization variability, such as with the QT variability index, the patients who experience ventricular tachycardia or ventricular fibrillation requiring ICD therapy can be relatively well identified among patients with remote AMI and severely depressed left ventricular function (Haigney et al. 2004). In the CARISMA study, which included post-AMI patients with somewhat better preserved left ventricular function, many HR variability parameters analyzed at 6 weeks after AMI were significant independent predictors of ventricular fibrillation or symptomatic sustained ventricular tachycardia (Huikuri et al. 2009, Figure 19.1). Furthermore, in the REFINE study, which included post-AMI patients with even better preserved left ventricular function than the CARISMA study, the combination of abnormal HR turbulence and T-wave alternans, predicted independently cardiac death or resuscitated cardiac arrest (Exner et al. 2007). The Risk Estimation Following Infarction Noninvasive Evaluation— ICD efficacy (REFINE-ICD) study is including post-AMI patients with LVEF from 36% to 49%, abnormal T-wave alternans, and impaired HR turbulence measured from 2 to 14 months after AMI. The study subjects are randomized 1:1 to prophylactic ICD treatment versus control therapy. The primary outcome measure of the study is mortality, and the secondary outcome measures are the quality of life and cost-effectiveness. The ancillary outcome measures include cardiac death, arrhythmic death, arrhythmic syncope, appropriate ICD therapies, inappropriate ICD therapies, system-related complications, and the influence of the type of ICD or AMI (ST-elevation/non-ST elevation) (Clinical Trial Registration Information: http://www.clinicaltrials.gov, NCT00673842). After further developments and standardizations, HR variability/turbulence, particularly when combined with other risk indicators, may become useful risk markers in selecting post-AMI patients for primary prophylactic ICD therapy. Before that ongoing or future large-scale studies, such as the REFINE-ICD study, should show that post-AMI patients who are risk stratified to ICD therapy based on HR variability–derived risk indicators benefit from the ICD therapy.

19.5 Conclusion

The current evidence is strong about the predictive power of many HR variability indexes, when measured either early or late after AMI. Future studies focusing on randomized trials using HR variability or HR turbulence as the basis for inclusion into the trial will reveal the clinical utility of routine measurement of HR variability/turbulence.

19.6 Summary

A large number of studies have shown that various measures of heart rate (HR) variability, measured mainly from 24-hour Holter recordings, can predict the future mortality of postinfarction patients. Both traditional statistical methods, such as time- and frequency-domain measures of HR variability and HR turbulence, as well as measures based on non-linear dynamics, such as fractal correlation indexes, have been used in risk stratification. Despite the predictive power of many HR variability indexes, the measurement of the HR variability after acute myocardial infarction (AMI) has not become a routine clinical tool. The lack of clinical utility is mainly due to the lack of studies showing that any therapeutic intervention could improve the prognosis of patients with impaired HR variability.

References

Bardy GH, Lee KL, Mark DB, Poole JE, Packer DL, Boineau R, Domanski M, Troutman C, Anderson J, Johnson G, McNulty SE, Clapp-Channing N, Davidson-Ray LD, Fraulo ES, Fishbein DP, Luceri RM, Ip JH. Sudden Cardiac Death in Heart Failure Trial (SCD-HeFT) Investigators. Amiodarone or an implantable cardioverter-defibrillator for congestive heart failure. *N Engl J Med* 2005;352:225–37. Erratum in: *N Engl J Med* 2005;352:2146.

Barthel P, Schneider R, Bauer A, Ulm K, Schmitt C, Schömig A, Schmidt G. Risk stratification after acute myocardial infarction by heart rate turbulence. *Circulation* 2003;108:1221–26.

Bauer A, Malik M, Schmidt G, Barthel P, Bonnemeier H, Cygankiewicz I, Guzik P, Lombardi F, Müller A, Oto A, Schneider R, Watanabe M, Wichterle D, Zareba W. Heart rate turbulence: Standards of measurement, physiological interpretation, and clinical use: International Society for Holter and Noninvasive Electrophysiology Consensus. *J Am Coll Cardiol* 2008;52:1353–65.

Bigger JT, Fleiss J, Steinman RC, Rolnitzky LM, Kleiger RE, Rottman JN. Frequency domain measures of heart period variability and mortality after myocardial infarction. *Circulation* 1992;85:164–71.

Bigger JT, Fleiss JL, Rolnitzky LM, Steinman RC. The ability of several short-term measures of RR variability to predict mortality after myocardial infarction. *Circulation* 1993;88:927–34.

Bigger JT Jr, Steinman RC, Rolnitzky LM, Fleiss JL, Albrecht P, Cohen RJ. Power law bahavior of RR-interval variability in healthy middle-aged persons, patients with recent acute myocardial infarction, and patients with heart transplants. *Circulation* 1996;93:2142–51.

Copie X, Hnatkova K, Staunton A, Fei L, Camm AJ, Malik M. Predictive power of increased heart rate versus depressed left ventricular ejection fraction and heart rate variability for risk stratification after myocardial infarction. Results of a two-year follow-up study. *J Am Coll Cardiol* 1996;27: 270–76.

Cripps TR, Malik M, Farrell TG, Camm AJ. Prognostic value of reduced heart rate variability after myocardial infarction: Clinical evaluation of a new analysis method. *Br Heart J* 1991;65: 14–19.

Dorian P, Hohnloser SH, Thorpe KE, Roberts RS, Kuck KH, Gent M, Connolly SJ. Mechanisms underlying the lack of effect of implantable cardioverter-defibrillator therapy on mortality in high-risk patients with recent myocardial infarction: Insights from the Defibrillation in Acute Myocardial Infarction Trial (DINAMIT). *Circulation* 2010;122:2645–52.

Exner DV, Kavanagh KM, Slawnych MP, Mitchell LB, Ramadan D, Aggarwal SG, Noullett C, Van Schaik A, Mitchell RT, Shibata MA, Gulamhussein S, McMeekin J, Tymchak W, Schnell G, Gillis AM, Sheldon RS, Fick GH, Duff HJ. REFINE Investigators. Noninvasive risk assessment early after a myocardial infarction: the REFINE study. *J Am Coll Cardiol* 2007;50:2275–84.

Fei L, Copie X, Malik M, Camm AJ. Short- and long-term assessment of heart rate variability for risk stratification after acute myocardial infarction. *Am J Cardiol* 1996;77:681–84.

Haigney MC, Zareba W, Gentlesk PJ, Goldstein RE, Illovsky M, McNitt S, Andrews ML, Moss AJ. Multicenter Automatic Defibrillator Implantation Trial II Investigators. QT interval variability and spontaneous ventricular tachycardia or fibrillation in the Multicenter Automatic Defibrillator Implantation Trial (MADIT) II patients. *J Am Coll Cardiol* 2004;44:1481–87.

Hartikainen J, Malik M, Staunton A, Poloniecki J, Camm AJ. Distinction between arrhythmic and nonarrhythmic death after acute myocardial infarction based on heart rate variability, signal-averaged electrocardiogram, ventricular arrhythmias and left ventricular ejection fraction. *J Am Coll Cardiol* 1996;28:296–304.

Hohnloser SH, Kuck KH, Dorian P, Roberts RS, Hampton JR, Hatala R, Fain E, Gent M, Connolly SJ. DINAMIT Investigators. Prophylactic use of an implantable cardioverter-defibrillator after acute myocardial infarction. *N Engl J Med* 2004;351:2481–88.

Huikuri HV, Castellanos A, Myerburg RJ. Sudden death due to cardiac arrhythmias. *N Engl J Med* 2001;345:1473–82.

Huikuri HV, Mäkikallio TH, Peng CK, Goldberger AL, Hintze U, Moller M. Fractal correlation properties of R-R interval dynamics and mortality in patients with depressed left ventricular function after an acute myocardial infarction. *Circulation* 2000;101:47–53.

Huikuri HV, Raatikainen MJ, Moerch-Joergensen R, Hartikainen J, Virtanen V, Boland J, Anttonen O, Hoest N, Boersma LV, Platou ES, Messier MD, Bloch-Thomsen PE. Prediction of fatal or near-fatal cardiac arrhythmia events in patients with depressed left ventricular function after an acute myocardial infarction. *Eur Heart J* 2009;30:689–98.

Huikuri HV, Stein PK. Clinical application of heart rate variability after acute myocardial infarction. *Front Physiol* 2012;3:41.

Iyengar N, Peng CK, Morin R, Goldberger AL, Lipsitz LA. Age-related alterations in the fractal scaling of cardiac interbeat interval dynamics. *Am J Physiol* 1996;271:R1078–84.

Jokinen V, Tapanainen JM, Seppänen T, Huikuri HV. Temporal changes and prognostic significance of measures of heart rate dynamics after acute myocardial infarction in the beta-blocking era. *Am J Cardiol* 2003;92:907–12.

Keeley EC, Page RL, Lange RA, Willard JE, Landau C, Hillis LD. Influence of metoprolol on heart rate variability in survivors of remote myocardial infarction. *Am J Cardiol* 1996;77:557–60.

Kleiger RE, Miller JP, Bigger JTJr, Moss AJ. The Multicenter Post-Infarction Research Group. Decreased heart rate variability and its association with increased mortality after acute myocardial infarction. *Am J Cardiol* 1987;59:256–62.

Laitio TT, Huikuri HV, Kentala ES, Mäkikallio TH, Jalonen JR, Helenius H, Sariola-Heinonen K, Yli-Mäyry S, Scheinin H. Correlation properties and complexity of perioperative RR-interval dynamics in coronary artery bypass surgery patients. *Anesthesiology* 2000;93:69–80.

Lampert R, Ickovics JR, Viscoli CJ, Horwitz RI, Lee FA. Effects of propranolol on recovery of heart rate variability following acute myocardial infarction and relation to outcome in the Beta-Blocker Heart Attack Trial. *Am J Cardiol* 2003;91:137–42.

La Rovere MT, Bigger JT Jr, Marcus FI, Mortara A, Schwartz PJ. Baroreflex sensitivity and heart-rate variability in prediction of total cardiac mortality after myocardial infarction. ATRAMI (Autonomic Tone and Reflexes After Myocardial Infarction) Investigators. *Lancet* 1998;351: 478–84.

Lipsitz LA, Goldberger AL. Loss of 'complexity' and aging. Potential applications of fractals and chaos theory to senescence. *JAMA* 1992;267:1806–09.

Maestri R, Pinna GD, Porta A, Balocchi R, Sassi R, Signorini MG, Dudziak M, Raczak G. Assessing nonlinear properties of heart rate variability from short-term recordings: Are these measurements reliable? *Physiol Meas* 2007;28:1067–1077.

Mäkikallio TH, Seppänen T, Airaksinen KE, Koistinen J, Tulppo MP, Peng CK, Goldberger AL, Huikuri HV. Dynamic analysis of heart rate may predict subsequent ventricular tachycardia after myocardial infarction. *Am J Cardiol* 1997;80:779–83.

Mäkikallio TH, Hoiber S, Kober L, Torp-Pedersen C, Peng CK, Goldberger AL, Huikuri HV. Fractal analysis of heart rate dynamics as a predictor of mortality in patients with depressed left ventricular function after acute myocardial infarction. TRACE Investigators. TRAndolapril cardiac evaluation. *Am J Cardiol* 1999a;83:836–39.

Mäkikallio TH, Koistinen J, Jordaens L, Tulppo MP, Wood N, Golosarsky B, Peng CK, Goldberger AL, Huikuri HV. Heart rate dynamics before spontaneous onset of ventricular fibrillation in patients with healed myocardial infarcts. *Am J Cardiol* 1999b;83:880–84.

Mäkikallio TH, Huikuri HV, Hintze U, Videbaek J, Mitrani RD, Castellanos A, Myerburg RJ, Moller M. Fractal analysis and time- and frequency-domain measures of heart rate variability as predictors of mortality in patients with heart failure. *Am J Cardiol* 2001;87:178–82.

Mäkikallio TH, Barthel P, Schneider R, Bauer A, Tapanainen JM, Tulppo MP, Schmidt G, Huikuri HV. Prediction of sudden cardiac death after acute myocardial infarction: Role of Holter monitoring in the modern treatment era. *Eur Heart J* 2005;26:762–69.

Moss AJ, Zareba W, Hall WJ, Klein H, Wilber DJ, Cannom DS, Daubert JP, Higgins SL, Brown MW, Andrews ML. Multicenter Automatic Defibrillator Implantation Trial II Investigators. Prophylactic implantation of a defibrillator in patients with myocardial infarction and reduced ejection fraction. *N Engl J Med* 2002;346:877–83.

Nolan RP, Jong P, Barry-Bianchi SM, Tanaka TH, Floras JS. Effects of drug, biobehavioral and exercise therapies on heart rate variability in coronary artery disease: A systematic review. *Eur J Cardiovasc Prev Rehabil* 2008;15:386–96.

Odemuyiwa O, Farrell TG, Malik M, Bashir Y, Millane T, Cripps T, Poloniecki J, Bennett D, Camm AJ. Influence of age on the relation between heart rate variability, left ventricular ejection fraction, frequency of ventricular extrasystoles, and sudden death after myocardial infarction. *Br Heart J* 1992;67:387–91.

Odemuyiwa O, Malik M, Farrell T, Bashir Y, Poloniecki J, Camm J. Comparison of the predictive characteristics of heart rate variability index and left ventricular ejection fraction for all-cause mortality, arrhythmic events and sudden death after acute myocardial infarction. *Am J Cardiol* 1991;68:434–39.

Odemuyiwa O, Poloniecki J, Malik M, Farrell T, Xia R, Staunton A, Kulakowski P, Ward D, Camm J. Temporal influences on the prediction of postinfarction mortality by heart rate variability: A comparison with the left ventricular ejection fraction. *Br Heart J* 1994;71:521–27.

Pedretti R, Etro MD, Laporta A, Sarzi Braga S, Carù B. Prediction of late arrhythmic events after acute myocardial infarction from combined use of noninvasive prognostic variables and inducibility of sustained monomorphic ventricular tachycardia. *Am J Cardiol* 1993;71:1131–41.

Peltola MA, Seppänen T, Mäkikallio TH, Huikuri HV. Effects and significance of premature beats on fractal correlation properties of R-R interval dynamics. *Ann Noninvasive Electrocardiol* 2004;9:127–35.

Peltola M, Tulppo MP, Kiviniemi A, Hautala AJ, Seppänen T, Barthel P, Bauer A, Schmidt G, Huikuri HV, Mäkikallio TH. Respiratory sinus arrhythmia as a predictor of sudden cardiac death after myocardial infarction. *Ann Med* 2008;40:376–82.

Peng CK, Buldyrev SV, Havlin S, Simons M, Stanley HE, Goldberger AL. Mosaic organization of DNA nucleotides. *Phys Rev* 1994;E49:1685–89.

Peng CK, Havlin S, Stanley HE, Goldberger AL. Quantification of scaling exponents and crossover phenomena in nonstationary heartbeat time series. *Chaos* 1995;5:82–87.

Perkiömäki JS, Bloch Thomsen PE, Kiviniemi AM, Messier MD, HuikuriHV. For the CARISMA study investigators. Risk factors of self-terminating and perpetuating ventricular tachyarrhythmias in post-infarction patients with moderately depressed left ventricular function, a CARISMA subanalysis. *Europace* 2011;13:1604–11.

Perkiömäki JS, Hämekoski S, Junttila MJ, Jokinen V, Tapanainen J, Huikuri HV. Predictors of longterm risk for heart failure hospitalization after acute myocardial infarction. Ann Noninvasive *Electrocardiol* 2010;15:250–58.

Perkiömäki JS, Huikuri HV, Koistinen JM, Mäkikallio T, Castellanos A, Myerburg RJ. Heart rate variability and dispersion of QT interval in patients with vulnerability to ventricular tachycardia and ventricular fibrillation after previous myocardial infarction. *J Am Coll Cardiol* 1997;30:1331–38.

Perkiömäki JS, Jokinen V, Tapanainen J, Airaksinen KE, Huikuri HV. Autonomic markers as predictors of nonfatal acute coronary events after myocardial infarction. *Ann Noninvasive Electrocardiol* 2008;13:120–09.

Perkiömäki JS, Zareba W, Daubert JP, Couderc JP, Corsello A, Kremer K. Fractal correlation properties of heart rate dynamics and adverse events in patients with implantable cardioverter-defibrillators. *Am J Cardiol* 2001a;88:17–22.

Perkiömäki JS, Zareba W, Kalaria VG, Couderc J, Huikuri HV, Moss AJ. Comparability of nonlinear measures of heart rate variability between long- and short-term electrocardiographic recordings. *Am J Cardiol* 2001b;87:905–08.

Perkiömäki JS, Zareba W, Ruta J, Dubner S, Madoery C, Deedwania P, Karcz M, Bayes de Luna A. IDEAL Investigators. Fractal and complexity measures of heart rate dynamics after acute myocardial infarction. *Am J Cardiol* 2001c;88:777–81.

Pikkujämsä SM, Mäkikallio TH, Airaksinen KE, Huikuri HV. Determinants and interindividual variation of R-R interval dynamics in healthy middle-aged subjects. *Am J Physiol Heart Circ Physiol* 2001;280:H1400–06.

Pikkujämsä SM, Mäkikallio TH, Sourander LB, Räiha IJ, Puukka P, Skytta J, Peng CK, Goldberger AL, Huikuri HV. Cardiac interbeat interval dynamics from childhood to senescence: Comparison of conventional and new measures based on fractals and chaos theory. *Circulation* 1999;100:393–99.

Sacha J, Barabach S, Statkiewicz-Barabach G, Sacha K, Müller A, Piskorski J, Barthel P, Schmidt G. How to select patients who will not benefit from ICD therapy by using heart rate and its variability? *Int J Cardiol* 2013b;168:1655–58.

Sacha J, Sobon J, Sacha K, Barabach S. Heart rate impact on the reproducibility of heart rate variability analysis. *Int J Cardiol* 2013a;168:4257–59.

Salo MA, Huikuri HV, Seppänen T. Ectopic beats in heart rate variability analysis: Effects of editing on time and frequency domain measures. *Ann Noninvasive Electrocardiol* 2001;6:5–17.

Sandrone G, Mortara A, Torzillo D, La Rovere MT, Malliani A, Lombardi F. Effects of beta blockers (atenolol or metoprolol) on heart rate variability after acute myocardial infarction. *Am J Cardiol* 1994;74:340–45.

Schmidt G, Malik M, Barthel P, Schneider R, Ulm K, Rolnitzky L, Camm AJ, Bigger JT Jr, Schömig A. Heart-rate turbulence after ventricular premature beats as a predictor of mortality after acute myocardial infarction. *Lancet* 1999;353:1390–96.

Schneider RA, Costiloe JP. Relationship of sinus arrhythmia to age and its prognostic significance in ischemic heart disease. *Clin Res* 1965;13:219.

Stein PK, Domitrovich PP, Kleiger RE. CAST Investigators. Including patients with diabetes mellitus or coronary artery bypass grafting decreases the association between heart rate variability and mortality after myocardial infarction. *Am Heart J* 2004;147:309–16.

Tapanainen JM, Thomsen PE, Kober L, Torp-Pedersen C, Mäkikallio TH, Still AM, Lindgren KS, Huikuri HV. Fractal analysis of heart rate variability and mortality after an acute myocardial infarction. *Am J Cardiol* 2002;90:347–52.

Vaishnav S, Stevenson R, Marchant B, Lagi K, Ranjadayalan K, Timmis AD. Relation between heart rate variability early after acute myocardial infarction and long-term mortality. *Am J Cardiol* 1994;73:653–57.

Whang W, Bigger JT Jr. Comparison of the prognostic value of RR-interval variability after acute myocardial infarction in patients with versus those without diabetes mellitus. *Am J Cardiol* 2003;92:247–51.

Wolf MM, Varigos GA, Hunt D, Sloman JG. Sinus arrhythmia in acute myocardial infarction. *Med J Aust* 1978;2:52–53.

Zareba W, Couderc JP, Perkiömäki JS, Berkowitzch A, Moss AJ. Heart rate variability and outcome in postinfarction patients with severe left ventricular dysfunction. *Circulation* 2003;108(suppl):3209(abstr).

Zuanetti G, Neilson JM, Latini R, Santoro E, Maggioni AP, Ewing DJ. Prognostic significance of heart rate variability in post-myocardial infarction patients in the fibrinolytic era. The GISSI-s results. *Circulation* 1996;94:432–36.

20

Beat-to-Beat QT Interval Variability and Autonomic Activity

Mathias Baumert

CONTENTS

20.1 Introduction

The QT interval of a body surface electrocardiogram (ECG), illustrated in Figure 20.1 [1], reflects the depolarization and repolarization processes across the ventricular myocardium 20.2 [2]. Since the depolarization process reflected by the QRS complex is relatively stable, the QT interval is clinically used to measure prolongation or shortening of the ventricular repolarization process. QT interval prolongation can be either congenital or acquired. The former is caused by a range of potassium or sodium ion channel mutations, while the latter is associated with a reduction in repolarization reserve that can be induced by pharmaceutical agents, hypokalemia, or hypomagnesemia. Both conditions have been associated with increased cardiac mortality [3]. Since the QT interval is dependent on heart rate, it is typically reported after correcting for it (QT_c), by using one of the many available correction formulas. QT_c has gained wide acceptance as a steady-state measure of ventricular repolarization.

Ventricular repolarization and, hence the QT interval duration, fluctuate from one heartbeat to the next, giving rise to so-called QT interval variability (QTV) [4]. During the last two decades, the study of QTV has received increasing clinical interest as elevated

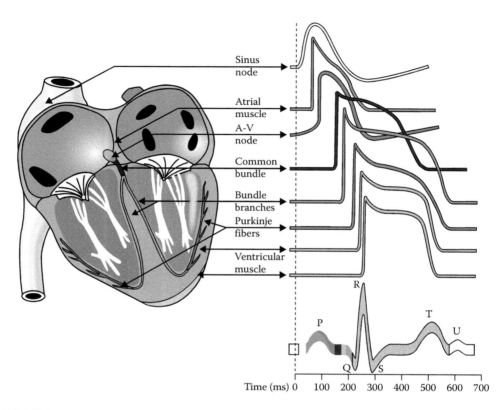

FIGURE 20.1
Electrophysiology of the heart. The different waveforms represent characteristic action potentials for each of the specialized cells found in the heart. The latency shown approximates that normally found in the healthy heart. (Image taken from Jaakko Malmivuo and Robert Plonsey. *Bioelectromagnetism: Principles and Applications of Bioelectric and Biomagnetic Fields*. Oxford University Press, 1995.)

QTV has been demonstrated in patients suffering from various cardiac conditions, including myocardial infarction and dilated cardiomyopathy [5–7]. Importantly, increased QTV was shown to be predictive of adverse cardiac events [8,9]. Significant research efforts have been undertaken to elucidate mechanisms that underlie the beat-to-beat fluctuations in QT interval and evaluate the clinical significance of QTV. One of the physiological variables that has been repeatedly linked to QTV is the activity of the sympathetic nervous system [10] and, therefore, the question has been posed whether QTV can be used as a noninvasive marker of sympathetic outflow directed to the ventricular myocardium. Since chronically increased sympathetic nerve activity is a key factor in the development of hypertension and cardiac disease and acute surges in sympathetic activity can trigger malignant arrhythmias in pathological cardiac substrates, a simple, noninvasive index of ventricular sympathetic outflow would be highly desirable. However, no such technique is currently available. Aside from microneurography, which facilitates the invasive measurement of sympathetic nerve activity in human muscle or skin tissue, noradrenaline spillover [11] and ^{123}I-metaiodobenzylguanidine (^{123}I-MIBG) scintigraphy [12] have been used to measure cardiac sympathetic activity and innervation, respectively, in humans.

In this chapter, I review the evidence for a relationship between QTV and sympathetic nervous system activity as reported in the literature and summarize our results obtained from the direct comparison between measures of sympathetic activity and QTV. First, I will address some of the technical considerations regarding the QT interval measurement from beat to beat.

20.2 Technical Considerations

20.2.1 Beat-to-Beat QT Interval Extraction

Under resting conditions during periods of stable heart rates, the beat-to-beat fluctuations in QT interval are rather small with a standard deviation of less than 5 ms. Consequently, high-resolution ECG sampled at a rate of 500 Hz or higher are recommended, combined with computerized high-precision ECG measurement. While the QRS complex can be automatically detected with relative ease, delineation of the T-end is generally challenging due to its typically slow transient character. Hence, the measurement error that is produced by conventional QT measurement algorithms such as threshold-based methods is in most circumstances too large to yield a reliable assessment of the beat-to-beat changes in QT interval. Consequently, template-based methods have been introduced to increase the accuracy of measurement. Instead of delineating the T-wave terminus based on some criteria for each beat individually, template beats are generated that comprise part of or the whole T-wave, which are subsequently compared and adapted to consecutive heartbeats, where the relative changes in template duration (*time stretching method* [7]) or time shifts in the template (*time shifting method* [13]) are used to measure QTV.

We recently introduced a template method that involves two-dimensional signal warping (2DSW) of ECG waveforms [14,15]. Briefly, a template beat is generated in an automated fashion based on aligning and averaging beats, by using the improved Woody's method [16]. The template is then mapped onto a $N \times M$ grid of *warping points*. Each of these warping points can be shifted in two dimensions, and the areas they encompass— including template waveform segments—are warped accordingly. Minimizing the Euclidean distance, the template waveform is warped such that it resembles the heartbeat under consideration as closely as possible. Fiducial points, including Q-onset and T-end, are marked on the template in a semiautomated way, and relative changes in fiducial points in the template due to warping are tracked to obtain a measure of beat-to-beat QTV. Figure 20.2 illustrates this procedure. The algorithm was proven to be very robust in the presence of noise and common ECG artifacts [15,17].

20.3 Measures of QTV

QTV is typically measured over either 5-minute time intervals or 256 heartbeats under quasi-stationary conditions. Several metrics have been proposed for the quantification of QTV. The most popular time-domain measures, which are also reported in this review, are summarized below:

- meanQT—average QT interval, uncorrected for heart rate
- sdQT—standard deviation of QT intervals

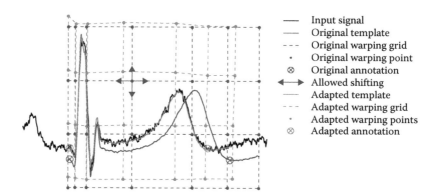

FIGURE 20.2
Illustration of the two-dimensional warping algorithm. The template beat (light gray) is mapped to a warping grid (light gray), which is adapted to the incoming beat (black) by moving the warping points such that the distance between template and incoming beat is minimized. The optimally fitted template and corresponding warping points are shown in dark gray.

- QTVar—variance of QT intervals
- QTVN—normalized QT variance, $\text{QTVN} = \dfrac{\text{QTVar}}{\text{meanQT}^2}$
- HRVN—normalized HR variance, $\text{HRVN} = \dfrac{\text{HRVar}}{\text{meanHR}^2}$
- QTVI—QT variability index, $\text{QTVI} = -\log \dfrac{\frac{\text{QTVar}}{\text{meanQT}^2}}{\frac{\text{HRVar}}{\text{meanHR}^2}}$, where meanHR and HRVar are average and variance of beat-to-beat heart rate time series, respectively

20.4 Sympathetic Nervous System Activity and QTV

20.4.1 Possible Physiological Mechanisms That Link QTV to Ventricular Sympathetic Outflow

Although the role of the autonomic nervous system (ANS)—in particular, the sympathetic branch—in generating and/or modulating QTV has not been fully elucidated, it is likely that the ANS acts at several levels via different pathways.

A significant portion of QTV is the direct consequence of heart rate variability and mediated via rate-dependent modulation of the action potential duration in ventricular myocytes. Thus, any vagal or sympathetic influences on the cardiac pacemaker region (sinoatrial node) would also have secondary effects on the QTV. Within ventricular myocytes, the sympathetic nervous system can principally act on L-type calcium channels and the slowly activating delayed rectifier potassium current (Ik_s). The former affects myocardial contractility while the latter has an effect on the repolarization process. Beta-adrenoceptor stimulation during Ik_s blockade was shown to increase variability in the cellular repolarization duration of canine myocytes [18], supporting the idea that an increase in ventricular sympathetic outflow may lead to an increase in the QTV.

At the tissue level, transmural differences in action potential duration affect the T-wave morphology in body surface ECG [19]. This may be altered during periods of sympathetic activation [20]. Heterogeneous distribution of β-adrenoceptors, regional arborization of sympathetic nerves [21], and differential cardiac sympathetic control [22] may contribute to spatial dispersion in action potential duration across the ventricles during periods of high sympathetic activity.

The existence of ventricular vagal innervation is now well established. Vagal nerve activity may alter the action potential duration of ventricular myocytes directly via the acetylcholine-activated K^+ current [23], or indirectly through accentuated antagonistic effects on the sympathetic nerve terminals, both pre- and postsynaptically [24].

20.4.2 Indirect Evidence on the Relationship between QTV and Cardiac Sympathetic Activity

A substantial number of interventional studies, using different autonomic stimuli, reported an increase of QTV during periods of heightened sympathetic nervous system activity.

Acute orthostatic stress is a frequently used paradigm in provocation tests for measuring cardiovascular autonomic responsiveness. The manoeuvre results in an immediate cardiac vagal withdrawal and sympathetic activation, and studies in normal subjects have shown increases in QTV in response to (graded) head-up tilt, sitting, or standing up (see Figure 20.3) [10,25–27], suggestive of a sympathetic and/or vagally mediated modulation of QTV. A study that reported increased QTV in response to sympathetic activation induced by acute hypoxia adds further evidence for the relationship between sympathetic nervous system activity and QTV in normal subjects [28]. A study on the spectral components of QTV in normal subjects recorded during interview stress and physical exercise, both of which increasing sympathetic activity, demonstrated increased low-frequency oscillations (10-second waves, observed as Traube–Hering–Mayer waves in blood pressure) in QTV [29]. A subsequent study by the same authors, in which QTV spectra were estimated during a mental stress test—while the atria was paced at a constant rate to exclude heart rate variability–driven QTV—confirmed the increase in low-frequency oscillations during stress and furthermore, suggest a direct, rate-independent influence of the sympathetic nervous system on QTV [30].

A number of studies involving physical exercise have demonstrated an increase in the ratio of QTV-to-HRV, expressed as QTVi [31–33], while QTV itself showed inconsistent

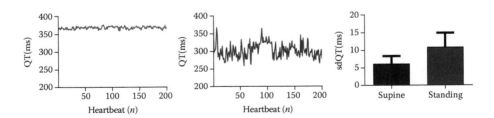

FIGURE 20.3
Example of beat-to-beat QT interval variability in a healthy subject measured in the supine position (left) and during standing (middle) as well as standard deviation of QT intervals (sdQT) obtained from 10 healthy subjects in the supine position and subsequently during standing. Group data are shown as mean values and standard deviations.

increase [33], suggesting that HRV reduction is the primary driver of QTVi increase. Possibly, a reduction in the signal-to-noise ratio of ECG recordings, which often occurs during exercise due to movement artifacts and muscle activity artifacts, may explain the inconsistent QTV change and render this stress paradigm less suitable for QTV measurement.

Aside from noninvasive interventions, pharmacological studies have been performed to explore the relationship between ANS activity and QTV. Several studies measured QTV in subjects with a normal ventricular myocardium in response to pharmacological β-adrenoceptor activation and showed consistently an increase in QTV [10,28,34,35]. Pharmacological β-adrenoceptor block showed no effect on QTV when measured during resting conditions [34,36], but a reduction in QTV when the effect of HRV was removed during atrial pacing [37]. Possibly, the activity of the sympathetic nervous system is too low during rest to exhibit a notable influence on QTV, or this influence may be masked by underlying HRV-driven QTV. Collectively, these studies strongly support the notion of a qualitative relationship between acute changes in sympathetic activity and QTV in normal subjects.

Two studies reported QTV in patients with panic disorder (PD) who were subjected to drugs, which affect the ANS. In patients with PD, the α_2-adrenergic antagonist yohimbine increased anxiety as well as QTVi, whereas α_2-adrenergic agonist clonidine reduced QTVi [38]. Response to β_1- and β_2-receptor activation with isoprotenerol was pronounced in patients with PD compared to normal subjects [39].

In cardiac patients, the response of QTV to acute autonomic stimuli appears to be blurred, but data are limited. In congestive heart failure patients, baseline QTVi was reported higher than in normal subjects, but the response to head-up tilt was impaired [26,40]. In another study in patients with heart failure, acute pharmacological β-adrenoceptor blockade had no effect on QTV [34]. In postmyocardial infarction patients, an anger recall test did not affect QTVi during β-adrenoceptor blockade [41]. Reasons for the impaired QTV response to acute changes in autonomic tone may be medications, chronic changes in autonomic tone, sympathetic dysinnervation, or a reduction in repolarization reserve.

Cross-sectional studies on β-blocker treatment suggest a link between ANS activity and QTV. In postmyocardial infarction patients who received β-blockers, QTV measured in ambulatory ECG was smaller than in patients who did not receive β-blockers, the former showing values similar to those of normal subjects [42]. This study provides evidence for sympathetic nervous system involvement in augmenting QTV, but importantly suggests that QTV, which may indicate pathological repolarization instability in these patients, can be reversed by attenuating the sympathetic influences. In patients with ischemic cardiomyopathy-related heart failure, β-blocker treatment over 1 year reduced QTVi [43].

20.4.3 Direct Evidence for the Relationship between Sympathetic Activity and QTV

Although the qualitative relationship between acute changes in sympathetic activity and QTV can be considered firmly established—at least in normal subjects as summarized above—the question remains whether it can serve as a coarse quantitative measure of sympathetic activity or help identifying subjects with sympathetic overactivity. We thus conducted correlation studies in which we compared metrics of the QTV with direct measures of sympathetic activity or innervation, employing the noradrenaline spillover technique and MIGB scintigraphy, respectively, as detailed below.

20.4.3.1 Cardiac Noradrenaline Spillover

Noradrenaline spillover measurement is a biochemical method for measuring organ-specific sympathetic nervous function. It exploits the relationship between sympathetic nerve firing rate and spillover of noradrenaline into its venous effluent [44]. It is based on isotope dilution, where the regional rate of spillover of noradrenaline into plasma can be determined during constant-rate infusion of radiolabeled noradrenaline:

$$\text{Spillover} = \left[\left(C_v - C_a \right) + C_a \cdot E \right] \cdot PF \tag{20.1}$$

where C_v and C_a are the plasma concentration of noradrenaline in regional venous and arterial plasma, E is the fractional extraction of tritiated noradrenaline, and PF is the organ plasma flow.

In the experiments, a coronary sinus angiographic catheter was introduced via the antecubital venous sheath and placed under fluoroscopic control in the coronary sinus for blood sampling to measure cardiac noradrenaline spillover. Coronary sinus blood flow was estimated from the double product (systolic blood pressure × heart rate). During the catheter study, participants received a tracer infusion of ^{3}H-labeled noradrenaline via a peripheral vein, after a priming bolus, for the measurement of noradrenaline kinetics by isotope dilution.

In a retrospective study of 12 patients with major depressive disorder (MDD; 5 males, 7 females; age 45 ± 15 years) and five patients with PD (3 males, 2 females; age: 32 ± 9 years), we compared QTV measured in high-resolution ECG (lead III, 1000 Hz, using PowerLab, AD Instruments, Australia) recorded during rest in the supine position over 5 minutes followed by cardiac noradrenaline spillover measurement [45]. Diagnosis was based on the Mini International Neuropsychiatric Interview (MINI) and the Composite International Diagnostic Interview (CIDI). The Hamilton Depression Scale and Hamilton Anxiety Rating Scale (HamD and HamA, respectively), the Clinical Global Impressions scale (CGI), and the Beck Depression Inventory (BDI-1) were used to monitor progress. All patients had Ham D>18; BDI>18; positivity for MDD and PD on MINI and CIDI; and assessment as having a significant major depression or PD as the primary illness on interview by a psychiatrist. Initial studies were performed within 10 days of a confirmed diagnosis of MDD/PD.

In a subsequent retrospective study of 23 patients with essential hypertension (17 males, 6 females; age 44 ± 12 years) and 9 normotensive (NT) subjects (7 males, 2 females; age 38 ± 13 years), we sought to explore the association between cardiac noradrenaline spillover and QTV, using the same experimental setup [46]. None of the patients had accelerated hypertension, clinical coronary artery disease, heart failure, a history of stroke, renal insufficiency, or diabetes mellitus. Previous use of antihypertensive therapy was reported in 11 hypertensive subjects. Antihypertensive therapy was discontinued for at least 4 weeks before the study. NT control subjects underwent careful clinical evaluation and serum biochemistry measurements to exclude renal and hepatic disease. None of the control subjects had a history of incidental disease or blood pressure above 140/85 mmHg.

To explore associations between QTV recorded in the supine position during rest and cardiac sympathetic activity, we investigated scatter plots and computed correlation coefficients between different metrics of QTV and noradrenaline spillover. In the group of patients with MDD and PD we did not observe any correlation, while in the study of hypertensive patients, a moderate yet significant positive correlation was observed between QTVN and cardiac noradrenaline spillover ($r^2 = 0.31$, $p = 0.001$). Subgroup correlation analysis, performed separately for the NT and the hypertensive group, showed a significant correlation between QTVN and cardiac norepinephrine (NE) spillover in hypertensive subjects ($r^2 = 0.38$, $p = 0.002$), but not in NT subjects. Further, QTVN was correlated with resting systolic BP (all subjects; $r^2 = 0.16$, $p = 0.02$). There was no significant correlation between QTVi and cardiac NE spillover.

These two studies represent the only investigations of QTV and directly assessed cardiac sympathetic activity available to date, using the spillover measurement technique. ECG recording obtained from normal subjects and patients with MDD and/or PD at rest do not support the idea of using resting QTV as an indicator of baseline cardiac sympathetic activity in subjects with normal cardiovascular function. Resting ECG recordings of hypertensive subjects, on the other hand, do suggest that a coarse indication of sympathetic (over-)activity may be obtained from QTV assessment. Given that our sample sizes were small and covered a limited range of cardiac noradrenaline spillover values and furthermore that only ECG lead III was available, which is prone to noise [47], the strength of association between QTV and spillover might have been generally underestimated. Measurement of ECG in the supine position during rest might not lend itself to assessment of sympathetic activity as in the absence of pathology or autonomic stimulus. In a subsequent study, we sought to assess ECG during standing, when cardiac sympathetic activity is elevated, using a cardiac imaging technique.

20.4.3.2 ^{123}I-MIBG Scintigraphy

Cardiac imaging using (^{123}I-MIBG) scintigraphy allows quantification of sympathetic innervation of the heart. ^{123}I-MIBG is taken up by sympathetic neurons due to its similarity to the noradrenaline molecule and can be observed with single photon emission computed tomography (SPECT). A reduction in cardiac ^{123}I-MIBG uptake is due to low ventricular β_1-adrenoreceptor density and/or noradrenaline uptake, indicative of sympathetic dysinnervation.

We retrospectively analyzed ^{123}I-MIBG data along with short-term ECG from 31 patients with type-2 diabetes mellitus with no history of cardiovascular disease, cancer, or psychiatric or other severe illness [48]. Exercise echocardiography studies were performed in all patients to verify normal ejection fraction (>50%) and the absence of coronary artery disease (i.e., no inducible wall motion abnormalities indicative of ischemia).

For ^{123}I-MIBG imaging, patients were premedicated with potassium perchlorate to block thyroid uptake of radioiodine. A standard camera with a low-energy, high-resolution collimator (Symbia, Siemens, Erlangen, Germany) was used in the acquisition of anterior planar and SPECT (32 projections for 50 seconds each) images 15 minutes (early) and 4 hours (delayed) following injection of ^{123}I-MIBG. Global cardiac uptake of ^{123}I-MIBG was calculated from both early and delayed planar images by the ratio of tracer activity (mean count per pixel) in the heart (excluding the cavity) and mediastinum. The delayed heart-to-mediastinum (H/M) ratio was primarily used in analyses and to define the presence of cardiac sympathetic dysinnervation (H/M ratio < 1.8). Cardiac sympathetic dysinnervation (i.e., a relative reduction of the SPECT signal) was identified in 16 patients.

Five-minute high-resolution ECG (lead II, 1 kHz, Powerlab, ADInstruments, Australia) was recorded in the supine position during rest. In a subgroup of 15 patients, ECG was also recorded for 5 minutes during standing, following a stabilization period of at least 2 minutes, and patients were instructed to maintain the position with minimal movement. Beat-to-beat QT variability was computed using the template stretching method described by Berger et al. [7].

During rest, HRV was significantly reduced in patients with cardiac sympathetic dysinnervation, while QTVN was comparable, which resulted in an overall increase of QTVi. The inverse association of the H/N ratio with QTVi was accompanied by a positive correlation with the denominator (HRVN), but no relation with the numerator (QTVN). Upon standing, QTVN was significantly higher in patients with cardiac sympathetic dysinnervation compared to patients with normal innervation, but HRVN was comparable, resulting in a significant overall increase in QTVi in patients with sympathetic dysinnervation. The H/N ratio was inversely correlated with standing QTVN, but not with standing HRVN.

Several important observations can be made from this study: (1) Sympathetic dysinnervation appears to be associated with increased QTV in diabetic autonomic neuropathy. The underlying mechanisms are not clear but may involve increased spatiotemporal dispersion of sympathetic modulation across the ventricular myocardium and/or increased variability in the action potential of cardiac myocytes. (2) The QT variability index, QTVi, that is, the ratio of QT variability to heart rate variability, designed to "normalize" QTV to HRV, may have equivocal interpretations. Measured in the supine position during rest in patients with diabetic autonomic neuropathy, it is reflective of vagal dysfunction and the associated reduction in HRV, while upon standing, characterized by vagal withdrawal and sympathetic activation, it quantifies sympathetically mediated aspects of cardiac autonomic neuropathy that directly affect QTV. Thus, interpretation of QTVi requires great care and should include individual appraisal of HRV and QTV values. (3) The quantitative association between QTV and sympathetic activity may become stronger during periods of sympathetic activation. Consequently, a measurement protocol designed to exploit QTV as a simple noninvasive marker of sympathetic activity may involve an autonomic stimulus, evoking sympathetic activation, such as an orthostatic stress test.

Since these observations are solely based on ECG recordings from diabetic patients with varying degrees of autonomic neuropathy, they might not be extrapolated to the general population or other pathologies.

20.5 Summary and Future Perspective

In this chapter, I have reviewed the evidence available for the association between cardiac sympathetic activity and QTV. While increased QTV during periods of sympathetic activation is a common finding in normal subjects across studies, there is insufficient data regarding the association between QTV and sympathetic activity in patients with cardiac pathologies. Possibly, other factors that contribute to ventricular repolarization and repolarization reserve may override this association. Aside from a change in cardiac substrate and autonomic tone, medication may play a significant role. Thus, comprehensive studies into the relation between sympathetic activity and QTV in cardiac disease are advocated to identify relevant factors.

There is a paucity of studies aiming to establish a direct relationship between sympathetic activity and QTV. Available data do suggest that QTV could be used as a quantitative measure of sympathetic activity, but further studies are required to confirm this relationship. Measurement modalities need to be refined and experimental protocols established. Outcomes are presumably better when conducting ECG measurements during periods of sympathetic activation, induced by orthostatic stress, for example. Precision of QT interval measurement, in particular, in conditions where the repolarization process is drastically altered and, consequently, ECG waveforms vary broadly, may need improvement.

In conclusion, assessment of QTV may provide a simple non-invasive tool for probing cardiac sympathetic (over)activity in subjects with normal hearts. With a lack of alternatives, it appears reasonable to investigate the QTV approach further.

References

1. Jaakko Malmivuo and Robert Plonsey. *Bioelectromagnetism: Principles and Applications of Bioelectric and Biomagnetic Fields.* New York: Oxford University Press, 1995.
2. Ilan Goldenberg, Arthur J. Moss, and Wojciech Zareba. QT interval: How to measure it and what is normal. *Journal of Cardiovascular Electrophysiology,* 17(3):333–336, 2006.
3. Arthur J. Moss. Measurement of the QT interval and the risk associated with QTc interval prolongation: A review. *American Journal of Cardiology,* 72(6):B23–B25, 1993.
4. Mathias Baumert, Alberto Porta, Marc A. Vos, Marek Malik, Jean Philippe Couderc, Pablo Laguna, Gianfranco Piccirillo, Godfrey L. Smith, Larisa G. Tereshchenko, Paul G A Volders. QT interval variability in body surface ECG: Measurement, physiological basis, and clinical value: position statement and consensus guidance by the European Heart Rhythm Association jointly with the ESC Working Group on Cardiac Cellular Electrophysiology. *Europace,* 18(6):925–44, 2016.
5. Muhammad A. Hasan, Derek Abbott, and Mathias Baumert. Beat-to-beat vectorcardiographic analysis of ventricular depolarization and repolarization in myocardial infarction. *PLOS ONE* 7(11):e49489, 2012.
6. Kenji Hiromoto, Hiroki Shimizu, Takanao Mine, Tohru Masuyama, and Mitsumasa Ohyanagi. Correlation between beat-to-beat QT interval variability and impaired left ventricular function in patients with previous myocardial infarction. *Annals of Noninvasive Electrocardiology,* 11(4):299–305, 2006.
7. Ronald D. Berger, Edward K. Kasper, Kenneth L. Baughman, Eduardo Marban, Hugh Calkins, and Gordon F. Tomaselli. Beat-to-beat QT interval variability novel evidence for repolarization lability in ischemic and nonischemic dilated cardiomyopathy. *Circulation,* 96(5):1557–1565, 1997.
8. Mark C. Haigney, Wojciech Zareba, Philip J. Gentlesk, Robert E. Goldstein, Michael Illovsky, Scott McNitt, Mark L. Andrews, and Arthur J. Moss. QT interval variability and spontaneous ventricular tachycardia or fibrillation in the Multicenter Automatic Defibrillator Implantation Trial (MADIT) II patients. *Journal of the American College of Cardiology,* 44(7):1481–1487, 2004.
9. Gianfranco Piccirillo, Damiano Magrì, Sabrina Matera, Marzia Magnanti, Alessia Torrini Eleonora Pasquazzi Erika Schifano Stefania Velitti Vincenzo Marigliano Raffaele Quaglione and Francesco Barillà. QT variability strongly predicts sudden cardiac death in asymptomatic subjects with mild or moderate left ventricular systolic dysfunction: A prospective study. *European Heart Journal,* 28(11):1344–1350, 2007.
10. Vikram K. Yeragani, Robert Pohl, VC Jampala, Richard Balon, Jerald Kay, and Gina Igel. Effect of posture and isoproterenol on beat-to-beat heart rate and QT variability. *Neuropsychobiology,* 41(3):113–123, 2000.
11. Bronwyn A. Kingwell, Jane M. Thompson, David M. Kaye, Grant A. McPherson, Garry L. Jennings, and Murray D. Esler. Heart rate spectral analysis, cardiac norepinephrine spillover, and muscle sympathetic nerve activity during human sympathetic nervous activation and failure. *Circulation,* 90(1):234–240, 1994.
12. Yoshihiro Imamura, Hiroshi Ando, Wataru Mitsuoka, Shougo Egashira, Hiroyuki Masaki, Toshiaki Ashihara, and Takaya Fukuyama. Iodine-123 metaiodobenzylguanidine images

reflect intense myocardial adrenergic nervous activity in congestive heart failure independent of underlying cause. *Journal of the American College of Cardiology*, 26(7):1594–1599, 1995.

13. Vito Starc and Todd T. Schlegel. Real-time multichannel system for beat-to-beat QT interval variability. *Journal of Electrocardiology*, 39(4):358–367, 2006.

14. Martin Schmidt, Mathias Baumert, Alberto Porta, Hagen Malberg, and Sebastian Zaunseder. Two-dimensional warping for one-dimensional signals conceptual framework and application to ECG processing. *IEEE Transactions on Signal Processing*, 62 (21):5577–5588, 2014.

15. S. Zaunseder, M. Schmidt, H. Malberg, and M. Baumert. Measurement of QT variability by two-dimensional warping. In *Cardiovascular Oscillations (ESGCO), 2014 8th Conference of the European Study Group on*, pp. 163–164. IEEE, 2014.

16. Aline Cabasson and Olivier Meste. Time delay estimation: A new insight into the Woody's method. *Signal Processing Letters, IEEE*, 15:573–576, 2008.

17. Mathias Baumert, Vito Starc, and Alberto Porta. Conventional QT variability measurement vs. template matching techniques: Comparison of performance using simulated and real ECG. *PLOS ONE*, 7(7):e41920, 2012.

18. Daniel M. Johnson, Jordi Heijman, Chris E. Pollard, Jean-Pierre Valentin, Harry JGM. Crijns, Najah Abi-Gerges, and Paul G.A. Volders. I-Ks restricts excessive beat-to-beat variability of repolarization during beta-adrenergic receptor stimulation. *Journal of Molecular and Cellular Cardiology*, 48(1):122–130, 2010.

19. Michael R. Franz, Klaus Bargheer, W. Rafflenbeul, Axel Haverich, and Paul R. Lichtlen. Monophasic action potential mapping in human subjects with normal electrocardiograms: Direct evidence for the genesis of the T wave. *Circulation*, 75(2):379–386, 1987.

20. Silvio H. Litovsky and C. Antzelevitch. Differences in the electrophysiological response of canine ventricular subendocardium and subepicardium to acetylcholine and isoproterenol. A direct effect of acetylcholine in ventricular myocardium. *Circulation Research*, 67(3):615–627, 1990.

21. Koichiro Yoshioka, Dong-Wei Gao, Michael Chin, Carol Stillson, Elizabeth Penades, Michael Lesh, William O'Connell, and Michael Dae. Heterogeneous sympathetic innervation influences local myocardial repolarization in normally perfused rabbit hearts. *Circulation*, 101(9): 1060–1066, 2000.

22. Antonio Zaza, Gabriella Malfatto, and Peter J. Schwartz. Sympathetic modulation of the relation between ventricular repolarization and cycle length. *Circulation Research*, 68(5):1191–1203, 1991.

23. Shin-Ichi Koumi and Andrew J. Wasserstrom. Acetylcholine-sensitive muscarinic k+ channels in mammalian ventricular myocytes. *American Journal of Physiology—Heart and Circulatory Physiology*, 35(5):H1812, 1994.

24. Marco Stramba-Badiale, Emil Vanoli, Gaetanom M. De Ferrari, Donatrlla Cerati, Robert D. Foreman, and Peter J. Schwartz. Sympathetic-parasympathetic interaction and accentuated antagonism in conscious dogs. *American Journal of Physiology* 260(2 Pt 2):H335–40, 1991.

25. Alberto Porta, Eleonora Tobaldini, Tomaso Gnecchi-Ruscone, and Nicola Montano. RT variability unrelated to heart period and respiration progressively increases during graded head-up tilt. *American Journal of Physiology—Heart and Circulatory Physiology*, 298(5):H1406–H1414, 2010.

26. Gianfranco Piccirillo, Marzia Magnanti, Sabrina Matera, Silvia Di Carlo, Tiziana De Laurentis, Alessia Torrini, Nicola Marchitto, Renato Ricci, and Damiano Magri. Age and QT variability index during free breathing, controlled breathing and tilt in patients with chronic heart failure and healthy control subjects. *Translational Research*, 148(2):72–78, 2006.

27. Katerina Hnatkova, Donna Kowalski, James J. Keirns, E. van Gelderen, and Marek Malik. Relationship of QT interval variability to heart rate and RR interval variability. *Journal of Electrocardiology*, 46(6):591–596, 2013.

28. Olivier Xhaet, Jean-Francois Argacha, Atul Pathak, Marko Gujic, Anne Houssiere, Boutaina Najem, Jean-Paul Degaute, and Philippe Van De Borne. Sympathoexcitation increases the QT/RR slope in healthy men: Differential effects of hypoxia, dobutamine, and phenylephrine. *Journal of Cardiovascular Electrophysiology*, 19(2):178–184, 2008.

29. Radu Negoescu, James E. Skinner, and Stewart Wolf. Forebrain regulation of cardiac function spectral and dimensional analysis of RR and QT intervals. *Integrative Physiological and Behavioral Science*, 28(4):331342, 1993.

30. R. Negoescu, S. Dinca-Panaitescu, V. Filcescu, D. Ionescu, and S. Wolf. Mental stress enhances the sympathetic fraction of QT variability in an RR-independent way. *Integrative Physiological and Behavioral Science*, 32(3):220–227, 1997.

31. Silke Boettger, Christian Puta, Vikram K. Yeragani, Lars Donath, Hans-Josef Muller, Holger H. Gabriel, and Karl-Jurgen Bar. Heart rate variability, QT variability, and electrodermal activity during exercise. *Medicine and Science in Sports and Exercise* 42(3):443–448, 2010.

32. Mark C. Haigney, Willem J. Kop, Shama Alam, David S. Krantz, Pamela Karasik, Albert A. DelNegro, and John S. Gottdiener. QT variability during rest and exercise in patients with implantable cardioverter defibrillators and healthy controls. *Annals of Noninvasive Electrocardiology*, 14(1):40–49, 2009.

33. Michael J. Lewis, D. Rassi, and A.L. Short. Analysis of the QT interval and its variability in healthy adults during rest and exercise. *Physiological Measurement*, 27(11):1211, 2006.

34. Sachin Nayyar, Kurt C. Roberts-Thomson, Muhammad A. Hasan, Thomas Sullivan, Judith Harrington, Prashanthan Sanders, and Mathias Baumert. Autonomic modulation of repolarization instability in patients with heart failure prone to ventricular tachycardia. *American Journal of Physiology-Heart and Circulatory Physiology*, 305(8):H1181–H1188, 2013.

35. Srikanth Seethala, Vladimir Shusterman, Samir Saba, Susan Mularski, and Jan Nemec. Effect of β-adrenergic stimulation on QT interval accommodation. *Heart Rhythm*, 8(2):263–270, 2011.

36. Giuseppe Piccirillo, Mauro Cacciafesta, Marco Lionetti, and Vincenzo Marigliano. Influence of age, the autonomic nervous system and anxiety on QT-interval variability. *Clinical Science*, 101:429–438, 2001.

37. Takanao Mine, Hiroki Shimizu, Kenji Hiromoto, Yoshio Furukawa, Tetsuzou Kanemori, Hiroaki Nakamura, Tohru Masuyama, and Mitsumasa Ohyanagi. Beat-to-beat QT interval variability is primarily affected by the autonomic nervous system. *Annals of Noninvasive Electrocardiology*, 13(3):228–233, 2008.

38. Vikram Kumar Yeragani, Manuel Tancer, and Thomas Uhde. Heart rate and QT interval variability: Abnormal alpha-2 adrenergic function in patients with panic disorder. *Psychiatry Research*, 121(2):185–196, 2003.

39. Robert Pohl and Vikram K. Yeragani. QT interval variability in panic disorder patients after isoproterenol infusions. *International Journal of Neuropsychopharmacology*, 4(01):17–20, 2001.

40. Nagaraj Desai, D.S. Raghunandan, Mallika Mallavarapu, Ronald D. Berger, and Vikram K. Yeragani. Beat-to-beat heart rate and QT variability in patients with congestive cardiac failure: Blunted response to orthostatic challenge. *Annals of Noninvasive Electrocardiology*, 9(4):323–329, 2004.

41. Damiano Magri, Gianfranco Piccirillo, Raffaele Quaglione, Annalaura DellArmi, Marilena Mitra, Stefania Velitti, Daniele Di Barba, Andrea Lizio, Damiana Maisto, and Francesco Barilla. Effect of acute mental stress on heart rate and QT variability in post-myocardial infarction patients. *ISRN Cardiology* 2012, 2012.

42. Yoshio Furukawa, Hiroki Shimizu, Kenji Hiromoto, Tetsuzou Kanemori, Tohru Masuyama, and Mitsumasa Ohyanagi. Circadian variation of beat-to-beat QT interval variability in patients with prior myocardial infarction and the effect of β-blocker therapy. *Pacing and Clinical Electrophysiology*, 29(5):479–486, 2006.

43. Gianfranco Piccirillo Raffaele Quaglione, Marialuce Nocco, Camilla Naso Antonio Moisè, Marco Lionetti, Silvia Di Carlo, and Vincenzo Marigliano. Effects of long-term beta-blocker (*metoprolol* or *carvedilol*) therapy on QT variability in subjects with chronic heart failure secondary to ischemic cardiomyopathy. *American Journal of Cardiology*, 90(10):1113–1117, 2002.

44. Murray Esler. Clinical application of noradrenaline spillover methodology: Delineation of regional human sympathetic nervous responses. *Pharmacology and Toxicology*, 73(5):243– 253, 1993.

45. Mathias Baumert, Gavin W. Lambert, Tye Dawood, Elisabeth A. Lambert, Murray D. Esler, Mariee McGrane, David Barton, and Eugene Nalivaiko. QT interval variability and cardiac norepinephrine spillover in patients with depression and panic disorder. *American Journal of Physiology—Heart and Circulatory Physiology*, 295(3):H962–H968, 2008.
46. Mathias Baumert, Markus P. Schlaich, Eugene Nalivaiko, Elisabeth Lambert, Carolina I. Sari, David M. Kaye, Murray D. Elser, Prashanthan Sanders, and Gavin Lambert. Relation between QT interval variability and cardiac sympathetic activity in hypertension. *American Journal of Physiology-Heart and Circulatory Physiology*, 300(4):H1412–H1417, 2011.
47. Muhammad A. Hasan, Derek Abbott, and Mathias Baumert. Relation between beat-to-beat QT interval variability and T-wave amplitude in healthy subjects. *Annals of Noninvasive Electrocardiology*, 17(3):195–203, 2012.
48. Julian W. Sacre, Bennett Franjic, Jeff S. Coombes, Thomas H. Marwick, and Mathias Baumert. QT interval variability in type 2 diabetic patients with cardiac sympathetic dysinnervation assessed by 123I-metaiodobenzylguanidine scintigraphy. *Journal of Cardiovascular Electrophysiology*, 24(3):305–313, 2013.

21

The Predictive Utility of Heart Rate Variability in Chronic Kidney Disease: A Marker of Patient Outcomes

Cara M. Hildreth, Ann K. Goodchild, Divya Sarma Kandukuri,
and Jacqueline K. Phillips

CONTENTS

21.1 Introduction

Autonomic dysfunction is highly prevalent in patients with chronic kidney disease (CKD). Sympathetic overactivity is commonly described (Kotanko, 2006; Grassi et al., 2012; Rubinger et al., 2013) with direct microneurograph recordings of muscle sympathetic nerve activity indicating that it is substantially elevated (Converse et al., 1992; Klein et al., 2001, 2003) and that this occurs early in the disease course (Grassi et al., 2011). Classical autonomic tests indicate that vagal outflow is also altered with impaired heart rate responses to administration of atropine,* respiration, table tilt, or the Valsalva maneuver[†] (for review

---

* Atropine: a nonspecific antagonist of muscarinic acetylcholine receptors. Inhibits parasympathetic control of the heart.
[†] Valsalva maneuver: a test used to examine autonomic control of the heart by examining the heart rate response (tachycardia) to forced expiration against a closed airway. In patients with autonomic dysfunction, no tachycardia is observed (Barbato, 1990).

see Robinson and Carr, 2002). The precise underlying cause for autonomic dysfunction is unknown and likely multifactorial. With respect to sympathetic overactivity, activation of the renal afferent nerves,[*] central and/or peripheral actions of angiotensin II,[†] and inhibition of brain nitric oxide synthase[‡] have been postulated as likely mechanisms (Kotanko, 2006). Notably, each of these postulated mechanisms have the capacity to impair vagal control of heart rate too (e.g., Felder, 1986; Ruggeri et al., 2000; Kawada et al., 2009). The resulting sympathetic overactivity and vagal insufficiency leads to altered sympathovagal balance at the level of heart in CKD and is a likely contributor to the increased risk of cardiac death (Herzog et al., 2008; Vaseghi and Shivkumar, 2008).

Heart rate variability (HRV) is widely measured in CKD patients as a means of examining autonomic regulation of the heart and is consistently reported as reduced, most notably in those receiving dialysis therapy (Axelrod et al., 1987; Hathaway et al., 1998a; Vita et al., 1999; Kurata et al., 2000; Furuland et al., 2008; Mylonopoulou et al., 2010; Celik et al., 2011). Interpreting HRV measures in CKD patients can be difficult due to the progressive nature of the disease, associated comorbidities such as cardiovascular disease and diabetes, the demographics of the patient population at risk for CKD and the potential effect of treatment on HRV. In this chapter, the impact of these different variables on HRV within the CKD population will be discussed with a view toward highlighting the predictive utility of HRV as marker of patient outcomes.

21.2 HRV and Its Relationship to CKD Progression

While it is largely appreciated that patients with CKD have reduced HRV, at what point within the development of CKD HRV begins to decline is as yet unknown. It has been repeatedly documented that HRV is negatively correlated with renal function, implying that as kidney function deteriorates, HRV reduces (Burger et al., 2002; Tang et al., 2012). Accordingly, the Renal Research Institute-CKD study (Chandra et al., 2012), a four center prospective cohort study of adults with stage 3–5 CKD (see Table 21.1 for description of CKD staging), and one of only a few studies to measure HRV in CKD patients as kidney function deteriorates, showed that HRV decreased as renal disease severity increased. In this study, standard deviation of the NN interval (SDNN),[§] standard deviation of the average NN interval (SDANN),[¶] very low-frequency (VLF),[**] and low-frequency/high-frequency (LF/HF)[††] power was lower in stage 5 non-dialysis CKD patients compared with stage 3 and 4 CKD patients (see Table 21.2), with stage 5 patients exhibiting lower estimated

---

[*] Renal afferent nerves: sensory nerves that project from the kidney to the sites within the central nervous system involved in cardiovascular regulation and respond to renal ischemia, changes in the ionic composition of the renal interstitium, decreases in renal perfusion pressure, and increases in renal artery, venous, and/or pelvic pressure (Ciriello and de Oliveira, 2002).

[†] Angiotensin II: a circulating hormone that is also produced locally within a number of tissues including the heart, brain and kidneys (Paul et al., 2006).

[‡] Nitric oxide synthase (NOS): an enzyme, which occurs in three different forms—eNOS (endothelial NOS), nNOS (neuronal NOS), and iNOS (inducible NOS)—responsible for producing nitric oxide from L-arginine.

[§] Standard deviation of the NN interval (SDNN): reflects all factors responsible for producing heart rate variability during the recording period.

[¶] Standard deviation of the average NN interval (SDANN): reflects changes in heart rate due to cycles of 5 minutes or greater.

[**] VLF: may reflect hormonal and thermoregulatory influences on heart rate

[††] LF/HF ratio: an approach used whereby LF power is divided by HF power in order to normalise for underlying vagal tone thereby revealing the sympathetically mediated oscillations in heart rate.

TABLE 21.1

CKD Staging Based on eGFR

CKD Stage	eGFR (mL/min/1.73 m^2)
1	≥ 90
2	60–89
3	30–59
4	15–29
5	< 15 (or on dialysis)

TABLE 21.2

Baseline HRV Measurements in Stage 3–5 CKD Patients

	Overall (*n* = 305)	CKD Stage 3 $30 \leq$ eGFR < 60 (*n* = 126)	CKD Stage 4 $15 \leq$ eGFR < 30 (*n* = 140)	CKD Stage 5 eGFR < 15 (*n* = 39)
Heart rate (obtained during Holter monitoring)				
Mean 24 hours (b.p.m)	73.5 ± 10.4	73.6 ± 10.6	73.5 ± 10.0	73.1 ± 11.6
Mean day/night difference	7.9 ± 9.7	8.0 ± 8.0	8.3 ± 7.4	6.1 ± 5.9
Time domain (ms)				
SDNN	107.4 ± 37.5	**107.6 ± 36.7**	**110.4 ± 37.4**	**95.7 ± 39.3**
SDANN	87.4 (25, 258)	**88.0 (25, 258)**	**91.7 (27, 202)**	**69.3 (34, 147)**
ASDNN	47.1 ± 26.1	41.0(12, 188)	42.5(12, 195)	37.0 (18, 187)
RMSSD	24.6(6, 267)	26.0(6, 267)	22.8(9, 259.5)	22.9 (8, 262)
Frequency domain (ms^2)				
VLF	1005.5 (36, 7532)	**1019.0 (520, 5908)**	**1084.0 (36, 6252)**	**589.0 (162, 7532)**
LF	310.0 (13, 11 977)	292.5 (13, 6688)	327.0 (16, 11 977)	241.0 (27, 7151)
HF	121.5 (5, 15 123)	141.0 (5, 11 247)	112.0 (16, 15 123)	102.0 (11, 11 445)
LF/HF ratio	2.5 (0.2, 14)	**2.3 (0.2, 12)**	**2.9 (0.2, 14)**	**2.1 (0.3, 9)**
Total power	1555.0 (118, 30 828)	1560.5 (132, 25 058)	1645.0 (118, 30 828)	1131.0 (306, 25 436)

Source: Reproduced from Chandra P et al., *Nephrology, Dialysis, Transplantation,* 2012 "by permission of Oxford University Press." Retrieved from http://ndt.oxfordjournals.org.
Continuous variables are reported as mean ± SD for normally distributed variables and median (min, max) for skewed variables. Significant differences for CKD Stage 5 versus Stage 3 and 4 are shown in bold ($p < .05$).

glomerular filtration rate (eGFR),* increased blood urea nitrogen and increased urine albumin to creatinine ratio, indicative of a greater reduction in renal function. Interestingly, not all indicators of poor renal function are consistently associated with reduced HRV, with proteinurea, an independent predictor for the development of end-stage renal disease (ESRD) (Iseki et al., 2003), reported by some as associated with reduced HRV (Poulsen et al., 1997; Wirta et al., 1999) and not by others (Tamura et al., 2008; Drawz et al., 2013).

---

* Estimated glomerular filtration rate (eGFR): a test used to estimate the amount of blood that passes through the glomeruli each minute, thereby indicating how well your kidneys are filtering blood. A decreasing eGFR indicates that renal function is worsening and is a measure used to classify the stage of CKD (see Table 21.1).

It has been suggested by some that this relationship is tied to levels of albuminuria,[*] with normal to mild albuminuria promoting a relationship between proteinuria (i.e., kidney damage) and HRV, while high levels of albumin mask the relationship (Drawz et al., 2013).

21.3 Covariates of Reduced HRV in CKD

In the Chronic Renal Insufficiency Cohort study (Drawz et al., 2013), when SDNN, estimated from standard electrocardiogram (ECG) recordings of 10-second duration, was stratified into the following quartiles: $< 8.5, 8.5$ to $< 14.9, 14.9$ to < 25.5 and greater than 25.5 ms, CKD patients whose SDNN estimates fell into the lower quartile, in addition to having a lower eGFR, were older, more likely to be hypertensive, have cardiovascular disease (i.e., coronary artery disease and heart failure) and/or diabetes, be anemic, and not exercise. In addition to this, increased body mass index, left ventricular mass index, smoking, higher C-reactive protein levels, increased high-density lipoprotein levels, elevated serum phosphorus levels, and the use of beta-blockers are associated with reduced HRV in CKD patients (Cashion et al., 2005; Brotman et al., 2010; Chandra et al., 2012; Suzuki et al., 2012). Thus, impaired renal function is not the only determinant of reduced HRV in CKD patients, exemplifying the complexity of the relationship between reduced HRV and CKD. The following covariates are of notable mention.

21.3.1 Diabetes

Perhaps the most significant covariate affecting HRV in CKD patients is diabetes. This is probably largely driven by the fact that cardiovascular autonomic neuropathy is a complication of diabetes leading to a functional denervation of parasympathetic activity and initially a relative increase in sympathetic activity, before sympathetic denervation also results (for review of cardiovascular autonomic neuropathy in diabetes see Kuehl and Stevens, 2012). This loss of autonomic regulation of heart rate results most often in a reduction in HRV. Accordingly, patients with either type I or type II diabetes exhibit reduced SDNN, RMSSD,[†] and HF[‡] power (Pagani et al., 1988; Bernardi et al., 1992; Singh et al., 2000; Giordano et al., 2001; Mylonopoulou et al., 2010; Jaiswal et al., 2013). As illustrated in Figure 21.1, CKD patients with diabetes exhibit a lower level of HRV (Hathaway et al., 1998a,b; Giordano et al., 2001; Mylonopoulou et al., 2010; Chandra et al., 2012), potentially driven by the fact that lower eGFR is more strongly associated with reduced HRV (lower SDNN and RMSSD) in diabetic than non-diabetic CKD patients (Drawz et al., 2013). Together this suggests that there is a compound relationship between CKD and diabetes on HRV, such that the presence of both diabetes and CKD has an additive effect on HRV resulting in a further reduced HRV in this patient population. This may explain why diabetic ESRD patients undergoing dialysis are at greater risk of mortality than non-diabetic ESRD patients (Locatelli et al., 2010; Verdalles et al., 2010).

---

[*] Albuminuria: presence of excessive amounts of the protein albumin in the urine. Can be used to detect patients with CKD that don't have reduced renal function (i.e., eGFR < 60 mL/min/1.73 m^2) and indicates that the kidneys are damaged (Johnson et al., 2012).

[†] Square root of the mean squared differences of successive NN intervals (RMSSD): a measure of short-term variations in heart rate that correlates with high-frequency oscillations in heart rate.

[‡] High-frequency (HF) power: represents vagal control of heart rate and is influenced by respiration.

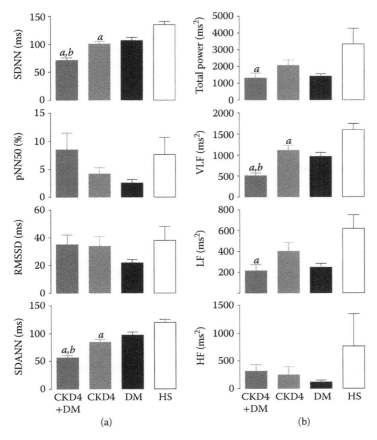

FIGURE 21.1

Differences in time-domain (a) and frequency-domain (b) estimates of heart rate variability (HRV) between stage 4 chronic kidney disease with diabetes (CKD4+DM), stage 4 chronic kidney disease patients without diabetes (CKD4), patients with diabetes mellitus (DM), and healthy subjects (HS). [a]$p < .05$ versus HS. [b]$p < .05$ versus DM. HF, high-frequency power; LF, low-frequency power; pNN50, proportion of successive pairs of NN intervals that differ by more than 50 ms; RMSSD, square root of the mean of the square of successive NN intervals; SDANN, SD of the averages of 5-minute NN intervals; SDNN, SD of all normal RR (NN) intervals; VLF, very low-frequency power. (Adapted from Mylonopoulou M et al., *Nephrology, Dialysis, Transplantation*, 2010 "by permission of Oxford University Press.")

21.3.2 Anemia

Anemia, a common feature of CKD patients (Horl, 2013), has a negative impact on autonomic function, leading to reduced parasympathetic function and a relative increase in sympathetic function (Connes and Coates, 2013). Accordingly, in anemic disorders such as sickle cell anemia, thalassemia, and iron deficient anemia, HRV is reported as reduced (Franzoni et al., 2004; Yokusoglu et al., 2007; Hedreville et al., 2014). The underlying cause of autonomic dysfunction in anemia is not well established, but may relate to aberrant respiratory neural drive or hypersensitive autonomic responses to hypoxia (Sangkatumvong et al., 2008a,b; Connes and Coates, 2013). Given that the peripheral chemoreflex, which responds to hypoxia, is tonically activated in CKD patients, contributing to the elevated level of sympathetic nerve activity (Hering et al., 2007), it is possible that similar mechanisms underlie the link between anemia and reduced HRV in CKD patients. In support, normalization of hemoglobin levels using epoetin* in stage 4 CKD patients with renal anemia resulted in an improvement in frequency-domain estimates of HRV (both total power [TP] and LF power) but not time-domain measures (Furuland et al., 2008).

21.3.3 Age

Within the general healthy population, HRV declines with age (van Dijk et al., 1991; Ziegler et al., 1992; Umetani et al., 1998; Fluckiger et al., 1999; Agelink et al., 2001) and as such, it is unsurprising that age is such a strong covariate. However, while age independently affects HRV, it is likely that it has a greater effect for CKD patients. In a group of CKD patients receiving hemodialysis aged 19–85, Di Leo et al. (2005) showed that a significant negative correlation between HRV (measured as LF power) and age existed (see Figure 21.2). While HRV also correlated with age in the healthy control subjects, the slope of this correlation differed significantly between the two groups, implying that age has a greater negative impact on HRV in CKD subjects.

Age is repeatedly reported as a determinant of HRV in adult CKD cases; however, it does not appear to be causally related to HRV in pediatric CKD cases. Analysis of HRV estimates taken from children enrolled in the Chronic Kidney Disease in Children study (Barletta et al., 2014), using a linear mixed-model, indicated that age was not a variable affecting HRV estimates. Whether this reflects differences in the underlying cause of kidney disease in pediatric versus adult cases and therefore a different pathophysiology is unknown. Certainly, in support of this theory, different factors are associated with a reduction in HRV in pediatric cases, with hypertensive CKD children exhibiting lower HRV than normotensive CKD children (Barletta et al., 2014), a pattern not observed in adult cases (Tamura et al., 1998; Kurata et al., 2000).

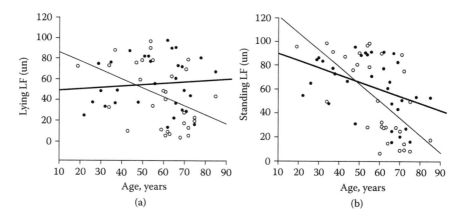

FIGURE 21.2
Comparison of linear regression models (age vs. low-frequency [LF] band value) obtained in controls (filled circle and thick line) and in uremics (open circle and thin line) on lying (a) and on standing (b) positions. There was a significant difference in the slope of regression line on lying ($p < .03$) and on standing ($p < .04$). Retrieved from http://www.nature.com/ki/index.html. (Reprinted by permission from Macmillan Publishers Ltd: *Kidney International* 67: 1521–1525, copyright 2005.)

---

* Epoeitin: stimulates the bone marrow to produce more red blood cells and is therefore a treatment used for anemia.

21.4 Prognostic Value of HRV in CKD

Regardless of the underlying etiology of reduced HRV in CKD patients, a reduction in HRV has repeatedly been shown to be associated with an increased risk of mortality, cardiovascular or renal outcome (Brotman et al., 2010; Chandra et al., 2014). The specific HRV parameters reported vary depending on the study design and not all HRV parameters have been shown to be associated with these endpoints. Most notably, a reduction in SDNN, SDANN, ASDNN,* TP, LF, and LF/HF ratio have been identified as independent risk factors (Fukuta et al., 2003; Oikawa et al., 2009; Chandra et al., 2012). Accordingly, Suzuki et al. (2012) demonstrated that hemodialysis patients who died due to all causes had exhibited reduced SDNN, SDANN, TI, VLF, LF, and LF/HF. Both the Renal Research Institute-CKD study (Chandra et al., 2012) and the Atherosclerosis Risk in Communities study (Brotman et al., 2010) demonstrated that a low LF/HF ratio was associated with a higher risk of deterioration in renal function, with the Atherosclerosis Risk in Communities study showing that this association remained even after correction for classical risk factors such as diabetes, hypertension, and low baseline renal function. Specifically, in hemodialysis patients that exhibit left ventricular hypertrophy, a LF/HF ratio greater than 1.9 is associated with greater survival (Nishimura et al., 2010). Both retrospectively and prospectively, it has been demonstrated that CKD patients (stage 3+) that died of coronary artery disease, peripheral artery disease, congestive heart failure, acute myocardial infarction or a cardiac arrest had shown reduced TP, VLF, LF, and LF/HF ratio compared with survivors (Fukuta et al., 2003; Cashion et al., 2005; Oikawa et al., 2009; Chandra et al., 2012). Lesser used indices of HRV, such as reduced triangular index† (Hayano et al., 1999; Fukuta et al., 2003), ultra-low frequency‡ (Fukuta et al., 2003), and scaling exponent α_1§ (Suzuki et al., 2012) have also been identified as potential predictors of an increased risk of mortality.

In a clinical setting, simple readily obtainable HRV estimates need to be utilized if HRV can realistically be used as a means of risk stratification for CKD patients. Perhaps the simplest of HRV measures is the time-domain estimate SDNN. A SDNN less than 50 ms has been reported to be associated with an increased risk of sudden death in CKD patients (Hathaway et al., 1998a, Hayano et al., 1999), while if the threshold is reduced to 75 ms, SDNN is also an independent predictor of all-cause and cardiovascular-related death (Oikawa et al., 2009). Nevertheless, it must be pointed out that while using a SDNN of 50 ms carries a good sensitivity (60%), negative predictive value (99%) and accuracy and specificity (83%), the positive predictive value is low (7%) (Hathaway et al., 1998a) and thus a number of false positives will be detected. Furthermore, not all changes to HRV may be reflected by a change in SDNN (Goldberger and West, 1987) and a greater number of frequency-domain measures than time-domain measures of HRV have been established to predict a clinical outcome for CKD patients (Chandra et al., 2012). Therefore, a low SDNN (75 ms or less) may serve as a good clinical screening tool to identify patients potentially at risk of an adverse outcome, who require wider HRV measurements to further stratify their risk and therefore require closer clinical monitoring.

---

* Mean of the standard deviation in all 5-minute segments of a 24-hour period (ASDNN or SDNN index): measures variability due to oscillations shorter than 5 minutes in duration.
† Triangular index: a geometrical method to estimate HRV, which gives the integral of the density of distribution of all NN intervals divided by the maximum density of distribution.
‡ Ultra-low-frequency power: reflects very long-term influences on HRV such as exercise.
§ Scaling exponent α_1: short-term fractal component used to quantify the complexity of heart rate.

Interestingly, and perhaps counter-intuitively, an increased level of HRV has also been shown to predict an increased risk of mortality in CKD patients. In the Chronic Renal Insufficiency Cohort study (Drawz et al., 2013), both low and high levels of SDNN and RMSSD were associated with an increased hazard ratio for all-cause mortality. This is consistent with that observed in the Rotterdam Study, where in elderly patients, both a decrease and an increase in HRV, measured as SDNN, was associated with an increased risk of cardiac mortality (Bruyne et al., 1999). The underlying cause of this relationship is unknown, but has been postulated to indicate an underlying dysfunction at the level of the sinoatrial node (Drawz et al., 2013).

21.5 Effect of Treatment on HRV

Given the association between reduced or increased HRV and an increased risk of both all-cause and cardiovascular-related mortality in CKD patients, there would appear a strong necessity to implement treatment strategies in CKD patients that have a positive effect on HRV.

21.5.1 Antihypertensive Therapy

Intriguingly, given the known association between blood pressure and HRV in the general population (Singh et al., 1998), mean blood pressure does not correlate with HRV estimates in CKD patients (Tamura et al., 1998; Kurata et al., 2000). This suggests that either hypertension is not driving the reduction in HRV in CKD patients or that the use of antihypertensive therapy, in and of itself, is reducing HRV. In support of the latter, there are some reports that the chronic use of beta-blockers is associated with reduced HRV in CKD patients (Chandra et al., 2012). This contrasts with the reported observations that use of beta-blockers is associated with an improvement in HRV in patients with chronic heart failure (Lin et al., 1999, 2004) and following myocardial infarction (Molgaard et al., 1993; Lurje et al., 1997). Furthermore, this finding is paradoxical given the fact that acute administration of propranolol results in an increase in the HF component of HRV, with albeit a nonsignificant increase in LF power also noted (Tory et al., 2004). The latter finding suggests that in CKD patients, a shift in sympathovagal balance toward sympathetic dominance is suppressing HRV and that by acutely inhibiting cardiac sympathetic tone, by blockade of beta-adrenoceptors, cardiac vagal tone is facilitated resulting in an improvement in HRV. The exact mechanisms underlying the negative effect of long-term beta-adrenoceptor blockade on HRV in CKD patients, however, is unknown.

Mixed reports exist with regard to the effects of angiotensin II inhibitors, another class of antihypertensive medications favored in CKD patients (Ripley, 2009; Kidney Health Australia, 2012) on HRV. In patients enrolled into the Renal Research Institute-CKD study, there was no association between the use of angiotensin converting enzyme inhibitors or angiotensin II receptors blockers and the level of HRV (Chandra et al., 2012). Conversely, others have shown that treatment with the angiotensin-converting enzyme inhibitor ramipril resulted in a 49% reduction in HRV (measured as SDNN) (Ondocin and Narsipur, 2006). Finally, treatment with the angiotensin II receptor blockers losartan, candesartan, or valsartan have been shown to have no effect on HRV (Shigenaga et al., 2009; Peters et al., 2014), while others have shown that treatment with olmesartan improves HRV (measured as SDNN) and weakens the correlation between glomerular filtration rate and

HRV (Sato et al., 2013). The latter finding may be the key to the wide variation in findings in relation to the use of angiotensin II inhibitors and HRV, with an improvement in renal function necessary for a positive therapeutic effect.

21.5.2 Lifestyle Modification

While the use of antihypertensive therapy has been shown to have variable effects on HRV, lifestyle modification through the incorporation of exercise, has a positive beneficial effect on HRV in CKD patients. Following a 10-month exercise program, involving up to 40 minutes of cycling followed by 30 minutes of muscle strengthening exercises performed three times weekly, Kouidi et al. (2009) demonstrated an improvement in both time- and frequency-domain measures of HRV in chronic hemodialysis patients (see Figure 21.3). Remarkably, the number of individuals with an SDNN less than 70 ms and exhibiting Lown

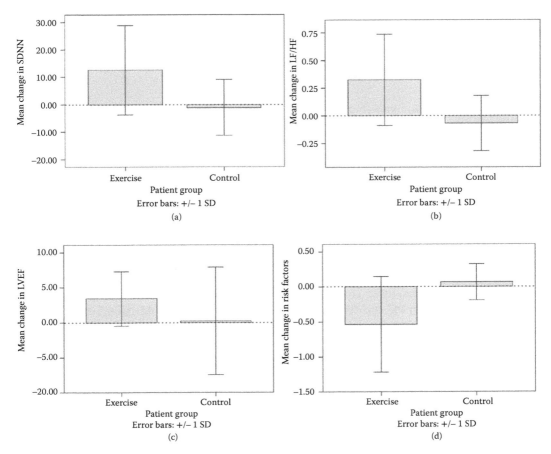

FIGURE 21.3
Bar charts of mean changes in (a) SD of the normal RR intervals (SDNN), (b) low-frequency (LF)/high-frequency (HF) ratio, (c) left ventricular ejection fraction (LVEF), and (d) risk factors over time in the two groups. Vertical line extends to ±1 SD. (Reprinted from *American Journal of Kidney Diseases*, 54(3), Kouidi EJ et al., Effects of exercise training on noninvasive cardiac measures in patients undergoing long-term hemodialysis: A randomized controlled trial, 511–521, Copyright (2009), with permission from Elsevier.)

class > II arrhythmias* decreased significantly. Given that a reduction in HRV is known to be associated with an increased risk of sudden cardiac death (La Rovere et al., 1998) and that a SDNN of 70 ms or less has specifically been shown to be associated with an increased risk of death in CKD patients (Hathaway et al., 1998a; Hayano et al., 1999; Oikawa et al., 2009), this finding strongly supports the utility of exercise as a therapeutic intervention to improve HRV and reduce cardiovascular risk in CKD patients. It is possible that shorter term incorporation of an active lifestyle will provide similar improvements in HRV, with Deligiannis et al. (1999), in an earlier study, showing that exercising three to four times per week for 6 months, involving 50 minutes of aerobic exercise, while providing no improvement in renal function or hematocrit levels, resulted in a marked improvement in HRV and reduction in the incidence of arrhythmias. In both the studies cited, however, HRV was not assessed during the training program and therefore, it is not known how soon an improvement is observed. Nevertheless, the fact that exercise can improve HRV in association with a reduction in the incidence of arrhythmias, in spite of the fact that there is no improvement in renal function or anemia, two variables independently associated with reduced HRV in CKD patients (Chandra et al., 2012; Drawz et al., 2013), strongly supports the incorporation of exercise as a therapeutic measure to improve HRV and reduce cardiovascular risk in hemodialysis patients.

21.5.3 Dialysis

Understanding how dialysis therapy affects HRV can be difficult due to the fact that dialysis therapy in itself can alter HRV as well as having long-term effects on HRV. When considering the acute effects (i.e., within the dialysis session and immediately following dialysis treatment), how HRV changes is variable and relates to the hemodynamic stability of the patient during the dialysis session.

In patients who are hemodynamically unstable and exhibit hypotension during the dialysis session, LF/HF ratio and LF power, but not HF power, decreases over the course of the treatment (Yamamoto et al., 2012). These changes in HRV are not gradual and more likely localized to the period of intradialytic hypotension. Barnas et al. (1999) demonstrated that in hypotension-prone patients, up until 10 minutes prior to the development of hypotension, LF/HF power remained unchanged. When hypotension was observed, LF/HF levels decreased below baseline and returned to baseline levels in association with a restoration in blood pressure. Thus, these changes in HRV may reflect autonomic changes precipitating and resulting from the sudden change in blood pressure. Additionally, baseline levels of HRV may reflect a predisposition to intradialytic hypotension, as dialysis patients that exhibit lower HRV estimates, when measured by both frequency (VLF, LF, and LF/HF) and time (SD and SDANN) domain methods, prior to treatment, exhibited intradialytic hypotension (Sato et al., 2001; Rubinger et al., 2004).

Conversely, in patients who experience intradialytic increases in blood pressure, how HRV changes can be clearly segregated on the basis of whether heart rate has increased or decreased with those exhibiting tachycardia showing an increase in HRV, as measured using frequency-domain analysis, while those exhibiting bradycardia showed no change

---

* Lown classification of arrhythmias: A grading system used to classify the degree of ventricular arrhythmia. Class 0 = no ventricular premature beats. Class I ≤ 30 ventricular premature beats an hour. Class II ≥ 30 ventricular premature beats an hour. Class III = presence of multiform ventricular extrasystoles. Class IVa = two consecutive ventricular premature beats. Class IVb = three or more consecutive ventricular premature beats. Class V = presence of R-on-T phenomenon.

in HRV (Rubinger et al., 2012). This dichotomy on the basis of heart rate response may explain why others, who don't report intradialytic heart rate responses, demonstrate no intradialytic change in HRV in hypertension-prone dialysis patients (Chou et al., 2006).

Mixed reports exist with respect to the effects of hemodialysis on HRV in hemodynamically stable patients, with some reporting that HRV declines (Rubinger et al., 2004; Tong and Hou, 2007), whereas others report that it improves (Celik et al., 2011; Yamamoto et al., 2012) during the course of the dialysis session. A number of factors relating to the dialysis conditions may impact on whether HRV improves and the extent to which it improves. When the dialysis solution is administered at 37°C, only an increase in LF/HF ratio is observed, whereas if the solution is chilled to 35°C then an increase in TP and LF power, and the LF/HF ratio is observed (Zitt et al., 2008). The choice of dialysis solution is also a determinant with administration of an icodextrin-based dialysis solution, allowing for better metabolic and fluid overload control, resulting in an increase in TP, LF, and HF power. In contrast, in those that receive a glucose-based dialysis solution, all HRV parameters declined (Orihuela et al., 2014). The different processes undertaken during a dialysis session also impact upon HRV. When the ultrafiltration and diffusion phases of dialysis session are isolated, at the end of the ultrafiltration phase, SDNN, SDANN, and RMSSD are decreased, with the reduction in SDNN positively correlated with the ultrafiltration rate. Throughout the subsequent hemodialysis session, these values return to baseline levels (Galetta et al., 2001).

Beyond the acute response, studies looking at the long-term effects of dialysis therapy show an improvement in HRV. At 3 months following commencement of dialysis therapy, HRV as estimated by time domain (SD, SDNN, and SDANN) improved (Mylonopoulou et al., 2010). Such improvements are also evident at 1 year post commencement dialysis therapy and are observed to a greater extent in patients receiving continuous ambulatory peritoneal dialysis compared with those receiving hemodialysis (Dursun et al., 2004) suggesting that more vigorous regulation of body fluid status and removal of uremic toxins results in a greater improvement in HRV. Supporting this, studies conducted over a 3-year follow-up period indicate that those with a Kt/V* value greater than 1.2 HRV improves. When in the range of 1–1.2 HRV remains mainly unchanged, while in those less than 1 HRV tends to decline (Laaksonen et al., 2000).

21.5.4 Renal Transplantation

The effects of renal transplantation on HRV are variable and certainly, there is no immediate improvement in HRV (Yang et al., 2010). While not consistently observed (Kurata et al., 2004; Parisotto et al., 2008), HRV does appear to improve over the longer term and by 4–6 months post-translation, HRV as measured by frequency-domain estimates is increased (Yildiz et al., 1998; Yang et al., 2010) and by 12 months, both time- and frequency-domain estimates are increased (Rubinger et al., 2009). Interestingly, the delay in HRV improvement does not appear to relate to any ongoing improvements in kidney function. Yang et al. (2010) who examined HRV in transplant recipients over a 6-month follow-up showed that while renal transplantation produced an immediate and sustained reduction in serum creatinine levels noted by 1 month post-transplantation HRV did not improve until 6 months post-transplantation despite the fact that there was no further reduction in serum creatinine levels

---

* Kt/V value: a measure of dialysis adequacy that expresses the volume of dialyser cleared during a dialysis session as a proportion of a patient's body mass made up of water. For dialysis to be adequate, a patient's Kt/V value should be greater than 1.2.

between 1 and 6 months post-transplantation. When patients are stratified on the basis of their pretransplantation HRV levels into patients with low HF power (< 3 In(ms^2)) and high HF power (≥ 3 In(ms^2)), only patients with low HF power showed an improvement in HRV by 6 months post-transplantation (see Figure 21.4). It must be noted, however, that a reduction in HF power, which is a measure of cardiac vagal function (Anonymous, 1996; Stauss, 2003), is not consistently observed in CKD patients (Vita et al., 1999). Nevertheless, early studies using classical tests to examine parasympathetic function, for example, assessment of the expiration/inspiration ratio, supine/standing ratio, and assessment of baroreflex function show that 6-month post-transplantation performance on these tests is improved (Agarwal et al., 1991). Whether similar functional improvements in sympathetic regulation of the cardiovascular system exist is debatable. While metaiodobenzylguanidine imaging* suggests an improvement in sympathetic innervation of the heart as early as 3 months post-transplantation, this does not correlate with any improvement in HRV (Kurata et al., 2004). Although argument exists as to whether the HRV parameters measured (LF and LF/HF) are sufficiently sensitive measures of sympathetic control of the heart (La Rovere et al., 1998; Stauss, 2003), which may explain this discordance, previous studies using more classical measures of sympathetic function (e.g. cold pressor test, blood pressure response to mental arithmetic, or loud noise and plasma noradrenaline levels [Agarwal et al., 1991]) show no improvement in sympathetic function at 6 months post-transplantation. Therefore, the variability that exists with regard to the timing of HRV improvement may relate to the underlying autonomic cause of reduced HRV, with parasympathetic dysfunction resolved at an earlier time point than sympathetic dysfunction.

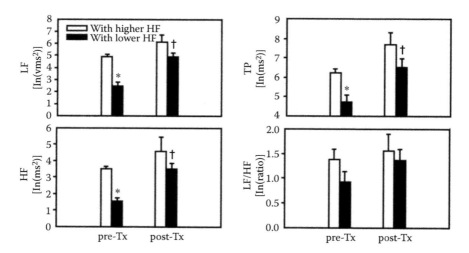

FIGURE 21.4
The power frequency determinations of low frequency (LF), high frequency (HF), total power (TP), LF/HF in end-stage renal disease (ESRD) patients undergoing hemodialysis (pre-TX) and 6 months after renal transplantation (post-Tx). In natural logarithm, variances are presented as mean $\pm$ SE. *$p < .05$ versus ESRD with HF 3 In(ms^2) before renal transplantation, †$p < .05$ versus ESRD patients with HF < 3 In(ms^2) before transplantation. (Reprinted from *Transplantation Proceedings*, 42(5), Yang, W.S et al., Heart rate variability during hemodialysis and following renal transplantation, 1637–1640, Copyright (2010), with permission from Elsevier.)

---

* Metaiodobenzylguanidine (MIBG) imaging: used to image cardiac noradrenaline reuptake and therefore the synaptic availability of noradrenaline at the heart. Reflects sympathetic neurotransmission.

21.6 HRV in Animal Models of CKD

Using the Lewis polycystic kidney (LPK) rat model, our group has used HRV to examine autonomic control of heart rate. The LPK is a rodent model of autosomal recessive cystic kidney disease resulting from a mutation in the never in mitosis gene a—related kinase 8 (*Nek8*) gene (McCooke et al., 2012). This rat model presents with renal cysts by 3 weeks of age, hypertension by at least 6 weeks of age that continues to increase through to 18 weeks of age in parallel with a progressive deterioration in renal function, which becomes significantly compromised by 12 weeks of age (Phillips et al., 2007; Salman et al., 2014). The majority of our work to date has used HRV to investigate autonomic regulation of the heart at 12 weeks of age following the establishment of hypertension yet prior to the development of renal failure. At this particular age, frequency-domain estimates of HRV do not differ in the LPK compared with its control, the Lewis rat, under conscious conditions (Hildreth et al., 2013a). Under anaesthetized conditions, however, all frequency-domain parameters (i.e., TP, VLF, LF, and HF powers) are reduced in the LPK (Harrison et al., 2010). The latter may suggest a greater vulnerability of the autonomic nervous system to general anesthetics in CKD and therefore, potentially, a greater risk of cardiac events during anesthesia.

While at 12 weeks of age, HRV parameters are not altered under conscious conditions, there is an overall decline in HRV as the kidney disease progresses in the LPK. Using radiotelemetry to obtain intra-arterial recordings of blood pressure in conscious LPK from 10 to 16 weeks of age, corresponding with the time frame over which renal function markedly deteriorates in the LPK (Phillips et al., 2007), and examining HRV using the pulse interval, we have demonstrated that the LF component of HRV only is reduced in the LPK (see Figure 21.5; Hildreth et al., 2013b). The lack of any change in HF power in the conscious LPK suggests that vagal control of heart rate, to a large degree, is preserved. Nevertheless, it is probable that sympathovagal balance is altered culminating in an overall decline in the ability of the autonomic nervous system to appropriately regulate heart rate. Supporting this notion, as renal disease progresses in the LPK, baroreceptor reflex control of heart rate declines (Hildreth et al., 2013b; Salman et al., 2014) and the changes in resting heart rate that result following injection of methylatropine, reflective of cardiac vagal tone, are mildly reduced, while that resulting following injection of atenolol, reflective of cardiac sympathetic tone, are greatly increased (see Figure 21.6). This latter finding brings forward an important cautionary note regarding the interpretation of LF power, which is regarded by some as an index of cardiac sympathetic tone, and that LF power may not reflect the degree of sympathetic tone present. This is particularly pertinent to CKD as a disease cohort as sympathetic overactivity is present both patients (Klein et al., 2001, 2003; Grassi et al., 2011) and the LPK rat (Phillips et al., 2007; Salman et al., 2014, 2015), whereas LF HRV power is consistently reported as reduced (Fukuta et al., 2003; Di Leo et al., 2005; Harrison et al., 2010; Suzuki et al., 2012; Hildreth et al., 2013b).

21.7 Concluding Remarks

HRV serves as a useful clinical marker of disease severity and outcome in patients with CKD/ESRD. The underlying cause of reduced HRV for CKD patients remains unknown and is complicated by the large number of covariates that are independently associated

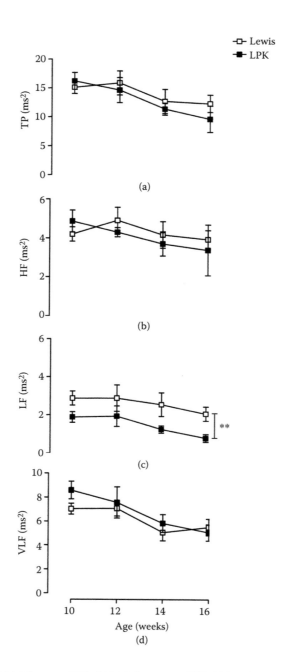

FIGURE 21.5
Fortnightly estimates of (a) total power (TP), (b) high-frequency (HF), (c) low-frequency (LF), and (d) very low-frequency (VLF) components of heart rate variability (HRV) in Lewis polycystic kidney (LPK) and Lewis rats at 10, 12, 14, and 16 weeks of age. Data are the mean $\pm$ SEM. $n = 4$–8 per group. $**p < .01$. (Figure taken from Hildreth, C.M et al., Temporal development of baroreceptor dysfunction in a rodent model of chronic kidney disease. 458–465, 2013. Copyright Wiley-VCH Verlag GmbH & Co. KGaA. Reproduced with permission.)

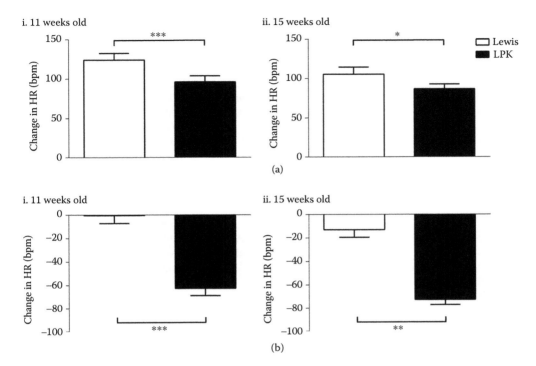

FIGURE 21.6
Comparative changes in heart rate (HR) in response to injection of methylatropine (2 mg/kg i.p.; a) and atenolol (1 mg/kg i.p.; b) in the Lewis and Lewis polycystic kidney (LPK) at 11 and 15 weeks of age. HR was recorded continuously over a 60-minute period following injection and averaged into 5-minute bins. The change in HR was calculated for each 5-minute bin relative to a 5-minute recording immediately prior to injection. Data were analyzed using a two-way ANOVA with strain and time as variables and data presented as the average change in HR over the 60-minute recording period. In both strains, regardless of age, methylatropine (a) produced an increase in HR, the magnitude of which was smaller in the LPK. Conversely, atenolol (b) produced a decrease in HR that was significantly greater in the LPK at both ages studied. $*p < .05, **p < .01, ***p < .001; n =$ minimum 6 per group.

with reduced HRV, the most notable being diabetes, older age and anemia. As HRV improves both in the long-term following dialysis therapy and renal transplantation, the kidney certainly places a driving role in instigating the autonomic dysfunction that contributes to the reduced HRV. Patients with SDNN estimates lower than 75 ms represent those most at risk of all-cause and cardiovascular-related mortality and those with estimates lower than 50 ms are at greater risk of sudden cardiac death. Using HRV to identify "at risk" patients may help to reduce mortality rates, through implementation of lifestyle modification, such as exercise, or more aggressive management of residual renal function.

References

Anonymous (1996). Heart rate variability: Standards of measurement, physiological interpretation and clinical use. Task Force of the European Society of Cardiology and the North American Society of Pacing and Electrophysiology. *Circulation* **93**, 1043–1065.

Agarwal A, Anand IS, Sakhuja V, and Chugh KS (1991). Effect of dialysis and renal transplantation on autonomic dysfunction in chronic renal failure. *Kidney International* **40**, 489–495.

Agelink MW, Malessa R, Baumann B, Majewski T, Akila F, Zeit T, and Ziegler D (2001). Standardized tests of heart rate variability: Normal ranges obtained from 309 healthy humans, and effects of age, gender, and heart rate. *Clinical Autonomic Research* **11**, 99–108.

Axelrod S, Lishner M, Oz O, Bernheim J, and Ravid M (1987). Spectral analysis of fluctuations in heart rate: an objective evaluation of autonomic nervous control in chronic renal failure. *Nephron* **45**, 202–206.

Barbato AL (1990). Bedside evaluation of the autonomic system. In *Clinical Methods: The History, Physical, and Laboratory Examinations*. Walker HK, Hall WD and Hurst JW (ed), Boston: Butterworths.

Barletta GM, Flynn J, Mitsnefes M, Samuels J, Friedman LA, Ng D, Cox C, Poffenbarger T, Warady B, and Furth S (2014). Heart rate and blood pressure variability in children with chronic kidney disease: A report from the CKiD study. *Pediatric Nephrology* **29**, 1059–1065.

Barnas MG, Boer WH, and Koomans HA (1999). Hemodynamic patterns and spectral analysis of heart rate variability during dialysis hypotension. *Journal of the American Society of Nephrology* **10**, 2577–2584.

Bernardi L, Ricordi L, Lazzari P, Solda P, Calciati A, Ferrari MR, Vandea I, Finardi G, and Fratino P (1992). Impaired circadian modulation of sympathovagal activity in diabetes. A possible explanation for altered temporal onset of cardiovascular disease. *Circulation* **86**, 1443–1452.

Brotman DJ, Bash LD, Qayyum R, Crews D, Whitsel EA, Astor BC, and Coresh J (2010). Heart rate variability predicts ESRD and CKD-related hospitalization. *Journal of the American Society of Nephrology* **21**, 1560–1570.

Bruyne MCd, Kors JA, Hoes AW, Klootwijk P, Dekker JM, Hofman A, van Bemmel JH, and Grobbee DE (1999). Both decreased and increased heart rate variability on the standard 10-second electrocardiogram predict cardiac mortality in the elderly: The Rotterdam study. *American Journal of Epidemiology* **150**, 1282–1288.

Burger AJ, D'Elia JA, Weinrauch LA, Lerman I, and Gaur A (2002). Marked abnormalities in heart rate variability are associated with progressive deterioration of renal function in type I diabetic patients with overt nephropathy. *International Journal of Cardiology* **86**, 281–287.

Cashion AK, Holmes SL, Arheart KL, Acchiardo SR, and Hathaway DK (2005). Heart rate variability and mortality in patients with end stage renal disease. *Nephrology Nursing Journal* **32**, 173–184.

Celik A, Melek M, Yuksel S, Onrat E, and Avsar A (2011). Cardiac autonomic dysfunction in hemodialysis patients: The value of heart rate turbulence. *Hemodialysis International* **15**, 193–199.

Chandra P, Sands RL, Gillespie BW, Levin NW, Kotanko P, Kiser M, Finkelstein F, Hinderliter A, Pop-Busui R, Rajagopalan S, and Saran R (2012). Predictors of heart rate variability and its prognostic significance in chronic kidney disease. *Nephrology, Dialysis, Transplantation* **27**, 700–709.

Chandra P, Sands RL, Gillespie BW, Levin NW, Kotanko P, Kiser M, Finkelstein F, Hinderliter A, Rajagopalan S, Sengstock D, and Saran R (2014). Relationship between heart rate variability and pulse wave velocity and their association with patient outcomes in chronic kidney disease. *Clinical Nephrology* **81**, 9–19.

Chou KJ, Lee PT, Chen CL, Chiou CW, Hsu CY, Chung HM, Liu CP, and Fang HC (2006). Physiological changes during hemodialysis in patients with intradialysis hypertension. *Kidney International* **69**, 1833–1838.

Ciriello J and de Oliveira CR (2002). Renal afferents and hypertension. *Current Hypertension Reports* **4**, 136–142.

Connes P and Coates TD (2013). Autonomic nervous system dysfunction: Implication in sickle cell disease. *Comptes Rendus Biology* **336**, 142–147.

Converse RL, Jacobsen TN, Toto RD, Jost CMT, Cosentino F, Fouad-Tarazi F, and Victor RG (1992). Sympathetic overactivity in patients with chronic renal failure. *New England Journal of Medicine* **327**, 1912–1918.

Deligiannis A, Kouidi E, and Tourkantonis A (1999). Effects of physical training on heart rate variability in patients on hemodialysis. *American Journal of Cardiology* **84**, 197–202.

Di Leo R, Vita G, Messina C, and Savica V (2005). Autonomic function in elderly uremics studied by spectral analysis of heart rate. *Kidney International* **67**, 1521–1525.

Drawz PE, Babineau DC, Brecklin C, He J, Kallem RR, Soliman EZ, Xie D, Appleby D, Anderson AH, and Rahman M (2013). Heart rate variability is a predictor of mortality in chronic kidney disease: A report from the CRIC Study. *American Journal of Nephrology* **38**, 517–528.

Dursun B, Demircioglu F, Varan HI, Basarici I, Kabukcu M, Ersoy F, Ersel F, and Suleymanlar G (2004). Effects of different dialysis modalities on cardiac autonomic dysfunctions in end-stage renal disease patients: One year prospective study. *Renal Failure* **26**, 35–38.

Felder RB (1986). Excitatory and inhibitory interactions among renal a cardiovascular afferent nerves in dorsomedial medulla. *American Journal of Physiology* **250**, R580–588.

Fluckiger L, Boivin JM, Quilliot D, Jeandel C, and Zannad F (1999). Differential effects of aging on heart rate variability and blood pressure variability. *Journals of Gerontology. Series A, Biological Sciences and Medical Sciences* **54**, B219–224.

Franzoni F, Galetta F, Di Muro C, Buti G, Pentimone F, and Santoro G (2004). Heart rate variability and ventricular late potentials in beta-thalassemia major. *Haematologica* **89**, 233–234.

Fukuta H, Hayano J, Ishihara S, Sakata S, Mukai S, Ohte N, Ojika K, Yagi K, Matsumoto H, Sohmiya S, and Kimura G (2003). Prognostic value of heart rate variability in patients with end-stage renal disease on chronic haemodialysis. *Nephrology, Dialysis, Transplantation* **18**, 318–325.

Furuland H, Linde T, Englund A, and Wikstrom B (2008). Heart rate variability is decreased in chronic kidney disease but may improve with hemoglobin normalization. *Journal of Nephrology* **21**, 45–52.

Galetta F, Cupisti A, Franzoni F, Morelli E, Caprioli R, Rindi P, and Barsotti G (2001). Changes in heart rate variability in chronic uremic patients during ultrafiltration and hemodialysis. *Blood Purification* **19**, 395–400.

Giordano M, Manzella D, Paolisso G, Caliendo A, Varricchio M, and Giordano C (2001). Differences in heart rate variability parameters during the post-dialytic period in type II diabetic and non-diabetic ESRD patients. *Nephrology, Dialysis, Transplantation* **16**, 566–573.

Goldberger AL and West BJ (1987). Fractals in physiology and medicine. *Yale Journal of Biology and Medicine* **60**, 421–435.

Grassi G, Bertoli S and Seravalle G (2012). Sympathetic nervous system: Role in hypertension and in chronic kidney disease. *Current Opinion in Nephrology and Hypertension* **21**, 46–51.

Grassi G, Quarti-Trevano F, Seravalle G, Arenare F, Volpe M, Furiani S, Dell'Oro R, and Mancia G (2011). Early sympathetic activation in the initial clinical stages of chronic renal failure. *Hypertension* **57**, 846–851.

Harrison JL, Hildreth CM, Callahan SM, Goodchild AK, and Phillips JK (2010). Cardiovascular autonomic dysfunction in a novel rodent model of polycystic kidney disease. *Autonomic Neuroscience* **152**, 60–66.

Hathaway DK, Cashion AK, Milstead EJ, Winsett RP, Cowan PA, Wicks MN, and Gaber AO (1998a). Autonomic dysregulation in patients awaiting kidney transplantation. *American Journal of Kidney Diseases* **32**, 221–229.

Hathaway DK, Cashion AK, Wicks MN, Milstead EJ, and Gaber AO (1998b). Cardiovascular dysautonomia of patients with end-stage renal disease and type I or type II diabetes. *Nursing Research* **47**, 171–179.

Hayano J, Takahashi H, Toriyama T, Mukai S, Okada A, Sakata S, Yamada A, Ohte N, and Kawahara H (1999). Prognostic value of heart rate variability during long-term follow-up in chronic haemodialysis patients with end-stage renal disease. *Nephrology, Dialysis, Transplantation* **14**, 1480–1488.

Hedreville M, Charlot K, Waltz X, Sinnapah S, Lemonne N, Etienne-Julan M, Soter V, Hue O, Hardy-Dessources MD, Barthelemy JC, and Connes P (2014). Acute moderate exercise does not further alter the autonomic nervous system activity in patients with sickle cell anemia. *PLOS ONE* **9**, e95563.

Hering D, Zdrojewski Z, Krol E, Kara T, Kucharska W, Somers VK, Rutkowski B, and Narkiewicz K (2007). Tonic chemoreflex activation contributes to the elevated muscle sympathetic nerve activity in patients with chronic renal failure. *Journal of Hypertension* **25**, 157–161.

Herzog CA, Mangrum JM, and Passman R (2008). Sudden cardiac death and dialysis patients. *Seminars in Dialysis* **21**, 300–307.

Hildreth CM, Goodchild AK, and Phillips JK (2013a). Insight into autonomic nervous system control of heart rate in the rat using analysis of heart rate variability and baroreflex sensitivity. In *Stimulation and Inhibition of Neurons*, vol. 78. Pilowsky PM, Farnham MMJ and Fong AY (eds.), pp. 203–223. New York: Humana Press.

Hildreth CM, Kandukuri DS, Goodchild AK, and Phillips JK (2013b). Temporal development of baroreceptor dysfunction in a rodent model of chronic kidney disease. *Clinical and Experimental Pharmacology and Physiology* **40**, 458–465.

Horl WH (2013). Anaemia management and mortality risk in chronic kidney disease. *Nature Reviews. Nephrology* **9**, 291–301.

Iseki K, Ikemiya Y, Iseki C, and Takishita S (2003). Proteinuria and the risk of developing end-stage renal disease. *Kidney International* **63**, 1468–1474.

Jaiswal M, Urbina EM, Wadwa RP, Talton JW, D'Agostino RB, Jr., Hamman RF, Fingerlin TE, Daniels S, Marcovina SM, Dolan LM, and Dabelea D (2013). Reduced heart rate variability among youth with type 1 diabetes: The SEARCH CVD study. *Diabetes Care* **36**, 157–162.

Johnson DW, Jones GR, Mathew TH, Ludlow MJ, Chadban SJ, Usherwood T, Polkinghorne K, Colagiuri S, Jerums G, Macisaac R, and Martin H (2012). Chronic kidney disease and measurement of albuminuria or proteinuria: A position statement. *Medical Journal of Australia* **197**, 224–225.

Kawada T, Mizuno M, Shimizu S, Uemura K, Kamiya A, and Sugimachi M (2009). Angiotensin II disproportionately attenuates dynamic vagal and sympathetic heart rate controls. *American Journal of Physiology Heart and Circulatory Physiology* **296**, H1666–H1674.

Kidney Health Australia (2012). Chronic Kidney Disease (CKD) Management in General Practice, Melbourne.

Klein IH, Ligtenberg G, Oey PL, Koomans HA, and Blankestijn PJ (2001). Sympathetic activity is increased in polycystic kidney disease and is associated with hypertension. *Journal of the American Society of Nephrology* **12**, 2427–2433.

Klein IHHT, Ligtenberg G, Oey PL, Koomans HA, and Blankestijn PJ (2003). Enalapril and losartan reduce sympathetic hyperactivity in patients with chronic renal failure. *Journal of the American Society of Nephrology* **14**, 425–430.

Kotanko P (2006). Cause and consequences of sympathetic hyperactivity in chronic kidney disease. *Blood Purification* **24**, 95–99.

Kouidi EJ, Grekas DM, and Deligiannis AP (2009). Effects of exercise training on noninvasive cardiac measures in patients undergoing long-term hemodialysis: A randomized controlled trial. *American Journal of Kidney Diseases* **54**, 511–521.

Kuehl M and Stevens MJ (2012). Cardiovascular autonomic neuropathies as complications of diabetes mellitus. *Nature Reviews. Endocrinology* **8**, 405–416.

Kurata C, Uehara A, and Ishikawa A (2004). Improvement of cardiac sympathetic innervation by renal transplantation. *Journal of Nuclear Medicine* **45**, 1114–1120.

Kurata C, Uehara A, Sugi T, Ishikawa A, Fujita K, Yonemura K, Hishida A, Ishikawa K, Tawarahara K, Shouda S, and Mikami T (2000). Cardiac autonomic neuropathy in patients with chronic renal failure on hemodialysis. *Nephron* **84**, 312–319.

La Rovere MT, Bigger JT, Jr., Marcus FI, Mortara A, and Schwartz PJ (1998). Baroreflex sensitivity and heart-rate variability in prediction of total cardiac mortality after myocardial infarction. ATRAMI (Autonomic Tone and Reflexes After Myocardial Infarction) Investigators. *Lancet* **351**, 478–484.

Laaksonen S, Voipio-Pulkki L, Erkinjuntti M, Asola M, and Falck B (2000). Does dialysis therapy improve autonomic and peripheral nervous system abnormalities in chronic uraemia? *Journal of Internal Medicine* **248**, 21–26.

Lin JL, Chan HL, Du CC, Lin IN, Lai CW, Lin KT, Wu CP, Tseng YZ, and Lien WP (1999). Long-term beta-blocker therapy improves autonomic nervous regulation in advanced congestive heart failure: A longitudinal heart rate variability study. *American Heart Journal* **137**, 658–665.

Lin LY, Hwang JJ, Lai LP, Chan HL, Du CC, Tseng YZ, and Lin JL (2004). Restoration of heart rate turbulence by titrated beta-blocker therapy in patients with advanced congestive heart failure: Positive correlation with enhanced vagal modulation of heart rate. *Journal of Cardiovascular Electrophysiology* **15**, 752–756.

Locatelli F, Del Vecchio L, and Cavalli A (2010). How can prognosis for diabetic ESRD be improved? *Semin Dial* **23**, 214–219.

Lurje L, Wennerblom B, Tygesen H, Karlsson T, and Hjalmarson A (1997). Heart rate variability after acute myocardial infarction in patients treated with atenolol and metoprolol. *International Journal of Cardiology* **60**, 157–164.

McCooke JK, Appels R, Barrero RA, Ding A, Ozimek-Kulik JE, Bellgard MI, Morahan G, and Phillips JK (2012). A novel mutation causing nephronophthisis in the Lewis polycystic kidney rat localises to a conserved RCC1 domain in Nek8. *BMC Genomics* **13**, 393.

Molgaard H, Mickley H, Pless P, Bjerregaard P, and Moller M (1993). Effects of metoprolol on heart rate variability in survivors of acute myocardial infarction. *American Journal of Cardiology* **71**, 1357–1359.

Mylonopoulou M, Tentolouris N, Antonopoulos S, Mikros S, Katsaros K, Melidonis A, Sevastos N, and Katsilambros N (2010). Heart rate variability in advanced chronic kidney disease with or without diabetes: Midterm effects of the initiation of chronic haemodialysis therapy. *Nephrology, Dialysis, Transplantation* **25**, 3749–3754.

Nishimura M, Tokoro T, Nishida M, Hashimoto T, Kobayashi H, Yamazaki S, Imai R, Okino K, Iwamoto N, Takahashi H, and Ono T (2010). Sympathetic overactivity and sudden cardiac death among hemodialysis patients with left ventricular hypertrophy. *International Journal of Cardiology* **142**, 80–86.

Oikawa K, Ishihara R, Maeda T, Yamaguchi K, Koike A, Kawaguchi H, Tabata Y, Murotani N, and Itoh H (2009). Prognostic value of heart rate variability in patients with renal failure on hemodialysis. *International Journal of Cardiology* **131**, 370–377.

Ondocin PT and Narsipur SS (2006). Influence of angiotensin converting enzyme inhibitor treatment on cardiac autonomic modulation in patients receiving haemodialysis. *Nephrology (Carlton)* **11**, 497–501.

Orihuela O, de Jesus Ventura M, Avila-Diaz M, Cisneros A, Vicente-Martinez M, Furlong MD, Garcia-Gonzalez Z, Villanueva D, Alcantara G, Lindholm B, Garcia-Lopez E, Villanueva C, and Paniagua R (2014). Effect of icodextrin on heart rate variability in diabetic patients on peritoneal dialysis. *Peritoneal Dialysis International* **34**, 57–63.

Pagani M, Malfatto G, Pierini S, Casati R, Masu AM, Poli M, Guzzetti S, Lombardi F, Cerutti S, and Malliani A (1988). Spectral analysis of heart rate variability in the assessment of autonomic diabetic neuropathy. *Journal of the Autonomic Nervous System* **23**, 143–153.

Parisotto V, Lima EM, Silva JM, de Sousa MR, and Ribeiro AL (2008). Cardiac sympathetic dysautonomia in children with chronic kidney disease. *Journal of Nuclear Cardiology* **15**, 246–254.

Paul M, Poyan Mehr A, and Kreutz R (2006). Physiology of local renin-angiotensin systems. *Physiology Reviews* **86**, 747–803.

Peters CD, Kjaergaard KD, Jensen JD, Christensen KL, Strandhave C, Tietze IN, Novosel MK, Bibby BM, Jensen LT, Sloth E, and Jespersen B (2014). No significant effect of angiotensin II receptor blockade on intermediate cardiovascular end points in hemodialysis patients. *Kidney International* **86**, 625–637.

Phillips JK, Hopwood D, Loxley RA, Ghatora K, Coombes JD, Tan YS, Harrison JL, McKitrick DJ, Holobotvskyy V, Arnolda LF, and Rangan GK (2007). Temporal relationship between renal cyst development, hypertension and cardiac hypertrophy in a new rat model of autosomal recessive polycystic kidney disease. *Kidney and Blood Pressure Research* **30**, 129–144.

Poulsen PL, Ebbehoj E, Hansen KW, and Mogensen CE (1997). 24-h blood pressure and autonomic function is related to albumin excretion within the normoalbuminuric range in IDDM patients. *Diabetologia* **40**, 718–725.

Ripley E (2009). Complementary effects of angiotensin-converting enzyme inhibitors and angiotensin receptor blockers in slowing the progression of chronic kidney disease. *American Heart Journal* **157**, S7–S16.

Robinson TG and Carr SJ (2002). Cardiovascular autonomic dysfunction in uremia. *Kidney International* **62**, 1921–1932.

Rubinger D, Backenroth R, and Sapoznikov D (2009). Restoration of baroreflex function in patients with end-stage renal disease after renal transplantation. *Nephrology, Dialysis, Transplantation* **24**, 1305–1313.

Rubinger D, Backenroth R, and Sapoznikov D (2012). Sympathetic activation and baroreflex function during intradialytic hypertensive episodes. *PLoS One* **7**, e36943.

Rubinger D, Backenroth R, and Sapoznikov D (2013). Sympathetic nervous system function and dysfunction in chronic hemodialysis patients. *Seminars in Dialysis* **26**, 333–343.

Rubinger D, Revis N, Pollak A, Luria MH, and Sapoznikov D (2004). Predictors of haemodynamic instability and heart rate variability during haemodialysis. *Nephrology, Dialysis, Transplantation* **19**, 2053–2060.

Ruggeri P, Battaglia A, Ermirio R, Grossini E, Molinari C, Mary DA, and Vacca G (2000). Role of nitric oxide in the control of the heart rate within the nucleus ambiguus of rats. *Neuroreport* **11**, 481–485.

Salman IM, Hildreth CM, Ameer OZ, and Phillips JK (2014). Differential contribution of afferent and central pathways to the development of baroreflex dysfunction in chronic kidney disease. *Hypertension* **63**, 804–810.

Salman IM, Phillips JK, Ameer OZ, and Hildreth CM (2015). Abnormal central control underlies impaired baroreflex control of heart rate and sympathetic nerve activity in female Lewis Polycystic Kidney rats. *Journal of Hypertension* **33**, 1418–1428.

Sangkatumvong S, Coates TD, and Khoo MC (2008a). Abnormal autonomic cardiac response to transient hypoxia in sickle cell anemia. *Physiological Measurement* **29**, 655–668.

Sangkatumvong S, Khoo MC, and Coates TD (2008b). Abnormal cardiac autonomic control in sickle cell disease following transient hypoxia. *Conference Proceeding IEEE Engineering Medicine and Biology Society* **2008**, 1996–1999.

Sato M, Horigome I, Chiba S, Furuta T, Miyazaki M, Hotta O, Suzuki K, Noshiro H, and Taguma Y (2001). Autonomic insufficiency as a factor contributing to dialysis-induced hypotension. *Nephrology, Dialysis, Transplantation* **16**, 1657–1662.

Sato R, Mizuno M, Miura T, Kato Y, Watanabe S, Fuwa D, Ogiyama Y, Tomonari T, Ota K, Ichikawa T, Shirasawa Y, Ito A, Yoshida A, Fukuda M, and Kimura G (2013). Angiotensin receptor blockers regulate the synchronization of circadian rhythms in heart rate and blood pressure. *Journal of Hypertension* **31**, 1233–1238.

Shigenaga A, Tamura K, Dejima T, Ozawa M, Wakui H, Masuda S, Azuma K, Tsurumi-Ikeya Y, Mitsuhashi H, Okano Y, Kokuho T, Sugano T, Ishigami T, Toya Y, Uchino K, Tokita Y, and Umemura S (2009). Effects of angiotensin II type 1 receptor blocker on blood pressure variability and cardiovascular remodeling in hypertensive patients on chronic peritoneal dialysis. *Nephron Clinical Practice* **112**, c31–40.

Singh JP, Larson MG, O'Donnell CJ, Wilson PF, Tsuji H, Lloyd-Jones DM, and Levy D (2000). Association of hyperglycemia with reduced heart rate variability (The Framingham Heart Study). *American Journal of Cardiology* **86**, 309–312.

Singh JP, Larson MG, Tsuji H, Evans JC, O'Donnell CJ, and Levy D (1998). Reduced heart rate variability and new-onset hypertension: Insights into pathogenesis of hypertension: The Framingham Heart Study. *Hypertension* **32**, 293–297.

Stauss HM (2003). Heart rate variability. *American Journal of Physiology* **285**, R927–R931.

Suzuki M, Hiroshi T, Aoyama T, Tanaka M, Ishii H, Kisohara M, Iizuka N, Murohara T, and Hayano J (2012). Nonlinear measures of heart rate variability and mortality risk in hemodialysis patients. *Clinical Journal of the American Society of Nephrology* **7**, 1454–1460.

Tamura K, Tsuji H, Nishiue T, Yajima I, Higashi T, and Iwasaka T (1998). Determinants of heart rate variability in chronic hemodialysis patients. *American Journal of Kidney Diseases* **31**, 602–606.

Tamura K, Yamauchi J, Tsurumi-Ikeya Y, Sakai M, Ozawa M, Shigenaga A, Azuma K, Okano Y, Ishigami T, Toya Y, Yabana M, Tokita Y, Ohnishi T, and Umemura S (2008). Ambulatory blood pressure and heart rate in hypertensives with renal failure: Comparison between diabetic nephropathy and non-diabetic glomerulopathy. *Clinical and Experimental Hypertension* **30**, 33–43.

Tang W, Li LX, Pei J, and Wang T (2012). Heart rate variability in peritoneal dialysis patients: What is the role of residual renal function? *Blood Purification* **34**, 58–66.

Tong YQ and Hou HM (2007). Alteration of heart rate variability parameters in nondiabetic hemodialysis patients. *American Journal of Nephrology* **27**, 63–69.

Tory K, Horvath E, Suveges Z, Fekete A, Sallay P, Berta K, Szabo T, Szabo AJ, Tulassay T, and Reusz GS (2004). Effect of propranolol on heart rate variability in patients with end-stage renal disease: A double-blind, placebo-controlled, randomized crossover pilot trial. *Clinical Nephrology* **61**, 316–323.

Umetani K, Singer DH, McCraty R, and Atkinson M (1998). Twenty-four hour time domain heart rate variability and heart rate: Relations to age and gender over nine decades. *Journal of the American College of Cardiology* **31**, 593–601.

van Dijk JG, Koenderink M, Zwinderman AH, Haan J, Kramer CG, and den Heijer JC (1991). Autonomic nervous system tests depend on resting heart rate and blood pressure. *Journal of the Autonomic Nervous System* **35**, 15–24.

Vaseghi M and Shivkumar K (2008). The role of the autonomic nervous system in sudden cardiac death. *Progress in Cardiovascular Diseases* **50**, 404–419.

Verdalles U, Abad S, Aragoncillo I, Villaverde M, Jofre R, Verde E, Vega A, and Lopez-Gomez JM (2010). Factors predicting mortality in elderly patients on dialysis. *Nephron Clinical Practice* **115**, c28–34.

Vita G, Bellinghieri G, Trusso A, Costantino G, Santoro D, Monteleone F, Messina C, and Savica V (1999). Uremic autonomic neuropathy studied by spectral analysis of heart rate. *Kidney International* **56**, 232–237.

Wirta OR, Pasternack AI, Mustonen JT, Laippala PJ, and Reinikainen PM (1999). Urinary albumin excretion rate is independently related to autonomic neuropathy in type 2 diabetes mellitus. *Journal of Internal Medicine* **245**, 329–335.

Yamamoto K, Kobayashi N, Kutsuna T, Ishii A, Matsumoto T, Hara M, Aiba N, Tabata M, Takahira N, and Masuda T (2012). Excessive fall of blood pressure during maintenance hemodialysis in patients with chronic renal failure is induced by vascular malfunction and imbalance of autonomic nervous activity. *Therapeutic Apheresis Dialysis* **16**, 219–225.

Yang YW, Wu CH, Tsai MK, Kuo TB, Yang CC, and Lee PH (2010). Heart rate variability during hemodialysis and following renal transplantation. *Transplantation Proceedings* **42**, 1637–1640.

Yildiz A, Sever MS, Demirel S, Akkaya V, Turk S, Turkmen A, Ecder T, and Ark E (1998). Improvement of uremic autonomic dysfunction after renal transplantation: A heart rate variability study. *Nephron* **80**, 57–60.

Yokusoglu M, Nevruz O, Baysan O, Uzun M, Demirkol S, Avcu F, Koz C, Cetin T, Hasimi A, Ural AU, and Isik E (2007). The altered autonomic nervous system activity in iron deficiency anemia. *Tohoku Journal of Experimental Medicine* **212**, 397–402.

Ziegler D, Laux G, Dannehl K, Spuler M, Muhlen H, Mayer P, and Gries FA (1992). Assessment of cardiovascular autonomic function: Age-related normal ranges and reproducibility of spectral analysis, vector analysis, and standard tests of heart rate variation and blood pressure responses. *Diabetic Medicine* **9**, 166–175.

Zitt E, Neyer U, Meusburger E, Tiefenthaler M, Kotanko P, Mayer G, and Rosenkranz AR (2008). Effect of dialysate temperature and diabetes on autonomic cardiovascular regulation during hemodialysis. *Kidney and Blood Pressure Research* **31**, 217–225.

22

Beat-to-Beat Variability of Cardiomyocytes

Helmut Ahammer, Brigitte Pelzmann, Klaus Zorn-Pauly, Robert Arnold, and Michael Mayrhofer-Reinhartshuber

CONTENTS

22.1 Introduction

Heart rate (HR) constantly changes on a beat-to-beat basis due to autonomic influences on the pacemaker process of the sinoatrial node. These changes can be quantified as heart rate variability (HRV). In principle, HRV is caused by complex nonlinear interactions between sinoatrial node cells and the autonomic nervous system. However, a certain degree of beat-to-beat variability (BBV) is also intrinsically present—not only on the level of isolated heart but although within the isolated sinoatrial node and even at the level of the single sinoatrial node cell (Lombardi and Stein 2011; Papaioannou et al. 2013; Zaniboni et al. 2014). Intrinsic BBV was also studied in spontaneously beating embryonic chick heart cells (Clay and DeHaan 1979) and neonatal rat ventricular cells (Ponard et al. 2007) since both show fluctuating beat-to-beat intervals. Diminished HRV is a common clinical phenotype expressed by critically ill patients and has been already proven as a valuable prognostic tool in human neonatal sepsis (Griffin et al. 2005; Moorman et al. 2011). Particularly, in clinical conditions associated with systemic inflammation like in multiorgan dysfunction syndrome and sepsis, a reduction in HRV and an increase in cardiac cycle regularity are crucial (Godin et al. 1996; Rassias et al. 2005). For instance, reduction in both variability and regularity could be observed in human volunteers that were subjected to endotoxemia (Godin et al. 1996). Currently, it is not well known whether a reduced HRV in sepsis rather reflects an altered input from the autonomic nervous system or a remodeling of the sinoatrial node cells. Experimental evidence suggests that a loss of interorgan communication may be important for HRV reduction in sepsis (Godin et al. 1996; Scheff et al. 2012). The pacemaker channel comprises an important final common pathway for autonomic HR regulation translating autonomic input into sinus node pacemaking. This mixed cation current (Na^+ and K^+) carried by HCN channels contributes to the diastolic depolarization in the action potential of sinoatrial node cells and is therefore a potential contributor to alterations in HR characteristics in sepsis. Sepsis is induced by lipopolysaccharide (LPS), an endotoxin and a major component of the outer cell wall of Gram-negative bacteria. We recently reported a massive reduction of HCN channel availability under elevated endotoxin levels (Zorn-Pauly et al. 2007; Scheruebel et al. 2014) possibly impairing the response of the pacemaker current to autonomic fluctuations. LPS was also shown to reduce intrinsic BBV. Contractility measurements in neonatal rat myocytes demonstrated a narrowing of BBV under the influence of LPS (Schmidt et al. 2007). Further, in measuring action potentials in spontaneously beating chick embryonic ventricular myocytes, we could show that LPS decreases (1) the firing rate and (2) the BBV by applying entropy as well as fractal estimators (Ahammer et al. 2013).

Measuring BBV of isolated cells *in vitro* instead of HRV *in vivo* provides standardized biological conditions and therefore interpretations of underlying mechanisms and functions may be easily determined. On the other side, HRV can most often be analyzed directly using standard electrocardiogram data streams, whereas BBV must be measured in an experimental setup. However, two data acquisition methods can be accomplished without extensive effort: transmembrane electrode measurement techniques and optical video capturing.

22.2 Methods

22.2.1 Cell Isolation

Ventricular myocytes were isolated from embryonic chick hearts as previously described and modified (Koidl et al. 1980; Pelzmann 1996). Hearts of 7-day embryos were removed, and the ventricles were chopped off, minced, and transferred to flasks containing 0.25% trypsin (bovine pancreas; Boehringer Mannheim, Deisenhofen, Germany) in a nominally Ca^{2+}- and Mg^{2+}-free Hanks' balanced salt solution (HBSS; in mM: 137 NaCl, 5.4 KCl, 0.34 Na_2HPO_4, 0.44 KH_2PO_4, 4.2 $NaHCO_3$, and 5 glucose, pH 7.4). The flasks were placed in a shaker bath at 37° C for 7 minutes. The resulting cell suspension was gently agitated with a pipette and filtered through a 100-μm mesh to dissociate the cells from tissues and cell clumps. HBSS supplemented with fetal calf serum (5% final concentration) was added to stop trypsin activity. The cell suspension was centrifuged at ∼100 g for 5 minutes at 4°C, the supernatant was discarded, and the cell pellet was resuspended in fresh trypsin-free HBSS two times. After the third centrifugation step cells were resuspended in cell culture medium (M199 [Sigma] supplemented with 4% fetal calf serum, 2% horse serum, and

0.7 mM glutamine, pH 7.4) to yield a density of 5×10^5 cells/mL. The cell suspension was transferred to plastic culture dishes that were incubated at 37° C in a water-saturated atmosphere of 95% air and 5% CO_2. Muscle cells were separated by this procedure from nonmuscle cells by the differential attachment technique due to the adherence of nonmuscle cells to the culture dishes. Aliquots (0.6 mL) of the cell suspension containing the nonadhesive cardiomyocytes were transferred after 0.5–2 days to cell culture dishes (Greiner, Austria) containing microscope slide coverslips. This procedure allowed the myocytes to adhere to the glass surface, where they could divide and form small clusters of cells. Experiments were performed on small clusters 12–36 hours after the cells were plated.

22.2.2 Electrode Measurements

Intracellular recordings of spontaneous action potentials were performed with glass micropipettes (microelectrodes). Glass capillaries with filaments were used to pull microelectrodes with a very small tip pore diameter of 0.3 µm or less in order to prevent ion exchange between the intracellular fluid and the pipette filling solution. Microelectrodes were filled with 3 M KCl and had a resistance of 10–30 MΩ. For action potential recording, the coverslip with attached myocytes was placed in an experimental chamber of an inverted microscope (Zeiss, Axiovert). Cells were superfused with extracellular solution (in mM: 137 NaCl, 5.4 KCl, 1.8 $CaCl_2$, 1.1 $MgCl_2$, 2.2 $NaHCO_3$, 0.4 NaH_2PO_4, 10 Na-HEPES, and 5.6 glucose, with pH adjusted to 7.4 with NaOH) at 36–37°C with a flow rate of 1.5 mL/min. Impalement of the microelectrodes was established by mechanical force, that is, by guiding the microelectrode with a hydraulic three-dimensional (3D) micromanipulator to the cell under the microscope until the microelectrode penetrated the cell membrane.

22.2.2.1 Signal Recording

Microelectrodes were connected to a battery operated amplifier (Electro 705, WPI, Sarasota, FL). The reference electrode for potential measurements was a chlorided silver wire immersed into the experiment chamber. Electrical signals were digitized using a USB-powered analog to digital converter (NI USB-6210, National Instruments, Austin, TX) with a sample rate of 50 kHz and a resolution of 16 bit. Online monitoring was performed with custom written software (LabVIEW, National Instruments, Austin, TX). Signal data were stored in a DADiSP (DSP Development Corporation, Newton, MA) compatible binary format.

22.2.2.2 Determining the Beat-to-Beat Interval from Electrode Measurement

Action potentials recorded from spontaneously beating cells showed a steep upstroke phase when the cell was activated. This upstroke from –20 mV to +20 mV allowed the determination of the instance of time at which a cell was activated by a simple threshold criterion. For this work, a threshold of 0 mV was used.

After detection of all consecutive beats within a signal recording, beat-to-beat intervals were calculated as differences in milliseconds between the actual beat and the previous beat.

22.2.3 Video Analysis

Microscopic techniques are commonly used in order to visualize biological tissues or cells. Beside aspects of magnification, illumination, and resolution, the most important parameter in order to visualize beating single cells is contrast. Obviously, contrast should be as high as possible. Several illumination techniques such as bright field illumination, axial illumination, oblique illumination, dark field illumination, and Rheinberg illumination show distinct values of contrast, but actually contrast of cells with thickness of about 10 μm is not very high for all of these techniques. Improved contrast can be achieved by specimen staining, especially by using fluorescence dyes, or by using phase contrast, polarized light, and differential interference contrast (DIC). Second to contrast, it is important to record images that show a decent intensity change, at least on a restricted area, for beating cells. Particularly, staining techniques of living cells are prone to intensity variations due to high interexperiment variabilities. Usually, polarized light configurations as well as DIC show less intensity changes and therefore, phase contrast seems to be very appropriate.

Using inverted microscopes and appropriate equipment to keep cells alive, it is usually very convenient to observe living cells at least for time spans of several minutes or even more. Digital cameras for still images as well as video cameras can be easily mounted using standardized mechanical interfaces, for example, C-mounts. Therefore, with microscopes, spontaneously beating cardiomyocytes can be investigated by manual inspection as well as by video recording. Obviously, manual inspection can only be used to determine the overall status or health of cells. Quantitative evaluations are very limited and particularly BBV cannot be treated or investigated satisfactorily. Otherwise, digital recordings of images or image sequences allow postprocessing and storage of data.

Taking and analyzing videos seems to be appropriate for BBV analyses but care has to be taken in order to set parameters properly. Modern equipment paired with user-friendly software allows the recording of videos without considering detailed settings, but certainly these videos most often cannot be used for quantitative evaluations. It is absolutely necessary to adjust parameters involved accordingly. The most important parameters are region of interest (ROI), recording length, frame rate, and data compression. A detailed description of these parameters follows, because they limit the huge range of equipment, which is offered by several manufacturers.

22.2.3.1 Region of Interest

The microscope's field of view depends on the magnification as well as additional optical elements such as mirrors or lenses in the optical path. Most often the field of view recognized by eye through the ocular lens is not the same size as the field of view of the digital camera, simply because of separated optical paths. The field of view of the camera may be smaller than the field of view of the ocular lens. However, this discrepancy should not be an issue as long as the camera captures the whole of a single cell's body or even more. If the field of view of the camera captures more than a single cell, it might be advisable to reduce this field. Otherwise, background material is recorded, increasing the amount of memory needed without adding useful information. Field of view can be reduced to the part of an image that shows the most prominent intensity change caused by cell contraction. Narrowing down a ROI very close to the strongest contracting area inside the field of view seems to be appropriate, but overall (slow) movement of a cell on the glass during the total recording time can lead to a relative displaced position of the ROI at the end of the recording. A compromise between memory consumption and high recording quality during the whole recording process must be found.

22.2.3.2 Recording Length

Standards for measuring of HRV were defined by the task force of the European Society of Cardiology and the North American Society of Pacing and Electrophysiology (Malik et al. 1996). Accordingly, short-term recordings should last 5 minutes and long-term recordings 24 hours. Naturally, HRV *in vivo* is not identical to BBV of cells *in vitro*, but nevertheless, a strong relation between these two measures is biologically obvious. Standards or regulations for *in vitro* assays do not exist and therefore it seems appropriate to fulfill at least the task force's standards if possible.

Short-term recordings of isolated cells can be performed routinely with the microelectrode technique (at least 5 minutes), but according to experience, long-term recordings cannot be achieved since the impalement of myocytes possibly impairs a cell's vitality. Video recordings offer the possibility of long-term recordings, but in practice, high-speed recordings of more than several minutes might lead to an enormous memory demand, which would be unmanageable. Details of frame rate settings will be described in the next section.

It might be worth considering a reduction of recording time to 5/2 or maybe 5/3 minutes because the resting HR of embryonic cardiomyocytes is often two to three times higher compared to human. With a recording length of 5 minutes and a resting HR of 1 Hz, a total number of 300 beats will be recorded, leading to 300 beat-to-beat durations or in other words to 300 data points for subsequent data analyses. A total of 300 data points is quite enough for conventional statistics such as mean, variances, and so on, but for nonlinear analyses, such as calculation of fractal dimensions or entropies, this number is rather low. Therefore, we conclude that the recording length of video analyses for BBV studies should preferably not be smaller than 5 minutes.

22.2.3.3 Frame Rate

The number of images taken per second for commercial videos or home entertainment must be higher than the human visual system can separately recognize. Then a smooth and fluid viewing experience is maintained. In order to fulfill this requirement, the European PAL and French SECAM systems work with 25 full images per second (50 half images/second) and the American NTSC format uses 30 full images per second (60 half images/second). There exist a vast number of subsystems implementing slightly changed specifications. Additionally, videos can be recorded by using several data format containers, with or without compression.

A frame rate of 25 Hz (25 full images/second) is undoubtedly quite enough to get an adequate subjective viewing experience, but for following quantitative and mathematical analyses, it is simply too low for analysis of BBV. Each single image must be considered as a single data point in between a beat and the next beat. In order to measure the beat-to-beat duration, it is absolutely necessary to get enough data points (images) between two beats. Assuming a resting beat rate of 1 Hz, the duration of one beat to the next beat is obviously 1 second. Since Shannon, we know that a sampling frequency of 2 Hz (500 milliseconds sampling time) is enough to reconstruct a continuous 1 Hz signal. Unfortunately, in the case of beat-to-beat durations and analyses of their variations, Shannon's theorem cannot be applied. It is mandatory to get the duration time of every single beat as accurate as possible and a sample frequency much higher than two times the average signal frequency is needed. For every beat, the time point (time stamp) of, for example, the maximal contraction of the cell must be determined. The difference between two time points gives the beat-to-beat duration. Assuming an accuracy of 1%, 100 images must be taken from one beat to the next. This leads to a sampling duration of 10 milliseconds or a sampling frequency of 100 Hz. Accordingly, this means a frame rate of 100 frames per second (fps). Table 22.1 shows some values for the video frame rate depending on accuracy of measurements and on the resting beat rate. Obviously, the frame rate demand increases further with increasing resting beat rate.

It can clearly be seen in the table that common video frame rates up to 30 Hz would lead to far too high errors. An accuracy of only 10% would lead to an error of 100 milliseconds at a resting beat rate of 1 Hz. An erroneous variation of 100 milliseconds for an average duration of 1 second is far too high in order to reputably investigate beat-to-beat variations.

In summary, a minimum frame rate of at least 100 fps for the video recording should be used and common frame rates of 25 Hz or 30 Hz should be avoided. Some low-cost devices can be operated with higher frame rates, maybe up to 150 Hz, but preferably, higher frame rates should be used and hence, only very expensive high-speed camera systems can be used.

Several systems, especially low-cost cameras, show an additional severe source of error, which must be mentioned. These cameras are usually connected to a computer (PC or laptop) via USB or FireWire interfaces. Video capturing software handles the camera settings such as the frame rate, recording time, ROI settings, and so on. Interactively, the recording can be started and after the preset time, the record stops automatically. Although it seems that low-cost systems are appropriate to record beating cells in order to investigate BBV, a closer look reveals their inadequacy. The main aspect that must be considered is the absolute time duration between two recorded images. Unfortunately, these time durations are not exact. The main reason is that a computer is not a measurement device; it is rather a multitasking information processing unit. A computer is steadily operating several tasks and it is not guaranteed that time intervals between captured images have exactly the same length.

Experiments with an USB-connected camera and a theoretical sampling time of 100 milliseconds showed sporadically erroneous image-to-image intervals of up to 160 milliseconds. This led to a smaller number of total recorded images, too. In brief, the physical and real-time interval between two subsequent images should have an exact value, but low-cost systems cannot ensure this demand. A varying or sporadically increased image-to-image interval might subjectively not be visible during viewing a video but introduces an artificial variation and statistics for beat-to-beat measurements. These variations and their statistics overlay with the physiological statistics and introduce errors, which must be avoided.

TABLE 22.1

Video Recording Frame Rates for Several Accuracies and Resting Beat Rates

	Resting Beat Rate		
Accuracy	1 Hz	2 Hz	3 Hz
10%	10 fps	20 fps	30 fps
1%	100 fps	200 fps	300 fps
0.1%	1000 fps	2000 fps	3000 fps

Note: fps, frames per second

Therefore, only high-speed camera systems ensuring exact image-to-image time durations are appropriate. The software should only provide an interactive graphical user interface (GUI) to set parameters and should trigger hardware, which records the images directly to a hard disk.

22.2.3.4 Data Compression

Consumer cameras for taking video as well as still images usually compress images in order to save storage space. Unavoidably, lossy compression formats, for example, JPEG and others, introduce color as well as intensity artifacts. These artifacts may prevent exact quantitative analyses, because very often calculations directly using gray values of an image are performed. As an example, the co-occurrence matrix of gray value pairs at a distinct distance can be used to calculate several statistical second-order parameters such as energy, entropy, correlation, homogeneity, and others. For such calculations, lossy compression should be avoided.

Fortunately, moderate compression artifacts are not crucial when videos are taken in order to determine the times from beat to beat of a beating cell. For measuring the time duration between two subsequent beats, it is necessary to find characteristic subsequent time points (images) with the most changing gray values. Local distributions of gray values are not important as an image is always treated as a whole. Having stated this, it must be mentioned that excessive compression should be avoided, as undesirable and disturbing gray value fluctuations may occur. Compression rates can be set manually (e.g., for the JPEG codec) and should be compared initially to uncompressed data evaluations.

22.2.3.5 Determining the Beat-to-Beat Interval from Video Streams

After recording a video with the required parameters and quality, video and signal analyses have to be applied to obtain the beat-to-beat intervals.

The aim of the video analysis is to perform the described data reduction, that is, to obtain a single one-dimensional (1D) time signal out of the huge amount of images of the recorded video.

If the analyzed video was perfect for analysis, straightforward and simple image calculations would produce satisfying results. The most obvious method would be to compare the pixel values of each frame with the corresponding pixel values of the first frame of the video, for example, for each frame to calculate the difference of each gray value to the value of the same pixel in the first frame and sum up over all absolute values of these differences. These types of procedures work fine for perfect videos in which the sample (cell) holds exactly its position and background, illumination, and so on do not change throughout the whole recording. However, problems arise due to deviations from this perfect recording, having their origins in a broad variety of different influences, which are described in detail in Section 22.2.3.2. To overcome these challenges, the following more advanced procedure was implemented in MATLAB®.

In a first step, the whole video, containing N images $I_i (i = 1 \ldots N)$, was divided into $k = 1 \ldots K$ shorter sequences (subsequences), denoted by $\{I_j^k\}$ and with j as image index of images inside the subsequence k. The subsequence lengths were manually chosen in a way that they contain at least one full beat. Within each of these subsequences k, our algorithm searched for two frames showing different states, one frame that represents the baseline, that is, no contraction, $B^k <$ and one that represents the maximum contraction of the cell, M^k. First, a difference image of these two images was calculated for each subsequence k:

$$D^k = \left| M^k - B^k \right|$$

From this difference image, all pixel positions $p = (x, y)$, where $D^k(p)$ shows an absolute value larger than a given threshold t_1, were determined:

$$P^k = \{p^k\} := \{p \mid D^k(p) > t_1\}$$

These pixels were used for calculating a 1D signal in the following manner.

From the baseline frame B^k of the actual subsequence k to the baseline frame B^{k+1} of the next subsequence, difference images of each frame of the subsequence k with the baseline frame were calculated:

$$D^k_j = \left| I^k_j - B^k \right|$$

Based on these difference images, a set of pixel positions belonging to $k-1$, k, or $k+1$ and having a value larger than a threshold t_2 were selected for the actual "measurement":

$$P^m = \{p^m\} := \{p \in \{P^{k-1}, P^k, P^{k+1}\} \mid D^k_j(p) > t_2\}$$

The values of D^k_j at these positions were summed up to obtain a single data point s^k_j of the signal:

$$s^k_j = \sum_{p \in P^m} \text{Gray value}(D^k_j(p))$$

The resulting time signal S^k for a subsequence k was then the set of all individual sums s^k_j:

$$S^k = \{s^k_j\}$$

To take into account the different numbers of pixels contributing to each subsequence and data point, all elements s^k_j of the set S^k were normalized with

$$s^k_j = \frac{s^k_j - \min(S^k)}{\max(S^k)}$$

Thus, the baseline had a value around 0 and the maximum value, that is, during maximum contraction, was 1.

Finally, this was calculated for all K subsequences to obtain a set of time signals:

$$S = \{S^{k=1}, \dots, S^{k=K}\}$$

With the time signals S, the beat-to-beat time intervals were extracted using signal analysis routines in intelligent quality management (IQM; Kainz et al. 2015). First, outliers in the time signal may be treated with mean or median filtering techniques. Then two different techniques were applied to determine the intervals. Results obtained by using a manually defined threshold were compared to results obtained by using a more advanced but still simple to implement moving average curve (MAC) algorithm (Lu et al. 2006). For this study, the manual threshold and also the offset value for the MAC algorithm were set to 0.5 for the normalized signals.

22.2.3.6 Quantitative Analysis of BBV

Electrode measurements as well as video analyses give 1D data point series of interbeat intervals. These time series can similarly be analyzed as *in vivo* measured normal-to-normal heartbeat intervals NN. Therefore, time-domain methods such as the standard deviation of the NN interval (SDNN) or the number of pairs of adjacent NN intervals differing by more than 50 milliseconds (NN50) can be calculated. Frequency-domain methods such as powers in distinct frequency ranges (very low frequency [VLF], low frequency [LF], and high frequency [HF]) or ratios of these (LF/HF) are appropriate, too.

Recently, nonlinear methods, such as calculations of entropies or fractal dimensions, have also become popular. Entropies measure disorder whereas fractal dimensions measure space-filling properties of the system under investigation. Both measures are useful in order to measure the complexity of a system by analyzing a measured 1D time signal. Although complexity is not exactly defined, it is widely accepted that it should have low values for very regular and deterministic systems and it should have higher values for more irregular (e.g., nonlinear) systems. For very irregular systems (e.g., random distributions), the concept of complexity is still not clear. The first group of concepts for complexity involves measures that show the highest value for randomly distributed signals. Contrarily, the second group of concepts shows very low values for highly irregular (random) signals. Although the second group of concepts may sound more intuitive and natural, the first group of concepts has far more concrete implementations and has very successfully been applied for several decades. Therefore, in order to not overcomplicate this study, we leave out the concepts of the second group.

Within the first group of complexity concepts, particularly the approximate entropy as well as the sample entropy should be mentioned (Lake et al. 2002). The sample entropy is an extension of the approximate entropy in order to avoid data point length dependencies. Therefore, approximate entropy should be avoided for electrode measurements, because individual records usually have different lengths. Video recordings can have constant data series lengths, but interstudy comparisons may suffer from this aspect, too. Therefore, calculation of the sample entropy should be preferred.

Fractal dimensions, also belonging to the first group of complexity concepts, can be calculated by performing phase space reconstructions or by direct time-domain methods. Direct time-domain methods seem to be preferable, because they are very well suited for short data point series. Phase space reconstructions, on the other hand, need a lot of data points and are most often very prone to noise. Higuchi (1988) proposed a very robust method to determine the fractal dimension by summing up differences of data points at distinct distances in between. Furthermore, it is well suited for short data point series.

22.3 Challenges

22.3.1 Electrode Measurements

For data analysis, signal recordings of at least 5 minutes are desired as stated above. During this period of time, the impalement of the microelectrode has to be stable to acquire usable data. Experience has shown that small movements of the cells due to the flow of extracellular bath solution as well as the contraction movement itself force the tip of the microelectrodes out of the cells and render the acquired data useless. After loss of impalement, it is not recommended to repeat the measurement with the same cell since obviously the cell membrane is damaged and the vitality of the cell cannot be guaranteed anymore. Hence, a new spontaneously beating cell has to be found and impalement of the microelectrode has to be repeated, which makes the procedure very time consuming.

22.3.2 Video Analysis

Although it seems straightforward and easy to implement, video analysis of beating cells is not that easy to accomplish. A single image out of a video stream can be interpreted as a time stamp of the temporal beating signal. Each single image gives only one single value of the current state of the cell and nothing more. Then, several of these single values are used to define a beat-to-beat interval. Data reduction is therefore enormous. A typical image of 500×500 pixels has 2.5×10^5 image pixels. Measuring with a minimum frame rate of 100 fps and an assumed average beat rate of only 1 Hz, we get on average 100 images per beat-to-beat interval. Therefore, 2.5×10^7 data points reduce to only one value for the beat-to-beat interval. For higher frame rates or higher beat rates, this reduction ratio is further increased. This enormous amount of data reduction involves sophisticated hardware as well as software algorithms. Minimum frame rates must be high enough in order to measure the beat intervals with high enough accuracy and therefore, high-speed capturing video recording systems are necessary.

The quality of the extractable data is strongly dependent on the quality of the recorded video. Hence, previous to any analysis of the video stream, creating optimal settings during the recording, for example, spatial and temporal constant illumination, is important.

Computational effort is often rather high in video analysis and depends among other things on the image size. Therefore, in a first step, the analyzed region in a video may be reduced by introducing a ROI, which contains only important data for analysis, that is, the cell or conglomerate of cells under investigation (sample), still keeping in mind a possible overall movement of the sample during recording time. These ROIs may either be set manually or automatically. Automated setting and possible adjustment of ROIs during the process of video analysis is difficult due to the different and changing shapes of the investigated samples and requires sophisticated image and video analysis algorithms. However, satisfying results can be obtained with a far less complex manual setting of a fixed ROI.

Several other challenges arise due to the experimental setup and the sample itself. To obtain a useful and reliable outcome, the following points have to be handled by the video analysis software:

1. The video may start during a contraction, that is, the first frame cannot be taken as a reference.
2. The sample may move (usually slowly) during the recording, for example, due to the flow of extracellular bath solution.
3. The video may suffer from jittering, for example, due to vibration of the sample, camera, etc. and digitalization effects (e.g., the border of the cell may "jump" from one pixel to its neighbor and vice versa).
4. The intensity of the contraction may vary, that is, the number of pixels from which the beats can be extracted may change during recording.
5. Small and moving impurities (dust or air bubbles) may be present in all or some parts of the video.

6. The stream of the extracellular bath solution may create flickering and brighter and darker areas due to optical effects.

Also after the conversion of the video into a time signal, problems have to be tackled. The extraction from the beat-to-beat intervals can be performed by applying different algorithms such as simple thresholding or MAC. The slope of each beat peak is finite and changes both within the peak and from peak to peak. Hence, the choice of method may influence the outcome. Therefore, the obtained results must be treated carefully and different methods should be compared for differences (e.g., by using different values for the manually set threshold or comparing a manually set threshold with MAC).

22.4 Discussion

The crucial and most challenging aspect of measurements with microelectrodes is the establishment of stable impalements over a long period of time. To improve stability, floating microelectrodes could be used. Therefore, the microelectrodes are not rigidly attached to the amplifier system but are attached with a thin silver wire (approximately 100 μm diameter) to the amplifier system. This allows the microelectrode to float with the contraction movement within a small range and ensures stable impalement. However, with this method, the microelectrode has to be positioned directly above the cell, which means at least partly blocking the optical path.

Another crucial aspect concerns data analysis. Beat-to-beat intervals have to be determined with high accuracy. The currently used simple threshold criterion to determine the activation time of the cell only performs reasonably when (1) the upstroke is steep enough and (2) the signal waveform is constant over the measurement period.

Video and signal analyses were used to convert the videos into time signals and extract beat-to-beat intervals subsequently. The most challenging aspects in video analysis were to get rid of the disturbing influences from the (slow) movement of the cells and the variations of contraction intensity during recording time.

These challenges were tackled by an algorithm that divided the whole video into shorter subsequences, in which pixels with maximum differences between minimum and maximum contraction were identified and used to extract the time signal for every subsequence individually. Subsequently, they were merged to obtain the full-time signal.

As mentioned previously in the context of measurements with microelectrodes, in the subsequent time signal analysis, the methods used to determine the beat-to-beat intervals from the time signals have certain performance characteristics that are only reasonable if the signals fulfill specific criteria (steep upstroke and similar shape of the beats).

Statistical analyses of BBVs can be performed by using identical algorithms for investigating HRVs. Conditions and requirements are quite similar and accordingly, interpretations and conclusions can be made similarly. Calculations of the sample entropy and the Higuchi dimension seem to be especially appropriate and probably will give reliable results.

However, future developments may strengthen on analyses, specially constructed for BBVs. Specialized algorithms could overcome limitations of varying signal lengths for electrode measurements or may include more of the huge amount of image data for video streams.

References

Ahammer, H., S. Scherubel, R. Arnold, K. Zorn-Pauly, and B. Pelzmann. 2013. Beat to beat variability of embryonic chick heart cells under septic conditions: Application and evaluation of entropy as well as fractal measures. In *2013 35th Annual International Conference of the IEEE Engineering in Medicine and Biology Society (EMBC)*, 5566–69. doi:10.1109/EMBC.2013.6610811.

Clay, J. R. and R. L. DeHaan. 1979. Fluctuations in interbeat interval in rhythmic heart-cell clusters—Role of membrane voltage noise. *Biophysical Journal* 28 (3): 377–89.

Godin, P. J., L. A. Fleisher, A. Eidsath, R. W. Vandivier, H. L. Preas, S. M. Banks, T. G. Buchman, and A. F. Suffredini. 1996. Experimental human endotoxemia increases cardiac regularity: Results from a prospective, randomized, crossover trial. *Critical Care Medicine* 24 (7): 1117–24.

Griffin, M. P., D. E. Lake, and J. R. Moorman. 2005. Heart rate characteristics and laboratory tests in neonatal sepsis. *Pediatrics* 115 (4): 937–41.

Higuchi, T. 1988. Approach to an irregular time-series on the basis of the fractal theory. *Physica D* 31 (2): 277–83.

Kainz, P., M. Mayrhofer-Reinhartshuber, and H. Ahammer. 2015. IQM: An extensible and portable open source application for image and signal analysis in java. *PLOS ONE* 10 (1): e0116329. doi:10.1371/journal.pone.0116329.

Koidl, B., H. A. Tritthart, and S. Erkinger. 1980. Cultured embryonic chick heart cells: Photometric measurement of the cell pulsation and the effects of calcium ions, electrical stimulation and temperature. *Journal of Molecular and Cellular Cardiology* 12 (2): 165–78. doi:10.1016/0022-2828(80)90086-3.

Lake, D. E., J. S. Richman, M. P. Griffin, and J. R. Moorman. 2002. Sample entropy analysis of neonatal heart rate variability. *American Journal of Physiology-Regulatory Integrative and Comparative Physiology* 283 (3): R789–97.

Lombardi, F. and P. K. Stein. 2011. Origin of heart rate variability and turbulence: An appraisal of autonomic modulation of cardiovascular function. *Frontiers in Physiology* 2 (December). doi:10.3389/fphys.2011.00095.

Lu, W., M. M. Nystrom, P. J. Parikh, D. R. Fooshee, J. P. Hubenschmidt, J. D. Bradley, and D. A. Low. 2006. A semi-automatic method for peak and valley detection in free-breathing respiratory waveforms. *Medical Physics* 33 (10): 3634–36.

Malik, M., J. T. Bigger, A. J. Camm, R. E. Kleiger, A. Malliani, A. J. Moss, and P. J. Schwartz. 1996. Heart rate variability standards of measurement, physiological interpretation, and clinical use. *European Heart Journal* 17 (3): 354–81.

Moorman, J. R., W. A. Carlo, J. Kattwinkel, R. L. Schelonka, P. J. Porcelli, C. T. Navarrete, E. Bancalari, J. L. Aschner, M. Whit Walker, J. A. Perez, C. Palmer, G. J. Stukenborg, D. E. Lake, and T. Michael O'Shea. 2011. Mortality reduction by heart rate characteristic monitoring in very low birth weight neonates: A randomized trial. *Journal of pediatrics* 159 (6): 900–906.e1. doi:10.1016/j.jpeds.2011.06.044.

Papaioannou, V. E., A. O. Verkerk, A. S. Amin, and J. M. T. de Bakker. 2013. Intracardiac origin of heart rate variability, pacemaker funny current and their possible association with critical illness. *Current Cardiology Reviews* 9 (1): 82–96.

Pelzmann, B. 1996. Die wirkung von bariumionen auf spontanaktivität und ionenströme isolierter embryonaler hühnerherzventrikelzellen. Doctoral dissertation, Graz, Austria: Karl-Franzens University.

Ponard, J. G. C., A. A. Kondratyev, and J. P. Kucera. 2007. Mechanisms of intrinsic beating variability in cardiac cell cultures and model pacemaker networks. *Biophysical Journal* 92 (10): 3734–52. doi:10.1529/biophysj.106.091892.

Rassias, A. J., P. T. Holzberger, A. L. Givan, S. L. Fahrner, and M. P. Yeager. 2005. Decreased physiologic variability as a generalized response to human endotoxemia. *Critical Care Medicine* 33 (3): 512–19.

Scheff, J. D., P. D. Mavroudis, P. T. Foteinou, S. E. Calvano, and I. P. Androulakis. 2012. Modeling physiologic variability in human endotoxemia. *Critical Reviews in Biomedical Engineering* 40 (4): 313–22.

Scheruebel, S., C. N. Koyani, S. Hallström, P. Lang, D. Platzer, H. Mächler, K. Lohner, E. Malle, K. Zorn-Pauly, and B. Pelzmann. 2014. If blocking potency of ivabradine is preserved under elevated endotoxin levels in human atrial myocytes. *Journal of Molecular and Cellular Cardiology* 72 (100): 64–73. doi:10.1016/j.yjmcc.2014.02.010.

Schmidt, H., J. Saworski, K. Werdan, and U. Müller-Werdan. 2007. Decreased beating rate variability of spontaneously contracting cardiomyocytes after co-incubation with endotoxin. *Journal of Endotoxin Research* 13 (6): 339–42. doi:10.1177/0968051907086233.

Zaniboni, M., F. Cacciani, and R. L. Lux. 2014. Beat-to-beat cycle length variability of spontaneously beating uinea pig sinoatrial cells: Relative contributions of the membrane and calcium clocks. *PLOS ONE* 9 (6): e100242. doi:10.1371/journal.pone.0100242.

Zorn-Pauly, K., B. Pelzmann, P. Lang, H. Mächler, H. Schmidt, H. Ebelt, K. Werdan, B. Koidl, and U. Müller-Werdan. 2007. Endotoxin impairs the human pacemaker current I_f. *Shock* 28 (6): 655–61.

23

Associations between Genetic Polymorphisms and Heart Rate Variability

Anne Voigt, Jasha W. Trompf, Mikhail Tamayo, Ethan Ng, Yuling Zhou, Yaxin Lu, Slade Matthews, Brett D. Hambly, and Herbert F. Jelinek

CONTENTS

23.1 Aim

In this chapter, we review and discuss the influence of genetic polymorphisms on heart rate variability (HRV). One of the first studies that investigated the heritability of HRV patterns compared age-matched twins. The successful correlation found between genetic markers and HRV opened the possibility of identifying further genetic risks for cardiovascular diseases (CVDs) by studying other genetic polymorphisms that may be associated with HRV.

23.2 Genetic Polymorphisms

Since the first mapping of chromosomes and their association with mutations in *Drosophila melanogaster* (Hunt 1910; Sturtevant 1913), the biomedical field has turned its attention to the effect of genetic polymorphism and their associated diseases. The identification of disease risk genes now allows for a possible earlier diagnosis based on genetic polymorphisms, especially if it is a single gene polymorphism, and a more informed prognosis. Many genetic polymorphisms are currently being used as direct targets for treatment of diverse diseases, but also need to be considered when prescribing medication, due to possible gene product interaction with the medication (Ma and Lu 2011).

Differences in the genetic sequence between individuals, or genetic polymorphisms, make up the foundation of diversity in biological organisms. Genetic polymorphisms require at least two variants in the population of a species, of which the least common one cannot be explained by recurrent mutations (Ford 1965). These polymorphisms have been studied using mostly restriction fragment length polymorphisms (RFLPs) and microsatellite markers. RFLP is based on the use of restriction enzymes, which cut the DNA sequence at a known position in order to compare the length of the sequence fragments between individuals (Botstein et al. 1980). RFLP was first used in 1983 for the mapping of the Huntington disease gene (Gusella et al. 1983). Micro- and mini-satellite markers (variable number of tandem repeats [VNTRs]) mark repetitive DNA sequences, which include repeated DNA motifs and have also been studied for gene mapping (Ellegren 2004).

Methods for genetic analysis have relied on polymorphisms for more than two decades, but the current focus has shifted to single nucleotide polymorphisms (SNPs). This is the most common type of genetic variation in humans and is defined as a position in the sequence with at least two variants. The rarer variant has a frequency of at least 1%. SNPs are quite common and can be found as 1:1000 base pairs (bp) in the human genome. They are used in clinical tests, forensics, and, as in the case of HRV, to identify genes related primarily to CVD, but have also been shown to be important in renal disease and psychosis (Wang et al. 1998). SNP mapping has become cheaper and more efficient with the development of new methods. Mapping started with Sanger DNA sequencing and is now moving on to alternative methods, such as pyrosequencing. Unlike Sanger sequencing, which is time-consuming, labor-intensive, and requires labeling, pyrosequencing is efficient and the time necessary for the detection of SNPs has been significantly decreased. This makes pyrosequencing an ideal method for the comparison of variants in large-scale screening tests. It is based on the detection of fluorescence in proportion to the correct number of nucleotides incorporated into the sequence (Fodor et al. 1991; Southern at al, 1992; Ronaghi et al. 1998).

23.3 Heart Rate Variability

HRV is the temporary variation between sequences of consecutive heartbeats. On an electrocardiogram (ECG), it is observed as the successive RR interval of adjacent QRS complexes. This variability is produced by continuous changes to the sympathetic and parasympathetic balance of heart rhythm (Nasimi and Hatam 2011). It is a reflection of the many physiological factors that alter the baseline rhythm of the heart.

HRV can be interpreted as a quantitative indication of the heart's ability to adapt to changes in the internal and external environment such as posture, anxiety, and weather conditions. The heart needs to quickly and efficiently respond to stimuli in order to compensate for any stressors that may impede normal bodily function. HRV analysis is a good measure of cardiac health and in some cases the state of the autonomic nervous system

(ANS), which is responsible for maintaining proper cardiac activity (Acharya et al. 2006). Abnormalities in HRV, however, can also be associated with brainstem pathology such as Parkinson's disease and cortical dysfunction, including depression and schizophrenia, as well as interactions between the peripheral and central nervous system, which through intricate neurological connectivity patterns lead to a change in ANS regulation of the heart (Baguley 2008; Russell 2010; Kemp et al. 2012; Barbieri et al. 2013; Schulz et al. 2015).

23.4 Techniques to Measure HRV

HRV can be evaluated from an ECG trace recorded from patients in a supine position. In this method, a continuous ECG is recorded and the QRS complex is detected. The first step in analysis is the removal of nonsinus beats and artefacts (Pumprla et al. 2002). After this editing, the RR intervals are recorded and various calculations can be made. The simplest method involves time-domain measures. Calculations include the mean RR interval, mean heart rate (HR), and the difference between the shortest and longest RR interval. The simplest variable to calculate is the standard deviation of the RR intervals (SDNN index). This can be achieved by plotting a histogram of the RR duration against the number of RR intervals. It is generally measured over a 2-minute to 24-hour time period and encompasses short-term high-frequency (HF) variations and low-frequency (LF) variations, providing a nonspecific, global measure of variation (Malik 1998). Another technique of measuring HRV is frequency-domain analysis. This is usually presented graphically by plotting the amount of variation in a recording on the y-axis against the frequency on the x-axis. The area under the curve at different frequencies is a quantitative measure of the amount of HF and LF cyclical variability in the recording This is a basic representation of how variance, also known as "power," distributes as a function of frequency (Pumprla et al. 2002) and encompasses short-term HF variations and LF power variations, providing a nonspecific, global measure of HRV (Malik 1998).

23.5 Neuropathies

Neuropathies result from functional disruption and pathologic changes in the nervous system. The molecular basis of neuropathies is complex and a number of pathological mechanisms are believed to be involved in the disease progression. These include disorders of polyol metabolisms, disorders of fatty acid metabolism, accumulation of glycated proteins, endoneuronal ischemia/hypoxia, destruction of nerve growth factors and axonal transport, immunological processes, and oxidative stress (Schönauer et al. 2011). Changes in the biochemical environment, in conjunction with genetic predisposition and environmental factors, can lead to peripheral as well as central nervous system neuropathy. Diabetes is an example of changes in the blood biochemistry possibly caused by hyperglycemia and oxidative stress, which affects peripheral ANS and peripheral somatic nerve function.

Environmental and genetic factors contribute to the onset and development of complications associated with diabetes, such as neuropathy, which leads to diffuse and widespread damage of peripheral nerves and small vessels (Vinik et al. 2003). The mechanisms for the development of diabetic neuropathies remain unknown, though the causes are most likely multifactorial and involve environmental and lifestyle factors, as well as genetic predisposition.

The widespread distribution of the ANS means that virtually all organs are affected by diabetic autonomic neuropathy, making the understanding of the genetic basis vital for improved methods of treatment and diagnosis (Witzel et al. 2015). The nerves innervating the cardiovascular system are usually affected first (Rolim et al. 2008), making it an option for a clinical marker for diagnosis. Autonomic neuropathy includes clinical symptoms such as resting tachycardia, postural hypotension, abnormal pupillary responses, gastroparesis, and impotence (Said 2007).

23.6 Cardiac Autonomic Neuropathy

Cardiac autonomic neuropathy (CAN) is a common autonomic dysfunction and plays a large role in both type 1 (T1DM) and type 2 diabetes mellitus (T2DM) complications, by contributing a significant cause of mortality through increasing cardiac arrhythmias and leading in many cases to sudden death (Pop-Busui 2010).

The T2DM patients inherit a variety of different genetic factors that together with environmental factors can be additive and increase the risk of complications such as diabetic CAN. However, not only long-term diabetic patients with lack of good glycemic control are affected. Patients with near optimal glycemic control have also been seen to develop complications, despite the application of risk management strategies (Kennon et al. 1999). This implies genetic factors contribute to the susceptibility for cardiovascular complications, such as genetic polymorphisms in candidate genes.

There are various noninvasive ways to measure CAN. Five cardiovascular reflex tests are most often used and known as the Ewing battery maneuver (Ewing et al. 1985). The Ewing battery, however, cannot be used if patients have cardiorespiratory disease and/or are extremely obese, frail, or arthritic.

Candidate genes, copy number, and genetic variants likely interact with epigenetic and microRNA systems to influence biological pathway products associated with disease risk. This involves association mapping to identify marker alleles present at different frequencies in cases possessing a trait versus control.

23.7 Genome-Wide Association

Genome-wide association studies (GWAS) apply a case-control approach, examining the genetic variants in a large number of individuals. This enables the identification of a variant that can be associated with a disease (Kuivaniemi et al. 2014). The focus lies on SNPs, which are inherited and therefore offer an ideal marker for mapping any genetic variation in individuals. This approach suffers from the limited ability to reach statistical significance as well as complications arising from the multitude of SNPs involved. A large number of participants are necessary for this approach, making it impractical for recruitment of participants if the disease is rare. Currently, in the diabetic field, GWAS has been applied to the studies of T2DM, retinal, and renal vascular complications (Hindorff 2014).

The alternative method for discovery of pathological genetic changes is the candidate gene approach. This method involves the genotyping of key genes, using SNP haplotypes, then testing the phenotype of the SNP haplotypes. The candidate gene approach takes advantage of information on gene location and function of the protein product. Positive association or linkage of the gene to the disease implies they are correlated.

23.8 Genetics in HRV

Interest in the genetic background of HRV increased when it was realized that many CVDs, such as blood pressure (BP) and steady-state HR, have a genetic background. In 1996, Voss et al. applied a twin study to the search for a genetic component in HRV and the influence of genetics on the different HRV measures. This provided clinicians with a phenotype for patients at risk for cardiac arrhythmia and evidence for the genetic heredity of HRV. However, the frequency-domain parameters included in the Voss et al. study were not linked to genetic differences or family background. Studies on HRV were expanded in the following years, with HRV turning into a more precise marker by introducing different HRV analysis methods and parameters that were more robust against the nonstationarity and nonlinearity inherent in the HR over time in order to assess the risk of CVDs, such as coronary heart disease (CHD). Reduced total HRV was linked to an increase in risk of sudden cardiac death (SCD) (Bigger et al. 1992). On this basis, Sinnreich et al. (1998) examined the familial association of HRV indices. The HRV indices had been determined using short-Holter recordings. They discovered a significant correlation between parent and offspring, providing further evidence for familial resemblance and a genetic contribution to individual differences in HRV.

Research continued to focus on the genetic background of HRV and soon the question arose of whether chronic diseases exacerbate the underlying genetic background of HRV. Uusitalo et al. (2007) focused on how environmental and somatic factors affected HRV in a population-based study in middle-aged men. Age contributed largely to a negative effect on HRV, except for LF/HF. Body mass index (BMI) and medication were also shown to influence HRV. With these findings, Uusitalo et al. were able to make a case for the influence of environmental factors on HRV, alongside the genetic aspects, which would be important to identify specific effectors on cardiac health.

Since the heredity of HRV had been demonstrated numerous times, it was and still is necessary for research to focus on the specific genes influencing HRV. Extensive rodent studies were able to identify the first batch of candidate genes. Kreutz et al. (1997) led the development in this field when they found a link between a locus on chromosome 3 in rats, thought to correspond to a K^+-channel, and HR regulation. Howden et al. (2008) delved deeper into rodent studies on HRV, despite the ambiguity which could be found in the literature between findings of genetics in HR regulation and HRV (Campen et al. 2002; Hoit et al. 2002; Tankersley et al. 2002; Tankersley et al. 2007). They based their study on inbred strains of mice and focused on the within- and between-strain differences in HR and HRV. With this, they were among the first to systematically examine the genetic factors involved and provided a basis for the study of the specific interactions between underlying pathways and genotypes in HR.

23.9 Candidate Genes Involved in HRV

23.9.1 Angiotensin-Converting Enzyme

Attention has largely been focused on genes encoding the angiotensin-converting enzyme (ACE). In diabetic neuropathy and HRV variability, it has been identified as a candidate gene in regard to its role in HRV. Differences in ACE concentration in plasma between individuals were linked to a major gene polymorphism (Rigat et al. 1990). ACE is a central player in the renin–angiotensin system (RAS) (Kennon et al. 1999), a cardiovascular regulatory system, which regulates cardiovascular function and BP (Nishikino et al. 2006). RAS has been shown to be elevated in patients with metabolic syndrome (MetS) (Sharma 2004), suggesting a link to CAN. ACE is involved in the activation of angiotensin II (Ang II), through which vascular contraction, renal function, fluid homeostasis, and sympathetic nerve activity are regulated. Ang II also leads to the production of reactive oxygen species (ROS), increasing oxidative stress and damaging NO synthases (Elton et al. 2010).

The polymorphism is associated with ACE levels found in the plasma of patients and refers to the presence (insertion, denoted I) or absence (deletion, denoted D) of a 287-bp sequence of DNA in intron 16 of the ACE gene (rs4340) (Gayagay et al. 1998). The highest levels of ACE can be found in the homozygous DD genotype, followed by the ID and II genotypes (Agerholm-Larsen et al. 2000). Though the successful inhibition of ACE in hypertension (HT) and CVD treatments has made it an obvious choice as a candidate gene to be studied for influence of genetic factors, it is unclear how the different ACE genotypes are associated with pathology. Positive association between the ACE polymorphism and carotid intima-media thickness has been reported in one study (Sayed-Tabatabaei et al. 2006), while being refuted in another (Islam et al. 2006). Part of the controversial nature of the ACE polymorphism is the fact that while it is intronic, which leads to its removal in the splicing process, it is still able to exert a functional effect in the form of higher plasma levels of ACE. Its absence drives the change in ACE plasma levels and proven by a number of studies, which were able to show that the ACE DD genotype exhibits higher rates of Ang I to Ang II conversion (Ueda et al. 1995; Buikema et al. 1996).

It is still unclear how the DD genotype is responsible for the higher levels of ACE observed and a number of explanations have been brought forward. In the 1990s, it was first suggested that the effect of the ACE I/D polymorphism may be the result of a linkage disequilibrium with another adjacent gene (Cambien et al. 1994). The degree of linkage disequilibrium between the D allele and some other variant of the gene could cause this upregulation (Schunkert 1997). Simultaneously, it was proposed that the higher levels resulted from different splicing patterns. ACE pre-mRNA would either include the sequence (insertion) or it would be absent (deletion) after differential splicing, altering the mature RNA and therefore modifying the final product (Rigat et al. 1990). The insertion itself could then change the splicing process of ACE precursor mRNA by interfering with the lariat formation step (Smith et al. 1989). Though the mechanisms are still unknown, it is believed that the observed genetic influence in serum levels of ACE is based on differences at the transcriptional level (Schunkert 1997). More recently, it has been proposed that the insertion/deletion itself is likely not to play a direct part in controlling ACE transcription, but rather forms a linkage disequilibrium with regulatory elements of the ACE gene (Schunkert 1997).

The influence of the genetic variation in ACE on HRV has mostly been studied in its relation to the effect it has on HRV measurements and analysis in combination with diabetes.

Diabetes is closely linked to CVD by accelerating atherosclerosis through an increase in oxidative stress, constant low-level inflammation, and endothelial dysfunction (Matheus et al. 2013; Maschirow et al. 2015). The DD genotype has been shown to be related to an increase in HRV and could hence be shown to be heritable (Busjahn et al. 1998). Yet, the I/D genotype does not influence HRV following a myocardial infarction (Steeds et al. 2002). The II genotype in T2DM was specifically associated with autonomic imbalance in HRV measures, denoted by a decrease in LF. Noting that HRV is also decreased significantly in subjects with CAN, the link between obesity, autonomic imbalance, and T2DM will be likely to make screening of HRV beneficial for patients. The assessment of genetic risk factors contributing to CAN adds another dimension to prognosis and treatment procedures.

In summary, the ACE I/D polymorphism is of growing interest in the field of clinical research. Its physiological consequences have been recognized as an important factor in the development of numerous CVDs. Various other studies have highlighted the interactions between gene polymorphisms and myocardial infarction, coronary artery disease, obesity, MetS, and most importantly in the context of this study, T2DM and CAN.

Unfortunately, the literature on the nature of the interaction between the ACE I/D polymorphism and CVD has been inconsistent when examined on a global scale. Still it can safely be concluded from these findings that ACE influences HRV in combination with diabetic status and consequential neuropathies (Marzbanrad et al. 2014). Diabetic and genetic status of the ACE gene has been shown to be significantly linked to the HRV measures: entropy, total power, LF power, SD1, SD2, RMSSD, and SDNN. This implies that genetic variants in genes, which are assumed to play a role in diabetic neuropathies, will need to be considered for their effect on HRV in consideration of a patient's pathological (diabetic) status (Marzbanrad et al. 2014).

23.9.2 Transcription Factor 7-Like 2 (TCF7L2) Gene Polymorphisms

TCF7L2 gene polymorphisms have shown a strong association with an increased risk of T2DM in European populations. Additionally, research suggests that certain TCF7L2 polymorphisms are specifically linked to CAN among other diabetes-related complications, including retinopathy and coronary artery disease.

TCF7L2 is a DNA-binding transcription factor that plays an important role in canonical Wnt signaling by binding β-catenin. Wnt signaling has defined roles in determining cell fate, survival, proliferation, and movement, and has a recognized function in embryonic development as well as carcinogenesis (Savic et al. 2011). Furthermore, and with particular importance to diabetes, Wnt signaling attenuates the synthesis of GLP-1 by intestinal L cells. GLP-1 is insulinotropic and also mimics insulin in glucose regulation, energy homeostasis, and food intake. Consequently, it is proposed that TCF7L2 gene variants may predispose individuals to T2DM by indirectly altering GLP-1 levels. Indeed, TCF7L2 polymorphisms are correlated with impaired GLP-1-induced insulin secretion and pancreatic β-cell function (Loos et al. 2007; Boccardi et al. 2010). However, direct links between HRV and this gene polymorphism have not yet been reported.

23.9.3 Choline Transporter—CHT1

The process of high-affinity choline uptake into cholinergic nerve terminals provides choline as a substrate for synthesis of the neurotransmitter acetylcholine (ACh) by the enzyme choline acetyltransferase (ChAT). Cholinergic neurons transmit signals to a variety

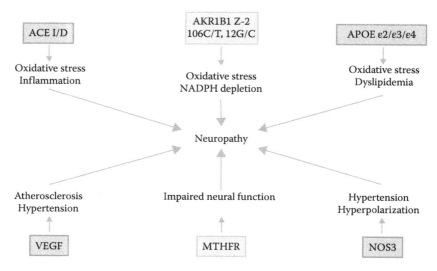

FIGURE 23.1
Effects of common genetic variants linked to diabetic neuropathies. (From Witzel, I. I. et al., *Front Endocrinol (Lausanne)*, 6, 88, 2015.)

of target cells in the central and peripheral nervous systems, and thus are involved in numerous biological processes, including the autonomic innervation of the heart. In the central and peripheral nervous systems, choline transporter (CHT) is expressed almost exclusively in cholinergic neurons (Black and Rylett 2012). Presently only one study has shown a link with a polymorphism in CHT and HRV (Neumann et al. 2005). Another study investigated the same polymorphism in diabetics with CAN; interestingly, a correlation was seen suggesting a role of CHT1 in CAN (Parson 2011).

23.9.4 Other Potential Polymorphisms That May Link to HRV

Figure 23.1 refers to a number of polymorphisms that have been linked to diabetic neuropathies that are known to be linked to CAN, by using methods other than HRV (Witzel et al. 2015). Thus, associations of polymorphisms of these genes with HRV should be investigated. These genes include the aldose reductase gene (AKRB1), apolipoprotein E (APOE), 5,10-methylene-tetrahydrofolate reductase (MTHFR), nitric oxide synthase (NOS3), and vascular endothelial growth factor (VEGF) (Witzel et al. 2015).

A number of other genetic polymorphisms that may influence HRV, but with tenuous evidence, have been identified in the literature and can be found in the Table 23.1.

23.10 The Future: Epigenetics in HRV

Focus has shifted from providing evidence for the genetic heritability of HRV to the specific genes involved in leading to interindividual differences. Naturally, the next step will be to study the influence of environmental factors in HRV and how they affect genes via

TABLE 23.1

Genes Linked to Heart Rate Regulation, Heart Rate Variability, and HRV-Related Cardiovascular Diseases

Gene	Polymorphism	Influences	References
Direct influence on HRV parameter			
CYP11B2 AT1R	C344T A1166C	LF/HF in supine position	Stolarz et al. (2004)
ApoE	Isoforms: E2, E3, E4	HRV change in mental stress	Ravaja et al. (1997)
Angiotensin II Receptor T1	A11666C	↑ SDNN	Mitro et al. (2008)
GSTT1 null	I105V	↓ HRV	Probst-Hensch et al. (2008)
AKAP 10	I646V	↑ resting HRV; ↓ HRV (SDNN)	Tingley et al. (2007)
LQT1, LQT4	To be identified	QTc interval with congenital long QT syndrome	Busjahn et al. (1999)
KCNH2 (HERG)	K897T	Max QT interval	Pietila et al. (2002)
Influence on heart rate regulation			
SCN2A	Locus: HR-SP1	HR regulation	Kreutz et al. (1997)
Influence on cardiovascular diseases			
NSD1	Reference Table 1	Congenital heart defects	Cecconi et al. (2005)
F12	C46T	↓ (c) FXII, myocardial infarction; coronary artery disease	Roldan et al. (2005)
ZC3H12A	To be identified	MCP1 induced protein; ischemic heart disease	Gombojav et al. (2008)
ET2	A985G	Hypertension	Sharma et al. (1999)
CAV3	To be identified	Cardiac myocyte hypertrophy	Cribbs et al. (2001)

AKAP 10, A kinase anchoring protein 10; ApoE, Apolipoprotein E; AT1R, type-1 angiotensin II receptor; CAV3, caveolin-3 muscle-specific protein; CYP11B2, aldosterone synthase; ET2, endothelin 2; F12, coagulation factor XII; GSTT1, glutathione S-transferase 1; HERG, human ether-a-go-go-related gene; NSD1, nuclear receptor SET domain containing gene 1; SCN2A, type-2 voltage-gated sodium channel; ZC3H12A, zinc finger CCCH type containing 12A.

epigenetics. Epigenetic changes have influenced how pathological conditions are perceived and treated. Mechanisms include histone modification, in which the amino end of the histones is changed through methylation, phosphorylation, and so on (Pinney and Simmons 2012), inducing activation or repression of transcription and DNA methylation, which can trigger gene activation as well as repression (Jayaraman 2012). These two mechanisms have the ability to influence each other, for example, methylation of Lysine 9 on histone 3 leads to an increase in DNA methylation. Noncoding RNAs, such as miRNAs, have also been identified as epigenetic gene regulators.

Epigenetic modifications have been shown to influence diseases such as diabetes, with maternal nutrition or gestational diabetes influencing the risk of diabetes in offspring (Jayaraman 2012; Pinney and Simmons 2012; Lehnen et al. 2013).

It can be safely assumed that in addition to continuing candidate gene studies, research on HRV will move on to the effects of epigenetics and focus on treating those with an epigenetic predisposition to the disease accordingly before the onset of complications.

23.11 Conclusions

The research focus on HRV will enable us to gain a better understanding of diabetic neuropathies and will help create a model to better understand the causes of diabetic neuropathies. Early subclinical detection of diabetic neuropathy, by assessing genetic predisposition as well as metabolic control and physiology of diabetic patients, is critical in facilitating early intervention and prevention of the potentially serious consequences of diabetic neuropathy. Current studies are still not informative enough and limited by a lack of reproducibility and insufficient statistical power. It will be necessary to increase the sample sizes in future studies in order to access current genetic risk factors. Once this has been achieved, the development of a pathway model will elucidate how these risk factors may be contributing to diabetic neuropathies by interacting in as yet unknown ways. The knowledge of genetic polymorphisms will also allow accurate quantification of T2DM risk in order to develop models of pathogenesis, which hold diagnostic and prognostic potential.

References

Acharya, R., R. V. Patwardhan, D. R. Smith, B. K. Willis, M. Fowler, and A. Nanda. 2006. Intraspinal synovial cysts: A retrospective study. *Neurol India* 54 (1):38–41.

Agerholm-Larsen, B., B. G. Nordestgaard, and A. Tybjaerg-Hansen. 2000. ACE gene polymorphism in cardiovascular disease: Meta-analyses of small and large studies in whites. *Arterioscler Thromb Vasc Biol* 20 (2):484–92.

Baguley, I. J. 2008. The excitatory:inhibitory ratio model (EIR model): An integrative explanation of acute autonomic overactivity syndromes. *Med Hypotheses* 70 (1):26–35. doi: 10.1016/j.mehy.2007.04.037.

Barbieri, R., L. Citi, and G. Valenza 2013. Increased instability of heartbeat dynamics in Parkinson´s disease. *Comp Cardiol* 40:89–92.

Bigger, J. T., Jr., J. L. Fleiss, R. C. Steinman, L. M. Rolnitzky, R. E. Kleiger, and J. N. Rottman. 1992. Frequency domain measures of heart period variability and mortality after myocardial infarction. *Circulation* 85 (1):164–71.

Black, S. A. and R. J. Rylett. 2012. Choline transporter CHT regulation and function in cholinergic neurons. *Cent Nerv Syst Agents Med Chem* 12 (2):114–21.

Boccardi, V., I. Ambrosino, M. Papa, D. Fiore, M. R. Rizzo, G. Paolisso, and M. Barbieri. 2010. Potential role of TCF7L2 gene variants on cardiac sympathetic/parasympathetic activity. *Eur J Hum Genet* no. 18 (12):1333–8. doi: 10.1038/ejhg.2010.117.

Botstein, D., R. L. White, M. Skolnick, and R. W. Davis. 1980. Construction of a genetic linkage map in man using restriction fragment length polymorphisms. *Am J Hum Genet* 32 (3):314–31.

Buikema, H., Y. M. Pinto, G. Rooks, J. G. Grandjean, H. Schunkert, and W. H. van Gilst. 1996. The deletion polymorphism of the angiotensin-converting enzyme gene is related to phenotypic differences in human arteries. *Eur Heart J* 17 (5):787–94.

Busjahn, A., H. Knoblauch, H. D. Faulhaber, T. Boeckel, M. Rosenthal, R. Uhlmann, M. Hoehe, H. Schuster, and F. C. Luft. 1999. QT interval is linked to 2 long-QT syndrome loci in normal subjects. *Circulation* 99 (24):3161–4.

Busjahn, A., A. Voss, H. Knoblauch, M. Knoblauch, E. Jeschke, N. Wessel, J. Bohlender, J. McCarron, H. D. Faulhaber, H. Schuster, R. Dietz, and F. C. Luft. 1998. Angiotensin-converting enzyme and angiotensinogen gene polymorphisms and heart rate variability in twins. *Am J Cardiol* 81 (6):755–60.

Cambien, F., O. Costerousse, L. Tiret, O. Poirier, L. Lecerf, M. F. Gonzales, A. Evans, D. Arveiler, J. P. Cambou, G. Luc et al. 1994. Plasma level and gene polymorphism of angiotensin-converting enzyme in relation to myocardial infarction. *Circulation* 90 (2):669–76.

Campen, M. J., Y. Tagaito, T. P. Jenkins, P. L. Smith, A. R. Schwartz, and C. P. O'Donnell. 2002. Phenotypic differences in the hemodynamic response during REM sleep in six strains of inbred mice. *Physiol Genomics* 11 (3):227–34. doi: 10.1152/physiolgenomics.00031.2002.

Cecconi, M., F. Forzano, D. Milani, S. Cavani, C. Baldo, A. Selicorni, C. Pantaleoni, M. Silengo, G. B. Ferrero, G. Scarano, M. Della Monica, R. Fischetto, P. Grammatico, S. Majore, G. Zampino, L. Memo, E. L. Cordisco, G. Neri, M. Pierluigi, F. D. Bricarelli, M. Grasso, and F. Faravelli. 2005. Mutation analysis of the NSD1 gene in a group of 59 patients with congenital overgrowth. *Am J Med Genet A* 134 (3):247–53. doi: 10.1002/ajmg.a.30492.

Cribbs, L. L., B. L. Martin, E. A. Schroder, B. B. Keller, B. P. Delisle, and J. Satin. 2001. Identification of the t-type calcium channel (Ca(v)3.1d) in developing mouse heart. *Circ Res* 88 (4):403–7.

Ellegren, H. 2004. Microsatellites: Simple sequences with complex evolution. *Nat Rev Genet* 5 (6): 435–45. doi: 10.1038/nrg1348.

Elton, T. S., S. E. Sansom, and M. M. Martin. 2010. Cardiovascular disease, single nucleotide polymorphisms; and the renin angiotensin system: Is there a microRNA connection? *Int J Hypertens* 2010. doi: 10.4061/2010/281692.

Ewing, D. J., C. N. Martyn, R. J. Young, and B. F. Clarke. 1985. The value of cardiovascular autonomic function tests: 10 years experience in diabetes. *Diabetes Care* 8 (5):491–8.

Fodor, S. P., J. L. Read, M. C. Pirrung, L. Stryer, A. T. Lu, and D. Solas. 1991. Light-directed, spatially addressable parallel chemical synthesis. *Science* 251 (4995):767–73.

Ford, E. B. 1965. *Genetic Polymorphism*. London: Faber and Faber.

Gayagay, G., B. Yu, B. Hambly, T. Boston, A. Hahn, D. S. Celermajer, and R. J. Trent. 1998. Elite endurance athletes and the ACE I allele—The role of genes in athletic performance. *Hum Genet* 103 (1):48–50.

Gombojav, B., H. Park, J. I. Kim, Y. S. Ju, J. Sung, S. I. Cho, M. K. Lee, H. Ohrr, J. Radnaabazar, and J. S. Seo. 2008. Heritability and linkage study on heart rates in a Mongolian population. *Exp Mol Med* 40 (5):558–64. doi: 10.3858/emm.2008.40.5.558.

Gusella, J. F., N. S. Wexler, P. M. Conneally, S. L. Naylor, M. A. Anderson, R. E. Tanzi, P. C. Watkins, K. Ottina, M. R. Wallace, A. Y. Sakaguchi et al. 1983. A polymorphic DNA marker genetically linked to Huntington's disease. *Nature* 306 (5940):234–8.

Hindorff, L., J. MacArthur, J. Morales, H. A. Junkins, P. N. Hall, A. K. Klemm, and T. A. Manolio. 2014. A catalog of published genome-wide association studies. https://www.genome.gov/gwastudies/.

Hoit, B. D., S. Kiatchoosakun, J. Restivo, D. Kirkpatrick, K. Olszens, H. Shao, Y. H. Pao, and J. H. Nadeau. 2002. Naturally occurring variation in cardiovascular traits among inbred mouse strains. *Genomics* 79 (5):679–85. doi: 10.1006/geno.2002.6754.

Howden, R., E. Liu, L. Miller-DeGraff, H. L. Keener, C. Walker, J. A. Clark, P. H. Myers, D. C. Rouse, T. Wiltshire, and S. R. Kleeberger. 2008. The genetic contribution to heart rate and heart rate variability in quiescent mice. *Am J Physiol Heart Circ Physiol* 295 (1):H59–68. doi: 10.1152/ajpheart.00941.2007.

Hunt, T. M. 1910. Sex limited inheritance in drosophila. *Science* 32 (812):120–122. doi: 10.1126/science.32.812.120.

Islam, M. S., T. Lehtimaki, M. Juonala, M. Kahonen, N. Hutri-Kahonen, K. Kainulainen, H. Miettinen, L. Taittonen, K. Kontula, J. S. Viikari, and O. T. Raitakari. 2006. Polymorphism of the angiotensin-converting enzyme (ACE) and angiotesinogen (AGT) genes and their associations with blood pressure and carotid artery intima media thickness among healthy Finnish young adults–The cardiovascular risk in young Finns study. *Atherosclerosis* 188 (2):316–22. doi: 10.1016/j.atherosclerosis.2005.11.008.

Jayaraman, S. 2012. Epigenetic mechanisms of metabolic memory in diabetes. *Circ Res* 110 (8):1039–41. doi: 10.1161/CIRCRESAHA.112.268375.

Kemp, A. H., D. S. Quintana, K. L. Felmingham, S. Matthews, and H. F. Jelinek. 2012. Depression, comorbid anxiety disorders, and heart rate variability in physically healthy, unmedicated patients: Implications for cardiovascular risk. *PLoS One* 7 (2):e30777. doi: 10.1371/journal.pone.0030777.

Kennon, B., J. R. Petrie, M. Small, and J. M. Connell. 1999. Angiotensin-converting enzyme gene and diabetes mellitus. *Diabet Med* 16 (6):448–58.

Kreutz, R., B. Struk, P. Stock, N. Hubner, D. Ganten, and K. Lindpaintner. 1997. Evidence for primary genetic determination of heart rate regulation: Chromosomal mapping of a genetic locus in the rat. *Circulation* 96 (4):1078–81.

Kuivaniemi, H., E. J. Ryer, J. R. Elmore, I. Hinterseher, D. T. Smelser, and G. Tromp. 2014. Update on abdominal aortic aneurysm research: From clinical to genetic studies. *Scientifica (Cairo)* 2014:564734. doi: 10.1155/2014/564734.

Lehnen, H., U. Zechner, and T. Haaf. 2013. Epigenetics of gestational diabetes mellitus and offspring health: The time for action is in early stages of life. *Mol Hum Reprod* no. 19 (7):415–22. doi: 10.1093/molehr/gat020.

Loos, R. J., P. W. Franks, R. W. Francis, I. Barroso, F. M. Gribble, D. B. Savage, K. K. Ong, S. O'Rahilly, and N. J. Wareham. 2007. TCF7L2 polymorphisms modulate proinsulin levels and beta-cell function in a British Europid population. *Diabetes* 56 (7):1943–7. doi: 10.2337/db07-0055.

Ma, Q. and A. Y. Lu. 2011. Pharmacogenetics, pharmacogenomics, and individualized medicine. *Pharmacol Rev* 63 (2):437–59. doi: 10.1124/pr.110.003533.

Malik, M. 1998. Heart rate variability. *Curr Opin Cardiol* 13 (1):36–44.

Marzbanrad, F., B. Hambly, E. Ng, S. Tamayo, S. Matthews, C. Karmakar, A. H. Khandoker, M. Palaniswami, and H. F. Jelinek. 2014. Relationship between heart rate variability and angiotensinogen gene polymorphism in diabetic and control individuals. *Conf Proc IEEE Eng Med Biol Soc* 2014:6683–6. doi: 10.1109/EMBC.2014.6945161.

Maschirow, L., K. Khalaf, H. A. Al-Aubaidy, and H. F. Jelinek. 2015. Inflammation, coagulation, endothelial dysfunction and oxidative stress in prediabetes—Biomarkers as a possible tool for early disease detection for rural screening. *Clin Biochem* 48 (9):581–5. doi: 10.1016/j.clinbiochem.2015.02.015.

Matheus, A. S., L. R. Tannus, R. A. Cobas, C. C. Palma, C. A. Negrato, and M. B. Gomes. 2013. Impact of diabetes on cardiovascular disease: An update. *Int J Hypertens* 2013:653789. doi: 10.1155/2013/653789.

Mitro, P., K. Mudrakova, H. Mickova, J. Dudas, P. Kirsch, and G. Valocik. 2008. Hemodynamic parameters and heart rate variability during a tilt test in relation to gene polymorphism of renin-angiotensin and serotonin system. *Pacing Clin Electrophysiol* 31 (12):1571–80. doi: 10.1111/j.1540-8159.2008.01228.x.

Nasimi, A. and M. Hatam. 2011. The role of the cholinergic system of the bed nucleus of the stria terminalis on the cardiovascular responses and the baroreflex modulation in rats. *Brain Res* 1386:81–8. doi: 10.1016/j.brainres.2011.02.056.

Neumann, S. A., E. C. Lawrence, J. R. Jennings, R. E. Ferrell, and S. B. Manuck. 2005. Heart rate variability is associated with polymorphic variation in the choline transporter gene. *Psychosom Med* 67 (2):168–71. doi: 10.1097/01.psy.0000155671.90861.c2.

Nishikino, M., T. Matsunaga, K. Yasuda, T. Adachi, T. Moritani, G. Tsujimoto, K. Tsuda, and N. Aoki. 2006. Genetic variation in the renin-angiotensin system and autonomic nervous system function in young healthy Japanese subjects. *J Clin Endocrinol Metab* 91 (11):4676–81. doi: 10.1210/jc.2006-0700.

Parson, H. K., M. W. Winchester, S. A. Neumann, and A. Vinik. I. 2011. Choline transporter gene variation is associated with diabetes and autonomic neuropathy in African Americans. *Acute and Chronic Complications*:2116, PO.

Pietila, E., H. Fodstad, E. Niskasaari, P. Pj. Laitinen, H. Swan, M. Savolainen, Y. A. Kesaniemi, K. Kontula, and H. V. Huikuri. 2002. Association between HERG K897T polymorphism and QT interval in middle-aged Finnish women. *J Am Coll Cardiol* 40 (3):511–4.

Pinney, S. E. and R. A. Simmons. 2012. Metabolic programming, epigenetics, and gestational diabetes mellitus. *Curr Diab Rep* 12 (1):67–74. doi: 10.1007/s11892-011-0248-1.

Pop-Busui, R. 2010. Cardiac autonomic neuropathy in diabetes: A clinical perspective. *Diabetes Care* 33 (2):434–41. doi: 10.2337/dc09-1294.

Probst-Hensch, N. M., M. Imboden, D. Felber Dietrich, J. C. Barthelemy, U. Ackermann-Liebrich, W. Berger, J. M. Gaspoz, and J. Schwartz. 2008. Glutathione S-transferase polymorphisms, passive smoking, obesity, and heart rate variability in nonsmokers. *Environ Health Perspect* 116 (11):1494–9. doi: 10.1289/ehp.11402.

Pumprla, J., K. Howorka, D. Groves, M. Chester, and J. Nolan. 2002. Functional assessment of heart rate variability: Physiological basis and practical applications. *Int J Cardiol* 84 (1):1–14.

Ravaja, N., K. Raikkonen, H. Lyytinen, T. Lehtimaki, and L. Keltikangas-Jarvinen. 1997. Apolipoprotein E phenotypes and cardiovascular responses to experimentally induced mental stress in adolescent boys. *J Behav Med* 20 (6):571–87.

Rigat, B., C. Hubert, F. Alhenc-Gelas, F. Cambien, P. Corvol, and F. Soubrier. 1990. An insertion/ deletion polymorphism in the angiotensin I-converting enzyme gene accounting for half the variance of serum enzyme levels. *J Clin Invest* 86 (4):1343–6. doi: 10.1172/JCI114844.

Roldan, V., J. Corral, F. Marin, J. Pineda, V. Vicente, and R. Gonzalez-Conejero. 2005. Synergistic association between hypercholesterolemia and the C46T factor XII polymorphism for developing premature myocardial infarction. *Thromb Haemost* 94 (6):1294–9. doi: 10.1160/TH05-06-0453.

Rolim, L. C., J. R. Sa, A. R. Chacra, and S. A. Dib. 2008. Diabetic cardiovascular autonomic neuropathy: Risk factors, clinical impact and early diagnosis. *Arq Bras Cardiol* 90 (4):e24–31.

Ronaghi, M., M. Uhlen, and P. Nyren. 1998. A sequencing method based on real-time pyrophosphate. *Science* 281 (5375):363, 365.

Russell, J., S. Hijazi, and L. Edington. 2010. Cardioavascular complications and sudden death associated with eating disorders. *Interet J Cardiovas Res* 7 (1).

Said, G. 2007. Diabetic neuropathy—A review. *Nat Clin Pract Neurol* 3 (6):331–40. doi: 10.1038/ncpneuro0504.

Savic, D., H. Ye, I. Aneas, S. Y. Park, G. I. Bell, and M. A. Nobrega. 2011. Alterations in TCF7L2 expression define its role as a key regulator of glucose metabolism. *Genome Res* 21 (9):1417–25. doi: 10.1101/gr.123745.111.

Sayed-Tabatabaei, F. A., B. A. Oostra, A. Isaacs, C. M. van Duijn, and J. C. Witteman. 2006. ACE polymorphisms. *Circ Res* 98 (9):1123–33. doi: 10.1161/01.RES.0000223145.74217.e7.

Schönauer, M., A. Thomas, S. Morbach, J. Niebauer, U. Schönauer, and H. Thiele. 2011. Cardiac autonomic diabetic neuropathy. *Diab Vasc Dis Res* 5:336–44.

Schulz, S., K. J. Bär, and A. Voss. 2015. Analysis of heart rate, respiration and cardiorespiratory coupling in patients with schizophrenia. *Entropy.* 17:483–501.

Schunkert, H. 1997. Polymorphism of the angiotensin-converting enzyme gene and cardiovascular disease. *J Mol Med (Berl)* 75 (11–12):867–75.

Sharma, A. M. 2004. Is there a rationale for angiotensin blockade in the management of obesity hypertension? *Hypertension* 44 (1):12–9. doi: 10.1161/01.HYP.0000132568.71409.a2.

Sharma, P., A. Hingorani, H. Jia, R. Hopper, and M. J. Brown. 1999. Quantitative association between a newly identified molecular variant in the endothelin-2 gene and human essential hypertension. *J Hypertens* 17 (9):1281–7.

Sinnreich, R., J. D. Kark, Y. Friedlander, D. Sapoznikov, and M. H. Luria. 1998. Five minute recordings of heart rate variability for population studies: Repeatability and age-sex characteristics. *Heart* 80 (2):156–62.

Smith, C. W., E. B. Porro, J. G. Patton, and B. Nadal-Ginard. 1989. Scanning from an independently specified branch point defines the 3′ splice site of mammalian introns. *Nature* 342 (6247):243–7. doi: 10.1038/342243a0.

Southern, E. M., U. Maskos, and J. K. Elder. 1992. Analyzing and comparing nucleic acid sequences by hybridization to arrays of oligonucleotides: Evaluation using experimental models. *Genomics* 13 (4):1008–17.

Steeds, R. P., J. Fletcher, H. Parry, S. Chowdhary, K. S. Channer, J. West, and J. N. Townend. 2002. The angiotensin-converting enzyme gene I/D polymorphism and heart rate variability following acute myocardial infarction. *Clin Auton Res* 12 (2):66–71.

Stolarz, K., J. A. Staessen, K. Kawecka-Jaszcz, E. Brand, G. Bianchi, T. Kuznetsova, V. Tikhonoff, L. Thijs, T. Reineke, S. Babeanu, E. Casiglia, R. Fagard, J. Filipovsky, J. Peleska, Y. Nikitin, H. Struijker-Boudier, T. Grodzicki, and European Project on Genes in Hypertension Investigators. 2004. Genetic variation in CYP11B2 and AT1R influences heart rate variability conditional on sodium excretion. *Hypertension* 44 (2):156–62. doi: 10.1161/01.HYP.0000135846.91124.a5.

Sturtevant, A. H. 1913. The linear arrangement of six sex-linked factors in Drosophila, as shown by their mode of association. *J Exp Zool* 14:43–59. doi:10.1002/jez.1400140104.

Tankersley, C. G., A. Bierman, and R. Rabold. 2007. Variation in heart rate regulation and the effects of particle exposure in inbred mice. *Inhal Toxicol* 19 (8):621–9. doi: 10.1080/08958370701353049.

Tankersley, C. G., R. Irizarry, S. Flanders, and R. Rabold. 2002. Circadian rhythm variation in activity, body temperature, and heart rate between C3H/HeJ and C57BL/6J inbred strains. *J Appl Physiol (1985)* 92 (2):870–7. doi: 10.1152/japplphysiol.00904.2001.

Tingley, W. G., L. Pawlikowska, J. G. Zaroff, T. Kim, T. Nguyen, S. G. Young, K. Vranizan, P. Y. Kwok, M. A. Whooley, and B. R. Conklin. 2007. Gene-trapped mouse embryonic stem cell-derived cardiac myocytes and human genetics implicate AKAP10 in heart rhythm regulation. *Proc Natl Acad Sci U S A* 104 (20):8461–6. doi: 10.1073/pnas.0610393104.

Ueda, S., H. L. Elliott, J. J. Morton, and J. M. Connell. 1995. Enhanced pressor response to angiotensin I in normotensive men with the deletion genotype (DD) for angiotensin-converting enzyme. *Hypertension* 25 (6):1266–9.

Uusitalo, A. L., E. Vanninen, E. Levalahti, M. C. Battie, T. Videman, and J. Kaprio. 2007. Role of genetic and environmental influences on heart rate variability in middle-aged men. *Am J Physiol Heart Circ Physiol* 293 (2):H1013–22. doi: 10.1152/ajpheart.00475.2006.

Vinik, A. I., R. Freeman, and T. Erbas. 2003. Diabetic autonomic neuropathy. *Semin Neurol* 23 (4):365–72. doi: 10.1055/s-2004-817720.

Voss, A., A. Busjahn, N. Wessel, R. Schurath, H. D. Faulhaber, F. C. Luft, and R. Dietz. 1996. Familial and genetic influences on heart rate variability. *J Electrocardiol* 29 Suppl:154–60.

Wang, D. G., J. B. Fan, C. J. Siao, A. Berno, P. Young, R. Sapolsky, G. Ghandour, N. Perkins, E. Winchester, J. Spencer, L. Kruglyak, L. Stein, L. Hsie, T. Topaloglou, E. Hubbell, E. Robinson, M. Mittmann, M. S. Morris, N. Shen, D. Kilburn, J. Rioux, C. Nusbaum, S. Rozen, T. J. Hudson, R. Lipshutz, M. Chee, and E. S. Lander. 1998. Large-scale identification, mapping, and genotyping of single-nucleotide polymorphisms in the human genome. *Science* 280 (5366):1077–82.

Witzel, I. I., H. F. Jelinek, K. Khalaf, S. Lee, A. H. Khandoker, and H. Alsafar. 2015. Identifying common genetic risk factors of diabetic neuropathies. *Front Endocrinol (Lausanne)* 6:88. doi: 10.3389/fendo.2015.00088.

Index

A

Milton Keynes UK
Ingram Content Group UK Ltd.
UKHW052023071024
449327UK00027B/2406